More advance praise for *An American Health Dilemma*

At last! The authors must be congratulated for having produced the first comprehensive, well-researched project that gives timely insights and understanding into racism as a major root cause for the ethnic health disparities that have plagued African Americans for the past several centuries.
RODNEY G. HOOD, M.D.
President, National Medical Association

An American Health Dilemma is a must read for every medical student, every medical historian, and every physician who cares about understanding the complexity of medicine.
RICHARD O. BUTCHER, M.D.
President, Summit Health Coalition
Past President, National Medical Association

Drs. Byrd and Clayton have made a major contribution to our understanding of the historical impact of race on health care in America. From slavery days to the modern age, the foundation for and consequences of unequal medical treatment are explored.
GARY C. DENNIS, M.D.
Past President, National Medical Association

Fresh insights abound and relationships hitherto ignored are shown to have great significance. The book is filled with new ideas. . . . While students of race and medicine may be especially grateful for this work, all of us will come away with a clearer view of the human condition and a rare insight into how we got to be the way we are.
WILLIAM H. GRIER, M.D.
Author of *Black Rage*

This is a must read book for clinicians and health policy scientists interested in the health of the African American community. Without an understanding of the historical roots of the problems faced by this community, it is very difficult to comprehend the current challenges. This is a wonderful book.
BENJAMIN P. SACHS, M.D.
Harold H. Rosenfield Professor of Obstetrics,
Gynecology, and Reproductive Biology
Harvard Medical School

Comprehensive and authoritative, *An American Health Dilemma: A Medical History of African Americans and the Problem of Race: Beginnings to 1900* takes the full measure of the field and makes its distinctive contributions to the widest possible audience. It will be the standard information, research, and reference source for many years to come. What a pedagogical gold-mine!
DR. ROBERT V. GUTHRIE
Professor Emeritus, Southern Illinois University at Carbondale,
Author of *Even the Rat Was White: A Historical View of Psychology*

Drs. Byrd and Clayton have undertaken a tremendous task in their examination of racism in human society. . . . The work deserves to be thoughtfully read by all persons concerned for an open society of justice and humanity.
L. J. BERNARD, M.D., F.A.C.S.
Distinguished Professor of Surgery Emeritus,
Meharry Medical College

Not only is *An American Health Dilemma* important for policy development, but it is exciting and readable. . . . It will open your mind, challenge your assumptions, . . . and it will be of interest to a wide audience, not only in the medical field, but also to historians, sociologists, urban experts, and all who have an interest in the future of the nation.
REVEREND EDWARD B. BLACKMAN
Civil Rights and Community Activist

✕✕ An American Health Dilemma

VOLUME ONE

A Medical History of African Americans and the Problem of Race: Beginnings to 1900

DISCARDED

W. Michael Byrd, MD, MPH
Linda A. Clayton, MD, MPH

With a Foreword by Dr. Robert J. Blendon

Routledge

NEW YORK   LONDON

Published in 2000 by

Routledge
29 West 35th Street
New York, NY 10001

Published in Great Britain by
Routledge
11 New Fetter Lane
London EC4P 4EE

A *Member of the Taylor & Francis Group*

Library of Congress Cataloging-in-Publication Data
Byrd, W. Michael.
    An American health dilemma : a medical history of African Americans
and the problem of race / W. Michael Byrd and Linda A. Clayton.
        p.   cm.
Includes bibliographical references and index.
Contents: [1] Beginnings to 1900.
ISBN 0-415-92449-9 (v. 1 : alk. paper)
    1. Afro-Americans—Health and hygiene—History.   2. Afro-Americans—
Medical care—History.   I. Clayton, Linda A.
II. Title.

RA448.5.N4 B97 2000   99-027882
362.1'089'96073—dc21   CIP

*To Sybil, Alice, Lois,
and our fathers*

Ⅹ Contents

⋊ *List of Figures and Tables*

Figures

Tables

)(*Foreword*

This book represents an extraordinary achievement by the authors, who have brought together in two volumes the history of the African American health experience in the United States and its broader historical perspective.

In particular, *An American Health Dilemma: A Medical History of African Americans and the Problem of Race* documents in the most detailed manner how, from the nation's earliest period, the African American population suffered severely from years of slavery, racial discrimination, segregation of health care facilities, denial of health professional education opportunities and gross underfunding of those opportunities that existed, and neglect of the most elementary health needs of their community. It traces, through successive generations, the major barriers that prevented African Americans from receiving the most basic medical care and public health services, and examines the resulting high rates of death, disability, and human suffering.

Of additional importance, this book is the first to chronicle in such detail the courage, leadership, ingenuity, and scientific and professional skills of generations of individual African American physicians and other health professionals who struggled against great odds to build a responsive health system that would meet the needs of those living in a segregated society, often in great poverty.[1] It also highlights many of the important and heretofore unrecognized contributions made by a diverse group of African American pioneers to the broader world of medical treatment and biomedical science.

This series is of such significance because it seeks to explain and document the historical factors behind today's huge disparities in the level of health between Whites and African Americans.[2] The fact that African Americans today live substantially shorter lives than Whites; die more frequently from cancer, heart disease, stroke, and diabetes; and see their infants die at nearly twice the rate of Whites is in part a result of their unique and tragic historical experience in America. Growing from this, African Americans today also remain less likely than Whites to have health insurance coverage and less likely to be treated by a physician when they are ill.

The need for this book grows from the understanding that these health disparities and their historical antecedents are not well recognized by the majority of Americans, particularly White Americans. In fact, beliefs today are almost the opposite of the reality portrayed in this work. Surveys show that the majority of White Americans believe that discrimination, past and present, is not a major reason for the social and economic problems African Americans face today.[3] They also show that most Whites are not aware that African Americans have a shorter life expectancy, a higher rate of infant mortality, more problems with access to health care, and a higher rate of being uninsured than Whites.[4] It is my hope that these two volumes will become textbooks in classrooms across the country and will help bridge this wide gap in knowledge of the extent of African American health problems and their roots.[5] These volumes should also serve as important texts for minority students seeking greater understanding of the many contributions made by leaders of the African American medical community across many centuries. If not for the publication of these volumes, many of those extraordinary health care achievements would have remained unknown even to those most concerned with these issues.

The bringing together of this huge body of work about the history of the African American health care experience in the United States required years of dedicated research under difficult circumstances. We are all indebted to W. Michael Byrd, MD, and Linda A. Clayton, MD, for their devoted commitment to bringing this history to the broader health and medical community. I hope their effort will result in a movement in this nation to provide the African American population with a more responsive and caring health system in the new century.

I am very pleased and privileged that this important work was conducted under the auspices of the Department of Health Policy and Management and the Division of Public Health Practice of the Harvard School of Public Health.

Robert J. Blendon, Sc.D.
Professor of Health Policy and Political Analysis
Harvard School of Public Health and the Kennedy School of Government

Boston, Massachusetts
February 2000

References

1. Cunningham RM Jr. Discrimination and the doctor. *Medical Economics* 1952; 29(1): 119–124.

2. U.S. Department of Health and Human Services, Centers for Disease Control and Prevention, National Center or Health Statistics. *Health, United States, 1999.* Hyattsville, MD, 1999; U.S. Department of Health and Human Services, Public Health Service, Agency for Health Care Policy and Research. *Health Statutes and Limitations: A Comparison of Hispanics, Blacks, Whites, 1996.* Rockville, MD, 1999; Collins KS et al. *U.S. Minority Health: A Chartbook.* New York: The Commonwealth Fund, 1999.

3. *The Washington Post,* Kaiser Family Foundation, Harvard University Survey Project. *The Four Americas: A Report on Government and Social Policy through the Eyes oif America's Multi-racial and Multi-ethnic Society.* Menlo Park, CA: Kaiser Family Foundation, 1999.

4. The Henry J. Kaiser Foundation. *Race, Ethnicity and Medical Care: A Survey of Public Perceptions and Experiences.* Menlo Park, CA, 1999.

5. Blendon RJ et al. How White and African Americans view their health and social problems: Different experiences, different expectations. *Journal of the American Medical Association* 1995; 273(4): 341–346.

)(*Acknowledgments*

This book is the culmination of many years of research, experience in academic medicine, and clinical practice. Without the aid and assistance of many individuals, institutions, and sponsors it could not have been completed. As foundation stones of intellect and inspiration we are all indebted to men like Drs. James McCune Smith, Martin Robison Delany, John Sweat Rock, George Whipple Hubbard, Robert F. Boyd, Charles Victor Roman, W. E. B. Du Bois, John A. Kenney, and General Oliver O. Howard, who laid the building blocks in the quest for justice and equity in health care for all people in the United States beginning in the nineteenth century. Often obscured by their high-profile abolitionist or academic careers, or buried behind the "veil" of racism, their accomplishments as health professionals deserve resurrection. Building upon these historical legacies and inspired contemporaneous leadership provided by scholars committed to progress in African American health, such as Drs. Hildrus Poindexter, W. Montague Cobb, Herbert Morais, Julian Lewis, William Darity, M. Alfred Haynes, and Paul Cornely, this book strives to continue their efforts. All of these often unacknowledged pioneers provided the energy and inspiration for this book.

Institutions that supported both authors as they worked on this project deserve recognition. Meharry Medical College in Nashville, the Harvard School of Public Health (HSPH) in Boston, the State University of New York Medical Center at Brooklyn, Boston's Beth Israel Deaconess Medical Center, and Boston's Roxbury Comprehensive Community Health Center and Dimock Community Health

Center hold permanent places in our hearts and souls. Other supportive institutions and organizations worthy of mention are the National Medical Association (NMA); the Congressional Black Caucus; the Summit Health Coalition in Washington; the Ennix-Jones Center of the First Baptist Church Capitol Hill in Nashville, Tennessee, while under the leadership of Reverend Ces' Cook; and the Black Churches and Black Colleges Network headquartered in Detroit, Michigan. Their assistance was critical in the realization of this project.

We will forever be indebted to AT&T, which funded our postdoctoral fellowships at Harvard. The Tennessee Managed Care Network and the Medical Care Management Company provided pivotal financial support, without which this project could not have been completed. The Harvard Pilgrim Health Care Foundation funded this project's bridge into multicultural medicine. The Robert Wood Johnson Foundation sponsored various projects on African American and disadvantaged minority health care that were indirectly related to the book. Without these corporate and institutional sponsors this work would not have been possible.

Special access to research resources was provided by Ms. Mattie McHollin and Ms. Cheryl Hamburg of the Kresge Learning Resource Center of Meharry Medical College; Ms. Beth Howse, Special Collections Librarian of the Fisk University Library; and Mr. and Mrs. Wolff and Ms. Madeline Mullin of the Rare Book Room of the Countway Library of Medicine of Harvard. The Widener, Lamont, and Tozzer libraries of Harvard provided rare and focused resources for the research. Special thanks are extended to Ms. Salena Abrams of the National Cancer Institute's (NCI) library and her colleagues at the National Library of Medicine who provided so much medical historical material. We will be forever indebted to these individuals and the professional staffs of these various institutions.

We are forever indebted to our editors. Mr. Ricardo Guthrie, our colleague during our Harvard training years, reemerged to become our "Maxwell Perkins" editorially on the entire book project. We cannot begin to articulate our sincere appreciation for Mr. Guthrie's overall role as consultant editor, researcher, and scholar in African American Studies during the latter phases of the project. A special note of appreciation is made for his exceptional ability to lend clarity and ease of reading to areas that were extremely complex, highly technical, or medically and scientifically oriented. We will be eternally grateful for his contribution. Mr. Kevin Ohe at Routledge was an advocate for the project who then orchestrated the book's progress through the complex publishing process.

Academicians who lent their expertise in preparing this manuscript include Dr. Lucius Outlaw, philosopher and international authority on race from Haverford College; Dr. Robert Robinson, Associate Director, Office of Smoking and Health of the Centers for Disease Control and Prevention in Atlanta; Dr. Michael Blakey, chief anthropologist at Howard University and director of the New York African Burial Ground Project; and Dr. Cassandra Simmons, associate dean for students while at HSPH. Other scholars who heard, analyzed, and helped shape some of the content of the project were Dr. Deborah Prothrow-Stith of HSPH; Dr. Claudia Baquet of the University of Maryland School of Medicine; Dr. Ces' Cook,

CEO of Faith-Based Centers of Excellence in Nashville; Dr. Leslie Falk, retired professor of family practice and nationally noted medical historian and health policy authority of Meharry; Dr. Charles Finch, of the Morehouse School of Medicine; Dr. Richard Allen Williams, author and founder of the Minority Health Institute in Los Angeles; Dr. B. Waine Kong, CEO of the Association of Black Cardiologists, Inc., in Atlanta; Mrs. Cheryl Hamburg, library director at Meharry; Dr. Robert Guthrie, noted academic psychologist and researcher; and Dr. Todd Savitt, medical historian of East Carolina University Medical School. Mrs. Joan Clayton-Davis, Program Manager of the Academy of Educational Development of Nashville, provided advice and encouragement, served as a sounding board, and read parts of our manuscript incisively and objectively. Her unwavering support and her comments and input were greatly appreciated. We thank Dr. Stephen Jay Gould, anthropologist at Harvard University, for sharing his library and expressing his interest and support for the project.

Many individuals have been sentinels of support and encouragement for this project. Some include Dr. Robert Jay Blendon and Dr. Deborah Prothrow-Stith of HSPH; Dr. Charles Johnson of Duke University, who was a bulwark of inspiration, encouragement, and support, serving in many ways as "father" of this project; Anthony Cebrun, J.D., M.P.H., whose indefatigable interest and support served as a spiritual beacon guiding this complex project to realization; the late Dr. Robert Hardy ("Bob"), our intellectual conscience, critic, policy analyst, and confidant—besides being a dear friend and spiritual support for both of us; Drs. Tamara Jones and Bryan Gibbs of the Division of Public Health Practice at the HSPH; Drs. Eric Buffong, Richard Butcher, Ezra Davidson, Avis Pointer, Tracy Walton, Mike Lenoir, Yevonnecris Veal, Gary Dennis, Patricia Hart, Gilbert Parks, Anita Jackson, and Calvin Sampson, all of the NMA; Mrs. Rosemary Davis, Ms. Ruth Perot, Dr. Noma Roberson, and Dr. Ces' Cook, who provided spiritual, intellectual, and material support throughout the project; Ms. Sheree Bishop, videographer Chris Rogers, nurse Sandy Hamilton, Mrs. Linda Williams, and Mrs. Mary Lou Cornett, who provided vital academic, technical, and graphics support; Congressman John Conyers, Congresswoman Eva Clayton, Congressman Louis Stokes, Congresswoman Donna M. Christian-Christiansen, Congressman Earle Hilliard, and Congressman Bobbie Scott of the CBC; Drs. David Satcher, throughout his tenures as president of Meharry, director of the Centers for Disease Control and Prevention in Atlanta, and as sitting Surgeon General; Louis Bernard, chairman of the Department of Surgery at Meharry Medical College; Dr. Audreye Johnson, of the Department of Sociology of the University of North Carolina; Mrs. Joyce Clayton of the University of North Carolina; and Dr. Henry Foster, who will always be our mentor and chief. Health journalist and social scientist Dr. Kirk Johnson lent immeasurable aid in the editorial preparation and structuring of both volumes. Drs. John Boyce and Louis Camilian of SUNY-Downstate Medical Center lent unremitting support during the late stages of the project while my father was ill. Their loyalty and sensitivity will never be forgotten. Other lifelong supporters whose friendship and support blossomed around us in Brooklyn were Drs. Cathy Roans and Reba Williams and the staff of

Kings County Hospital Center. Ruth Browne, Director of the Arthur Ashe Institute of Urban Health at SUNY-Downstate Medical Center, and her family provided pivotal support during our time in Brooklyn. We also thank Dr. Lemuel Evans of the National Career Institute, who always encouraged our work.

Providers of indirect, but critical, support were Mrs. Ruth Baker and members of our family in Fort Worth, without whom the lead author could not have survived the stresses in his life, and Mrs. Lois Henderson, a linchpin of our extended family, who served as a life-sustaining force for both authors. We will be forever indebted to our brothers (Larry, Burley, Walter, Douglas, and Donald), sisters (Joan, Maxine, Doris, Alice, and Judy), nieces, nephews, cousins, other family members, and friends who gave their encouragement and support—without which this project would have been impossible.

The authors also acknowledge the special support provided by Mr. Ziad Obeid and the staff of the Division of Public Health Practice of HSPH. Ms. Scarlett Bellamy and Ms. Knashawn Hodge, of the Department of Biostatistics at HSPH, provided irreplaceable biostatistical support and expertise. We thank the staff and personnel of the Department of Health Policy and Management at HSPH, especially Ms. Elizabeth Marshall, Marilyn, and Ms. Dawn Linehan Elliot. The Computer Lab at HSPH, especially Sydney and Phillipe, lent invaluable assistance. The resources of Harvard University's massive library and research infrastructure were freely utilized. Meharry Medical College Library, the National Library of Medicine, Fisk University Library, and several private libraries were also used. Without the support of these institutions and their staffs, preparing this book would have been much more difficult. The audiovisual departments at Meharry Medical College, the Beth Israel Deaconess Medical Center of Boston, and Chromatics of Nashville lent invaluable aid and assistance in preparing visual material for the book.

Others who provided valuable support include Dr. Ben Sachs, Dr. Susan P. Pauker, Dr. Gabrielle Bercy-Roberson, Kerby Roberson, Esq., Dr. Ken Edelin, Dr. David Harris, Ms. Seleste Harris, Mrs. Sylvia Watts-McKinney and the staff of the African Meeting House, Mr. Jim Scott, Mrs. Jackie Jenkins Scott, Rev. Ed Blackman, Mrs. Sandra Blackman, Rev. Ozzie Edwards, Rev. Carolyn Corey, Mrs. Darlene Pope, Mrs. Ervina Jarrett, Mrs. Marilyn Thomas, Mrs. Carol Taylor, Mr. Monroe "Bud" Mosley, Ms. Dianne Kenney, Dr. John A. Kenney, Jr., Mrs. Sherry Pajari-Joseph, Mr. Randal Rucker, Mrs. Beatrice Riley, Mrs. Vina Fils-Amie, Mrs. Phyllis Cater, Mr. Elmer Freeman, Dr. Gillian Barkley, Ms. Anita Hamilton, Mr. Phillip Aquan, Mr. Raymond Offley, Mr. Luis Osorio, and our neighbors at the Bulfinch. We also thank our Boston and Fort Worth physicians—especially Drs. Jacques Carter, Clinton Battle, Mary King-Rankin, Kevin Dushay, Bruce Furie, Peter Gross, Walter Bagleman, Jerlin Dixon, and Marie Francouer—as well as our University of California at San Diego heart and lung team, including Ms. Connie Watt, Maureen Cavanagh, R.N., David Garcia, N.P., and Drs. Stuart Jamieson, William Auger, Kim Kerr, Naohide Sakakibara, Israel Sarfov, and Mark Fuester, who kept both of us alive and well to complete this project. If other major contributors have been omitted we extend our heartfelt apologies.

✗ Preface

In the wake of a 1991 U.S. Senatorial election in Pennsylvania, an American public consensus evolved. Senator Harris Wofford's upset victory over heavily favored Republican candidate Richard Thornburgh crystallized the public mood that the country was in the throes of a national health crisis. Moreover, most Americans felt that this crisis required major reform of the health system.[1] Some characteristics of this health crisis, which we refer to as the "mainstream" health crisis, were runaway health care cost inflation;[2] a health system consuming 14 percent of the gross domestic product (GDP);[3] an $800 billion national health care budget—twice the per capita expenditure of other health systems by 1992 and exceeding $1 trillion by 1994;[4] 37 million uninsured Americans and 40 to 50 million more underinsured;[5] and insecurity among all Americans, including the middle and upper classes, about future access to basic health services.[6] This mainstream health system crisis was defined, and perceived, primarily as a crisis in costs, financing, and access.[7]

In response to this health crisis, between 1992 and 1994 newly elected President William Jefferson Clinton launched a campaign for the most comprehensive health system reform ever attempted in the United States. His attempt at reform not only failed but also became an epic political disaster.[8] After the fiasco, the mainstream crisis worsened, with the quality of care showing signs of deterioration and the ranks of the uninsured growing to at least 40 million, according to the American Hospital Association, with projections to top 45.5 million by the time of the next presidential election in 2000.[9]

But this mainstream health crisis is not the only problem. Forgotten in the national health crisis debate is an older, more ominous, culturally driven health crisis afflicting African American and other poor populations.[10] Its separateness and silence historically reflect both the nation's faulty approach toward racial problems and the current wave of polarization and denial that is distorting U.S. public policy dialogue regarding race and class.[11] Major aspects of the *African American health crisis* were forced into the health system establishment's consciousness with the mid-1980s release of the Malone-Heckler Report, which detailed the wide and deep racial health disparities plaguing the U.S. health system.[12]

Some characteristics of this African American health crisis include persistent segregation of the health system along race and class lines;[13] race- and class-based inequities and inequalities endemic to each structural component of the health system, the origin of which is over 375 years old;[14] significant race- and class-based health outcome and health status disparities—many of which are worsening;[15] and an African American health insurance crisis wherein 25 percent of African Americans are uninsured, at least 25 percent are underinsured, and another 25 percent depend solely on stigmatized and inferior government insurance (Medicaid or public aid) for basic health services. This contrasts with 12.4 percent of White Americans uninsured, with estimates of another 15 percent underinsured and 6.8 percent covered by Medicaid.[16]

The stubborn persistence of the race- and class-based health system conundrum can be explained on the basis of a medical-social culture hundreds of years old that is heavily laden and burdened by race and class problems compounding continued social and economic deprivation. These factors interactively impact and contribute to the adverse health status and outcomes of African American and poor populations.[17] Many manifestations of these health system cultural problems exist. First is a generalized assumption and projection that poor health status and outcomes for Blacks and the poor are "normal" and acceptable.[18] Second, Blacks and the poor are marginalized at all levels of the health system, from patients to providers.[19] Third, there is a "blind spot" among the general public as well as policy makers regarding the practical and symbolic significance of the alienation and segregation of Black and poor patients from the mainstream health system. Thus, it is seldom emphasized by health policy makers and health providers that the majority of African American and poor patients are forced to utilize city hospitals, community health centers, public health departments, and emergency rooms (ERs) instead of the mainstream system.[20] These institutions—many of which provide yeoman service against great fiscal and logistical odds—are traditionally underfunded, understaffed, and overutilized, with substandard physical plants and equipment. Fourth is the historical tradition of self-serving behavior by Eurocentric organized medicine, the health profession's education systems, and the hospital associations in the United States, which often ignore the special problems of Blacks and the poor in the health system.[21] Fifth is a refusal to address the inequitable representation of the nation's racial and ethnic minorities in the health professions in lieu of compelling evidence that Black and poor populations are more likely to be served—and in a higher quality manner—by such professionals.[22] Sixth is an ongoing resurgence of the application of scientific racist principles to Black and disadvantaged minority populations in the United States.[23] Finally, racially and ethnically divided health professions have factions that are often contentious, conflicting, and contemptuous of each other.*[24]

In the course of our professional development, we became deeply attuned to these problems. The formal beginning of this project at Meharry Medical College in Nashville, Tennessee, in 1988 was a product of a natural evolutionary process. After graduating from medical school, the lead author from Meharry (1968) and the coauthor from Duke University in Durham, North Carolina, (1975), both independently desired to know more about African American health. As medical students we learned about the medical, scientific, and technical aspects of the tremendous health deficits affecting Blacks on a disease-by-disease basis. What was missing from the curriculum was instruction on medical and public health remedies to understand and correct these inequitable health status, health system structural, and outcome deficits. As is the case with virtually all medical schools, Meharry and Duke lacked formal training in the structure or functioning of the health care delivery system with respect to various patient populations. They were far removed from explaining how race and class considerations and interactions impeded Black health from rising above levels that have long since disappeared in other developed countries.[25] Why African Americans were treated differently, often poorly, in this health system was a nagging question. Moreover, poor Black health status and outcome scarcely raised an eyebrow within the medical and health establishments.

After completing a military tour in Vietnam and a residency in obstetrics and gynecology in 1975, the lead author committed himself professionally to an inner-city, private, predominantly African American medical practice. Black physicians practicing in such settings are exposed to the naked health care system discrimination based on race and class experienced by their patients. As profit-driven "private" hospitals market their services to patients with financial means and formidable health insurance, they "cream skim" patient populations, often creating policies that automatically exclude Black, poor, and Hispanic patients.[26] These patients are automatically forced into publicly financed health facilities or into charity care. Because of the composition of their practices, minority physicians—who disproportionately practice in poor neighborhoods— have high numbers of Medicaid, uninsured, and poor patients. As a result, they

---

*The National Medical Association (NMA) and the American Medical Association (AMA), for example, are often diametrically opposed in philosophy and ideology regarding health needs, health care/services, and health rights of disadvantaged populations. Of numerous health professions that often divide along lines of "Black caucuses" or separate organizations, these are the most prominent examples.

are often excluded or purged from hospital staffs and health maintenance organization (HMO) provider lists as a form of economic credentialing and managed care's avoidance of indigent or severely ill patients. Unfair, discriminatory, often economically driven HMO and hospital staff peer review thwarts quality assurance mechanisms, transforming them into tools to decrease the number of non-paying, extremely sick, and poor patients (categories disproportionately overrepresented in Black and disadvantaged minority communities) utilizing the HMO and their affiliated hospitals.[27] On the professional level, Black, Hispanic, and dark-skinned foreign physicians, who Paul Starr referred to as the "medical profession's third world," are often subjected to these troubling scenarios in the course of caring for their patients.[28]

Confronting these realities led to heavy involvement in health policy issues at the local and regional levels, including the lead author serving as a consultant with the National NAACP and the Southern Christian Leadership Conference (SCLC) and as an advisor to health care crusader Edith Irby Jones, M.D., of Houston, Texas. During her tenure as first woman president of the NMA, the lead author's career moved in academic and health policy directions. Soon after testifying before the U.S. Congress about racial discrimination in the health professions in 1985, opportunities to move into health policy and academic medicine at the regional level and, later, at Meharry Medical College became available.[29]

Dr. Clayton was one of the early African American graduates of Duke University Medical School. Before joining Meharry's medical faculty in 1984 as the first director of Gynecologic Oncology, she had completed her ob-gyn and gynecologic oncology training at Duke, codirected the Southeastern Trophoblastic Disease Center, served as gynecologic oncologist at major teaching hospitals, and completed a Visiting Professorship at the University of Dundee in Scotland. She was providentially placed as the director of the Cancer Control Research Unit at Meharry between 1988 and 1991. Perplexed, regarding minority and disadvantaged patient health policy issues, until her collaborative work with the lead author in the Cancer Unit, she sought a deeper understanding of the African American health experience. During her training at Duke she observed that Black cancer patients seemed to be sicker, presented at later stages in their disease processes, and fared worse than White patients. Although the unique and progressive policies then in effect at the wealthy Duke University Medical Center shielded her from most of the blatant race- and class-based barriers and inequities rife in the U.S. health system, after leaving that protected and atypical environment these problems became apparent to her. She also had the good fortune of working in the universal British health delivery system for one year in Dundee, Scotland, where she observed that all patients, including her cancer patients (who are expensive to care for), received screening, early detection, and state-of-the-art therapeutic interventions without excessive delay regardless of the ability to pay. The vast differences in access to health care dictated by race, class, and the ability to pay in the U.S. health system became even clearer to her at Meharry.

The authors first worked together at Meharry's Ob-Gyn Department and Cancer Control Research Unit in 1988. The research, patient care protocols, and consultations initially focused on the cancer crisis in the Black community. Cooperative work with the director, and later coauthor of this book, who had broad, national experience in cancer research focusing primarily on the Black/White differences in cancer incidence and outcomes, deepened our mutual concerns about African American and disadvantaged health. Based on contacts and collaborations with the National Cancer Institute, our newly forged team launched innovative cancer projects building on the work of Drs. LaSalle D. Leffall and Jack White, which detailed Black/White differences in cancer.* One of our innovative and unprecedented projects focused on resurrecting the African American cancer experience from slavery to the present.[30] Moreover, as a team, in cooperation with the NMA and the Drew-Meharry-Morehouse Consortium Cancer Center, we developed the only extant video available, as well as accompanying documentary evidence and reports, about the African American experience in the health delivery system.[31] After creating and publishing several important scientific articles, projects, and lectures on African American health issues, we agreed that more knowledge and training was needed if we were to positively influence the struggle in national health policy.

Attracted by Dr. Robert Jay Blendon's pioneering and progressive work in health policy and management and following the counsel of our mentors Drs. William Darity and M. Alfred Haynes,** we attended the Harvard School of Public Health. While there our ideas, perspectives, and projects were highly praised and warmly received. After earning M.P.H. degrees in 1992 we were subsequently asked to remain at Harvard to complete our research and write two books focusing on the African American health experience.

This work is intended to continue the efforts begun by pioneer and contemporary scholars of African American health such as W. E. B. Du Bois, Hildrus Poindexter, Paul Cornely, Julian Herman Lewis, Herbert Morais, W. Montague Cobb, William Darity, M. Alfred Haynes, and Richard Allen Williams. Some of these giants are still active and assisted in the preparation of this book. We were blessed by their encouragement and oversight as the project unfolded. These

---

*Drs. LaSalle D. Leffall and the late Jack White are surgeons and mentors based at the Howard University Medical School whose research and careers focused on ameliorating the African American cancer crisis.

**Drs. William Darity and M. Alfred Haynes are trained public health researchers, consultant-managers, and educators whose careers focused on ameliorating health disparities suffered by African American and other deprived populations.

volumes may begin providing a basis for reexamination of the American health system and equitable reform, which is a goal dominating the careers and lives of three previous generations of African American health professionals and scholars. If this book sheds new light on the race and class dilemmas plaguing America's health delivery system, the struggle and sacrifice will have been worthwhile.

Boston, Massachusetts
Winter 2000

✕ Introduction

*Of all the forms of inequality, injustice in health is the most shocking
and the most inhuman.*

THE REV. MARTIN LUTHER KING, AT THE SECOND NATIONAL
CONVENTION OF THE MEDICAL COMMITTEE FOR HUMAN RIGHTS,
CHICAGO, MARCH 25, 1966

*Factors affecting health include socioeconomic status, biology, and
environment. . . . [I]n a racist society such as ours, the effect of race is
all-encompassing. Race not only affects socioeconomic status, biology,
and physical environment; it also affects the way health care institutions
function to provide services. Independent of economics, race affects
access to care. Independent of economics, race affects the type and
quality of health care treatment received. Consequently, to improve the
health of African-Americans, it is not sufficient merely to remove
economic barriers to access. To improve the health of African-
Americans, health care institutions must be more than affordable. They
must be just.*

VERNELLIA R. RANDALL, *HEALTH MATRIX:
JOURNAL OF LAW-MEDICINE*, 1993

On the Origins of a Race- and Class-Based System

The impetus for this work is based upon the African American* health experience. The Black experience has been affected, if not dominated, by the issue of
race in Western culture and English North America (often referred to as the
American colonies)—now known as the United States. Therefore, the concepts
of "race" and "racism" deserve exploration. Since the late nineteenth century, a
bevy of historians and social scientists including, but not limited to, W. E. B. Du

---

*Traditionally, ethnic Americans have been designated with hyphenated names such as "African-
Americans," "Native-Americans," "Asian-Americans," etc. This implies that a person from outside the
U.S. would not recognize these other racial and ethnic groups as true Americans without this specific
designation. In contrast, "European Americans" (usually called White), are presumed to be U.S. citizens, thus, maintaining a position of power linguistically. The authors will refer to all racial and ethnic groups as equals according to regions from which their original ancestors migrated: Native (no
need to migrate) Americans, European Americans, African Americans, Asian/Pacific Islander Americans, Hispanic/Latino Americans, etc. See (Freuend, 1989) and (Randall, 1994) in the endnotes.

Bois, Frank Tannenbaum, C. Vann Woodward, Herbert Aptheker, Stanley Elkins, Kenneth Stampp, Steven Steinberg, Eugene Genovese, Gunnar Myrdal, E. Franklin Frazier, John Hope Franklin, Vincent Harding, Andrew Hacker, William Julius Wilson, and Manning Marable have analyzed the social, class, and ethnic implications of the race problem in the United States. Though unable to replace race as an independent variable, class and ethnic considerations and debates have immeasurably enriched and strengthened the scholarship and understanding surrounding race both qualitatively and quantitatively. No other group's experience approaches the negativity of African American's 246 years of chattel slavery (64.74% of the Black experience), 100 years of legal segregation and apartheid (26.31% of the Black experience), and less than one generation of *de jure*, though not *de facto*, freedom (8.95% of the Black experience) (see Table I.1). Thus, race becomes both a nexus and a tool for investigating and evaluating the profound sociocultural and medical-social problems that have been benchmarks of the U.S. health system.

This book takes several approaches toward answering questions and addressing issues surrounding race and racism relative to medicine and health care in America. First, it performs a history-based examination and evaluation of the U.S. health delivery system from an African American perspective. Second, a reassessment of the relationship between the medical profession and issues of race and racism in Western culture and the United States is undertaken. Third, the book evaluates the impact of race on the disparate health status and outcomes of African Americans and places race and racism in the context of their operational roles as key variables that must be factored into the complex equation necessary to solve the "American health dilemma." Fourth, the book offers a series of explanatory hypotheses that clarify and help explain the results of the ongoing relationships between race, the biomedical and other life sciences, health, and healthcare delivery in the United States from their ancient Afro-European beginnings.

America's changing sociocultural milieu, evidenced by Gunnar Myrdal's *An American Dilemma* (1944), raises the inevitable question of whether the nation lives according to its creeds. Awareness of the United States's "Negro problem" and its inconsistencies with America's "wider personal, moral, religious and civic sentiments and ideas,"[1] surfaced with Myrdal's book. Commonly held beliefs grounded in Enlightenment, Protestant, Christian, and legal values emphasizing "liberty, equality, justice and fair opportunity for everybody,"[2] buttressed by Christian ideals of human brotherhood and the Golden Rule, constituted an American Creed. Though the moral obligation imposed by the creed had been flouted for centuries, Myrdal forced an acknowledgment of the conflict between the creed and the attitudes and beliefs of Whites regarding African Americans as well as the way African Americans were treated by White Americans. This "American dilemma" extended, and still applies, to health and health care—thus an "American health dilemma."

Table I.1   African American Citizenship Status from 1619 to 1999

Time Span	Citizenship Status in Years	Percent [%] of U.S. Experience	Citizenship Status*	Comments
1619–1865	246	64.74%	Chattel slavery	Abolition of Atlantic Slave Trade [1808]. Black influx stopped. Black immigration since, scant.
1865–1965	100	26.31%	Virtually no citizenship rights	Thirteenth, 14th, and 15th Amendments virtually nullified. Legal segregation implemented 1896.
1965–1999	34	8.95%	Most citizenship rights	School desegregation [1954], Civil Rights Act [1964], Voting Rights Act [1965] passed. Apartheid, discrimination, institutional racism in effect.
1619–1999	380	100.00%	The struggle continues	SUM TOTAL

By Thomas Marshall's criteria citizenship carries three distinct kinds of rights relative to the State: [1] *civic rights*, including legal equality, free speech, free movement, free assembly, and organizational and informational rights; [2] *political rights*, including the right to vote and run for office in free elections, and; [3] *socioeconomic rights*, including the right to have a job, collectively bargain, unionize, and access social security and welfare if necessary. WM Byrd/LA Clayton, 1999

Sources:
Brinkley A. *The Unfinished Nation: A Concise History of the American People.* New York: Alfred A. Knopf, 1993.
Higginbotham AL. *In the Matter of Color: Race and the American Legal Process, The Colonial Period.* New York: Oxford University Press, 1978.
Kluger R. *Simple Justice: The History of* Brown v. Board of Education *and Black America's Struggle for Equality.* New York: Alfred A. Knopf, Inc., 1976. Paperback Edition. New York: Vintage Books, 1977.
Marable M. *Race, Reform, and Rebellion: The Second Reconstruction in Black America, 1945–1990.* Revised Second Edition. Jackson: University Press of Mississippi, 1991.
Marshall TH. *Citizenship, Social Class, and Other Essays.* Cambridge, England: Cambridge University Press, 1950.

Contemporary students of this health dilemma ask whether Blacks and the poor are to be considered worthy by politicians and the health establishment of equitable health care and health status requisite to full participation in a post-modern, representative democracy. While other disadvantaged ethnic American groups suffer disparate health outcomes for which race plays some part, African

Americans deserve specific studies because they are the oldest, and largest, minority group in the United States both numerically and chronologically*[3] and have the most oppressive race-based health history in the country. Representing the flash-point of the nation's health dilemma for more than 300 years, they also serve as excellent surrogates for the experiences of other minorities.

This investigation presents many Western scientific and cultural icons in a new light. In most instances their positive contributions are well known and beyond the scope of this inquiry. However, many of them played major roles and had great influences on the evolution of race and racism in Western science, society, medicine, and health care through lectures, research, publications, and their prestigious intellectual and social status. Any pursuit of objectivity on race and racism requires that their entire contributions are displayed, scrutinized, and analyzed objectively and without intellectual, scientific, ideological, or personal bias. Any negative aspersions or impressions the reader draws as a result of this objective examination is not the intent of the authors.

This volume begins by examining the concept of race and its intimate relationships with the Western biomedical sciences, scientific racism, and health care. In order to trace the evolution of scientific racism and document how it negatively impacts Black health care, health delivery, and health outcome, the authors expose its origins within the matrix of Western culture and its civilizations. Much of the early investigation focuses on Greece, the Near East, Africa, and Western Europe. Direct historical connections are made between scientific racism and unethical experimentation and exploitation on Blacks, the misuse of science for the pseudo-scientific documentation of racial biological and intellectual inferiority, the acceptance of poor Black health status and outcome as "natural," and a tradition of exclusionary policies relative to acceptance of people of African descent into medical educational programs and the prestigious health professions in general.

According to psychological and policy mechanisms suggested by authorities as varied as Joel Kovel, James H. Jones, Allen Chase, and Robert Jay Lifton, scientific racist processes involved in classifying Blacks as subhuman freed the White medical and health establishments to accept a matrix of adverse health phenomenon listed earlier and, thus, not to consider Black health on the same plane as White health. This "difference" has been used historically and contemporaneously, in overt and covert forms, as justification for nihilistic and substandard health care, health delivery, and subsequent poor health outcomes.

Both volumes of *An American Health Dilemma* explore the U.S. and its predecessor health systems by tracing and examining five major evolutionary currents within those systems. Utilization of these currents, which could be viewed as

---

*Of the non-indigenous groups populating the U.S. presently, over half the ancestors of African Americans were here by 1780. The similar median date for the arrival of European American ancestors is about 1890. Not until the 1840s did Europeans constitute more American arrivals than Africans.

major themes, assist in dissecting and analyzing the medical-social corpus of predecessor-Western and, later, U.S. health systems—revealing their race and class defects in the process. Such an approach effectively reveals and demonstrates this dilemma's operational mechanisms from its history-based roots to its present configuration, which is deeply imbedded within and permeates the U.S. health system and its culture. It becomes obvious that the peculiar matrix of issues surrounding the nexus of race, which also have profound class overtones, must be appropriately addressed if justice and equity in health care are to be obtained for all Americans. The five major evolutionary currents of study include: (1) the sociocultural milieu in which the U.S. health system evolved and developed as it approached the $1.5 trillion megastructure we see today, along with the major events surrounding race and racism and their direct and indirect effects on health and health care delivery in the United States; (2) the evolution and configuration of a race- and class-based U.S. health system to include its structure, institutions, organization, and administration; (3) an assessment of the historical continuum of race- and class-based health disparities that manifest as Black/White differences in access to health care, childhood and adult disease patterns, disability, quality of life, years of potential life lost, and death rates; (4) the evolution of the White medical profession with special focus on its dominance of the health system, its history-based racism, public health posture, and medical-social impact; and (5) the evolution and development of the Black medical profession focusing on its unique and often untold story of Black health advocacy, its unique and singular commitment to the public health and service needs of Black and disadvantaged patients, struggles against professional discrimination and abuse, community leadership, and, on occasion, heroism. Such an inquiry, by necessity, involves examining phenomena such as Black/White differences in health outcome; racial discrimination in the health system at the patient, institutional, and professional levels and its adverse effects on Black health in this country; and the pervasiveness and persistence of the ideology of White supremacy and dominance within the U.S. health delivery system at the professional, patient, and health policy levels.[4]

Due to the complexity, depth, density, and breadth of the endeavor, the first volume of *An American Health Dilemma* spans the period from antiquity to 1900. Abuse, exploitation, and ethical turpitude characterizing many aspects of this historical journey have poisoned roots stretching back into the ancient depths of Western medicine and science. This inquiry suggests that White America's strongest, almost anomic, driving forces regarding Black health have been indifference and neglect—except when direct self-interests were served. Volume One reveals the roots of these attitudes dating back beyond West Africa, the Atlantic slave trade, and the Virginia and Massachusetts colonies in English North America to Western civilization's ancient Middle Eastern, Mediterranean, and Northern African roots. Therefore, much of the ancient story involves Egypt, sub-Saharan Africa, the Middle East, Greece, and the rest of Europe. During the English Colonial period, policy developed that Blacks and Whites would continue to receive separate and unequal health care—a continuation of a 250-year-old tradition established by the Atlantic slave trade. This volume further demonstrates that in the wake of the Civil War, African Americans were severed from the traces of the paternalistic stewardship of the inferior "slave health subsystem" that, although generally inconstant and inconsistent, was an organized infrastructure in some areas of the South. With Blacks left alone after the Civil War experiencing unprecedented death rates, Freedmen's Bureau legislation incorporated provisions for the establishment of clinics, hospitals, and medical schools for freedmen all over the southern United States. By the turn of the century, Blacks, in response to segregation and discriminatory caste status in the health system, developed self-help health programs through civil rights and other community organizations; established the National Medical Association (NMA) in 1895, which because of legal and forced segregation was an almost exclusively Black health professions organization composed of physicians, dentists, and pharmacists; opened a network of Black clinics and hospitals; established African American medical, dental, pharmaceutical, nursing, and other allied health professions schools along with a medical journal; and established the foundation for a Black medical profession that could function independently and alongside a dominant White medical profession with limited interaction between the two. The millennia-long story covered in the first part of the book provides the background for understanding and assessing some of the most important health policy issues affecting the U.S. health system for more than 375 years—the problems of race and class. If an equitable system is to be developed in the future, these issues must be openly acknowledged and objectively examined.[5]

The second volume of *An American Health Dilemma* covers the period from 1900 to the failed Clinton health reform. The turn of the century is a natural dividing point of this extensive inquiry. Many U.S. health system contours that are recognizable today had emerged by 1900. Not only was the country developing into a world power by the turn of the century, but health system markers demonstrating the nation's racial health dilemma were also clearly discernible. The U.S. health system committed itself ideologically and institutionally to segregation and discrimination based on race at all levels. This included the delivery system, health professions educational system, and health policy infrastructure. Tacit in these decisions was an institutionalized refusal, whether formal or informal, to share the beneficence of Western medical progress with African Americans, except under White, self-serving preconditions that were often exploitive (e.g., excess medical demonstration, unethical surgery, exploitive research). By 1900 there was a nationally shared commitment, whether official or not, to erect a "mainstream" health system to serve the White majority. Alongside this burgeoning infrastructure was an inferior charity and publicly supported rump "non-system" composed of a few public hospitals (most major U.S. cities never built public hospitals), intermittently available public clinics (in most areas of the South where most Blacks lived, few public facilities were available to African

Americans prior to the Civil Rights Era), and charity programs for Blacks and the poor. By the turn of the century, institutionalization of separate medical professions segregated by chasms of race, separate educational institutions, and an official White regulatory power structure was already in place. One palpable result of these developments was the erection of a racially separate, hardscrabble health subsystem owned, managed, and operated by Blacks attempting to meet the overwhelming health needs of their community. All of these occurrences orchestrated a national health policy dictating that dual and unequal health care for the races and classes was predetermined, acceptable, and inevitable in the United States.[6]

The second volume continues an investigation of the evolution of the multitiered and unequal health system that grew into the present $1.5 trillion health infrastructure and explores how this system promoted and perpetuated history-based divisions along race and class lines and how it maintained undercare of the underprivileged. As we enter the twenty-first century, the tensions and clashes between the European American and African American medical professions, which have yet to be integrated into one professional body, will be revealed—perhaps for the first time. This volume demonstrates that the Black medical profession has, since its inception, had egalitarian ideological, medical, and public health commitments of service to the entire community as one principal reason for its existence. The White medical profession has never entirely shared this philosophy. The evolution of a loose network of largely eleemosynary, previously despised, health care institutions into a massive, corporate-dominated, hospital infrastructure is examined in light of the system's persistent race and class problems. The meteoric rise of the health insurance industry to a position of dominance since the 1930s is also discussed. As this industry orchestrates the present market-based commercialization of health care and health services along with the corporate takeover of the health system, the medical-social implications of these transformations for Black and underserved populations warrant analysis.[7]

After World War II, in lieu of the generalized medical progress in the United States, an elaborate system of tiered and unequal health care delivery expanded upon the foundations of an already racially segregated, dual,* and unequal health care structure. The second volume helps the reader understand that the health system's time-based trend away from overt racist mechanisms and florid class segregation have done little to lessen the effects of maintaining the disparate quality levels between the "haves" and "have-nots," or those disadvantaged by color and class-based designations in the United States. Acceptance and resignation to race- and class-based duality based on financing mechanisms and "market forces" instead of

---

*By this period the "dual" health system, rigidly organized based on race, could be more easily viewed as a complex multitiered organizational structure based on race, class, medical-social custom, and health-financing mechanisms. African Americans remain in the lower tiers. *Dual* and *multitiered* will continue to be used interchangeably.

overt social caste and dependency designations (e.g., the "worthy" or "unworthy poor") has permeated the fabric of the contemporary U.S. medical-social and health culture. This phenomenon is especially detrimental to African Americans—who, despite several cycles of national prosperity since World War II, continue to suffer the worst health status and outcomes of all U.S. racial and ethnic groups. Moreover, access to quality health care and services in the system continues to be limited both qualitatively and quantitatively for Blacks. As the U.S. health system continues to evolve and develop in terms of separate and unequal traditions established during slavery, the reader will understand and comprehend why race-based health disparities are inevitable and largely predetermined. Nothing short of specific, directed, corrective actions will reverse the trend. Paul Starr's observation, that "Social structure is the outcome of historical processes,"[8] is reaffirmed. He reminds us that to "understand a given structural arrangement . . . one has to identify the way in which people acted, pursuing their interests and ideals under definite conditions, to bring that structure into existence."[9] Contemporary aspects of Volume Two underscore the fact that failure to acknowledge, understand, address, and then correct systematic inequalities and outcomes related to the race and class problems in the U.S. health system threatens the constitutional and biological viability and competitiveness of entire racial and ethnic subpopulations.[10]

Goals and Objectives

Unlike many scientific projects, the goals and objectives of this book grew out of gut-wrenching, palpable, human needs. Previous health system projects, programs, policies, and paradigms relating to African American and poor populations throughout U.S. history have often been the results of serendipity or ideals and values such as White self-interest, paternalism, and Social Darwinism. In contrast, ethereal scientific hypotheses or abstract theoretical paradigms were not necessary for us to respond appropriately to the negative health manifestations of policies, ideals, and values that adversely impact African American health.

The overarching goal of this inquiry is to expand the knowledge base concerning the health experience of African Americans and other health-disadvantaged groups. By achieving this goal, developing strategies and policies for improving the health status and outcomes of these populations toward parity with other Americans could finally be realized. Some of the following are objectives used to accomplish this goal. They focus on questions the authors hope to answer with new knowledge and perspective gained throughout the study. Other objectives expand the health policy knowledge base regarding African American and disadvantaged group health by utilizing methods drawn from the social sciences, history, epidemiology, and public health.

The authors' impressions regarding Black health corroborate those of W. E. B. Du Bois, Herbert Morais, W. Montague Cobb, and Mitchell Rice and Woodrow Jones that any rational understanding of the contemporary African American health experience must begin with a racial-historical analysis and perspective. The authors intend to build upon and expand the work of these, and other, investigators. Although only Morais openly stated his intention to examine the Black health experience from a racial perspective, the others regularly did so. Early unfocused demographic racial health data compiled by the U.S. Bureau of the Census was often used to denigrate and disadvantage African Americans.* The first specific and scientifically balanced efforts to delineate the African American health experience began with Du Bois during the closing decade of the nineteenth century. His Philadelphia and Atlanta University studies were expanded and codified with the groundbreaking *The Health and Physique of the Negro American* released in 1906. The U.S. Bureau of the Census released monographs containing information on Black health after World War I and during the 1930s. Julian Lewis's *The Biology of the Negro* in 1942 was followed by a series of detailed monographs on African American health by W. Montague Cobb, titled *Medical Care and the Plight of the Negro* (1947), *Progress and Portents for the Negro in Medicine* (1948), and *The Black American in Medicine* (1981). Morais's 1967 effort *The History of the Negro in Medicine* was released under the auspices of The Association for the Study of Negro Life and History. Although not highly publicized, these writings serve as good beginnings for comprehending the African American health story.

With this background in mind, the first objective of this inquiry is to provide information that chronologically reconstructs the health experience of people of African descent in the U.S. and its predecessor health systems. This objective—to expand the health experience knowledge base—relates a human story, much of which has never been completely told. It is a portrayal of both a people and a group of patients forced to receive health care in a system that since Colonial times has been largely hostile toward them. Health providers who served Black patients—physicians, nurses, or traditional healers—are included. Institutions, both antagonistic and supportive, are described and placed in more realistic and all-inclusive contexts than in previous texts. To accurately document and portray the facts, epidemiologic, health services, public health, and health policy information have been included whenever possible. However, this is not an attempt to simply produce a numerical and tabular compilation of Black health statistics and outcomes—especially in the earlier parts of the book. Illustrations are utilized to enhance all of these efforts. Pursuit of this objective is, by necessity, intertwined with the development and evolution of Western health and life sciences—along with the medical profession. The development of a culturally competent and proficient health delivery system that values and respects the diverse racial, ethnic, and cultural populations it serves requires an understanding and appreciation of the African American health experience. There must also be a clear understanding of the historical relationship between race, medicine, and health care in the United States.

---

*Nineteenth-century data from the 1840, 1860, 1870, 1880, and 1890 censuses were misused to predict Black inferiority, dysfunction, and eventual extinction. Some of these flawed analyses caused scandals and controversy.

Before undertaking the first objective of reconstructing the African American experience in the health system, the authors wrestled with the concept of "race." We believe a review of this concept is necessary to understand the content and fully appreciate the scope of the book. As Haverford College philosophy professor Lucius Outlaw says, race "is a constitutive element of our common sense and thus is a key component of our 'taken-for-granted' valid reference schema"[11] that we live with and use every day. Much intuitive information on the subject, often inaccurate, along with frank misinformation and disinformation, abounds. Moreover, the relationship between the health sciences, the medical profession, and race has only been sketchily spelled out in the past. The first two chapters, "Race, Biology, and Health Care in the United States: Reassessing a Relationship," and "Race, Medicine, and Society: From Prehistoric to English Colonial Times," provide background for interested students on the relationships between race, the life sciences,* and health care. These chapters systematically delineate and clarify *race–medicine* and *race–health care* relationships that have existed in Western culture from its scientific beginnings. They also expose the effects race may have had, directly or indirectly over time, on the health status and outcomes of people of African descent. By necessity, this relationship, which has origins in antiquity, is examined through its various permutations in Egypt and the Middle East, Greece, Western Europe, English North America, and, later, the United States.[12]

The second objective of this project is to analyze the U.S. health system from the perspective of African American and health-disadvantaged populations. With the help of structural paradigms and methodologies drawn from the social sciences and public health, this analysis encompasses both historical and contemporary time frames. It includes analyses of relevant health events, institutions, and personages in the history of the Western healing sciences and medicine that affected the health and health care of Africans and African-descended people. Understanding the process, which began in antiquity, is critical to comprehending the depth and contemporary health aspects of America's race and class dilemma. Some methods drawn from the disciplines of public health and the social sciences are conventional, while others are new. One of the new tools, to which we previously alluded, is the five major evolutionary currents for studying the U.S. health system. This tool is coordinated with other modern analytic models whenever possible. The contemporary analytic model that will be most utilized is labeled "multicomponent analysis." Its lineage goes back to Florence Wilson and Duncan Neuhauser's work at the Harvard School of Public Health. The method divides the mammoth $1.5 trillion health infrastructure and medical-industrial complex into ten major components,**

---

*Life sciences is an inclusive term designating all branches of science (i.e., biology, medicine, anthropology, epidemiology, or sociology) that deal with living organisms and life processes.

**The ten components are health care institutions; health professions personnel; the pharmaceutical, medical supply, and medical appliance industries; health education and research infrastructure; ambulatory care facilities; health care financing industry; federal government and health care; state and local governments and health care; voluntary health agencies; and the review and control infrastructure.

making it easier to comprehend and analyze. Such an approach has several advantages: It imposes the discipline required to fully catalog all the necessary details for analysis and reform; it encourages dissecting out each component while highlighting its functions and impact in relation to the rest of the system; and it encourages factoring in the results of the interactions between the various components before reaching conclusions. Therefore, component analysis of the U.S. health system critically facilitates meaningful health planning, policy formulation, and reform while factoring in the chronological evolution of the health system. For the first time this analysis will include relevant and newly discovered health-related data not only from the conventional health sciences but also from many other academic, social, and political disciplines. This is consistent with our goal to deepen the understanding, increase the corpus of fact-based data, and broaden and change the foundations upon which race and class-based health policy analyses, debates, and decisions are grounded.

The third objective of *An American Health Dilemma* is to describe the African American health experience, placing it, whenever possible, in quantitative public health terms. Much of this effort focuses on demographics and descriptive epidemiology. State and local health department reports, U.S. and state government census data, insurance company tables, and academic proceedings and presentations such as the Atlanta University Studies are included, analyzed, and discussed to paint a picture of the standards, trends, and indicators of Black health status and outcomes throughout various periods of history. Wherever possible, qualitative and quantitative information will be utilized as tools to interpret past and present African American health disparities, interactions, and relationships with the health system. Such information is also used to predict future prospects of African Americans relative to their health and relationships to the health system.

Race-based health information is juxtaposed against institutional performance, health policy determination, and public health considerations, often for the first time. The third objective expands the understanding of, and renders more accurate perceptions regarding, African American health experiences. This objective is accomplished through the inclusion of remote and recent epidemiologic data, contemporary and remote descriptive health statistics, and current and historical health information that have been reanalyzed by means of newer and more sophisticated biostatistical methods. Charts, tables, and graphs are used to facilitate and enhance project goals and objectives whenever possible.

A fourth objective of this study is to reach some conclusions about the "American health dilemma" based on the African American health experience and to offer suggestions for corrective actions and meaningful health reform. This could lead the nation toward accomplishing the goal of African American and other health disadvantaged groups attaining justice and equity in health care for the first time in our history. These recommendations can be meaningfully based on realistic appraisals of U.S. health system performance relative to Black and poor patients. Other objectives are to introduce individuals and events into the story through the use of vignettes and mini-biographies to illuminate relevant and important health-related experiences, people, and places that have affected, or reflect upon, African American or poor people's health. Inclusion of these narratives and short personal biographies of these often obscure, but important, figures, places, or events clarifies and adds a human touch to our narrative.

Attempts to accomplish these goals and objectives continue throughout both volumes of this work. Incorporation of information from this book, derived from African American and disadvantaged ethnic American viewpoints, supplies a new perspective on U.S. health reality. Revealing reinterpretations of health data form a new basis for health policy formulation. Helping generate a more realistic and inclusive epistemology regarding the knowledge base about U.S. health and health care should serve to make the nation's present and future health policies stronger, fairer, and more likely to succeed.[13]

Methodology

Though able to serve as a scientifically sound contribution to the growing medical-social and public health literature, this book is written in an informational prose style. It is intended to communicate the substance of this important and interesting topic to any literate audience. In fact, the broader the dissemination of the message conveyed in this work the more likely health reform in America, whenever it does occur, will follow a wholesome, just, and equitable course inclusive of all Americans.

In a book of a technical nature like this one, specialized language is sometimes unavoidable. Technical and scientific terminology is used only when necessary to make points that cannot be conveyed in any other way. When the technical languages of disciplines such as biology, anthropology, psychology, biostatistics, health policy and management, or medicine interfere with lay understanding, adequate explanations are included either in the text or in appropriate footnotes for the reader's convenience. Illustrations are also used to lend clarity. The reader should not be encumbered by having to retrogress or look up items to comprehend or move forward in the text.

It is also necessary to include certain lists and tables, often containing technical data. These items are clearly labeled with necessary explanations such that any audience could master the material. Footnotes and material at the base of the table are designed with this in mind.

In the interests of convention, convenience, and logic, this book is organized into chapters. Each chapter after the background focuses on a particular period in African American health history and for pedagogic reasons is written as an autonomous unit. This is consistent with the basic premises, goals, and objectives of this study. Opening chapters on race and *racial thought* in the sciences as academic and sociopolitical subjects are included to orient the reader and provide background on these volatile and often misunderstood subjects. These inquiries on race focus on the relationship between race and the Western bio-medical sciences and health care from antiquity to the modern era. This approach facilitates understanding of the relationship between the social structure of the health system and its historical development as we trace the African American experience.

Voluminous notes at the end of each volume facilitate the dissemination of information and the incorporation of material into curricular form. In a ground-breaking work exploring new areas of academics in tension-filled areas such as race and multicultural history in America, extra documentation may prove less disturbing than leaving issues open ended or open to question. A comprehensive Bibliography and an Index appear at the end of the book.

Like any study entering uncharted territory, some limitations must be acknowledged. A major limitation is one that has bedeviled African American scholarship since this country was founded. That is one of limited resources. Another limitation common in the American system is a paucity of scholarly sources and references about Black health in either the historical or contemporary literature. The historically perceived lack of importance attached to the subject is reflected by the scant literature devoted to it. Moreover, the few references that are available are seldom kept in most libraries. Thus, the authors have had to rely heavily upon personal reference material carefully collected over the years in addition to their use of mainstream libraries such as the Countway Medical Library and other libraries in the Harvard University System, the National Library of Medicine, Meharry Medical College Library and Archive, and the Fisk University Library. This makes the road difficult for scholars trying to retrace or expand upon this work.

Much of the material in this study breaks new ground. It is either new to the health care literature or has been compiled, analyzed, and reinterpreted in an unprecedented manner. Moreover, in order to resurrect much of the Black medical history it has been necessary to consult other source materials such as biography, sociology, or general history. Although these new compilations and reinterpretations clarify much of the African American medical-social and historical experience, they resurrect areas of unfamiliar scholarship and generate hotbeds of potential controversy. For these unique reasons, to lessen the potential for controversy and decrease the material's veracity being questioned, some of the text may seem overdocumented, occasionally repetitive, or overburdened with endnotes and footnotes compared to conventional studies. Similar criticisms have been suggested regarding recent Black revisionist scholarship published by Van Sertima, Charles Finch, Martin Bernal, and St. Clair Drake.[14] As the uproar over the reception of their work proves, any scholarship involving the reassessment of American concepts of race, Western history, or American history calls forth contentiousness, defensiveness, and avoidance of allegations of intellectual dishonesty.[15] Clearly, since African American scholarship is often viewed with skepticism in today's scholarly circles, this study, while of overarching importance, might not be considered mainstream.

Background for Reassessing Race, Class, and Health Care in the United States

From the perspective of practicing African American physicians forged in the 1960s' crucible of a segregated South, it was becoming clear to many by the late 1970s that America's health care system was moving in directions that could threaten the Black population. By the late 1980s the deleterious effects of more than a decade and a half of health policies emphasizing privatization, commercialization, and cut-throat competition had eroded hard-won progress African Americans had made during the 1960s Civil Rights Era in health care. Contemporary evidence of the African American health crisis generated by this competitive era in health policy manifests today as wide, deep, race-based health disparities and an erosion of African American longevity for the first time in the twentieth century.[16] Indeed, *The Report of the Secretary's Task Force on Black and Minority Health*, also known as the Malone-Heckler Report, the most comprehensive modern report revealing the health status of disadvantaged minorities, had sent a thunderclap throughout the health system establishment.[17] Its release by the U.S. Department of Health and Human Services (DHHS) during a conservative Republican administration in 1985 and 1986 forced grudging acknowledgment of a Black health crisis and predicted that, without directed and concentrated efforts, African American morbidity, mortality, and survival rates in relative, and sometimes absolute, terms would perpetuate the then 365-year-old racial health deficits.[18]

President Bill Clinton's 1994 effort to rapidly reform the entire $1.1 trillion U.S. health care system by 1996 failed. The failure had little to do with the racial issues affecting the health system, for these went largely unmentioned and virtually unaddressed. His failed effort followed the unanticipated temporary ascent of health reform as a national priority during the 1992 presidential elections. The stage had been set by the 1991 Wofford Senatorial election in Pennsylvania. Harris Wofford's upset victory, fueled by the public's deep concern over a health care system that they felt demanded a complete overhaul, demonstrated to the political establishment that health was a high-priority national agenda item. But the uprising had more to do with unresolved history-based economic and class problems plaguing the U.S. health system. Although the movement was mediated by the middle class, much of the energy fueling the political demand for health care reform emanated from blue-collar working class and poor European Americans in Pennsylvania. After recovering from the shock of this revolt, which continued through the 1992 presidential elections, the health care establishment, mass media, and politicians immediately began framing this mainstream 1992 health crisis in terms of financing, costs, and access. They characterized the crisis as a combination of runaway health care costs; insecurity among all Americans, including the middle and upper classes, about future access to basic health services; and large and growing blocs of uninsured and underinsured Americans.[19] This mainstreaming of what actually is a race- and class-based health crisis has nearly obliterated the muted discussions about the African

American dilemma the health establishment had been forced to acknowledge since the 1986 release of the Malone-Heckler Report.[20]

During the ensuing health care debate virtually none of the front-running reform plans (of the more than 100 eventually submitted, approximately 10 were front runners), including President Clinton's, created a truly level playing field for African American and poor people.* Commercial interests, instead of public health needs, dominated. The President's plan was slightly more equitable than most of the others. However, framing of health care reform in terms of a market-based takeover of the health system offered a frightening prospect for most Blacks and the poor. The President's reform proposal, based on a paradigm called "managed competition," would have required a massive government bureaucracy to oversee the new commercially dominated system, thus triggering criticism over its costs.[21]

For African Americans these developments represented both threats and opportunities. African Americans have always been aware of the U.S. health system's race and class problems through their traditional interface with the system.[22] Ominously, much of the national health care reform debate occurred with little acknowledgment that African Americans have survived the worst health status, suffered the worst health outcomes, and been forced to utilize the worst health services of any other racial or ethnic group in the U.S. for nearly four centuries. However, the activities of the Summit '93 Health Coalition** and the NMA† seemed to heighten awareness of some blocs within the African American community about the importance of participating in the health care reform debate. Another important result of the failed health reform is that it alerted the Congressional Black Caucus (CBC) to the lack of a permanent formal institutional source of health policy recommendations focusing specifically on African American or disadvantaged patients and broadened their health policy commitment to corrective actions. None of the nation's 25 schools of public health, and only one—the Joint Center for Political and Economic Studies‡—of hundreds of privately funded, highly influential policy organizations

---

*The Wellstone-McDermott, Conyers plan, HR 1200, a universal, government financed, unitary system plan—because of its uniform financing mechanisms and one layer of care for all—came closest to a "level playing field" for all Americans; it was the sole exception.

**The Coalition was a consortium of more than 155 minority and progressive organizations supporting egalitarian health reform spearheaded by the Congressional Black Caucus Foundation, the NMA, National Dental Association, NAACP, National Association of Black County Officials, National Black Caucus of State Legislators, National Caucus and Center on Black Aged, Inc., and the National Pharmaceutical Association.

†The NMA is a predominantly African American medical professional association founded in 1895. Born out of American professional segregation and discrimination in medicine, and with a tradition of advocacy for Black and disadvantaged patients, it represents approximately 16,000 physicians.

‡The Joint Center for Political and Economic Studies, Inc., is a national, nonprofit, tax-exempt institution founded in 1970. Located in Washington, DC, it focuses on and conducts research on public policy issues of special concern to Black Americans. Eddie Williams is the CEO.

or agencies consider African American constituencies as their principal focus. Although the Joint Center for Political and Economic Studies delves quite professionally into health care as its priorities permit, there are no specialized health policy entities with full-time dedicated staff serving as constant sources of African American/disadvantaged patient health policy.* While organizations like the Children's Defense Fund and the Office of Minority Health have definite and important roles in addressing some focused minority health issues, their missions do not include serving as full-fledged, multifaceted, health policy organizations emphasizing the representation of African Americans along with other disadvantaged populations.

If national health reform—designed to meet the needs of all Americans—occurs, it would be one of the largest social transformations in U.S. history. It would involve more than 14 percent of the gross domestic product (GDP), 2.1 million nurses, over 600,000 physicians, 6,200 hospitals, 1,200 insurance companies, and one-seventh of the nation's economy. Harvard Health Policy Professor Marc Roberts calls it "the largest industry in the country."[23] For this to occur without the inclusion of the specific needs and perspectives of African Americans and similarly underserved groups (e.g., Native Americans, Hispanic Americans, women, other disadvantaged minorities, poor Whites, persons with disabilities) brings American democracy into question. Theda Skocpol warns that recent defeat of President Clinton's efforts at health reform increased the "ever-deeper skepticism about the capacity of U.S. democracy to deal with our widely shared problems."[24] It also reinforces the need to reassess the relationship between race and class problems and the performance of the American health care system. The survival of entire populations hangs in the balance.

Yet when journalists and health policy makers mention poor Black health outcomes at all, they continue to project them as stemming almost exclusively from a "culture of poverty" perspective that presumes defective health habits.[25] Indeed, many erroneously attribute aspects of the "dual" health crisis to the Black community's highly publicized problems with drug abuse, violence, and AIDS.[26] In many cases, the actual causes are less titillating than they are commonly portrayed. Whether sensational or mundane, the inappropriate responses to the health ailments that disproportionately affect the Black community are deeply imbedded in the structure and culture of America's health care system. Such chronic problems are not amenable to simple reforms of health financing and insurance markets based on classical economic theories. Although health promotion and disease prevention (HPDP), along with the correction of race-based socioeconomic problems, will ultimately be necessary to completely eliminate the racial health deficit, equalization of the health delivery system represents an

---

*The few health policy institutions with the potential to positively influence African American and disadvantaged minority health, such as the Minority Health Institute of Los Angeles, the Summit Health Coalition of Washington, DC, the Arthur Ashe Institute of Urban Health at SUNY-Downstate, and the Policy Institute of Harlem Hospital, are limited in scope and influence due to funding and support constraints.

irreplaceable first step. In fact, without an equitable health delivery system, approaching equality in health will be impossible, and many aspects of the HPDP models and programs will be ineffective.

The reality is that poor African American health status and outcomes are not aberrations—they are pervasive and systemwide. They are reflections not only of the poor performance of the health system but also of poor nutrition, being forced to live in toxin-exposed environments, poor housing, poor health habits, and health-risky behaviors. Blacks are suffering excess disease-related morbidity and mortality from chronic diseases like heart disease, hypertension, strokes, and diabetes; are suffering more than 90,000 excess deaths* annually; and are suffering cancer, childhood, and infant mortality rates as high as those in many developing countries.[27] While at least 10 to 15 percent of this poor health outcome can be *directly* related to the poor performance of the health care delivery system, some 80 percent of the excess mortality stems from treatable and chronic health conditions or preventable disease processes, which indirectly reflects the poor performance of the health care delivery system, as evidenced by a lack of immunizations, inability to afford to purchase medications or to keep medical appointments, and/or physician refusal to see patients because of their poverty or insurance status.[28] Basic issues of accessibility, affordability, availability, acceptability, and adaptability of health care, increasingly existing in the realm of rhetoric, seldom exert a pragmatic influence on health policy. These aspects, along with the cultural competence of providers, are glossed over by both media and a majority of print sources.[29] The race- and class-biased performance of the health care system is widely accepted. Indeed, it has been part of the status quo for over 380 years, despite wide agreement that health care is a human right. Describing the evolution of the present dual and unequal health system and the incorporation of attitudes and policies accepting of disparate health services and outcome based on race and class in the U.S. health system subculture is another focus of this book.[30]

One tier of this inferior health care subsystem, a loose network of public hospitals, government-run health clinics, and inconstant charity organizations (the public health sector), is increasingly the sole provider for a large proportion of the nation's population. Growing numbers of the poor—which includes almost one-half of the nation's racial minorities—and the increasing proportion of the nation's elderly poor and "new poor"** that depend on this public health care sector, are being systematically deprived of basic health services because of

---

*Excess deaths in the Black population are the number of deaths due to a particular condition above the level that would have occurred if Blacks had experienced the same age-, sex-, and cause-specific mortality rates as Whites. See Manton KG, Patrick CH, Johnson KW. Health differentials between Blacks and Whites: Recent trends in mortality and morbidity. In: Willis DP, ed. *Health Policies and Black Americans.* New Brunswick, NJ: Transaction Publishers, 1989, pp. 129–199; esp. 163.

**The "new poor" consists of a combination of the growing numbers of the working poor, chronically unemployed, and the elderly falling into poverty due to health expenses or inadequate pensions. Many of these working poor are nuclear families with one or two working parents employed in the burgeoning service and part-time sectors, which often do not provide health insurance.

shrinking public budgets and facilities and the recent dynamics of the health insurance and managed care markets. Deborah Prothrow-Stith, in her *Division of Public Health Practice: Strategic Planning Document,* cited William Keck and Douglas Scutchfield's warning regarding market force effects on the poor if new strategies were not forthcoming:

> [I]t is likely that Medicaid reimbursements to health departments will diminish as current health department Medicaid clients are forced to enroll in managed care, with a resultant decrease in the capacity of health departments to cross-subsidize health services for the growing number of the uninsured. . . . [I]t is also likely that managed-care organizations will either fail to meet the needs of many of their enrollees or be forced to duplicate services currently based in health departments.[31]

A diminishment in financing and quality of care for the poor is anticipated. This is exacerbated by the fact that the burgeoning commercial sector of the U.S. health system grudgingly accepts poor, high-risk populations only if sufficient profits can be squeezed out of providing minimal care for them.[32]

All of these developments contribute to, and accelerate, the undermining of the public health care sector. The current subsistence—almost starvation—level defunding of the Health and Hospitals Corporation (HHC) in New York City is one dramatic example.[33] The refugees of this war on poor patients have been forced to emigrate to Medicaid managed care or to the "netherworld" tier of the health care system (or receive no care at all). Once there, patients face a maze created by the numerous strategies these various tiers of the system use to avoid financial losses incurred from caring for disadvantaged patients. These include patient "dumping," cost-shifting, service denials, "cream skimming" populations for financially attractive patients, and emergency room (ER) care denials, shifting services and service sites, and closures. An increasingly popular tactic is the outright refusal of service to ill patients except in dire emergencies at the point-of-service, which is emblematic of the threatened viability of many Medicaid managed care or netherworld services to poor or uninsured patients. The market-dominated ethos that permeates the U.S. health care system rarely condemns such practices.[34]

In addition to this shrinking public health care sector, the netherworld health care system where patients go anticipating that they will receive free care is growing. Medically indigent health consumers, most of whom are employed, unlike Medicaid or public aid patients, usually have absolutely no health insurance coverage. This is the last domain of the growing ranks of the uninsured and underinsured, the working poor, and the homeless. Their ranks are growing predictably and constantly as the contemporary capitalist economy shifts from its "postindustrial" to "information age" configuration: Jobs migrating to suburbs or overseas, increasingly unavailable requisite training for employment to blocs of the population, chronic unemployment for a permanent underclass becoming public policy by default, and a job market shaped by arbitrary standards and tests.[35]

The netherworld health system emanates from the nation's hospital emergency rooms or urgent care facilities. The characteristics of this health care resemble the term itself. It is ephemeral, episodic, inconstant, fragmented, and inconsistent. Care in these settings is unbelievably expensive, although for a complex matrix of reasons, money seldom changes hands. For patients, these conditions make obtaining quality services—or sometimes any services at all—a crap shoot. Such characteristics are largely due to availability based on the largess and whim of the private sector—which shrinks, restructures, obliterates, or phases out these services whenever it desires. Depending on the mood of providers, results of the last senior management meeting, or exigencies of the market (e.g., advertising and public relations considerations, public perceptions regarding rendering of community service, excess profit availability), service provision often unpredictably disappears or relocates. Thus, dependent patient populations often get the runaround. These characteristics render the netherworld health system incomplete and inferior qualitatively. It is a natural consequence of patients forced to become beggars in a commercial health system. This netherworld tier exists alongside the public health care sector in some areas and stands alone in other regions of the United States where publicly funded health facilities are nonexistent. Near-worship of the "religion" of private entrepreneurship in the United States has given corporate entities operating the health care system virtual life-and-death power over underserved populations.[36] These phenomena contribute to the substantial growth of the netherworld subsystem throughout the 1980s and 1990s in contrast to the declining publicly funded health care sector. Declining interest and community support have led to vital public hospitals and community health centers being closed, sold off to private capitalists, or subjected to Draconian funding cuts. But the future of even the netherworld subsystem is now in question as privatization and corporate takeovers proceed.[37]

The studied silence surrounding Black health creates a frightening public policy scenario for America's oldest, largest, nonindigenous racial group. Without decent health care the prospect of high rates of constitutional defectiveness (because of absent or late prenatal care, the persistent presence of very low and low birth weight babies, etc.), elimination from intellectual and economic competition because of disease and illness (e.g., late detection of childhood visual and hearing defects, exposure to brain-damaging illnesses due to lack of immunizations), mounting numbers of excess deaths caused by chronic and treatable diseases (e.g., untreated or uncontrolled hypertension, untreated or uncontrolled diabetes, uncontrolled asthma), and compromised social productivity and viability are no longer beyond the realm of imagination or possibility. Health policies that dictate poor health outcomes are with us. Whether health policies with these implications are to become intentional and institutionalized in the future is the issue we must confront. We have reached a place in our history in which we espouse a color-blind society. With such ambitions, the time is past wherein the health delivery system remains a burden impeding the social progress of African Americans.

The Black health crisis poses particularly disturbing medical-social and ethical dilemmas to the White medical and health care establishments. White Americans have made several quasilegal declarations over recent decades claiming access to decent health care as a right. These declarations have no legal or entitlement authority.[38] Nevertheless, the concept of health care as a human right has become stronger with the acceptance of the human capital* perspective regarding social policy. Since World War II the "right to health care" has become incorporated into the unwritten American creed—another major concern within the national consciousness as recent events have demonstrated.[39] Nevertheless, although most health experts acknowledge that the U.S. health care delivery system does not provide health care to all Americans in a fair, just, or sometimes ethical manner, meaningful policies for corrective action are few. This conflict between what the nation espouses and what it actually practices poses a multifaceted dilemma. Demographic analyses demonstrate the strong racial overtones of this dilemma; structural analyses corroborate the impression.[40]

Quiet contemplation seems to have replaced the cacophonous national health care debate that raged between 1992 and 1994. Nevertheless, the dialogue on health policy continues to reflect unrealistic frames of reference for disadvantaged minorities. It neither represents nor speaks for the majority of African Americans; it considers almost exclusively the concerns of White, middle-class, fully employed Americans with nuclear families. This segment of the population, along with a small elite, constitutes one-half to two-thirds of the patients who use America's health care system. Events are rapidly deeding silent control of the health system to a privileged corporate oligarchy. Yet the unrepresented lower third, which includes most African Americans, may turn out to be the critical segment for public policy. Their inclusion or exclusion in the health care system may represent one of the challenges that decides the fate and future of this nation and its representative democracy. The specter of second rate political and economic status compounded by social unrest looms in the U.S. future if problems like these remain unaddressed.

The evolutionary threads of this major medical-social problem are similar to the origins of the problems Gunnar Myrdal pointed out in his classic *An American Dilemma*.[41] In this monumental work Myrdal documented the conflicts between the nation's ideal, epitomized by the American creed (reification of hard work, meritocracy, equal opportunity, fair treatment of all citizens), and the U.S. realities of racial segregation, discrimination, and domination by White society.

---

*The human capital perspective is a social scientific methodology wherein an attempt is made to place a money value directly on life. If life or productivity is lost because of premature death or illness, the costs to society can be calculated. See Holland WW, Detels R, Knox G, eds. *Oxford Textbook of Public Health* (Vol. 2, *Methods of Public Health*). 2nd ed. Oxford: Oxford University Press, 1991, pp. 301–302.

He viewed this problem as deeply implanted in the hearts and souls of the American public, which explains many of its persistent obsessional characteristics noted by later scholars such as Joel Kovel, Andrew Hacker, and Studs Terkel.[42] Myrdal articulated this gut-wrenching conflict and its place in the American psyche in this oft-quoted statement:

> *It is there that the interracial tension has its focus. It is there that the decisive struggle goes on. . . . Though our study includes economic, social, and political race relations, at bottom our problem is the moral dilemma of the American—the conflict between his moral valuations on various levels of consciousness and generality. The "American Dilemma". . . is the ever-raging conflict between, on the one hand, the valuations preserved on the general plane which we shall call the "American Creed," where the American thinks, talks, and acts under the influence of high national and Christian precepts, and, on the other hand, the valuations on specific planes of individual and group living, where personal and local interests; economic, social, and sexual jealousies; considerations of community prestige and conformity; group prejudice against particular persons or types of people; and all sorts of miscellaneous wants, impulses, and habits dominate his outlook.[43]*

Many of the health issues Myrdal pointed out in his 1944 work remain unaddressed today. Thus, his title still rings hauntingly true in health care more than 50 years later.

In contrast to previous decades when highly trained and nationally respected Black health policy makers such as Paul Cornely, W. Montague Cobb, William Darity, and M. Alfred Haynes allied with civil rights and African American service organizations to crusade for Black health progress, little such leadership exists today.[44] Moreover, many of the Black institutions within whose walls these men functioned—Black medical schools, civil rights organizations, and institutions of higher learning—are financially hobbled or are in the throes of being dismantled.

African American health advocates are conspicuous by their absence or lack of orientation to Black health needs in recent debates. Perhaps Black scholars and intellectuals have surrendered to the problem pointed out by James Anderson in *The State of Afro-American History: Past, Present, and Future*:

> *Instead of treating slavery and the black presence as fundamental dimensions of the growth of the American republic, authors . . . treat them as adjuncts to the American experience, aberrations of Jeffersonian democracy, and thus not a central part of the real American pageant.[45]*

The problem Anderson points out is pervasive in public health. Today's cadre of trained Black health professionals is either silent about the health crisis in the African American community as they pursue other agendas or marginalized when they speak up. The few who do investigate, research, and articulate these issues usually go unrecognized, unfunded, underfunded, or are even ostracized by mainstream professionals. Therefore, the majority of African American biomedical, health services, or health policy researchers—by choice, by chance, or by avoiding what appears to be a sure route to professional failure—concentrate their energies and training on endeavors that will benefit the mainstream rather than underserved patients. For many reasons that will become evident throughout the book, the least healthy group in America is being ill-served and remains virtually unrepresented at the upper echelons of policy making in the waves of health care reform and our current national transformation toward corporate-dominated managed care.

Necessity clearly dictates a different perspective on health care and health policy, based on African American needs and experiences. Such an infusion of newly resurrected and critically analyzed information, often revealed for the first time and with a minority perspective, may generate new and creative ideas, institutional interest, and leadership in the African American and health policy communities. In a contemporary health care reform debate that is data driven, good intentions and lofty medical ethics are not enough. The nation needs factual information about African American health and reputable databases that answers deficiencies created by the omissions and distortions of the past and the insensitivities and indifference of the present. *An American Health Dilemma* begins to fill some of these gaps.

Despite the massive body of facts and events surrounding the relationship between race, medicine, and health care examined and assessed in this book, many experts in the U.S. health delivery system contend, covertly or overtly, that race is not a significant factor in American health or health care. Some of these analysts choose strictly "materialistic"* and/or financial approaches to health care that, in effect, deny America's racial past. By adopting these approaches, medical-social and evolutionary events that structured America's health system are negated. Reifying** numerical, mechanistic, scientistic models ignores the social complexities of U.S. or Western cultural, historical, or social reality (the inclusion of which constitutes a constructionist approach to the problem). It perpetuates the myth that Western science has been completely objective and absent sociocultural bias.[46] The results of these flawed reductionist† and materialistic approaches compounded by inappropriate framing of the problem are tantamount to the misuse of

---

*Materialism is a doctrine that pursues ends connected with bodily pleasures, or the possession of material goods, or of things such as money, considered a means of obtaining such pleasures or goods. This is often contrasted with idealism, the pursuit of ideals that may be high-flown but are likely to be impossible to achieve in practice.

**Reifying is the fallacy of converting abstract concepts into entities. A prominent example is the recognition of the importance of the wondrously complex and multifaceted set of human capabilities comprising mentality. Intelligence, a shorthand symbol for this complex set of behaviors, is reified and transformed into a unitary "thing" capable of being expressed as a single number—the IQ.

†Reductionism is the method of thinking wherein everything is organized and explained in terms of its smallest, most basic, elements (e.g., the gene explains all dimensions of human beings including

the scientific method, the perpetuation of history-based "blind spots" regarding race and health in America, and perpetuating the continuum such that little corrective action takes place. These deleterious mechanisms have already impacted U.S. health policy and, subsequently, the health status and outcomes of African American and other disadvantaged ethnic American populations.

One weighty piece of evidence documenting the negation of race as a health system factor is an analysis of a late 1980s' U.S. government report on the nation's health published in a 1990 issue of the highly respected British medical journal *The Lancet*. In that review D. S. Greenberg noted that little is being done about the fact that African Americans still experience morbidity and mortality rates that were long ago eliminated in other industrial nations. The concepts of race and racism as possible explanatory hypotheses for these outcomes were implicated but not explored. Greenberg cites race-based health disparities as both a failure of the U.S. health care system and an ethical dilemma. "The issue of minority health . . . has held a high place on the rhetorical agenda of recent presidential administrations," Greenberg states. "Lacking, however, are both the needed financial resources and a willingness to abandon some of the political hallucinations that persist in the politics of minority health improvement," he concludes.[47]

Highlighting the need for a book examining these issues was the failed 1994 debate over national health reform. Participation of individuals representing African American and disadvantaged populations was scant and belated. The subsequent silent transformation of the health system into corporate, managed care directions following the defeat of health reform by the 103rd Congress is also a continuing concern with financial and ideological implications. The nexus of concern involves exclusion or underservice in the face of the African American community's legitimate health needs and concerns. Dialogue between U.S. health system policy makers and the variegated communities they serve is necessary to develop specific policies and programs ameliorating centuries-old health status and outcome disparities. Negation represents a persistent pattern over the past decade and a half by major institutions in the health delivery and medical establishments—who frame the 380-year-old African American health deficits almost entirely in nonracial terms. The result is devastating. Sorely needed research is prevented or vitiated, flawed and ineffective health care institutions and policies are preserved, and poor and disparate race-based health care outcomes remain the norm.[48]

Reports are issued that utilize methodology ignoring the effects of structural inequities and institutional racism in health delivery, biotechnology, and health education systems and how they impact the health outcomes of African Americans. Many of these analyses focus on "culture of poverty" deficits—laziness, ignorance about health, noncompliance with medical advice, poor work habits—in the victims as the primary explanations for their poor health outcomes and dysfunctional

---

their physical makeup and behaviors, so everything can ultimately be explained on the basis of atoms). It disregards factors such as the historical, hierarchical, or nonmaterial.

relationships with the health delivery system. Reports not openly downplaying race as a dominant factor in the production of these racial health disparities frame them in racially neutral terms.[49] Others view health insurance reform as a panacea or feel that socioeconomic status or class is the main issue, not race. Reports with these perspectives emanating from such influential sources as the National Research Council, the National Academy of Sciences, the National Academy of Engineering, the National Institute of Medicine, and the American Cancer Society project the impression that race is no longer a significant factor in American health care.[50]

Attempts to redefine these historical race-based health disparities in purely materialistic, reductionist, and, therefore, unrealistic terms risk not addressing the problems at all. Greenberg in *The Lancet* suggests that the racial positions adopted by the health care establishment are both irrational and insensitive. This reinforces James H. Jones's impression that the U.S. medical profession, and the biomedical research establishment that it has erected over the past century, has a "blind spot" when it comes to understanding the detrimental effects its racial attitudes and practices have on Black patients and national health policy.[51] Television features, documentaries, popular press, and media releases of the 1990s focusing on the relationship between race and unethical experimentation exemplified by the Tuskegee syphilis experiment, which included interviews with White medical researchers, reaffirmed Jones's conclusions.[52] Larry R. Churchill in *Rationing Health Care in America: Perceptions and Principles of Justice* details how the Puritan ethic, rugged individualism, the Horatio Alger legend, and similar aspects of the American character help drive the unjust rationing of American health care. These national character traits create social distance, generate cynicism, and encourage victim blaming within the nation's middle and upper classes regarding the poor and less fortunate in the health system. Sniderman and Piazza in *The Scar of Race* also perceive the rise of new forms of U.S. racism disguised as some of the traditional American values such as hard work, self-reliance, and individual initiative. These mechanisms exacerbate the system's historical race problems in health delivery. It is disconcerting and chilling how these American character traits that drive inequitable health care rationing overlap with postmodern forms of racism. Social scientists like William Ryan explain how middle-class American ideologies and cultural norms suggest that subsequent health disparities are the fault of the victims rather than inequitable and biased health care and sociopolitical systems.[53] These and other analyses demand that race be considered a key factor in any accurate portrayal of the U.S. health care system. Thus, the explanatory significance of race in African American health care delivery, health status, and outcome deserves both thorough reexamination and detailed reassessment.[54]

PART I

The Background

CHAPTER ONE

Race, Biology, and Health Care in the United States: Reassessing a Relationship

Race is a major factor in American life. Of all the factors that adversely affect the health status and outcomes of African Americans, race is one of the major contributors. The roots of the problem can be traced back thousands of years to the very origins of Western life sciences and the health subculture. But racial effects on health outcomes are often ignored and obscured by the very medical and health establishments that purport to aid those afflicted. So impressed were Louis Knowles and Kenneth Prewitt with the effects institutional racism had on the health and health care of African Americans that they included a chapter, "Why White Americans Are Healthier," in their pioneering book *Institutional Racism in America* (1969). The federally sponsored Kerner Commission Report of 1968, the *Report of the National Advisory Commission on Civil Disorders*, also cited the absence or inadequacy of health care based on race as one of the major precipitating factors in the epidemic of urban race riots sweeping the United States during the 1960s. Only now are medical and health policy researchers beginning to reexamine earlier assumptions.

During the 1980s a team led by leading health economist Eli Ginzberg conducted surveys and investigations focusing on the public health care sector (city and county hospitals, hospital and public clinics, and health departments) in a representative sample of the nation's major cities. Their conclusions were startling. African American and other economically disadvantaged groups disproportionately utilized the public health care sector for most of their health-related needs. The Ginzberg team's testimony before the U.S. Congress in 1994 indicated that health care for African Americans and the poor has not substantively changed since the 1960s and might be deteriorating.[1]

To comprehend the relationship between race and health care in the United States, what is actually known about race and its relationship to biomedical and other life sciences and health care must be analyzed and exposed while examining some of the modern concepts about race in Western society. An intellectual history of race can guide our inquiry and increase understanding of what is known about the concept in Western culture. A deeper and more comprehensive reckoning of the modern relationships between race and the life sciences, along with how the contemporary relationships evolved, necessitates a historical examination. Exploring concepts of race and racism and their connections to medicine and health care in U.S. and predecessor Western cultures is a critical goal of this inquiry. Through this examination the relationship between race and Western biomedical and other life sciences can be clearly and comprehensively drawn for the first time.

Race operates in society today more explosively and confusingly than ever before. Many factors confuse and reignite this ever smoldering social issue. They include, but are not limited to, the loss of the dominant society's patience with African Americans and the Civil Rights Movement; the efficacy of the more subtle racialist mechanisms of economic and social domination and discrimination; a relatively new and modern racialist mechanism built around the erection of a European American culture-based, IQ- and achievement test-oriented "meritocracy" favoring groups with access to privileged environments and quality education and training; the emergence of political and religious conservative movements with their traditions of religious and racial intolerance; the emergence of aggressive feminist and newly empowered Latino and Asian American groups competing with African Americans for limited jobs, training and educational opportunities, and political positions previously allocated for non-Europeans and women; and the lack of political, economic, and ideological commitment by the nation's European American leaders to openly address and alleviate the impact of racism in U.S. society. All these potent forces threaten to overpower the interests of America's oldest and largest minority* group.

For a variety of reasons, racial and ethnic polarization seems to be intensifying. How does race affect contemporary U.S. society—particularly health care? As evidenced by persistent race-based health disparities and segregation in the health care system, a new "hostile and unequal" racial climate profoundly affects African American health and health care.[2] (See Table 1.1.)

---

*The designation "minority" connotes subordination. Referring to African Americans, Asian/Pacific Islander Americans, Indian/Native/Eskimo Americans, and Hispanic/Latino Americans as "ethnic Americans," who now constitute 24.36% of the U.S. population, is preferable. However, because the usage of "minority" is pervasive and most commonly understood, the authors will utilize both terms interchangeably. See Randall (1993) in note 1 for this chapter in the Notes section (at the end of the book) and the *1990 U.S. Census* for further references.

Table 1.1   Racial Comparison of Health Data through Early 1990s

Health Parameters	Black–White Comparison	Comments/Significance
Longevity	Blacks live 5 to 7 years less than Whites.	The "Gold Standard" of health system performance: Black males continue the free fall in longevity that started in 1984; Black–White gap widening since 1984.
	Black life expectancy 69.2 years compared to 76 years for Whites.	Black life expectancy at lowest point since 1981 and 0.4 years shorter than the 1986 edition of Table 1.1.
Excess deaths	Blacks suffer 91,490 annually; 37% of Black deaths are "excess."	Almost 4 of 10 Black deaths are "extra"; if death rates for races were equal, these deaths wouldn't occur; excess deaths have increased 53% since 1984.
Death rate (deaths per 100,000 [10^5] population)	Black death rate of $783.1/10^5$ is $1.6 \times$ the White rate.	The ultimate sign of health system failure; misses huge amounts of morbidity (pain and suffering); death rate for Blacks now higher than 1982 rate.
Infant mortality rate (death in first year of life per 1000)	Black IMR of 17.7 per 1000 live births is $2.2 \times$ the White rate.	A major indicator of health status and a measure of general living standards of a population; Black rate worse than Cuba's, Puerto Rico's, or Costa Rica's; Black–White disparity widening since 1970s; rose in 1989.
Death rate 25- to 44-year-olds (per 100,000 [10^5] population)	Black rate of $373.6/10^5$ is $2.5 \times$ the White rate.	Huge number of person-years lost; responsible for a larger portion of poverty and matriarchal families plaguing Black communities; Black–White disparities widening since 1982.
Selected (leading) causes of death (National Vital Statistics System)	Blacks lead in 14 of 16 categories.	Many of these deaths preventable with known, basic, cost-effective medical treatments.

(continued)

Table 1.1 *continued*

Health Parameters	Black–White Comparison	Comments/Significance
Neonatal morality Black rate[a]	1987–89 Black rate at 12.1/103 live births, with Black–White ratio of 2.28.	Reflects prepregnancy health and prenatal, intrapartum, and neonatal care; racial gap is increasing; the rate rose in 1989; 1989 disparity between Black and White newborn death rates at widest point since 1950.
Low-birth-weight infants (<2500 gm)	Black rate of 13.51% is 136% more than White rate.	Racial discrepancy widening; leading killer and primary source of lifelong disability; Blacks presently experiencing 1950s White rates; Black rates higher than 1980; racial disparity widening.
Very low birth weight (<1500 gm)	Black rate of 2.95% is 3.2 × the White rate.	Physical and mental handicaps often impair survivors; racial discrepancy widening in recent years; Black rate increasing for last 20 years.
Perinatal mortality rate[b]	Black rate of $17.1/10^3$ live births is 111% higher than White rate.	Reflects quality of obstetrical care; is a valid indication of *infant morbidity*.
Post-neonatal mortality (death from day 29 to 364 per 1000 [10^3] live births)	Black rate of $6.4/10^3$ live births is more than 2 × White rate.	Reflects quality of health care for children; prevention and treatment of controlled, treatable diseases; this parameter, getting worse for past 2 years, has reached 1985 levels.
Maternal deaths by race	Black rate of $18.6/10^3$ live births is 3.4 × the White rate; amounts to almost 40% of US total.	Reflects lack of access to obstetrical care; current figures probably an undercount; 75% of these deaths are preventable; Black rate higher than 1982 levels.
Immunization rates (Black children)	69.1% immunized against DPT[c]; 56.5% immunized against polio by age 2 (ranks 56th internationally).	Black children still die, lose vision and hearing, and suffer brain damage from these easily preventable diseases; more children died from

(continued)

Table 1.1   *continued*

Health Parameters	Black–White Comparison	Comments/Significance
		measles in 1990 than in any year since 1971.
Child deaths by race (deaths per 100,000 [10^5] children)	Black rate 30 to 50 percent higher than White rate.	Many of these deaths preventable by immunizations, early diagnosis and treatment; more of these children are being locked out of the health delivery system daily.

<table>
<tr><td>Age</td><td>Black</td><td>White</td></tr>
<tr><td>1–4</td><td>79.65</td><td>46.05</td></tr>
<tr><td>5–14</td><td>34.7</td><td>24.65</td></tr>
</table>

Health Parameters	Black–White Comparison	Comments/Significance
Childhood anemia	One-fifth to one-third of Black children are anemic.	Easily diagnosed and treated with basic child care; reflects poor nutrition; adversely affects school performance.
Toxic lead levels	15–20% of Black urban children may have toxic lead levels.	The first thing lost is intellectual function; most of these children are probably undiagnosed and untreated; probably being mislabelled as retarded or "slow learners."
Childhood tuberculosis	Blacks 4 to 5 × the White rates.	Children's health programs are being cut despite this.
Dental care	40% of Black children <17 years old have never seen a dentist.	Two-thirds of Black children haven't seen a dentist in the past year, programs are being cut daily.
Prevalence Rates		
Diabetes	33% more common in Blacks.	Programs providing care for chronic diseases being cut annually.
Hypertension	Blacks: 34.05% prevalence. Whites: 20.6% prevalence.	Programs providing care for chronic diseases being cut annually.
Heart disease	1.5 × more common in Blacks.	Programs providing care for chronic disease being cut annually.
Stroke deaths	Black rate 1.93 × White rate.	Largely preventable with good, outpatient medical care; African American access for this care is declining.

(continued)

Table 1.1 *continued*

Health Parameters	Black–White Comparison	Comments/Significance
Diabetes death rate	Black rate 1.43 × White rate.	Largely preventable with good, outpatient medical care; African American access for this care is declining; Black–White discrepancy widening.
Heart disease death rate	Black rate 1.43 × White rate.	Largely preventable with good, outpatient medical care; African American access for this care is declining; Black–White discrepancy widening.
HIV infection	Black Male rate 3 × White rate; Black female rate 9 × White rate.	Rose from 15th to 11th leading cause of death; 25% of cases are in African Americans; 55.8% and 54.6% of AIDS cases/AIDS deaths respectively in children were Black between 1984 and 1991.
Pneumonia and influenza death rate	Black rate 1.5 × White rate.	Preventable by access to good medical care, treatment, and timely hospitalization; access for Blacks and the poor is being curtailed.
Nephritis, nephrosis, and nephrotic syndrome deaths	Black rate 3 × White rate.	Largely preventable with good, outpatient medical care and timely hospitalization; access for Blacks and the poor is being curtailed.
Persons unable to carry on major activity because of chronic conditions, according to race	Percent of Black Americans (6.5%) with this form of disability is 80% to 90% higher than White Americans.	This is a measure of the "walking wounded" due to illness; the B/W disparity not improving for a decade; Black rate increasing slightly since 1985.
Cancer incidence	Black: 27% increase White: 12% increase	Reflects increased environmental, toxic exposure, poor diet, and high-risk lifestyle; gap widening.

(continued)

Table 1.1 *continued*

Health Parameters	Black–White Comparison	Comments/Significance
Cancer mortality increase (since 1950)	Blacks: 50% increase Whites: 10% increase	Rates were even in 1950 when there was little treatment; Black access to early diagnosis and treatment being curtailed annually.

[a]Neonatal mortality refers to the death of an infant during the first 28 days of life.
[b]Number of stillbirths plus neonatal deaths per 1,000 live births.
[c]DPT refers to the standard diphtheria-pertussis-tetanus immunization vaccine.

Sources:

American Cancer Society. *Cancer Facts and Figures for Minority Americans: 1986, 1991.* New York: American Cancer Society, 1986.

American Cancer Society. *Cancer Facts and Figures—1988, 1992.* New York: American Cancer Society, 1988.

Byrd WM, Clayton LA. An American health dilemma: A history of blacks in the health system. *Journal of National Medical Association* 1992, 84:189–200.

Children's Defense Fund. *Black and White Children in America: Key Facts.* Washington, D.C.: Children's Defense Fund, 1985.

Cunningham FG, MacDonald PC, Gant NF. *Williams Obstetrics.* 18 Edition. Norwalk, Conn.: Appleton and Lange, 1989.

Haynes MA. The Gap in Health Status between Black and White Americans. In *Textbook of Black-related Diseases,* edited by RA Williams, 1–30, New York: McGraw-Hill, 1975.

Jaynes GD, Williams RM. eds. *A Common Destiny: Blacks and American Society.* Washington, D.C.: National Academy Press, 1989.

Mahaffey KR, Annest J, Roberts J, Murphy R. National Estimates of Blood Lead Levels: United States 1976–1980: Association with selected demographic and socioeconomic factors. *New England Journal of Medicine* 1982, 307:573–579.

National Center for Health Statistics. *Health Status of the Disadvantaged Chartbook/1990.* Hyattsville, Md.: Public Health Service, 1991.

National Center for Health Statistics. *Prevention Profile. Health United States, 1991.* Hyattsville, Md.: Public Health Service, 1992.

National Center for Health Statistics. *Advance Report of Final Mortality Statistics, 1989. Monthly Vital Statistics Report;* vol. 40 no. 8 supp. 2. Hyattsville, Md.: Public Health Service, 1992.

Physician Task Force on Hunger in America. *Hunger in America: The Growing Epidemic.* Middletown, Conn.: Wesleyan University Press, sponsored by the Harvard School of Public Health, 1985.

United Nations. *Demographic Yearbook 1983–1988.* New York: United Nations, 1988.

US Department of Health and Human Services. *Report of the Secretary's Task Force on Black and Minority Health,* vol. 1. *Executive Summary.* Washington, D.C.: US Government Printing Office, 1985.

US Department of Health and Human Services. *Nutrition Monitoring in the United States: Progress Report.* DHHS Pub. No. (PHS) 86-1255. Washington, D.C.: US Department of Health and Human Services, 1986.

World Health Organization. *World Health Organization Statistics Annuals.* Vols. *1985–1990.* Geneva, 1985–1990.

On Race: Examining an Enigma

A deep and probing inquiry on race is necessary for all of these reasons. One pre-requisite is to factor in the effects of the centuries-old relationship between race, Western medicine, science, and health care. A core of modern scholars such as philosopher-ethicist Cornel West; social scientists Thomas Pettigrew, Paul Snider-man and Thomas Piazza, Joe R. Feagin and Melvin P. Spikes, Douglas S. Massey and Nancy A. Denton, St. Clair Drake, William Julius Wilson, Robert W. Terry, and Timothy Maliqalim Simone; social commentators like Ellis Cose and the late Marlon Riggs; and racial theorists and philosophers such as Patricia Turner and Lucius Outlaw have recently attempted to disentangle the new and complicated mix of race relations in the United States. Their efforts at clarification are often complex and challenging. For the purposes of this study, a fresh and all-inclusive investigation of the ancient classical Greek, Arabic, and Western European socio-cultural and biomedical dimensions of race is still needed. Obtaining a deeper understanding of race as a social and scientific concept in Western culture demands that we establish some fundamental ground rules for analysis and com-prehension of how race operates in the U.S. health system and society.[3]

The origins of the word *race* are disputed and may derive from Arabic, Latin, or German sources. It seemingly predates the sixteenth- and seventeenth-century beginnings of modern Western science and the formal study called "racial thought." Initial English use of the word may have been in a 1508 poem by William Dunbar in which he referred to "bakbyttaris of sindry racis" (backbiters of sundry races).[4] The word *race* appeared in formal English literature in 1580 according to *Webster's Dictionary* and other sources. *Webster's* definitions of race are broad and so variegated they become somewhat nebulous. The first defini-tion is "a breeding stock of animals," alluding to current biological definitions. *Webster's* also defines race as "a family, tribe, people, or nation belonging to the same stock" and as "a class or kind of people unified by community of interests." This accumulation of various definitions demonstrates the broad range of intel-lectual territory necessary to cover the concept of race in the modern era. The word simultaneously refers to a biological term, a means of classifying different groups of people possessing common characteristics, and a sociocultural con-cept. Moreover, all of these usages are correct and proper in this modern era of racial thought.[5]

The word *race* has many connotations. Initially intended as a means of clas-sifying various branches of the human family, the ambiguity the word evokes is symptomatic of its variegated definitions and multifaceted meanings. It is capable of triggering as much, if not more, emotion or violence than any word or concept in contemporary Western civilization. The perverted usages and causes with which the term has been identified and associated throughout Western history, often with negative overtones, help explain the emotionally charged and volatile effects it registers on the Western psyche. Until recently race was used as the justification for differential treatment for groups of human beings; however, objective and scientific criteria for establishing biological differences between races have proved more imagined than real. This has led some scholars and scientists, such as Ashley Montagu, Jacques Barzun, and Allan Chase, to label "race" a dangerous *myth* that should be discarded by Western culture. Although biologically man is now considered a polytypic species—the races constituting the major subspecies—past and present inbreeding renders even this definition imprecise and absent clear divisions.

In zoology, *race* is defined as a variety or subspecies—a partially isolated breeding population with some differences in gene frequencies from related populations yet still entirely capable of interbreeding. Traditional racial classifications based on factors such as skin color, hair texture, intelligence, and physical features, although genetically and biologically insignificant, are still perpetuated by those who would justify social prejudice or political oppression. *Racism* is an excessive and irrational belief that race is the primary determinant of human traits and capacities and that racial differences produce inherent superiority or inferiority of a particular race, while *racialism* is the doctrine that race has a preponderant influence on the origin, development, and rank of various human societies. *Race prejudice* is a set of irrationally based, negative attitudes against certain groups on the basis of race.

Some contemporary scholars view race as a sociocultural concept driven by and mediated through racism. Racism is, in this modern sense, a set of prejudicial attitudes, behaviors, and social structures and mediators that differentiates, dominates, discriminates, oppresses, and subordinates individuals based on race. This book focuses on the effects of race and racism on the U.S. medical profession, health delivery system, health professions educational-research infrastructure, and the health status and outcomes of African Americans. While race operates as an independent variable throughout U.S. society, obtaining access to quality health care in the United States generates a unique matrix of interrelationships between race, economics, employment, education, and health.* This book's heavy emphasis on historical events and health care as a social process is necessary to help the reader understand that the health care system did not evolve in isolation but is a product of historical, sociocultural, economic, and political events and processes. For these reasons this menu of related issues are explored and discussed throughout the text to contextualize the operative mechanisms that define race, medicine, and health care in the United States. References to positive applications of race and racialism by both African and European Americans—including sociocultural phenomena such as Kwanzaa, Black pride, Black

---

*Other Western industrialized countries do not demand full employment, privileged economic status, or requisite educational or training status to ensure their citizens' full-fledged participation in the health care system.

nationalism, Afrocentric cultural identity, Black art, or African American studies—have long been the subject of other inquiries.[6]

One broader definition of racism that incorporates its institutional dimensions can be found in Robert Terry's *For Whites Only* (1992). Joe Feagin and
Melvin Spikes also outline a comprehensive definition in their more recent book
Living with Racism: The Black Middle-Class Experience (1994). These authors
use the term *racism* "to refer not only to the prejudices and discriminatory actions
of particular white bigots but also institutionalized discrimination and to the
recurring ways in which white people dominate black people in almost every
major area of this society."[7] These important revisions in taxonomy and epistemology—though not factoring in the effects of Black racism,* however—were
driven by the acknowledgment that although many European Americans have
adopted superficially egalitarian rhetoric during recent decades, "many whites
want interpersonal solutions *apart from societal changes.*"[8] This shift was so obvious to Robert Terry since the 1960s that he reexamined his conceptualization of
racism and now describes and defines *societal* and *individual* racism as his basic
categories. His most recent and more comprehensive definition of racism, which
emphasizes improving both "interpersonal relations and societal restructure,"
reads:

> Racism exists when one race/color group intentionally or unintention-
> ally refuses to share power, distributes resources inequitably, maintains
> unresponsive and inflexible institutional policies, procedures, and prac-
> tices, and imposes ethnocentric culture on any other race/color group for
> its supposed benefit, and justifies its actions by blaming the other
> race/color group.[9]

Thus, many contemporary views of racism incorporate important institutional
aspects of the problem, as suggested by Knowles and Prewitt in their classic *Institutional Racism in America* (1969)—a work precipitated by the 1968 Kerner
Commission Report on the causes of the urban race riots.[10]

Historically speaking, adverse outcomes due to racism in the United States
range from lynching, to racially motivated physical and emotional abuse; to chattel slavery; to medical abuse and exploitation (including overutilization of Blacks
for medical demonstration and experimentation purposes); to legalized racial
segregation and discrimination; to economic and social oppression, deprivation,
and exploitation. The mediators of racism in the United States are the engines

---

*Some authorities feel that since racism is strongly rooted in power relationships and the dominant
institutions in Western society are shaped according to White interests and organized symbolically
around whiteness, there can be no Black racism. However, even exponents of this extreme view con-
cede that Blacks, being human, are fully capable of prejudicial or bigoted behavior that could be
adduced as a Black racist response.

that drive and produce the adverse outcomes related to race prejudice (arising out of antipathetic attitudes and feelings, primarily—mental states that do not affect the external world unless acted upon). The shift from the older mediators of emotion-filled and psychologically mediated "gut" or overt racism to more subtle mediators of contemporary racism is a critical development of this century.

Over the past 50 years scholars of racial studies have explored the dynamics of race and racism in behavioral as well as chronological contexts. Changing contexts and definitions render the evaluation of the impact of race on a person or social event a direct function of the time and place in which it occurred. For example, when Yeats wrote in the nineteenth century

> *Many times man lives and dies*
> *Between his two eternities,*
> *That of race and that of soul,*
> *And ancient Ireland knew it all*[11]

the poet used "race" in the traditional sense, referring to a form of Irish lineage. Using race as a referent to an ethnic group or a national population was common in the nineteenth century. In certain contexts, such as being a member of the Irish race during that period, the term did not have the negative connotations and dire consequences that it did when applied to enslaved Africans during the same era.

Whether racism and racist behavior is an ancient or contemporary phenomenon is another chronological issue. French anthropologist Claude Lévi-Strauss believed that an unsophisticated, ethnocentric form of racism existed in primitive groups dating from prehistoric times. Differences in appearance were important. St. Clair Drake detailed the history-based antagonism against black as a concept and skin color in Western culture. (See Figures 1.1 and 1.2.) Lévi-Strauss contends that tradition was extended through the Golden Age of Greek culture (ca. 500 BC) until at least the Age of Discovery when Spaniards sent out "[c]ommissions of investigation to discover whether or not the natives had a soul."[12] Lévi-Strauss reported that the great philosophic and religious systems devised by Buddhist, Christian, Islamic, Stoic, and Kantian or Marxist doctrines—relatively recent players on the historic stage—all imperfectly articulate the concept "that all men are naturally equal and should be bound together in brotherhood, irrespective of race or culture."[13] Our later investigations corroborate the substance, if not all the details, of his hypothesis.

Michel Leiris, another French anthropologist, presents an alternative hypothesis that the virulent form of modern racism with which most Americans are familiar arose within the framework and context of the Atlantic slave trade between the fifteenth and nineteenth centuries. Africanist scholars Basil Davidson and Ali Mazrui agree there was a Western cultural intensification of anti-Black racism accompanying the Atlantic slave trade. Leiris observed that a milder

Figure 1.1 Names of Colors as Verbal Symbols with Multiple Referents

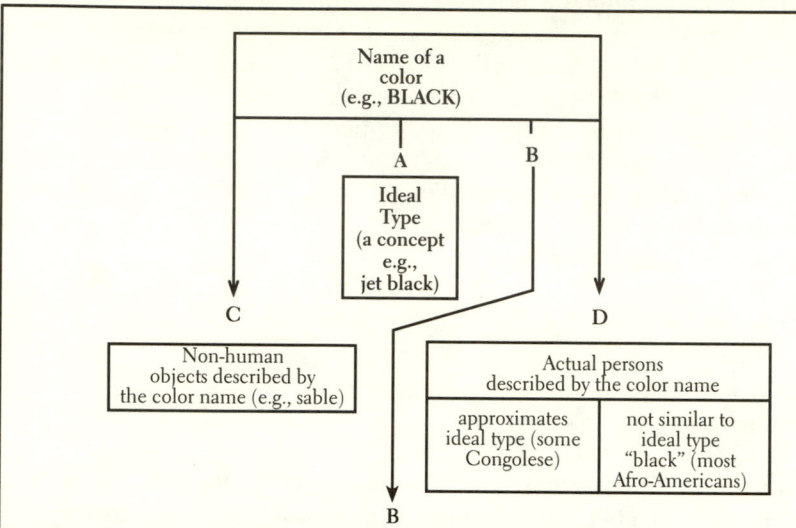

A number of referents with word "BLACK"					
Positive value		Neutral value		Negative value	
"Black is Beautiful" or "Black is spiritually powerful"or "in the black" (accounting)	Black Beauty, a horse in a story — Black Madonnas in Europe	"Black as Night" or black as absence of color in color spectrum	color of an auto or a dress — "Black Holes" in space	"Black is Evil" or "Black is Ugly"	Black cat in European folklore — Some devils — Some human races
abstract concept	empirical referent (in a context)	abstract concept	empirical referent (in a context)	abstract	empirical referent (in a context)

1. The term *Black*, in the chart above, has as referents
   [A] an ideal type concept of what *"Black"* is
   [B] a number of referents that are imputed to the word, "Black," and that presumably evoke emotions, sentiments, etc. (connotations)
   [C] inanimate objects described by the name of the color
   [D] individuals or groups of people referred to by the color name; they may, or may not, approximate the ideal type in actuality.
2. The critical question is, "When one referent of the color name is a characteristic or group of characteristics, is it possible that these characteristics are not necessarily imputed to *people* who may be called by the color name?" Is it possible that a distinction is drawn between color to designate abstract qualities and color to designate skin color?

St. Clair Drake points out the color black has positive, neutral, and negative value in Western culture. A large percentage of these referents are negative and are often applied to Black people in many contexts.

Figure 1.2   **Attitudes Expressed in Initial Contact between Individuals of Different Racial Groups**

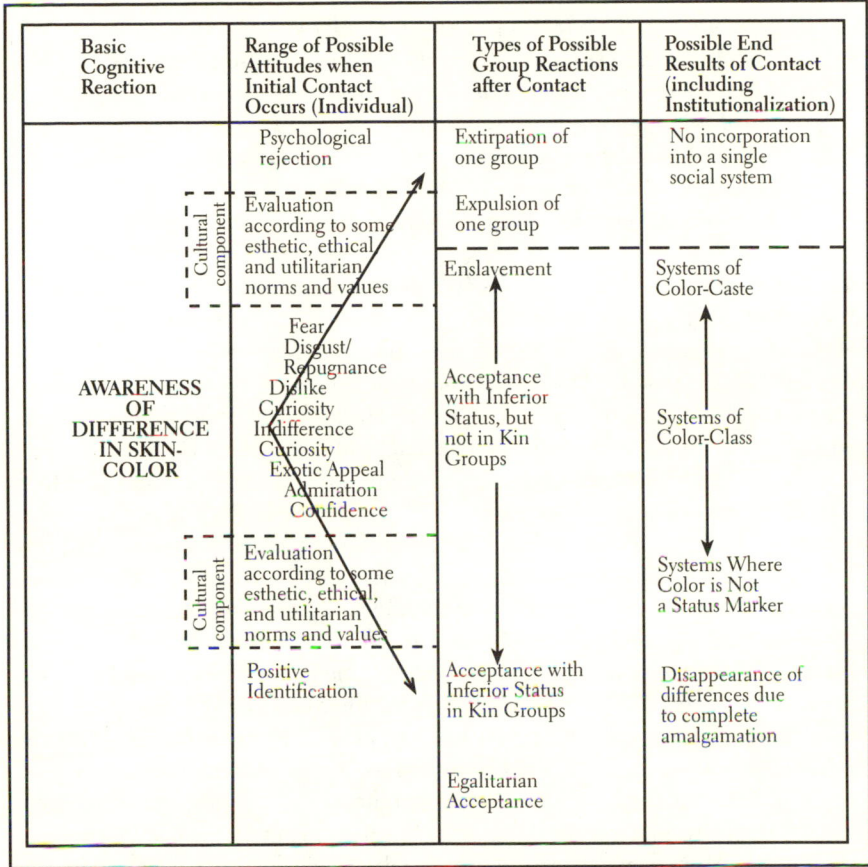

Basic Cognitive Reaction	Range of Possible Attitudes when Initial Contact Occurs (Individual)	Types of Possible Group Reactions after Contact	Possible End Results of Contact (including Institutionalization)
	Psychological rejection	Extirpation of one group	No incorporation into a single social system
Cultural component — Evaluation according to some esthetic, ethical and utilitarian norms and values		Expulsion of one group	
		Enslavement	Systems of Color-Caste
AWARENESS OF DIFFERENCE IN SKIN-COLOR	Fear, Disgust/ Repugnance Dislike Curiosity Indifference Curiosity Exotic Appeal Admiration Confidence	Acceptance with Inferior Status, but not in Kin Groups	Systems of Color-Class
Cultural component — Evaluation according to some esthetic, ethical, and utilitarian norms and values			Systems Where Color is Not a Status Marker
	Positive Identification	Acceptance with Inferior Status in Kin Groups	Disappearance of differences due to complete amalgamation
		Egalitarian Acceptance	

St. Clair Drake places racial behavior in both individual and institutional contexts.

form of ethnocentric-based racism existed prior to this period. However, he was prescient in recognizing the destructive potential of the most recent forms of science-based racism in the 1950s when he stated, "[T]he crowning paradox is that, to provide a rational justification for their blind prejudice, appeal is made to our age's gods—science and scientific objectivity."[14]

Pierre L. van den Berghe, in *Race and Racism* (1967), contrasts the racism of slavery with more modern forms—labeling the former "paternalistic racism" and the latter "competitive racism." In the paternalistic version, slaves were viewed as "childish, immature, irresponsible, exuberant, improvident, fun loving, good humored, and happy-go-lucky; in short, as inferior but lovable 'children' as long as they stay 'in their place.'"[15] Kevin Reilly concurred with van den Berghe:

> *This is the racism of the great slave plantations, celebrated by its defend-*
> *ers in Latin America and the Southern states as a world where master*
> *and slave confronted each other as real, living, breathing, thinking*
> *human beings. Here social distance allowed for extreme intimacy, as*
> *well as the extreme brutality that often accompanies such intimacy.*
> *Miscegenation was accepted, and often encouraged. The ruling class*
> *mixed its prejudice with oaths of love, service, and loyalty. The slaves*
> *either internalized the values of their masters, and (like Uncle Tom)*
> *loved their masters, or they rebelled viciously and with dignity, only to*
> *be annihilated for their fundamental breach of social order.*[16]

Such paternalistic societies of masters and slaves supposedly duplicated the father–child relationships of families, thus explaining and clarifying van den Berghe's "paternalistic" terminology. Based on absolute authority, mutually understood "rules" were practiced by both master-father and slave-child. Brutality, always a dangerous undercurrent, was unleashed when the social order built upon custom, habit, and acceptance was breached, and "bad" slaves were beaten or killed.

This contrasts strongly with van den Berghe's "competitive racism," which dominated race relations in the urban North before the Civil War and the entire country afterward. These environments were highly competitive with an almost "floating antagonism" wherein the poor White was pitted in direct competition against newly freed Blacks for employment, upward social mobility, and financial aggrandizement. As Kevin Reilly observed in *The West and the World*, "The poor whites could no longer accept the slaveowner's image of blacks as good children or pets."[17] As the poor Whites began exercising their newfound political and economic power after the Civil War, they saw Blacks as "aggressive, insolent, 'uppity,' clannish, dishonest, underhanded competitors for scarce resources and challengers of the status quo,"[18] in van den Berghe's words. Politicians, financiers, planters, and community leaders exploited this natural antagonism and economic tension to pit Whites and Blacks against each other. This interracial economic competition and the environment it created spawned rising tides of racism. In such environments, little sympathy could be generated regarding the plight of African Americans—health care problems or otherwise. The intimate and symbiotic relationship between van den Berghe's economically derived competitive racism model, Terry's power-mediated racism, and the contemporary "aversive" and "metaracist" racism paradigms defined by psychiatrist Joel Kovel crystallizes within the market-driven, capitalistic economic environment coalescing in the United States. This potent mix of racist mechanisms and economic competition has spawned sociological environments that have favored the perpetuation, and even intensification, of race-based social and economic inequalities.[19]

According to Terry, these pervasive mediators of modern racism can be conceptualized and viewed in terms of the current mechanisms of White social dominance and discrimination. These mediators include (1) *power*, the unfair distribution or disproportionate capacity by the dominant White/Anglo group to make and enforce decisions; (2) differentially controlling *resources* such as money, education, information, and political influence by the dominant racial group; (3) establishing societal *standards* according to dominant White/Anglo definitions, automatically marginalizing other group norms; and (4) incorrectly defining *problems* by the dominant White/Anglo group such that perceptions and solutions are distorted, inappropriate, manipulatable, and dysfunctional. In the health arena, these principles can be applied to the health system's historical and contemporary configurations. According to these theories, racism in the United States can be understood as a system of European American dominance affecting African Americans in the U.S. health system.[20]

Another important and useful psychologically and behaviorally derived model of modern racism is detailed in *White Racism: A Psychohistory* (1970). Utilizing psychological and behavioral contexts, Kovel examines mediating components of racism, such as unfair power control, unfair control and distribution of resources, preservation of White/Anglo standards, and defective problem definition. His analysis is strongly based on history and focuses on European Americans as the source and the perpetrators of U.S. racism and racial discrimination. Kovel reiterates, in two versions of his model (1984), the fundamental principle that racism "is the tendency of a society to degrade and to do violence to people on the basis of race . . . by whatever meditations may exist for this purpose."[21] The new, more plastic and subtle, forms of violence are equally as, if not more, devastating to African Americans and other ethnic groups as the older forms. European Americans of particular socioeconomic statuses, classes, and ethnic backgrounds continue to have greater access to financial, educational, and political resources. European American behavioral standards are the norms by which other groups are judged. Deviation from these standards leads to marginalization. When discussions about social problems like racism and discrimination take place, Whites often speak in terms of the "Black," "Hispanic," or "Native American" problems, according to Terry, Kovel, and Simone. Specious problem definition incorrectly lays the blame for the problems at the feet of the victims of White racism. As Terry, Kovel, and Simone reiterate, anti-Black and non-White racism is fundamentally a White problem.[22]

Kovel and other students of psychology and behavior who have studied the evolution of racism in the United States allege that the old-fashioned *dominative* racism based on direct physical oppression and sexual obsession has yielded to more modern forms such as *aversive* racism and *metaracism*. Kovel defines *aversive racism* as "the racism of coldness . . . belong[ing] to bourgeois life, proper, being that form of racism characteristic of the North, stable urban zones of segregation and suburbs."[23] This racist mechanism is characterized by dominant group avoidance (Whites) with isolation of the subordinate group (Blacks) in unobtrusive enclaves (the urban ghetto). It explains White flight to the suburbs and the creation of inner-city Black ghettos with all the attendant problems of segregation, isolation, and inequality. In contrast to both dominative and aversive racism, metaracism is "the racism of technocracy, i.e., one without psychological mediation as such, in which racist oppression is carried out directly through economic and technocratic means."[24] It is the last stage of racism that remains when racial passions have been washed away. Metaracism pervasively represents pure racism because it is systematic and independent of individual factors. This racism, for example, maintains unequal public school funding through inequitable taxation and funding mechanisms. Rich, White suburbs are able to raise adequate funding for their schools with lower tax rates levied on their prodigious property tax bases. Inner-city, African American, and poor districts with impoverished tax bases levy higher tax rates but still cannot adequately fund public schools. State funding for public education designed to equalize these disparities perpetuates inequalities by ensuring distribution to rich and poor districts rather than distribution according to disparity levels. In some instances, rich districts are awarded bonuses for participating in the program. The gap between rich and poor districts in many states is thus widened. Black public school children, who are disproportionately confined to poor public schools, are then blamed for lower "achievement" test scores when they have inadequate numbers of books, dilapidated and cramped quarters, and inadequate numbers of qualified teachers. Therefore, Whites do not have to directly discriminate against Black or poor children. This more subtle, equally racist, mechanism—rarely understood—accomplishes the same result. These structural educational inequalities between White and Black children have been buttressed by the federal courts.[25] Because it incorporates the most advanced forms of domination and is the most detached from the older, hate-filled, odious forms of racism leading to discrimination and overt and covert violence, Kovel predicted that metaracism might be the dominant mode of racism in postmodern,* late capitalist U.S. society.[26]

There is a plethora of evidence that Kovel's prediction about metaracism becoming the dominant racist mode has been realized. Metaracism disguises its racist oppression through the seemingly benign laws of economics—free-market competition or "survival of the fittest" in the marketplace, for example. It can also transform itself to create an idealized and arbitrary "meritocracy" through the imposition of White, culture-based tests and examinations for entry (e.g., IQ, SAT, GRE, LSAT, and the MCAT for entry into graduate, medical, or professional schools). Advancement in modern society is often based on successful scoring on such tests— but the unequal educational, training, or social environments available for disadvantaged ethnic American groups usually prohibits successful competition. Metaracism can assume an anti-racist veneer, exemplified by the recent utilization of anti-discrimination and affirmative action laws to protect European Americans from minority "takeovers" of a job market dominated and administered by Whites.

Postmodern is a "family resemblance" term used in a variety of contexts (politics, art, music) as a critique of Enlightenment values mounted by liberal-communitarian and neopragmatist persuasions, as a relaxation of the pretense of high-modernist culture, and for a laid-back pluralism of styles.

It may wear the costume of cold objectivity while weeding out African Americans and other disadvantaged minorities and securing privileged White enclaves in the job market, governmental agencies, and educational institutions on the basis of disingenuously defined standards of "quality." Its chameleon-like qualities are well adapted to the postmodern, late capitalist world. It changes and transforms itself to suit the challenges of the day (e.g., through mediation by economic discrimination—"redlining" Black neighborhoods by banks or denying Black access to decent housing through real estate mechanisms), reversing anti-racist intent (e.g., by devising reverse discrimination strategies or using anti-discrimination laws to protect Whites) and disguising itself and its motives behind the seemingly inherent genetic inferiority of non-Whites (the red herring of the IQ controversy).

Perpetuation of segregated, poorly funded, and sometimes inferior health facilities in inner-city or rural poor areas are health system examples. The transformation of the health system to a market economy is a mechanism that incorporates metaracism (intentionally or unintentionally) with the potential to intensify race and class inequities in the already disparate health infrastructure. The health care needs of African Americans, other ethnic minorities, the poor, and underserved populations do not significantly affect the decisions dictating the course of U.S. health policy.[27]

The imposition of cut-throat competition and a market economy ethos and methodology on the health care system has the potential to devastate Blacks. Huge health care corporations generate powerful market forces as they threaten the takeover of the entire U.S. health system. These private entities are unrestrained by public accountability and are owned and run by elite, White, male-run corporations. Racism and the equitable delivery of health care are either not a part of, or rank very low on, the agenda of these corporations. In commercial market-based systems, the poor automatically get less. Institutions charged with the care of low-income populations are either public or less desirable investments. They are the first considered for closure. All of these mechanisms are thus factor-loaded against Blacks and the poor. The creation of a commercial health system could transform into another metaracist mechanism for the promotion and perpetuation of a dual and unequal, race-based health delivery system in the United States.

The Evolution of a Racially Unequal Health System

The roots of inequitable and unequal health care and health systems for Blacks stretch back to slavery, but the modern mechanisms described here are different. The old dominative racism of legally segregated and inferior, or nonexistent, facilities has been supplanted by the metaracist mechanisms built around market forces, which place a premium on those who can afford health care. Since World War II, health services for Blacks (three-fourths of whom are either uninsured, underinsured, or totally dependent on diminishing government and public aid health insurance programs) and the poor have been shaped and dictated by several factors. Most important are the lack of fully trained, culturally competent physicians of quality willing to serve African Americans; the lack of adequate numbers or distribution of quality private or public outpatient health care facilities to serve the Black community; a U.S. tradition of underfunding and restricting the activities and delivery functions of health departments and other publicly funded health facilities; personal and/or institutional racial discrimination within the health care system; African American dependency for inpatient and primary health care on a loose and inconstant (many urban U.S. communities do not have public hospitals) network of underfunded, overcrowded, deteriorating public and voluntary hospitals; the inadequacies of episodic, sometimes absent, charity health services to plug gaps in the public health care sector or to meet vital Black community needs; and nonexistent or meager funding at local, state, or federal levels for the health care rendered to indigent, disadvantaged, or working poor patients. After a short period of improvement between 1965 and 1975 because of an infusion of funding and concern about the inferior health subsystem, deterioration of the limited health care systems for the poor resumed in the new "competitive" and privatized health system environment. Ginzberg described the impact of market forces in the health system on hospitals that care for Chicago's largely Black and poor inner-city population in a 1994 *Journal of the American Medical Association* article:

> *Chicago's capacity for inpatient care of the indigent deteriorated significantly over the decade as 11 voluntary hospitals in the inner city had to close largely as a result of the rising numbers of uninsured patients admitted through their emergency rooms and the substantial relocation of their earlier middle-class clientele.*[28]

He also noted Cook County Hospital's "steadily declining capacity and quality of care" as emblematic of the collapse of Chicago's public health care sector. A systemic national problem escalates as public hospital and health care systems are gutted through defunding, sell-outs to for-profit chains, and closures. Against this backdrop, new racial concepts outlined by Robert Terry and Joel Kovel serve as strong analytic and explanatory tools for what has occurred, and is occurring, in U.S. society and the U.S. health system.[29]

The components of American society that have affected and often determined the health of African Americans—the medical profession, the health care financing industry, the medical education system, federal and state governments, the health delivery system, and, increasingly, the health policy infrastructure—have also been, and continue to be, affected by these harmful social forces. Their medical-social importance in addressing racial differentials in health status, outcomes, and delivery has grown exponentially in recent decades with the promulgation of more effective medical interventions and therapies. Their potential for contributing to adverse health outcomes of African Americans and increasing the divergence in health outcomes between Blacks and European Americans also has grown. As lily-White-owned* and -operated health care corporations co-opt control of health care financing and distribution in the United States and dominate government participation in health care, their influence can be expected to increase. Utilizing Terry's and Kovel's racial/analytical tools can enable us to tease out and dissect the causes and effects of race and racism in the health delivery system in the United States. Exposing how this dysfunction affects the health status and outcome of African American and other health-disadvantaged groups can bring about corrective actions and cures for the historic malaise caused by race in the U.S. health system. These major contemporary definitions and concepts of racism inform and guide our investigation of race and medicine in the United States. A background discussion on their origins and evolution follows.[30]

Race Explored: A Life Sciences/Health Care Perspective

The reasons for clarifying and reassessing the relationships between race, the life sciences, and health care are compelling and clear. If we are to correct a problem, we must first understand it. An objective, external, constructionist, and comprehensive approach toward understanding and explaining the relationship between race, medicine and the other life sciences, and health care in the United States, to our knowledge, has never been undertaken. Objectivity and documentation are implicit in the goals and objectives of such a project. Pursuit of the biomedical-scientific story of U.S. health care and relating it to the sociopolitical, medical-historical, medical-social, and public health dimensions as they relate to race in the United States, particularly the African American experience, can produce both new understanding and a sound foundation of explanatory hypotheses and databases upon which to build toward future amelioration of the system's race and class problems.

To understand the contemporary and confusing contexts regarding race in U.S. society, one must digress through the intellectual and scientific history of the subject itself. Seeking the ancient origins of race and class designations in Western civilization, especially as they affect health, requires examination of ancient health systems and practices. Examining classical Greek, Roman, and Arabic cultures bridges the biomedical sciences and health professions to the concept of race in Western culture. Western medicine and the biomedical and other life sciences not only have been major contributors to the corpus of scientific and pseudoscientific knowledge about race, but they have also strongly guided and influenced the social acceptance and impact of race and racialist thought on Western societies. There are, therefore, compelling reasons for examining what is traditionally known about race in holistic Western cultural terms. However, certain caveats apply. Due to the

---

*"Lily-White" refers to its unique informal usage: "Excluding or seeking to exclude Black people." Source: *The American Heritage Dictionary*, 3rd ed., s.v. "lily-white."

overwhelming volume and variety of the material dealing with race in Western culture, a multifaceted approach of investigation is needed. Be it "myth" or a "badly abused concept," as suggested by various experts on the subject, race has held an almost morbid fascination in Western culture's scholarly circles.

Racially based Jewish persecution and the Holocaust, experienced before and during World War II, shook the scholarly world out of its complacent notion that racism was declining toward insignificance. The documented rise in racialist feelings and thought before the midpoint of the twentieth century is undeniable. The African American Civil Rights Movement took place within another cataclysm of racial strife and violence during the 1960s. Disturbing racial signs and symptoms have again resurfaced in the United States in the 1980s and 1990s. Events in Britain, France, Germany, Rwanda and Burundi, and Bosnia, Herzegovina, and Kosovo indicate the generalized deterioration in race relations that may continue for the foreseeable future.

The formal corpus of information on race has been accumulating for 400 years. The next section in this chapter, "Race: An Intellectual History," begins to organize and systematize our inquiry. Because health and health care have been inextricably linked with the medical profession and the biomedical sciences, the section "Race: A History of Science Perspective" examines the relationships between race, biology and the other life sciences, and health care. A digression to the ancient Mesopotamian, Egyptian, Greco-Roman, and Arabic roots of Western biomedical and medical-social knowledge bases will also be instructive. Since the mid-twentieth century, for a variety of reasons, there has been an explosive interest and proliferation in scholarly based racial and racially related studies in the United States. To secure a full understanding of the often confusing racial phenomena threatening to rip apart the U.S. social fabric as we enter the twenty-first century, a political-economic discussion, with race as a nexus, follows. The section entitled "Race, Class, Ethnic Politics, and Health Care" describes the new political economy of race, including the social welfare agenda, the equal treatment agenda, and the race-conscious agenda as these relate to health care. Background material to lend perspective is included to help readers understand the racial dimensions of present and future U.S. health policy events. It also reveals causative factors surrounding the 1994 defeat of President Clinton's attempt to reform the health system. Although his plan had many characteristics of an "avoidance reaction"—regarding a direct confrontation with the race issue in health care—it contained egalitarian efforts to universalize and equalize health care for all Americans. Lastly, developments in *critical theory* on race are presented to evoke legal and social strategies for resolving the U.S. race problem.[31]

While *race* can be a politically and emotionally charged word, it is universally acknowledged that all races of mankind are members of the species *Homo sapiens* ("wise man"). Biologically, a species is defined as "a reproductive community of populations (reproductively isolated from others) that occupies a specific niche in nature."[32] This definition by renowned bird taxonomist and field biologist Ernst

Mayr, which has been almost universally adopted, strikes at what matters most in the evolutionary sense — the genotype. Instead of attempting to classify animals on the basis of ephemeral characteristics such as skin color, hair texture, or feather colors or patterns, the true test of species membership is the reproduction of fertile offspring. Successful breeding leads scientists who are seriously interested in biological species differentiation to focus on genotype. Members of a species such as *Homo sapiens* differ from each other. For anyone interested in racial differentiation, understanding biological variation is a significant consideration. Variations can be either individual or geographic. Within local populations, individuals vary in sex, age, weight, color, height, and numerous other characteristics. Some of these variations are discontinuous, like sex, or continuous, like height or weight. Every population demonstrating such variations is called *polymorphic*. Interestingly, differentiating these variations on the basis of genes would be impossible. Pat Shipman amplified the unity of the human species in *The Evolution of Racism*, suggesting that "humans are so closely related to chimpanzees — over 99 percent of our genes are held in common with the chimpanzee — that the differences among the human races are swamped by the tremendous genetic unity among them."[33] Biologically, differences such as skin color, hair texture, nasal architecture, and skull configuration, markers humans put so much stock in socially, are actually trivial. The genetic unity between species members is much stronger. As Milner relates in *The Encyclopedia of Evolution*:

> [T]here is more variability between individuals in a given local population than between the averages of widely separated populations. For instance, there is much more variability between black Africans than between some kind of "average" African and European. Further, if most of the world's humans were wiped out, and the only surviving group was a thousand tribesmen in a remote mountain forest of New Guinea, that small, isolated population would contain 99% of the human genes and variations that exist.[34]

These findings explain why so many authorities maintain that genetic differences between individuals *within* races proves to be greater than the demonstrable genetic differences *between* races.[35]

Geographic variation can be even more confusing. As one goes farther away from one population in a species and encounters other populations within that species, variations can become striking. When one uses these interspecies variations to identify members of various geographic populations taxonomically, these differentiated populations can be called *subspecies*. However, such categorization is for convenience only (most taxonomists avoid naming subspecies). It is also arbitrary considering the discordance (the tendency to vary) of characters. For example, good characteristics for subspecies divisions, like skin color and blood groupings, often do not correlate. In many instances, they disagree entirely.

African tribes can have direct blood group correlations with White European populations and be totally unrelated to neighboring African tribes. Races can be arbitrarily categorized as subspecies of *Homo sapiens*. Thus, *Homo sapiens*, having two or more subspecies (Mongoloid, Negroid, and Caucasoid), is a *polytypic* species. This in no way negates the fact that these subspecies contribute to a larger interbreeding population that has no clear and fixed boundaries. As James C. King details in *The Biology of Race:*

> Subspecies are not discrete, isolatable units with fixed boundaries. They are merely partially differentiated pieces of one continuous unit, the species. No system of classification, no matter how clever, can give them a specificity and a separateness they do not have.[36]

Stephen Jay Gould further discounts racial, or subspecies, distinctness, noting that "humans move about and maintain the most notorious habits of extensive interbreeding. . . . [W]e interbreed wherever we move, breaking down barriers and creating new groups."[37] History copiously documents racial intermixture resulting from exploration, war, slavery, and travel. This reality of racial intermixture undercuts virtually all racial superiority and eugenics* theories, which have traditionally been grounded on the assumption of "racial purity," preservation of pure racial types, and avoidance of "mongrelization" of so-called pure races. Even the contemporary genetic-based IQ theories have such implicit assumptions. Advances in genetics, including mapping the human genome, are making these admittedly compromised biological divisions less relevant by verifying that more than 99% percent of genes are shared by the entire species *Homo sapiens*.[38]

Approaching race from another scientific direction based on modern genetics, an examination of what is popularly referred to as the "Eve hypothesis" is illuminating. Scientists such as Rebecca Cann applied contemporary genetics techniques to DNA carried in mitochondria (a tiny structure within the cell) instead of other various body proteins. Mitochondrial DNA is believed to be inherited solely through the maternal line. Although the data are complicated because of the subtlety of genetic variability of mitochondrial DNA among human beings and the difficulty of defining races due to extensive interbreeding among various populations, two important conclusions are emerging. Results suggest a relatively recent and single-population origin for the modern human races. This female, or discrete population, ancestor was of African (Negroid) lineage. The deluge of methodological criticisms and challenges from geneticists and paleoanthropologists cannot deflect these findings. If this theory is borne out, other racial analyses may prove moot. If the entire human population is the offspring of a single pair (or small group) of dark-skinned African predecessors who

---

*Derived from the Greek word for "wellborn," eugenics pertains to racial improvement by boosting the birth rate of the wellborn to the levels where they *speedily* prevail over the less suitable strains or socially less wellborn classes.

lived less than 250,000 years ago, what happens to theories of racial subspecies? The theory that the entire human species migrated out of Africa is not so far-fetched — exploding many myths about racial origins.

Having long since broken the confines of biology-based debates, most behavioralists and social scientists now view the "race problem" as a series of prejudicial attitudes and "behavior problems" that produce negative outcomes for particular groups that are discriminated against. These adverse outcomes are mediated by sociocultural constructs, institutions, and concepts based and structured on judgments and stereotypes supplemented by folk concepts (common sense), which are triggered by genetically transmitted physical characteristics such as skin color, hair texture, and thickness of the nose and lips (phenotypic appearance).[39]

While Black racial, intellectual, and biological inferiority have been Western assumptions in the scientific and lay cultures for more than 1,000 years,[40] there have been recent signs of attitudinal change regarding this mythology. Some of today's better-trained physicians and biomedical and biological scientists acknowledge racial differences as simple variations within the species *Homo sapiens*. This view is also gaining wide acceptance in the social and behavioral science communities. Such rethinking is increasingly prominent as legitimate sciences debunk biological racial differences, and social and behavioral sciences render sociocultural concepts built around race more objective. Nevertheless, divisive IQ, hereditarian, and sociobiological arguments continue to emanate from America's academic, medical, and health delivery communities, albeit in lesser volume than in previous scientific eras.[41] This evolutionary change in opinion in the scientific community has not escaped the attention of the popular media, which is beginning to portray race as a social construct.[42]

During what has been both a scientific and social transformation, race has largely been reconceptualized as an aspect of *ethnicity*, which views the differences in people as a function of sociology and culture rather than biology. This transformation has not been smooth. Ethnicity has not completely replaced race, and the attempted transformation from a biological to a sociological construct has been marred by controversy generated by racial IQ myths and lingering allegiances to biological determinism. Nor has overt race prejudice disappeared. For example, the most recent science-based defense of separate origins of the human species based on race, racial hierarchies of intelligence and civilization, and denigration of the African origins and development of humanity was Carlton Coon's *The Origin of Races* in 1962 and its sequel *The Living Races of Man* (1965). King noted that these were followed by Oxford University cytologist John R. Baker's scholarly volume *Race* (1974), which "concludes . . . by rating the human races on their innate capacity for originating civilization and ethical standards and finds the African blacks in last place."[43] The controversial and divisive *The Bell Curve* (1994) by Murray and Herrnstein resurrected old material and set off a new round of debates on Black inferiority in intelligence based on IQ testing. The so-called genetic basis of these differences brings into question the avalanche of biological and genetic data on the unity of the species *Homo sapiens*. That flawed tomes such as these could raise questions about the veracity of masses of scientific evidence documenting the unity of the human species in many people's minds is emblematic of the treacherous scientific and medical-social environments in the United States. Dorothy Nelkin and Laurence Tancredi in *Dangerous Diagnostics: The Social Power of Biological Information* (1989); Troy Duster in *Backdoor to Eugenics* (1990); Stephen Jay Gould in *The Mismeasure of Man* (1981); R. C. Lewontin, Steven Rose, and Leon J. Kamin in *Not in Our Genes* (1984); and Ruth Hubbard and Elijah Wald in *Exploding the Gene Myth* (1993) warn both scientific and lay publics of the current threats presented by the scientific information proliferation surrounding the subjects of genetics and biological determinism. Moreover, inherent dangers in the directions some of this science is going and the uses to which it is applied—criminology, insurability determination, cloning, hiring discrimination, searches for homosexual genes, genetic engineering, eugenics, research on racial "genes" for cancer, intelligence, violence, and criminality— are largely unappreciated. Therefore, though most of the negative information on race that influences U.S. social and political practices emanates from social scientists, there is still a significant scientific racist viewpoint within the biomedical and behavioral science communities.[44]

Virtually all agree that the transformation of a health culture tainted by sociocultural and scientific racism* is long overdue. For too long, scientific racism has provided important bases and energizing mechanisms for unfair and inequitable—and ultimately irrational—health and public policy and health system services in the world's richest representative democracy. Nevertheless, observers such as D. S. Greenberg, Marc Roberts, Robert Blendon, Eli Ginzberg, and the authors of this book question whether the United States is prepared to deal with aspects of the race and class problems plaguing its health system. Objective efforts to answer the question of whether America is "ready"—public opinion indicators are ambiguous, complex, and uncertain—add another layer of confusion. These indicators necessitate a continuing dialogue along racial lines in the United States. The persistence of discrimination in health, perpetuation of wide and deep race-based health status and outcome disparities, and recent failures to reform the U.S. health system in an equitable manner dictate that health care for African Americans continues to be responsibly framed in racial and civil rights** terms.

---

*The classical definition of scientific racism is the perversion of scientific and historical facts to create the myth of two distinct races of mankind. The first race consists of a small, healthy, wealthy, educable elite, while the second race is a far larger population of poor or nonwealthy, vulnerable, and allegedly uneducable by virtue of hereditarily inferior brains. The authors add anti-Black racism as one special branch of scientific racism with a set of unique and accentuating characteristics such as color prejudice, sexual imagery, and religious prejudice.
**Beginning with the pre–Civil War efforts of Black health crusaders like James McCune Smith and Martin Robison Delany, African Americans have had to crusade for health care as a civil right. Organizations such as the Afro-American League, the Niagra Movement, the NAACP, the NMA, and the National Urban League have continued these traditions.

The major socioeconomic and political dimensions directly and indirectly related to reforming the health system toward equity and equality are presented later in the section entitled "Race, Class, Ethnic Politics, and Health Care."[45]

Most observers agree that the potential health care implications of a dynamic driven by, and based upon, genetically or biologically determined racial inferiority, a variant of Feagin's *ideological racism,** are profound. However, similar "inevitability" and "uncorrectability" conclusions based on human deficiencies could be grounded in "culture of poverty" viewpoints related to noncompliance and moral turpitude taken to their extremes. Thus, the inferior social status imposed on particular racial or ethnic groups could be utilized by policy makers to justify deficient health services. Poor health status and outcome data could be rationalized on the basis of either racial or genetic "predispositions" or "unfitness" rooted in the notions of the "culture of poverty." Elevated disease or mortality rates, even compromised intelligence (measured by contemporary White culture-based standards such as IQ and "achievement" tests) due to disease-related causes (e.g., central nervous system lead toxicity, prematurity and low birth weight, rubella, congenital measles, congenital syphilis), could be viewed nihilistically as genetically, biologically, or even culturally predetermined occurrences based on race or class. For example, the poverty-stricken mother who did not present to the prenatal clinic to be treated for undiagnosed syphilis because of a lack of health insurance or cash to pay for the visit was thus "destined" to have a significant chance of delivering a brain-damaged infant. Such reasoning creates the circular dynamic William Ryan refers to in his work on "victim blaming." Nihilistic health policies and behaviors resulting from victim blaming could also serve as mechanisms and partial explanations for stubbornly persistent health status, outcome, and service utilization disparities seen from one race to another ("race-based"**). Victim blaming may also explain the disturbing indifference to the health circumstances of Blacks and other minorities. It could be an undercurrent that helps explain the dogged determination the U.S. leadership demonstrates to perpetuate the multitiered and unequal U.S. system, the inferior layers of which are disproportionately made up of African American and other disadvantaged groups. Such maldistribution of vitally needed health care services is no longer defensible and demands substantive corrective measures. In lieu of the confusion and ethical inconsistencies, authorities as diverse as the United Nations, social scientist Andrew Hacker, and social commentators such as Studs Terkel and Ellis Cose

---

*Ideological racism refers to an ideology that considers a group's unchangeable physical characteristics to be linked in a direct, causal way to psychological or intellectual characteristics and that, on this basis, distinguishes between superior and inferior racial groups. Source: Feagin JR, Feagin CB. *Racial and Ethnic Relations*. 6th ed. Upper Saddle River, NJ: Prentice Hall, 1999, 6.

**Some health statistics in the United States are collected on the basis of demographics such as age, sex, race, income, education, and socioeconomic status. This allows for calculable trends and disparities along and between each demographic variable.

recognize that race is a problem with the potential to tear American society asunder. Its potency is documented by incidents as varied as the brutal beating of Rodney King by policemen in Los Angeles, California, in 1991; the extermination of more than six million Jews in the Holocaust 60 years ago; the apartheid systems that existed until just recently in both the United States and the Republic of South Africa; the belated response of the United States and Europe to the ethnic cleansing atrocities in Bosnia and Herzegovina in 1995 and Kosovo in 1999; and the current growing antagonism between racial and ethnic groups demonstrable in the United States.[46]

Race: An Intellectual History

Race is a very complex subject. The growth of knowledge about what specialists call race and racial relations has been both voluminous and formidable over the years. Michael Banton, a British scholar specializing in the discipline that he refers to as *racial thought,** has attempted to systematize and rationalize this previously confused discipline by identifying organizing principles derived from the philosophy of science and applying them to this aspect of intellectual history. Therefore, before plunging into this formidable subject, an effort to organize its intellectual history and to systematize the study of race seems worthwhile. This is especially vital to a work examining the surprisingly intimate relationship between race, biology and the other life sciences, and health care in Western culture and, ultimately, the United States.

The authors of this book have observed, and Michael Banton has corroborated, that the corpus of racial thought is composed of massive bodies of variegated information from the disciplines of biology, medicine, psychology, history, genetics, biostatistics, sociology, anthropology, ethnology, ethology, linguistics, archaeology, paleontology, chemistry, and geology. Examination of the history of this eclectic field reveals that scholars have devoted large portions of, if not their entire, intellectual careers to the pursuit of knowledge in this field for over 400 years. Although the task may seem daunting, the importance of race and racial relations in this study of the U.S. health system dictates that we obtain a basic background in the fields that combine to make up the discipline of racial thought.

Precursors of the modern concepts of race and racism affected the fields of philosophy, natural philosophy,** and medicine as early as the dawn of recorded

---

*Although Banton's term for the discipline is "racial thought," the authors prefer "racial studies" and will use the terms interchangeably.
**Roots of this terminology date back to ancient times, when all fields of knowledge were branches of philosophy. All fields of inquiry having to do with the natural world were called "natural philosophy." Biology, botany, chemistry, physics would not break off from the natural philosophy branch of philosophy until the establishment of modern scientific disciplines in the eighteenth and nineteenth centuries.

history and Western civilization. The nature and effects these ancestors and precursors of racism had on science and its antecedents dating from ancient Mesopotamian, Egyptian, Greco-Roman, and Arabic times are examined in much greater detail later. However, the formal and systematic study of race as an academic discipline in Western European civilization can conveniently and arbitrarily be thought of as beginning in the sixteenth and seventeenth centuries. The word *race* did not enter the English language until the early sixteenth century.[47] Contributions that could be considered specific to the field were by necessity limited until the concept of race was accepted as a concrete entity in European language and thought.

Building upon Banton's work, the division of the history of racial thought into three periods is useful. Such an approach has several advantages. It lends organization and clarity to what otherwise may seem to be a chaotic amalgam of information from disparate and seemingly unrelated academic disciplines. It allows various investigators and their contributions to be placed in a scientific, epistemological, and chronological context. Works have more meaning when we are aware of the scientific world in which they occurred. The social influence some of these works exerted becomes clearer; lines of influence in academic and social circles and whether certain works had permanent impact are comprehensible when juxtaposed to historic and future scientific and social environments. Omitting specific characters, milestones, and events allows the value and impact of the scientific ideas and discoveries themselves to be scrutinized and evaluated. Other obvious advantages of an intellectual history approach are that it allows the value and appropriateness of contributions to be evaluated in light of competing contemporary and future work and also avoids many problems with "presentism."*

The three periods Banton refers to can be labeled the period of "racial lineage," the period of "racial type," and the "sociocultural period of race." The first period, designated as racial lineage, stretches from the dawn of modern science in the sixteenth century to the beginning of the nineteenth century. An almost natural accompaniment to the general increase in scientific knowledge about the varied forms of life and the many proposals on how to classify and interpret their diversity was a growth of knowledge and curiosity regarding what we call race. Studies on humans driven by scientific questions comparable to those being performed on various animal species, variants, and breeds were inevitable. During this period of racial thought, the concept of "lineage" was dominant. As Banton remarks, "From the sixteenth to the nineteenth centuries, in English, the principal use was that of race as lineage, to refer to a group of persons, animals, or

---

Presentism is an intellectual fallacy created by interpreting everything literally in the context of present knowledge bases and social conditions. This approach negates the effects exerted by different social forces present during different historical periods (e.g., the term *race* has had many meanings over time and referred to national groupings, tribal groups, and ethnic groups, according to many nineteenth-century European and American scholars).

plants, connected by common descent or origin."[48] Thus, race during this period was largely a descriptive term dividing the natural world of human beings into lines of descent from more primitive predecessors. Most of the scientific inquiries on race were attempts at descriptive and empirical data accumulation driven by questions of lineage. This view of descent conveniently tied in with the then-dominant Biblical view of cosmology and was strongly related to the ancient Great Chain of Being theory. Grounded in the philosophical concepts of "good-ness" and "continuity,"* this Great Chain theory, which dated from the Greek Platonic dominance of the Western intellectual world during the fifth century BC, hypothesized that all forms of life were related hierarchically to more primitive predecessors. (See Figure 1.3.) These relationships were fixed and immutable. *Scala naturae* ("Scale of Nature")** was a refined version of the theory. As Herbert Wendt remarked about the meaning and implications of the Great Chain theory on the natural sciences in *From Ape to Adam:*

> Nature, then, was no longer thought to be in a continual state of flux, as Heraclitus had taught, but was a system in which everything had its divinely ordained place, classification and purpose—a great "chain of being" which extended in strict linear gradation from lowest to highest. All types and forms were mere copies of external and immutable ideas; they were as eternal and unchanging as the ideas from which they were derived. An unbridgeable gulf was formed between man, the pinnacle of Creation, who had been made in the image of God, and the rest of the world, separating them completely.[49]

This hierarchy was permanent, unchangeable, and had existed since the Creation. The theory was also consistent with the Biblical description of Adam and Eve. Based on these Divine Creation theories man could still think of himself as being separate and distinct from the animal kingdom.

This hierarchical relationship extended to races, skin color, and sexual characteristics in the Judeo-Christian religious traditions embodied in Noah's curse of his son Ham's descendents. The curse consisted of black skin and other derogatory characteristics according to White physical and moral standards.

---

*Platonic "goodness" included the assumption not only that all things are known but also that the causes of their existence and reality are also known. Aristotle's concept of "continuity" was a continuation of Plato's "fullness" and, later, Christian "plenitude," wherein the "perfect" universe overflowed with diverse life forms ranging from simple to complex. This necessary aspect of perfection generated a natural hierarchy.

**Aristotle's *scala naturae* was actually a revision of Plato's Chain of Being. It represents the primacy of a metaphysical assumption over perceived reality. Aristotle, a professional naturalist, knew there was no perfect continuity of either inorganic or organic being. Substantial breaks and gaps could be included in his *scala naturae*. Nevertheless, with these caveats in mind, they can be used interchangeably.

Figure 1.3   The Great Chain Theory

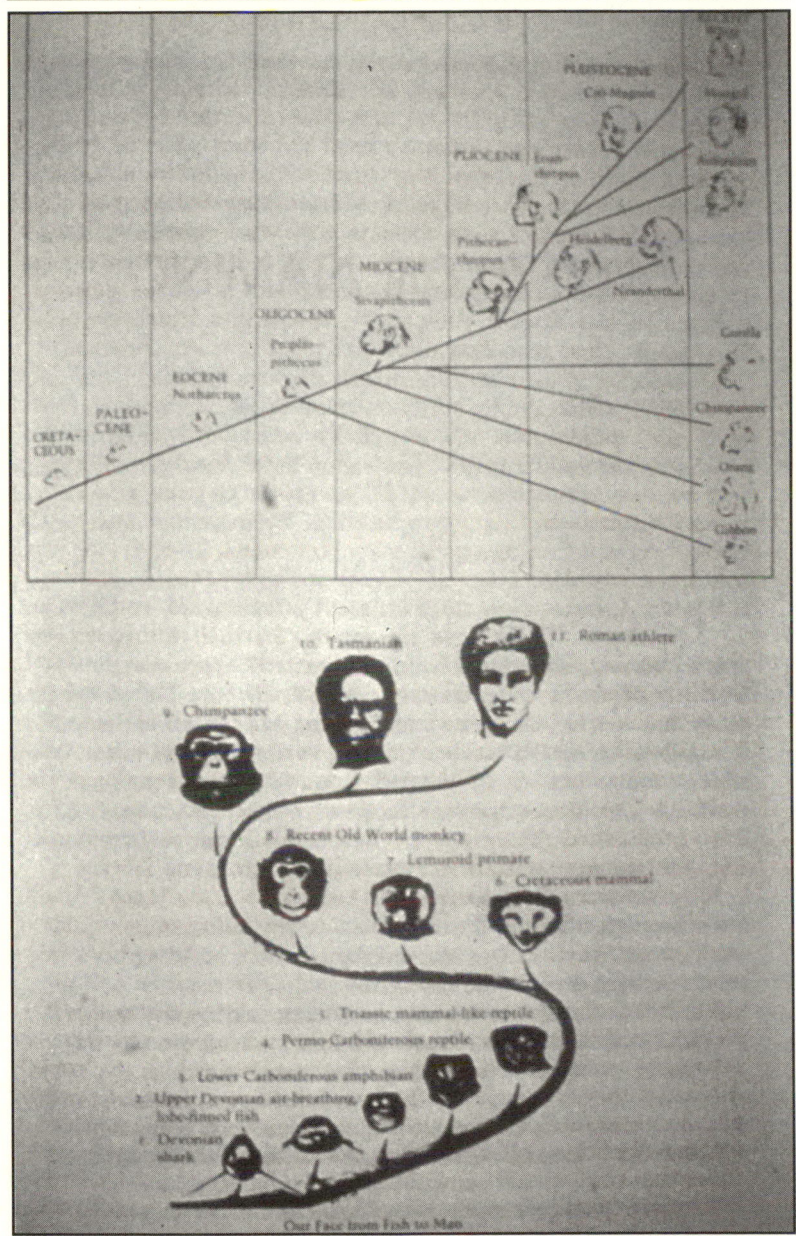

Dating from the era of Greek Platonic dominance of the Western world in the fifth century BC, the "Great Chain Theory" hypothesized that all forms of life were related hierarchically to more primitive ancestors. Racism crept into these classifications as White, Nordic races were viewed as the pinnacle of human evolution.

> "It must be Canaan, your firstborn, whom they enslave. . . . Canaan's
> children shall be born ugly and black! . . . Your grandchildren's hair
> shall be twisted into kinks . . . [their lips] shall swell." Men of this race
> are called Negroes; their forefather Canaan commanded them to love
> theft and fornication, to be banded together in hatred of their masters
> and never to tell the truth.[50]

Thus, religious-based physical and social characteristics designating Blacks as
inferior, ugly, and cursed were added to negative imagery and connotations
already surrounding slavery and the idea that "black" represented dirt while
"white" represented purity, which dates back to antiquity.

The pinnacle of the Great Chain classification was the white European
male, with other "lesser" beings such as Blacks and other non-Whites below
them. (See Figure 1.4.) As Milner noted in *The Encyclopedia of Evolution:
Humanity's Search for Its Origins:* "Racism is embedded in the Chain of Being;
the idea was used to rank the various races into 'higher' and 'lower.' Of course,
the white Europeans who devised it were at the top."[51] The 2,000-year-old Great
Chain tradition, which became natural scientific dogma, went unchallenged
until the Renaissance beginnings, and Enlightenment development, of empirical approaches to science that we are familiar with today. Nevertheless, by the
end of the period (between 1800 and 1900), due to the scientific influence and
work of physicians and natural philosophers, the "single line" evolution of man
was questioned. Whether man descended from a single line, *monogenesis,**
which corroborated the Biblical concept, or was created as separate and distinct
species, *polygenesis,*** which explained the marked differences in the races and
supported geological and archaeological data, was the debate that occupied the
early natural philosophers in the field for more than two centuries. As Banton
stated, "In this phase the dispute was whether all humans descended from Adam
and Eve."[52] Thus, the first great controversy within the field of "racial thought"
had strong religious implications and overtones. It was a dominant debate in both
the natural sciences and racial thought well into the nineteenth century. As
empirical data and taxonomic foundations in racial thought matured, the
groundwork for the second period emphasizing race as "type" was laid.[53]

During the seventeenth and eighteenth centuries the first attempts to classify
man scientifically by physician–natural scientists occurred. These efforts represented important developmental stages in the scientific method—namely, taxonomic classification. This preceded the period of *racial typology* in racial studies,
which lasted throughout the nineteenth century. Details relating the scientific
and historical events along with the participants involved fall under the purview

---

Monogenism proposed that all races of men originated from a single source. This scientific viewpoint upheld the scriptural unity of all peoples in the single creation of Adam and Eve.
**Polygenesis* proposed that human races were separate biological species. Proponents of this theory
often alleged that the scriptures were allegorical and that races of man arose from different Adams.

Figure 1.4   Zeus, an Ibo, and an Orang-outang: Comparisons

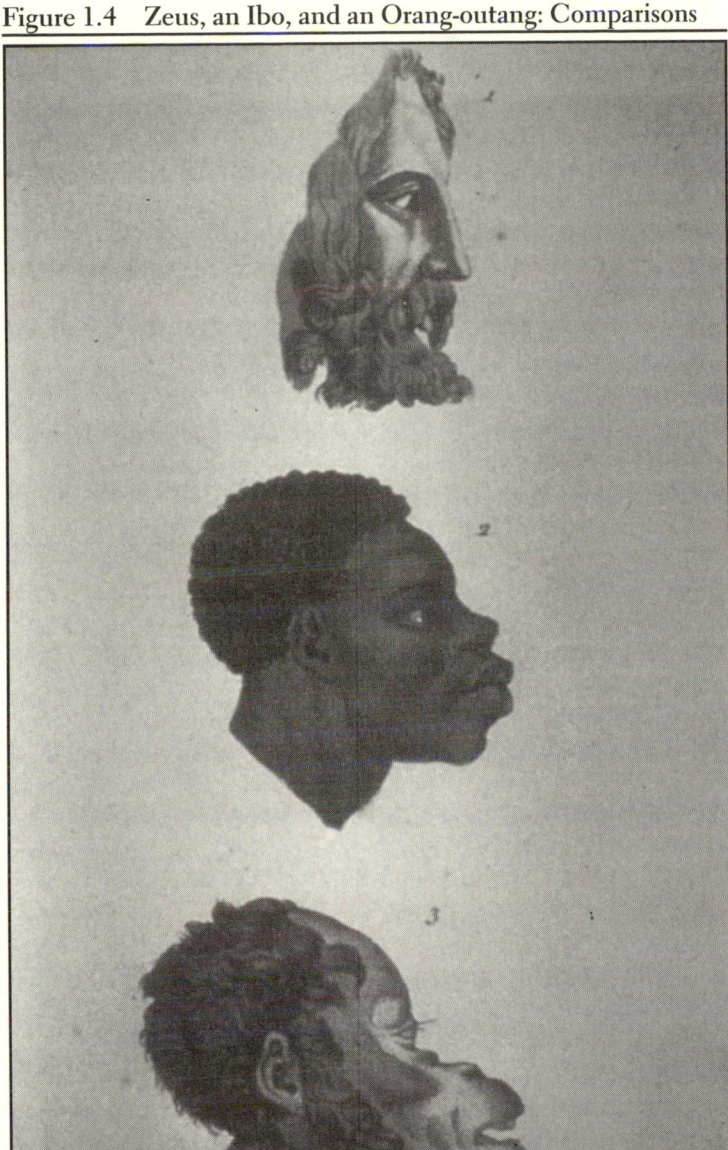

By the late eighteenth century, biological White superiority and Black inferiority were Western scientific assumptions. This 1801 illustration comparing the races and ranking Blacks below White Europeans was printed in Histoire naturelle du genre humain by Julien Joseph Virey. This scientific textbook, which was used in medical schools, was eventually reprinted in English as *The Natural History of the Negro Race* in 1837.

of history of science rather than intellectual history and are reviewed later. In addition to taxonomic advances, quantification, numerical tabulation, and statistical methods assumed important roles in scientific methodology during the Enlightenment. Thus, measurable and quantifiable parameters emerged as the new criteria for the classification and assessment of the races (see Figure 1.5). Skin color, hair length and texture, and physiognomy were early criteria. Anthropometry, the science of measuring various body parts and dimensions, seemed applicable to the brain and its contiguous structures (the cranium and facial bones). Craniometry thus became the leading racial criteria of the age. Another nineteenth-century science, phrenology, which lent itself to graphs and measurement, also grew in popularity during the early part of that century.*

From a scientific perspective a true conclusion requires true premises. However, quantitative measures such as facial angles, cranial capacities, and skull contours and dimensions did not correlate with the variables (intelligence, character traits, civilizing traits) they were supposed to measure. As evidence of their shortcomings piled up over time, these "sciences" increasingly proved to be scientifically useless. Despite their loss of scientific veracity, these pseudoscientific measures to define racial differences continued to be used well into the twentieth century.

By the nineteenth century European encounters with and domination of a wide variety of non-White people with drastically different cultures over the preceding three centuries had raised questions and intensified the interest in racial inquiry. Acceptable answers to many of these questions, framed in logical terms, seemed to originate in the natural sciences. Thus, *biological determinism* based on the "new science," a logical offshoot of these events, arose. Biological determinism theorizes that shared behavioral norms, and the social and economic differences between human groups—primarily races, sexes, and classes—arise from inherited, inborn distinctions. Social potential, even destinies, are determined by the genetic "cards" an individual is dealt at conception and is, thus, a reflection of biology. However, biological differences between individuals, such as skin color, height, weight, or brain size, cannot be used to predict a human being's potential. The empirical, quantitative "new science" branched out from the old philosophy-based "natural science" largely based on observation, description, and logic. Methods carved out by scientific pioneers such as Copernicus, Galileo, and Newton created the scientific disciplines of astronomy and physics considered to be the models of the scientific method. Early in the nineteenth century racial typology measurement and quantification had become the scientific fashion. As Gould

---

Physiognomy is the estimation of one's character and mental qualities by a study of the face and general bodily carriage. *Craniometry* was a pseudoscience based on the correlation of various measurements of the skull with brain size, intelligence, and personality and character traits in humans. As a quantitative so-called science it reached its zenith of authority and popularity in the nineteenth century. *Phrenology* was a popular pseudoscientific fad of the nineteenth century purporting to "read" human character with "scientific" accuracy from bumps on the skull.

Figure 1.5   A Table of Racial Comparisons of Cranial Capacities

Cranial Capacities

I. Noachites.

	Men Cubic Cent.	Women Cubic Cent.	Average Cubic Cent.	Authority
570 Europeans, mostly of S.W. Europe,	1,576	1,395	1,485	Broca.
38 Europeans,*			1,534	Morton.*
293 Britons, Anglo-Saxons, Swedes, Irish, Netherlanders			1,482	Davis
901 Noachites, mean capacity,			{1,500 1,486*	

II. Mongoloids.

	Men Cubic Cent.	Women Cubic Cent.	Average Cubic Cent.	Authority
22 Chinese,	1,518	1,383	1,450	Broca.
21 Chinese,			1,452	Davis.
18 Mongols			1,421	Morton.
12 Eskimo,	1,539	1,428	1,488	Broca.
7 Asiatic Eskimo,			1,488	Dall, etc.
6 N. W. American Eskimo,			1,270	Dall.
101 Greenland Eskimo,			1,250	Bessels.
126 Eskimo, mean capacity,			{1,372 1,286*	
61 Chinese and Mongols, mean capacity,			{1,441 1,442*	
187 Mongoloids, mean capacity,			{1,403 1,338*	

III. Negroes.

	Men Cubic Cent.	Women Cubic Cent.	Average Cubic Cent.	Authority
85 Negroes, W. Africa,	1,430	1,251	1,345	Broca.
79 Negroes of Africa,			1,364	Morton.
12 Dahoman Negroes,			1,452	Davis.
176 Negroes, mean capacity,			{1,387 1,360*	

IV. Australians.

	Men Cubic Cent.	Women Cubic Cent.	Average Cubic Cent.	Authority
18 Australians,	1,347	1,181	1,264	Broca.
15 Australians,			1,295	Davis.
			1,279	

As the author of this scientific textbook said, "Of all the measurements of the head, the capacity of the cranium is shown by observation to be most intimately connected with racial character." A compilation of the data of Paul Broca, MD; Samuel George Morton, MD; and a researcher named Davis, these impressive-looking measurements, some of which were erroneously compiled and totally unrelated to what they were purported to measure (e.g., good character, morality, and intelligence), were included in university and medical courses throughout the Western world.

states, "Craniometry was the leading numerical science of biologic determinism during the nineteenth century."[54] The climate was ripe for the dominance of the "American School" of anthropology, which was largely based upon the pseudoscientific discipline of craniometry and strongly emphasized elaborate cranial dimensions and measurements in its racial classifications. Through impressive numbers of methodologically flawed, unconsciously biased, and outright dishonest experiments, scientific texts, and statistical reports throughout the nineteenth century, the racial hierarchy, with "superior" Whites on top and Blacks and other non-Whites on the bottom, had been preserved. Both Blacks and Native Americans—through lengthy, detailed papers and books laden with statistically tabulated quantitative data—had been "proven" biologically inferior. This avalanche of information, much of which later proved to be scientifically unsound and unscientifically manipulated, influenced the national debate over slavery and Native American public policy. So-called "scientific" data were deemed important enough to be included in university and medical school curricula in the United States and Europe. European and American ideology and sociopolitical policies toward foreign exploration-expropriation, chattel slavery, political domination, and international economic exploitation of non-White people were strongly influenced and modulated, if not shaped, by these "scientific" laws and findings. Thus, for non-European peoples of different races, science had profound, mostly negative, worldwide sociocultural and political effects. The most prominent and obvious domestic example of this new application of "scientific" data" was that much of the material bolstered "natural and irrefutable" Southern justifications for Black chattel slavery.[55]

During the nineteenth-century period of racial typology, other factors came into play that altered the contours of the field of racial thought before the new century dawned. The most important was the general acknowledgement and widespread acceptance of the theory of evolution emanating from England after 1859. It dominated natural and social scientific thought by the 1890s. By the late nineteenth century this scientific movement had almost discredited the Creationist-driven, monogenesis-polygenesis arguments that raged earlier in the period. New evolutionary and geological theories required huge blocks of time that Biblical explanations did not provide. Evolution also required answers about poorly understood inheritance and genetic mechanisms that would not be clarified until the early twentieth century. Moreover, evolutionary theories planted seeds of inquiry that began investigating and addressing scientific questions about biological determinism based on race, the inheritance of acquired characters,*

---

*The theory of *acquired characters* is the erroneous theory, often called the "use and disuse" theory and attributed to naturalist Jean Baptiste Lamarck (1744–1829), that states that if an animal strived in a particular direction, for instance, a short-necked giraffe trying to reach leaves high on trees, its constant reaching would lengthen its neck. Its offspring would have slightly longer necks.

and the unit character mechanism of inheritance.* These unproven mechanisms were inappropriately used to explain the heredity of complex behaviors such as intelligence and criminality. But the cadre of originators of evolutionary theory proved prescient because the scientific evidence that appeared by the late nineteenth century disproved simplistic genetic mechanisms such as acquired characters and unit character genetic inheritance. These examinations raised questions about whether evolution itself was theory or fact; about the origin of life, sex, language, and phyla; about whether evolution offered "proof" or tautology regarding the origin of species; and later, about the relationship between genetics (later DNA) and phenotype.** The new science of genetics addressed these questions and, thus, had a profound effect on the field of racial thought.

Late nineteenth-century scientists posited theories of inherited criminality and intelligence with strong linkages to particular "races," such as Gypsies, Jews, and Blacks. Psychologists measured cognitive abilities and the ability to learn. They dubbed it intelligence. All of these discoveries, with their racial and gender associations, were offered as proof of justification for a "new science," strongly based on the new discipline of biostatistics and encouraging good human breeding—eugenics. As intelligence was scientifically linked to genetics, Blacks, Jews, women, recent U.S. immigrants, and non-Whites were tested and declared inferior. Genetic breakthroughs in the late nineteenth and early twentieth centuries demonstrated that biological human potential characteristics such as intelligence and morality were diffusely distributed throughout the species *Homo sapiens* and were not limited to particular groups (races, sexes, classes); that learned behaviors acquired during a person's lifetime were not passed to future generations; and that complex behaviors such as intelligence and criminality resulted from numerous factors, only a few of which could be said to be biological. It became increasingly clear that mainline eugenics theories, gender inferiority theories, and racial inferiority theories were belief systems and prejudices—not science. Thus, the departure of these areas from legitimate science was apparent to important members of the scientific community by the early twentieth century. It was also clear that legitimate science could neither prove nor support the concept of White superiority or racial hierarchies based on biological mechanisms or the inheritance of genes. Scientific bases of female inferiority were also being undermined. Nevertheless, untested facets of evolutionary theory, when applied to humans and extended into areas of inquiry its originators had not intended, were cleverly distorted by pseudoscientific race and class theoreticians to support and promulgate social prejudices well into the twentieth century.[56]

---

*The *unit character mechanism of inheritance* is the erroneous theory, popular around 1900, that each gene was believed to carry instructions for a particular trait. This was applied to complex behaviors and concepts such as intelligence and criminality.

**The *phenotype* is the physical body or expression of an individual's genetic code.

Despite the weight of scientific evidence accumulated by the early twentieth century, vestiges of these pseudoscientific movements survived. Now largely grounded in perversions of French efforts at intelligence testing and popular "survival of the fittest" social theories as we approach the twenty-first century, they linger as folk concepts, conservative sociopolitical movements, arbitrary IQ "meritocracy" crusades, continuing controversies surrounding Black inferiority, and remnants of the eugenics movement. Old racial arguments and biological deterministic paradigms explaining social status and outcome differences based on unproven concepts such as gloom-and-doom predictions of overpopulation by the unfit leading to eventual extinction of humanity and survival-of-the-fittest dogma from political scientists had been seriously challenged by a growing corps of well-trained biomedical scientists, social scientists, and psychologists. Their arguments, based on the scientific study of sociology, class problems, population theory, political economics, genetics, psychosocial behaviors, and agricultural science, emanated from burgeoning U.S. university and foundation systems of higher learning. The intellectual clashes and debates resulting from the introduction of these new scientifically based class, socioeconomic, and psychological arguments centered on social Darwinism, race, and racism. These debates enriched and objectified the corpus of racial thought immeasurably. Thus, the ground shifted under the discipline of racial studies into areas increasingly defined by the limits of science-based sociocultural and behavioral studies. The twentieth-century phenomena of the constructionist sociocultural and behavioral aspects of race gaining importance over the previous reductionist* attributes of biological and physical racial differences marked the beginning of the dominance of the "sociocultural period of race." The reader may find this brief intellectual history of racial thought helpful, providing additional clarity and insight into this eclectic discipline.[57]

Race: A History of Science Perspective

Western medical progress has been inextricably linked to scientific progress. Precursors of Western scientific medicine stretch as far back as ancient Mesopotamian, Egyptian, Greco-Roman, and Arabic eras. As Paul Starr observed in *The Social Transformation of American Medicine*: "Modern medicine is one of those extraordinary works of reason: an elaborate system of specialized knowledge, technical procedures, and rules of behavior."[58] U.S. society has conferred

---

Constructionist refers to the socially formed dimensions of an inquiry. Such an inquiry includes elements such as the history, social dimensions, and culture shaping a subject. *Reductionism* is the belief, very prevalently used in science, that the whole of reality consists of a minimal number of entities or substances. The major methodological reductive triumph of recent years is the demonstration that the classical unit of heredity, the gene, is a macromolecule—deoxyribonucleic acid, or DNA.

unprecedented levels of power and authority upon the medical profession and rewarded physicians as purveyors of scientific medicine, which is viewed as one of the quintessential works of reason and the foundation of medical progress. As a result, until recently the profession and its functionaries have been charged with the creation and administration of the nation's health system. Unfortunately, they have unconsciously, and sometimes consciously, burdened the system with their history-based human frailties of race and class prejudices and discrimination.[59]

We begin this discussion with a broad-based history of science investigation, simultaneously reassessing the relationships between race, medicine, and health care from its ancient Mesopotamian and Egyptian precursors. Building on this foundation, the Greco-Roman and Arabic roots of Western biomedical science's relationship to race and the Atlantic slave trade becomes clearer. Revealing the subsequent evolution of the U.S. health system in English North America, including its relationship to more than two centuries of Black chattel slavery, offers perhaps the singular tool capable of exposing and unraveling the profound effects of race on American life sciences, health, and health care. Such an investigation is a useful and necessary prerequisite to studying and clarifying present manifestations of this complex and multifaceted relationship. Grudgingly acknowledged is the fact that the medical and biological sciences have made major historical and contemporary contributions to negative definitions and usages of race in Western scientific, political, and lay minds. Moreover, there is a little-known and tortured history of the relationship between a science-based biomedical system that declared people of African descent inferior and subhuman while simultaneously being charged with providing their health care. Overcoming the ethical and public health tensions generated by this strange dynamic may be the litmus test of whether the United States is capable of creating a just and ethical health system equitably serving all Americans regardless of race, ethnicity, or socioeconomic status as we enter the twenty-first century. Despite commonly held beliefs, in this arena science has not proven to be completely objective and value free. Western science, especially in the biomedical and health policy-related fields, has amply displayed the biases and prejudices of its practitioners.

Although there are two millennia of precursors, most of modern science's contributions to the field of racial thought took place after the seventeenth century. A great deal of racial science has been both negative and theoretically flawed and has later proven to be scientifically inaccurate and worthless. The reasons for the obscurity of the important relationships between race, Western science, health policy, and ethical issues are multiple. Truth-seeking forces an examination of some of the ethical shortcomings of Western science that have not been widely discussed within or outside scientific circles. Such an investigation exposes scientific practices to widespread public scrutiny. Scientific discourse that has traditionally been conducted as formal and closed professional exercises is made more accessible. Elite social and informal "good ole boy" networks that usually conduct scientific and history of science investigations, for a number of reasons, have not shed much light on the social and scientific racist dimensions of Western culture's scientific activities. The Tuskegee experience was, thus, no aberration.[60] Its occurrence was directly related to a number of traditional practices within the American scientific community, including, but not limited to, disproportionately focusing on poor and disadvantaged groups for medical experimentation and demonstration; closed and often racially exclusive academic faculties and fraternities; a U.S. tradition of channeling the lion's share of scientific funding through privileged, elite, White institutions; and refusal to accept as mainstream the research and perspectives of African American and ethnic American scholars. With this background, open examinations of U.S. and other Western scientific processes from a variety of racial and ethnic perspectives should be viewed as positive developments.[61]

The general approach most often utilized in the fields of medical history, health history, and the history of science obscured Western science's negative contribution to society and its ability, intentionally or unintentionally, to legitimize scientific racism. The traditional U.S. history of science perspective is a "positivist"* one. This tradition emanated from Auguste Comte (1798–1857), a nineteenth-century French philosopher and mathematician, and was shepherded by George Sarton (1884–1956)—the Belgian-American science historian. It usually emphasized the "march of progress" or descriptions of selfless scientific heroes. Much of the classical American history of science was written by historians of this positivist school based on the assumptions that:

a. *History (i.e., the past, H_1) is an objective reality that is the unchangeable object of interest to the historian.*

b. *It is the task of the historian to reconstruct the past as it actually was, i.e., [to] give a true description of the course of events of the past. But it is not his task to interpret or evaluate the occurrences of the past or to draw conclusions about the present or future on the basis of history.[62]*

This approach had changed by the 1980s. As Helge Kragh observes in *An Introduction to the Historiography of Science*: "The positivist view of history has little credibility today."[63] Besides being positivist much American history of science has been internalistic, which is described by Kragh as focusing "on science as an isolated, autonomous system and on the great geniuses who are the bearers of this system."[64] This perspective largely ignores the place of science as a discrete activity in the larger, social world, which is characteristic of the externalistic approach. The internalistic viewpoint thus vitiates scientific history of its social, ethical, or cultural meaning. Adding the rich textures and contours of the entire social fab-

---

*The philosophy of *positivism* contends the only real knowledge is factual reality, or knowledge of things having objective existence.

ric to which science contributed its part is the primary advantage of the externalistic over the internalistic approach. Both positivist and internalistic approaches to the history of science seldom lend themselves to realistic or objective accountings of very human, sometimes socially culpable, scientific events. Such approaches to science invite and have virtually automatic, if inadvertent, effects of shielding scientific activity from scrutiny and from tests of social responsibility or accountability. Physician and biomedical scientific participation in unethical scientific, forced sterilization, and euthanasia experiments in several modern Western nations such as Germany and the United States have been well documented.[65] When these flaws are combined with the closed, scientific innercircle, structural characteristics shared by most U.S. scientific disciplines, there is little wonder much of American scientific and science-driven activity, of which health care is an extension, demands reexamination and, indeed, outside scrutiny. Adverse effects such as these are exacerbated in the United States by the sociologically and racially homogeneous composition of the U.S. biomedical scientific professions. Understandably, the effects race and racism have had on the biological and medical sciences have been studied to a very limited extent. Their effects have been little acknowledged and thus remain largely unappreciated.[66]

Evaluation of the nation's health history reveals that race and racism have adversely impacted U.S. health care education, health policy, public health, health care delivery, and health care institutions and infrastructures relative to African American health care status and outcome for nearly four centuries.[67] Although the poor racial health outcomes are obvious, most of the problems and mechanisms driving the disparities remain almost hidden by the health infrastructure, the media, and in the public perception.[68] Defining the nature and effects of this multidimensional, chameleon-like concept of race as it relates to health care in America is one of our major objectives. Shedding the light of objective scrutiny into this often dark corner of American institutional life could serve as a giant step leading to measures that might resolve America's racial health dilemma.

Race, Medicine, and Science: Ancient Relationships

Physical differences in the human species have been recognized since the earliest recorded history. Skin color, a prominent and obvious trait, emerged as a major racial determinant in early Egyptian and Greco-Roman times. Evidence dates from at least 1350 BC in Egyptian tomb paintings. In learned writings and plastic arts, preserved in libraries and museums throughout the world since the Greek Golden Age, Greek ideals of beauty have dominated the Western world. There were positive images associated with blackness, such as Prester John, the Noble Ethiopian King of legend, and "Isis the Black," the most dominant goddess in ancient Egypt who personified all that was good and moral while serving as a fecundity and fertility symbol. Between the seventh and fourteenth centuries a tradition of denigrating Black images and portraying Africa and Africans as abnormal, inferior, even dangerous, was discernible. This imagery persists in Western culture and continues to adversely affect attitudes of European Americans toward African American and other minority populations. The health care arena has not been spared the effects of this cultural trend. Investigating manifestations of this process in the life sciences and healing arts is part and parcel of this inquiry.[69]

The Greeks brought change. Greek philosophers introduced empiricism, objectivity, and logic to the world. Since then they have shaped many facets of Western learning and laid the foundations of the modern scientific method. The apogee of the Greek contribution of empiricism, objectivity, and logic to Western culture—all by-products of rationality—is embodied in the works of Plato (428–348 BC) and Aristotle (384–322 BC), the "fathers of modern science." Joseph Harris, Jean Devisse, H. P. Wassermann, and St. Clair Drake agree that Plato and Aristotle were influenced, directly and indirectly, by the contemporary Greek culture around them. Early historians, geographers, and natural philosophers such as Herodotus (484–425 BC), Pliny the Elder (AD 23–79), Solinus, Diodorus, and Poiseidonios (135–51 BC) created the sociocultural and intellectual milieu for early antecedents of science and scientific racism to thrive. Sir Moses Finley documented Herodotus's contribution to a prominent "we–they" viewpoint, which he felt later evolved into racism, regarding slaves in the Greco-Roman world: "Most Greeks and Romans . . . neither philosophers nor theorists . . . went on cheerfully believing, with Herodotus, that . . . slaves as a class were inferior beings, inferior in their psychology, by their nature."[70] Sir Moses Finley and St. Clair Drake describe definite relationships between Greco-Roman slavery and the eventual origins of Western racism and prejudice in *Ancient Slavery and Modern Ideology* and *Black Folk Here and There*.[71] Historians such as Herodotus, considered the father of history, "sowed seeds of racial prejudice that shaped black-white images for centuries to come," according to Joseph Harris.[72] Harris states, "He frequently referred to Africans as 'barbarians,' and characterized the people of Lybia* by saying, 'their speech resembles the shrieking of a Bat rather than the language of Men.'"[73] Pliny the Elder discussed Africans, who "by report have no heads but mouth and eies [*sic*] both in their breast," and others "who crawled instead of walking."[74] Solinus, a third-century geographer, described Ethiopians in his *Collection of Wonderful Things* as "Aethyop, of the filthy fashion of the people of that countrey."[75] Statements like these from Western intellectual icons were not considered racist until recent reexamination and reevaluation. Learned men did not need to voice overt racial prejudice to poison the racial atmosphere. When these negative attributes

---

*Lybia and *Africa* were used interchangeably to refer to the modern-day African continent by scholars until AD 600.

became associated with difference and dark skin, the anti-Black racial dynamic was automatically set in motion.[76]

The Classical Greek period (500–250 BC) is the juncture when power, history, and science converged—borrowing David Theo Goldberg's model—to create "the preconceptual grounds of racist discourse."[77] The preconceptual elements that he describes "include classification and order, value and hierarchy; differentiation and identity, discrimination and identification; exclusion and domination, subjection and subjugation, entitlement and restriction, and . . . violence and violation."[78] Goldberg's formulation is a significant tool for clarifying the ties between science and racism in Western culture. Goldberg's model is also critical to understanding how race and racism evolved and matured so that they function in modern contexts—including in the U.S. health delivery system. It also clarifies how these markedly heterologous scientific and social concepts evolved, combining and interacting in such a way as to produce negative and unified medical-social endpoints—racially conditioned health status and outcomes. Fleshing out themes alluded to and implied in Arthur O. Lovejoy's earlier work *The Great Chain of Being* (1936), the elements of Goldberg's model integrate perfectly into the historical Greek setting that sowed the seeds of scientific racism.

The first cluster of elements—*classification and order, value and hierarchy*—fit easily into the scientific method and "typological thinking" that Plato and Aristotle established. As Haverford College philosopher Lucius Outlaw pointed out in the *Anatomy of Racism,* "Plato and Aristotle . . . were the precursors of such thinking: the former with his theory of Forms; the latter through his classification of things in terms of their 'nature.'"[79] As Goldberg noted, "Classification is basically the scientific extension of the epistemological drive to place phenomena under categories."[80] He also observed, "The impulse to classify data goes back at least to Aristotle."[81] The capacity for rationality is considered a mark of humanity; thus, Goldberg states, "The race represented by the classifiers was considered to stand at the hierarchical apex."[82] The classifiers referred to—demonstrating signs of their well-known ethnocentrism—were the Greeks themselves. Based on these then-revolutionary concepts, these men were founding what we know as modern science.

The roots of Aristotle's *Scala naturae* theory, a naturalist's version of Plato's Great Chain of Being, posited that a perfect universe must constitute a continuous, ascending series of beings or things. While these philosophical and theoretical concepts were developed prior to the formal definition of racism as we know it today, these philosophers taught that there were gradations or scales of men, with Blacks, slaves, and other non-Whites at the lower end of the scale. It is unlikely that such thought processes and hierarchical principles were not transmitted into clinical decision making and health services. Thus, people considered a lower order of humanity, or similar to animals, were more than likely treated differently. The influence of these classification systems has persisted for 2,500 years.

Most of the terms contained in the second cluster of Goldberg's elements—
differentiation and identity, discrimination and identification—blend easily into
the empirical methodology of early science and later events of the seventeenth
and eighteenth centuries. Moreover, Goldberg's paradigm blends harmoniously
into the historical process of social differentiation between the slave and free populations and the various racial groups that took place in Greek society at that
time. This process was described by Jean Devisse, St. Clair Drake, Frank Snowden, and Sir Moses Finley.

The last two clusters of Goldberg's elements—*exclusion and domination, subjection and subjugation* and *entitlement and restriction, violence and violation*—
describe the movement of the racially nondiscriminatory early Greek society to
the markedly more oppressive, slave-based, class- and caste-divided Greco-Roman
societies dominant from the Greek Golden Age through the Roman Empire. His
breakthrough concepts also describe the social uses to which Renaissance scientific breakthroughs, in what we would label today the biomedical sciences,* were
applied. Biologically oriented racial sciences performed functions as eclectic as
validating White superiority myths, justifying the exploitation and extermination
of Northern and Southern American Indian populations, and justifying antebellum slavery in the Southern United States.[83]

Plato and Aristotle's philosophic attitudes about black skin color, and other
physical racial differences, became highly deterministic. As Wassermann
observed about Aristotle's attitude about Blacks in *Ethnic Pigmentation*, "He considered the Ethiopian a cross between a gorilla and a man."[84] This helps explain
why, whether purposefully or inadvertently, Plato and Aristotle planted the seeds
of scientific and anti-Black racism. Ancient writers had attributed differences
such as dark skin color to mythological events. The "burnt faces" of people they
named "Ethiops" resulted when Phaeton, the son of Helios the sun god, drove
his chariot wildly through the sky. According to the legend he drove too close to
the sun in some places and too close to the earth in others. In the process he purportedly scorched the earth, creating deserts and blackening the faces of some
men. This mythological approach to explaining natural phenomenon changed
in Greek culture. As St. Clair Drake observed:

> After the fifth century B.C., Greek rationalists, questioning the authen-
> ticity of the myths, began to develop an environmental theory that
> became characteristic of classical Greek explanations of differences as
> taught by most of the philosophers.[85]

---

*Allusions to "biomedical sciences" is not a presentist flaw, but a matter of convenience here. Though
most of these separate disciplines had not been formally recognized until the twentieth century, they
include, but are not limited to, the sciences of biology, anatomy, chemistry, biochemistry, pharmacology, physiology, botany, ethnology, anthropology, evolutionary biology, genetics, and molecular biology.

Thus, Greek intellectuals like Aristotle and Hippocrates (?c. 460–377 or 359 BC) hypothesized that climate and associated environmental changes were responsible for physical differences in the races. Therefore, the dark skin of the Ethiopian, as virtually all Negroid peoples were called then, was a result of overexposure to the sun. However, this initiated a dangerous trend, as Drake pointed out: "[T]he Greek explanation of the origin of skin color differences opened the door to deterministic theories that intermixed physical characteristics with personality traits."[86] For instance, hot climates were also thought to predispose toward heightened sexuality. As Church Fathers accepted environmentalist theories, which were developing alongside symbolic systems based on Zoroastrian, Manichaean, and Judeo-Christian myths,* black skin came to be equated not just with inordinate sensuality, but also with evil generally.[87]

Slavery is probably as old as civilization itself. For both Blacks and Whites, strong connections between slavery and presumed Black inferiority persist in Western culture. Prophetically, this connection was also reinforced by the Greeks during the era in which the foundations of modern science were begun. Plato and Aristotle, mirrors of a Greek society that characteristically thought in pejorative and narrow ethnic terms, were also chief perpetrators of racism in their analysis of slaves as inferior beings. Drake, Devisse, Finley, and others noted that during this period of Greek society the majority of Blacks were either slaves or servants. Because Plato and Aristotle ranked slaves and Blacks at the bottom of the scale of man and openly stated that Blacks were ape-like, they thus actively instigated and perpetrated racism. David Brion Davis summed up Plato's writings about slaves by stating, "a people with a capacity and ardent desire for freedom, as evidenced by their political institutions, could not legitimately be slaves."[88] Plato further stated that "a 'slavish people' lacked the capacity not only for self-government but also for the higher pursuits of virtue and culture."[89] World-renowned classicist and professor of ancient history at Cambridge University, Sir Moses Finley, clarified his position on the intimate "we–they" distinction Greeks and Romans made between themselves and slaves and the origins of racism:

> *A second element, a logical consequence of the slave-outsider equation, is racism, a term I insist on despite the absence of the skin-colour stigma; despite the variety of peoples who made up the ancient slave populations; despite the frequency of manumission and its peculiar consequences. The issue is not of a concept of "race" acceptable to modern biologists or of a properly defined and consistently held concept, but of*

---

*These three doctrines share a common thread of the cosmic struggle between Good symbolized by Light and Evil by Darkness. Mani, in AD 230 and 274, extended the concept to include the idea that various groups and individuals have different amounts of light to lift them from the Darkness. Manichaeanism and Zoroastrianism were Persian in origin, while the legends of Nimrod, son of Cush, Darkness, and Evil stem from the Judeo-Christian tradition.

> *the view commonly taken in ordinary discourse, then as now. There were Greek slaves in Greece, Italian slaves in Rome, but they were unfortunate accidents; ideological expressions were invariably formulated around "barbarians," outsiders, who made up the large majority in reality.*[90]

The racial implications of perceived slave inferiority was compounded by the fact that virtually all Greek slaves were foreigners and that most Blacks encountered by Greeks were slaves.[91] Devisse spoke to the real-life effects the ideologies and practices within Greco-Roman and early Christian societies had on the contradictory nature of Western racism:

> *In the last analysis the condemnation of slavery, in the monotheistic religions as well as in the Greek and Roman worlds, was at the discretion of the group that possessed privileged status: it was not the result of a universally respected principle, and in day-to-day affairs the generosity of proclaimed principles gave way to de facto inequality. Everything shows that from ancient times this is the way life was, and that we must not allow ourselves to be misled by the texts. This social inequality bred prejudice and raised barriers.*[92]

Based on these circumstances, including the sociocultural realities of their day, Plato and his disciple Aristotle speculated and codified in prescientific thought the notion that all slaves were inherently inferior and less intelligent and that Black slaves were the worst of the lot.[93]

The next major influence on the intimate relationship between the biomedical sciences and racial thought in Western civilization was the work of the immortal Roman physician Galen. Born in the Greek city of Pergamon in Asia Minor during the height of the Roman empire in AD 130, his influence on Western medicine should not be underestimated. As Bender stated:

> *Galen's writings and teachings—marked by brilliant observation and wise therapeutic application as well as colossal error and insufferable dogmatism—dominated medical thinking and practice for fifteen hundred years—an occurrence unique in the world experience.*[94]

As one adoring medical history treatise referred to him, he was "Galen, Influence for Forty-Five Generations."[95] Guthrie recalled, "Throughout the dull-witted early Middle Ages his views were not only accepted without question, but anyone who dared to differ was treated as a heretic."[96] Galen published voluminously about dietetics, pathology, therapeutics, pharmacy, anatomy and physiology, hygiene, medical philosophy, and the Hippocratic commentaries. Although it was not appreciated for over 1,000 years, he made major mistakes in all these areas.

However, Galen cannot be blamed for medicine's leaders following him blindly. Not until 1,400 years later would Vesalius correct his mistakes in anatomy and Harvey overthrow his incorrect dogma on the circulation of the blood. Although he left a discernible human legacy, with obvious major professional and personal shortcomings, he is ranked in the pantheon with the other Greek demigod of medicine, Hippocrates, of whom we know virtually nothing personal. Guthrie called Galen "The Medical Dictator," but only Haeger and Nuland accurately referred to his enormously acerbic and contentious persona. One of Galen's legacies that is seldom recounted was his huge contribution to the myth of Black racial inferiority and scientifically derogatory Black medical-racial differences. Galen's writings and teachings on Black racial inferiority—and his writings on myriad other medical subjects—were accepted as unquestionable fact by 45 generations of Western and Arabic physicians.[97]

Many Greek scholars espoused racial tolerance and stressed the unity and brotherhood of mankind. Unfortunately, the most influential physician in the Western medical tradition, Galen, wrote and taught in a manner alien to most Greco-Roman intellectual traditions. As Drake observed:

> Writing between A.D. 122 and A.D. 155, he produced a textbook on anatomy that profoundly influenced medieval Islamic and Christian medical practice. His works included a list of traits he claimed were found combined together in black men exclusively . . . stating that blacks inherited defective brains.[98]

David Brion Davis catalogued this list of traits in *Slavery and Human Progress*:

> This catalog of ethnic stereotypes included blackness of skin and kinky hair; thin or sparse eyebrows; wide nostrils; thick lips, sharp, white teeth; "chapped" hands and feet; an offensive odor; eyes with large black pupils; inferior intelligence; and an oversized penis.[99]

Perhaps the most noteworthy negative aspect of Galen's writings was underscored by Drake, who noted, "For the first time . . . a Greek philosopher appeared who associated the concept of a cognitive deficit with the Negro phenotype."[100] This was Galen. He also listed "merriment" as a trait, but in a most damaging assertion noted by both Davis and Drake, he said that feature "dominates the black man because of his defective brain, whence, also the weakness of his intelligence."[101] As Drake noted, "This is perhaps the earliest statement on record alleging that Blacks have an organically based cognitive deficit."[102]

Galen had worked for several years as physician for the gladiators, and he probably did encounter some Black athletes with certain of these physical traits. Most of these so-called "physical traits" described by Galen were, in fact, artificial and dictated by the alien cultures of the African gladiators. Some African groups he described actually did sharpen their teeth, lending them a "pointy" appearance; some African pastoral people anointed their bodies with pungent oils, rendering themselves "smelly" in the process. There were very tall males from certain parts of Africa that might indeed have possessed long penises or worn penile sheaths, accounting for Galen's observation regarding their genitals. But his attribution of this entire menu of traits, some of which were groundless and derogatory, to the entire Black population was inexcusable and was indicative of his prejudices and his arrogant and contentious personality.[103]

Given Galen's exalted status the probability is high that his writings, including his views on race, were taken seriously by other physicians and Church Fathers for at least the 1,200 years that his medical views were considered sacrosanct throughout the Occident and the Middle East. A presumption of widespread influence is likely in light of a Roman "cultural context that produced the fundamentally racist ideas of Julian the Apostate and Galen the physician."[104] Davis documents that "Arab writers, especially the physicians who wrote manuals on the slave trade, elaborated on the ten traits of African blacks that had originally been specified by Galen, the most celebrated medical authority of antiquity."[105] Clearly, this affected the practice of medicine regarding people of color throughout the Roman empire and what became Europe, North Africa, and the Middle East for hundreds of years.

The degree of influence Galen's teachings and attitudes had on the inferior "slave health sub-system," described by Finley in *Ancient Slavery and Modern Ideology*, cannot be measured at this time. Some of the medical-social aspects and dimensions of this ancient dual and unequal system of health delivery are discussed later.[106] Drake hypothesized that the adverse effects of Galen's racism were probably more wide-ranging than the health system: "Galen's demeaning of Blacks, with its strong racist potential . . . may have influenced attitudes and stereotypes . . . that men of learning developed toward Negroes."[107] Devisse corroborated Drake's impression of Galen's wide-ranging racist effects on Western culture. His research extended these unfortunate influences beyond the Roman and Muslim worlds and far into the future:

> Western European writers were equally zealous in copying Galen. From the seventh to the fourteenth century they handed on (explicitly or implicitly) this vision of Africa, according to which it was a land of geographic, physiological, and intellectual abnormality. The cultural heritage of antiquity, distorted and amplified by its heirs, predisposed those latter to regard Africa as dangerous and the African as subhuman.[108]

Clearly, one demonstrable development is that the negative effects of Galen's racist teaching on Western intellectual culture in the fields of medicine and philosophy cannot be taken lightly.[109]

The period designated historically as the Roman Empire lasted roughly from 500 BC to AD 500. During that era the notion of Black racial inferiority, though not a dominant theme among the Romans, had already found its way into Western intellectual and everyday life.[110] During the second half and subsequent dissolution of the Empire after the first century AD, an increasingly important Christian religious movement responded to increasing anti-Black theological and social phenomena. Led by Christian and Jewish theologians such as Saint Paul, Philo Judeus, and Saint Augustine (AD 260–340), the Christian Church began accommodating, although not subjugating, Church doctrine to anti-Black beliefs incorporated in the Canaan and Ham legends (which ascribed incestuous and other negative characteristics to a dark-skinned son of Noah); the growing theological and social influence of the Persian and Middle Eastern Zoroastrian and Manichaean doctrines of binary opposition and competition between light = purity = white skin color versus darkness = evil = black skin color; and growing anti-Black social attitudes and behaviors in the late-Roman multiethnic society associated with the erosion of ancient and generally favorable Black Ethiopian and Kemit myths and legends, supplemented by the increasing association of black skin color with slave status. Despite the writings and practices of a medical profession dominated by Galen, the contribution of biomedical sciences to precursors of racial thought was probably a minor factor in the growing mythology about Black inferiority. Nevertheless, from the perspective of people of African ancestry, it can be safely stated that Galen was the wrong medical scientist who came along at the wrong time because the science of the era was not substantial enough to disprove his racist speculations and dogma.[111]

Galen, the last dominant physician of the classical medical tradition, represented the last shining star of a Roman medical profession and science that had always been dominated by Greeks. After Galen's death in AD 200 the last of the classical tradition of physicians fortuitously made gargantuan efforts to preserve the medical knowledge generated by Greek predecessors. Oribasius (AD 325–403), physician to the much-maligned Julian the Apostate (c. 331–363),* wrote a digest of medicine and surgery in 70 volumes, of which 25 have been preserved along with a popular work on first aid, *Euporista*. Another sixth-century Byzantine physician, Aetius of Amida, a city on the River Tigris, wrote a 16-volume comprehensive medical work, *Tetrabiblion*, which was highly esteemed by Renaissance physicians and later by eighteenth-century Dutch physician Hermann Boerhaave (1668–1738). Alexander of Tralles (AD 525–605) contributed many works based on the masters that were later treasured at Selerno and other medieval medical schools. Paul of Aegina (AD 607–690), the last physician of the classical tradition, wrote a seven-volume comprehensive medical work, *Epitome*, which was later praised and preserved by the Arabs. As Guthrie observed, "[T]he Arabs . . . preserved and perpetuated the knowledge of Greek medicine during the ensuing centuries."[112] In that all of these works were strongly influenced by Galen, they

---

*Julian the Apostate was a Roman emperor of the Eastern empire who attempted to reinstate paganism after Constantine's conversion a half century earlier. He was also cited as having racist ideas.

deserve reassessment to specifically evaluate the degree to which racist material from Galenic texts was incorporated and how influential such material may have been on both the medical and social practices of eras that followed.

With the fall and dissolution of the Roman empire by AD 600, European medicine, along with European culture in general, fell into a lengthy period of backwardness and superstition. After the dissolution of the Greco-Roman world, Western classical knowledge and intellectual traditions were rescued, preserved, and perpetuated by both the Christian Church and Arab Moslem cultures.[113]

Race, Medicine, and Science: The Middle Ages

The 1,000-year period between the fall of Rome to the Goths in AD 476 and the beginning of the Renaissance in 1400—or 1453 if the fall of Constantinople is taken as the historical milestone—is beset with confusing terminology. The first five centuries are sometimes referred to as the Age of Faith. This refers to the rising influence of the Christian Church in the social and political vacuum created by the collapse of the Roman Empire. An alternative term denoting this period, the Dark Ages, alludes to the high levels of anti-rationalism and spiritualism that accompanied the loss of Classical and Greek learning after Rome fell. This was accompanied by the erosion of academic life and rampant illiteracy. Other historians refer to the first half of this 1,000-year period as the Early Middle Ages. The second half of this period, stretching from approximately AD 900 or 1000 to the fifteenth century, is called the Middle Ages, the Late Middle Ages, or the Medieval Period, depending on the reference.

The course of the biomedical sciences of the era was shaped by the social forces of the time. These include, but are not confined to, the rise of the Christian Church with its accompanying monastic movement, the decay and collapse of the Hellenistic and Classical Roman culture, and the rise of Islam after AD 632 and its scientific dominance after the tenth century. These social forces are important relative to their perpetuation of Galenic and Arabic traditions, with their potentially racist impact on biomedical science, medicine, and other areas of natural philosophy.[114]

During the waning days of the Roman Empire, including the first half of the Byzantine Period (the fourth to fifteenth centuries), economic collapse of the agricultural and commercial systems triggered by chronic warfare, depopulation of the countryside, repeated epidemics and plagues, and repeated invasions by Germanic tribes threatened to obliterate the intellectual and academic foundations of Classical Greco-Roman civilization. However, several factors converged to prevent the permanent disappearance of Greek medical knowledge. An increasingly influential Christian Church, in the midst of a struggle between its Eastern and Western branches over the development of an orthodoxy, reached back to early followers of Christ such as St. Peter and St. Paul (who were physi-

cians) by emphasizing the "Healing Mission of Christ." Healing had been prominently mentioned in the Gospels of Matthew, Mark, Luke, and John. In addition,
Christ's parable of the Good Samaritan, a model of the benevolent Christian performing good works out of compassion for his fellow man, strongly influenced
the development of the concept of "Christian charity." As medical historians
Lyons and Petrucelli observed: "Its relationship to the treatment of disease helped
establish a nexus between the developing Church and concern for the sick."[115]
These factors had led to the establishment of Christian hospitals in Rome,
Edessa, Cappadocia, and Bethlehem within two centuries of Constantine declaring himself Christian in AD 324 and establishing Christianity on an official basis
at the Council of Nicea in AD 325.[116]

The growing doctrinal schism between the Eastern and Western branches of
the Christian Church, the former ruled by an emperor and the latter by a pope,
led to a final division of what, geographically, had been the Roman Empire by
AD 1054. Inflexible religious doctrines of the Eastern Christian church presaged
an important event that inadvertently helped preserve Hippocratic and Classical medical traditions. Expulsion of the patriarch of Constantinople, Nestorios
(d. circa 451), as a heretic by the Council of Ephesos in AD 431 forced the migration of his sect, the Nestorians, to Edessa in upper Mesopotamia. The Nestorians
founded an influential medical school, which survived there until AD 489 when
the long arm of the Church once again had the sect expelled. The tolerant King
of Persia allowed the group asylum in his capital, Jundi Shapur. The Nestorians
again founded a hospital and medical school that affiliated with the university
located there. The medical school flourished and became world famous. The
University of Jundi Shapur was a leading intellectual center serving as an intellectual crossroads and interchange point for Persian, Greek, Alexandrian, Jewish,
Hindu, and Chinese scholars. The university not only survived Arabic capture in
AD 636, but it also flourished even more as the incubating institution of Arabic
medicine. As Majno related in *The Healing Hand: Man and Wound in the
Ancient World*:

> All the while, the Nestorians were performing a huge bibliographic task:
> translating Greek books into Syriac, the language of the university. Hip-
> pocrates and Galen were among their first translations. Then Muslims
> worked at Arabic translations of the Syriac. Eventually a large body of
> Greek literature became available in Syriac and Arabic.[117]

This circuitous route travelled by the Nestorians explains many developments in
the preservation of Western knowledge. (See Figure 1.6.)

As Mohammed's religion spread from Persia to the Pillars of Hercules,
including the Balkans, parts of Italy, and the Iberian peninsula, Latin translations
of Classical works pollinated and fertilized European learning and universities by
the tenth century. Knowledge transfers such as those at Jundi Shapur explain why

Figure 1.6   The Preservation Route of Western Medical Knowledge
from the Fifth through the Tenth Centuries

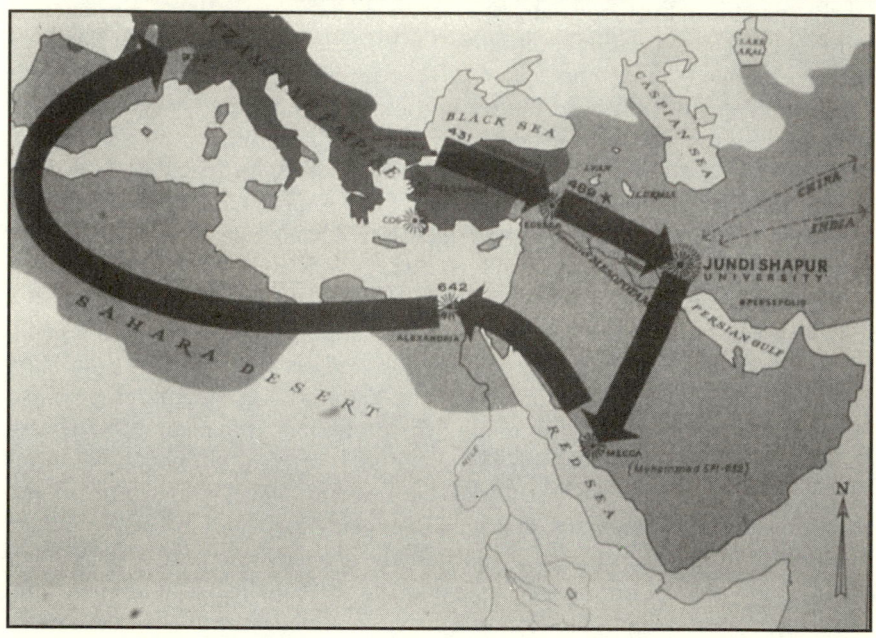

Classical Greco-Roman medical knowledge, which had been derived from Egypt and the Middle East, would not have survived had it not been for the Arabic preservation. From Gundi Shapur to dissemination over the Islamic world and, finally, through the Christian monasteries and early medieval medical schools, Western medical knowledge remained alive.

many Greek medical works have come down to us as Latin versions of translations from Arabic and Syriac texts. It also explains why the great Arabic physicians—Rhazes, Avicenna, and Albucasis—spoke the words of the Greek masters while adding their own Hindu and other Eastern healing influences to the corpus of Western medical knowledge. Through an indirect route, previous Classical and Christian-based medical and philosophical writings about racial inferiority were transported and transferred into the corpora of Western medicine and philosophy through the works of Galen, Classical Greeks, and Judeo-Christian scholars.[118]

Another major factor affecting the transmission of the Western Classical and Greek medical traditions was the monastic movement. From its northern African origins following the hermetic desert-based tradition of withdrawing from worldly society, the monastic movement in the Eastern Church affected the entire Christian world in general and medicine specifically. Monks prepared themselves for the hereafter by living an isolated existence of ascetic mysticism. Under leaders like Pachomius (d. 348), a North African hermit who improvised the first set of monastic rules, monks began banding together. In the Roman-dominated

Church, pioneers like St. Benedict of Nursia (480–554) emphasized living in religious communities and committing themselves to lives of service to the Church for their own salvation. Benedictines emphasized another Byzantine trait, that of copying and preserving old Classical manuscripts—including medical materials. This tendency, combined with the aforementioned Christian charity hospital traditions, served to involve monasteries heavily in health care and medical training. For example, Aurelius Cassiodorus's (480–573) career was integral in transforming the Benedictine monks into a medical order:

> [A]*fter serving as private secretary to Theodoric the Great, [he] entered the Benedictine order and recommended the study of Latin translations of Hippocrates, Galen, Diascorides. . . . [W]ithin a short period, the provision of medical care had become integral to the Benedictine order.*[119]

And so, for five centuries in the West, or until the Dark Ages ended in the eleventh century, monasteries served as the centers of organized medical care. There is no evidence that the Christian clerics involved in the preservation of Greek and Classical Western medical traditions, largely from the Benedictine and Augustinian orders, added to older racist intellectual trends. Although prominent monks such as Aurelius Cassiodorus, who had served as private secretary to Theodoric the Great,[120] preserved works that were racist, such as Galen's, whether the racial content was embellished or edited is never mentioned and deserves further scholarly investigation. By the end of the Dark Ages, other forces emerged to influence the medical training process, types of health care institutions, and the delivery of medical care.[121]

Some of the most influential participants in preserving the lineage of Western Hippocratic medical traditions often receive scant attention by Western historians. This introduces another racial dimension into the odyssey through Western scientific history. Due to Eurocentric or racist influences, many traditional historical treatises downplay, if not entirely ignore, the Moorish Western scientific contribution. Some scholars such as Jose V. Pimienta-Bey believe these contributions were ignored by historians because the Moslem conquerors of the Iberian peninsula—often referred to as Moors—under their leader Tariq in 711 were African. Many would be considered Negro by contemporary U.S. standards. Subsequent Moslem invasions reinforcing Islamic dominance on the peninsula were by African tribes known as the Almoravids and Almohads (these two dynasties dominated from the mid-eleventh to mid-thirteenth centuries), who had higher percentages of Black African lineage than the original invaders. By the tenth century the Iberian peninsula, which we now refer to as Portugal and Spain, flourished, becoming the most sophisticated society in the Western world from economic and cultural standpoints. The importance of the Moorish contribution to Western science is heightened by the fact that after the tenth century Cordoba became the center of the Moslem intellectual and cultural world. As Pimienta-Bey wrote in *Golden Age of the Moor:*

> *Western scholarship has characteristically dragged its feet on the issue of the historical significance of the Moor. . . . [T]he Moor's largely obscure fate . . . is not due to his insignificance in the history and development of Western civilization, but, rather, to the judgement passed upon him out of jealousy at his great influence!*[122]

In his opinion, the downplaying of Muslim importance in Western scientific history "is intentional. For behind Europe's 'Scientific Enlightenment,' we find many . . . Muslims. In fact, we find that the very foundation and structure of 'Western' Science and Academe is built upon the erudition of these people known as Moors."[123] Nevertheless, more recent scholarship has acknowledged the Arabic contribution to the Western medical tradition. As Guido Majno wrote: "The Roman Empire broke up. The flame of Greek medicine flickered, but never died out. . . . [T]he first revival occurred in Persia between the fifth and tenth centuries."[124] Arab physicians not only preserved Western medical traditions but also added substantially to them. The many political-economic reasons for this are pointed out by Nancy Sirasi in *Medieval and Early Renaissance Medicine:*

> *The most important developments in medicine between the seventh and the eleventh centuries took place not in rural, thinly populated, and economically underdeveloped Christian western Europe but in the environment of the flourishing cities, developed commercial economies, and lively intellectual milieus of the Muslim societies of the Middle East and the Iberian peninsula.*[125]

Moreover, as Pimienta-Bey remarks about physicians *(hakims)* in Arabic culture, "[P]hysicians . . . were considered the most vital of scientists and of greater importance than philosophers. The physician was the life-saver . . . because of the direct life-saving application of the medical sciences."[126] Some of the leading Arabic medical encyclopedists known to the West include, but are not limited to, Rhazes (AD 850–932), Haly Abbas (Ali ibn' ul-Abbas, d. AD 994), Avicenna (AD 980–1037), Albucasis (AD 936?–1013), Avenzoar (AD 1091?–1162), Averroës (AD 1126–1198), and the most famous Jewish physician in Arabic medicine, Maimonides (AD 1135–1204).

Another important function that Arabic medicine gave the Western profession was an elevation of status into a highly respected intellectual pursuit. This held true, at least in academic centers and communities throughout Islam, and in some parts of Arabic society in general. This trend carried over into the Medieval university system inaugurated in Europe in the tenth century and led eventually to the full professionalization of medicine in Western Europe centuries later.[127]

One Arabic medical figure, Rhazes, acquired great wealth practicing medicine, but was so generous with the less fortunate that he died penniless. Although this practice of assisting the unfortunate for future blessings continues to be practiced in Moslem culture generally, no distinct medical tradition seemed to spring from Rhazes' example. Of his 237 books on medical subjects as eclectic as alchemy, anatomy, physiology, and ethics, much was lost. He spent a great deal of time compiling the theories of Hippocrates, Galen, and others and left a celebrated work summarizing the medical and surgical knowledge of his time, *Al-Hawi (Liber Continens)*. In his *Almansor*, Rhazes was less dogmatic and more clinically oriented than Avicenna and other Arab physicians. Haly Abbas in his *Pantegni* and *Liber regius* and Avicenna in his *Canon* presented orderly synopses of the whole of medical knowledge largely based on Galen's teachings. Through this mechanism many Arabic physicians perpetuated racist ideology by their inclusion of the writings of Aristotle and Galen. Had that transfer not occurred, Galen's racial views may not have been passed down to us. However, as scholars Gordon, Devisse, and Lewis have observed, an indigenous anti-Black scholarly tradition flourished in the highly timocratic, medieval Islamic world. Murray Gordon stated in *Slavery in the Arab World*:

> [N]egative attitudes displayed by Arabs toward blacks were rooted in feelings of racial prejudice and cultural superiority. . . . [M]any Arabs were of the view that blacks were racially inferior people, a point of view that found expression in the writings of a number of early Arab writers and scholars. While some Arab scholars wrote about blacks in a compassionate way, a larger number revealed critical, if not outright hostile, feelings.[128]

Arabist scholar Bernard Lewis remarked, "[S]ome of the great thinkers of medieval Islam, such as Avicenna . . . agree in regarding the black as inherently inferior and designed by God to serve the rest of mankind as slaves."[129] Therefore, widely influential physicians in Arabic medicine, including the great Avicenna, added anti-Black prejudices of their own to the corpus of Western medicine.[130]

Avicenna and Haly Abbas both hailed from the Eastern Caliphate, in Persia, where the earliest flame of Arabic scholarship in medicine burned brightest. However, as Lyons and Petrucelli observed, "Cordoba in the West became more prominent in Islam as the caliphate in Baghdad lost influence."[131] The Western Caliphate on the Iberian peninsula contained the most Negroid Muslim population. Albucasis, court physician to the Andalusian Caliph al-Hakam II, was the major Muslim writer on surgery and strongly influenced Western medicine with his three-volume medical and surgical encyclopedia *al-Tasrif*. The surgical section of this work contained the first illustrated, systematic text on the subject. Avenzoar, Seville-born son of a Jewish physician, was a major influence over the medical and alchemical teachings of medieval European medical schools. He conducted original research and was one of the few Arabic medical scholars who studied and rejected much of the dogma of Aristotle and Galen. Despite his independent thinking, his *Kitab al-Taysir* and *Iqtisad*, both of which were translated into Latin and other European languages, were used as medical texts in European medical schools for hundreds of years.

Averroës, who some contend was of Black Moor lineage, was a pupil of Aven-zoar's who grew famous as a physician, philosopher, and mathematician. His encyclopedic medical text *Al-Kullyat fi-al-Tib [Generalities on Medicine]* was translated into Latin under various titles, including *Colliget* and *Correctorium.* According to Pimienta-Bey, in regard to the latter textbook, "[T]he mastery of this text was required for a medical degree at Bologna."[132] As Davis and Drake note, many of these Arabic texts were based upon the works of Galen, and they transmitted prominent and offensive Black racial inferiority stereotypes.[133] How much these racialist ideas permeated and affected the medical practices based on them is fruit for further study.

The fact that these Arab physicians were leaders in medical science was no accident. Many social, political, and scientific factors were involved. As Sirasi observed, "Arabic authors had access to many more works of Galen — in which there was a marked logical and philosophical component — as well as to much of the corpus of Greek philosophy, notably the works of Aristotle unknown in the West before the twelfth century." Therefore, linkages between medicine and philosophy, which had been strongest in antiquity, remained stronger in Arabic medicine. Being highly respected academics and professionals, Arabic physicians had access to lucrative patronage. Affiliations with royal courts and rich universities yielded rewards with time and resources to conduct research, write, and publish results.[134]

From an African perspective an unfortunate social evolution took place in the Moslem world during the interval between the seventh-century spread of Islam and the Renaissance in Western Europe. It manifested as increasing levels of anti-Black racism in Islam in general and on the Iberian peninsula in particular. This phenomenon manifested on several levels. Some causative factors were the increasing influence of the religious mythology from Judeo-Christian, Persian, and Moslem sources; the changing political economy of the Mediterranean world, which had the effect of protecting White Christians and Moslems from relegation to slave status; the increasing politico-military vulnerability and subjugation of Black Africans; and the changing social climate denigrating black skin and associating it with slavery. As Lewis and Sanders remark, by the tenth century slavery was imposed almost exclusively on Black people throughout Islam.[135] These phenomena affected Moslem medicine and health care in that Moslem medical manuals prominently included Galen's teachings on Black inferiority. As Devisse notes, "The blacks were real people, known although not very well, even though Galen's prejudices still influenced the minds of all the heirs of ancient cultures."[136] These racist pseudoscientific doctrines had already entered the mainstream Moslem, and later Western, medical corpus. Those studying these Arabic medical manuals, which were used by European physicians until well into the seventeenth century, must have been influenced by the racist doctrines contained therein. The prevalence and intensity of these effects on Moslem medical care deserve further study.[137]

Another force affecting the preservation, production, and dissemination of Western medical science was the medieval university movement. Sirasi described some of the factors involved:

> [R]apid development of western European society . . . took place between about 1050 and 1225 . . . often referred to as the "twelfth-century Renaissance," a population increase, economic growth, urbanization, the development of more sophisticated forms of secular and ecclesiastical government and administration, the growth of professional specialization and of occupations requiring literacy, the multiplication of schools, and the enlargement of philosophical, scientific, and technical learning were interwoven and interdependent phenomena. All had a marked impact on the study and practice of medicine.[138]

Increasing medical activity associated with the changes noted here, increased wealth among burgeoning middle and upper classes, and the demand for sophisticated and technical pedagogy triggered the opening of European medical schools such as those in Salerno in southern Italy (ninth century), Montpellier in southern France (ninth century), Paris (late twelfth century), Bologna (eleventh century), and Padua (early thirteenth century).

Close pedagogical ties to the Moslem medical traditions continued through direct transfer or cultural interchange. The former mechanism is exemplified by the multilingual academic physician Constantine the African (c. 1010–1087). He travelled throughout Syria, India, Egypt, and Ethiopia absorbing Moslem and Eastern medical traditions and accumulating medical manuscripts. Upon returning to his native Carthage he was accused of practicing magic and escaped to Salerno and later Monte Cassino in 1076. He translated texts from the medicine of the Eastern (primarily Islamic) world and from classical Greco-Roman texts. This monumental expansion of the database augmented the already widely known excellence of the medical school at Salerno. In other instances, contact with Eastern and African medicine, usually transmitted by way of the Islamic medical tradition, was more indirect.

It was not accidental that the medical school at Salerno was located close to Sicily, a Moslem outpost for centuries. Interaction with Moslems and Moors, as occurred at Montpellier in southern France, also spilled over into the medical schools throughout Europe. The Church's response to the Moslem influence, the growth of commercial medical practice, and the rise of nonmonastic centers of medical learning as a result of the economic explosion was to augment the transfer of western European medical practice out of the clerical sphere. Prohibitions such as the Council of Tours (1163), which discouraged monks from practicing medicine, were early examples of many subsequent restrictions. Church rules in 1219 forbade clergy from absenting themselves from clerical duties for medical or legal education, and in 1298 further modifications were made on what had by then become restrictive Canon Laws on the monks practicing medicine.[139]

Alterations in the Western European and Mediterranean racial climate in which the Middle Ages knowledge transfer of Western medicine occurred were important antecedents to Renaissance events. Until the Age of Discovery, there was limited contact between the races on the European continent itself except in the areas contiguous with the Moslem world such as the Iberian peninsula, Sicily and southern Italy, Constantinople, Cyprus, and Italian ports such as Venice and Genoa. These were all foci of the increasingly Black African slave trade. Although European slavery before the Renaissance declined, Davis notes:

> Throughout the Iberian Peninsula the religious wars kept slavery alive as a vital institution, with an unbroken continuity from Roman times to the revival of the Mediterranean trade. . . . [I]f chattel slavery all but disappeared on the feudal manors of Europe, it flourished at such urban seats of learning and civilization as Cordova and Constantinople.[140]

In lieu of Sanders's and Davis's impression that Iberian and Mediterranean bondage was becoming an exclusively Black African slavery in the years approaching the Renaissance, for the rest of Europe, as the institution of slavery subsided, a period of intense cultural isolation from Black Africa ensued. This period of cultural isolation, as Devisse pointed out, intensified anti-Black beliefs and attitudes based on religious legends, myths, and travelers' tales. Moreover, Spanish and Portuguese Christians, primed by more than 700 years of religious warfare with predominantly non-White and Africanoid peoples on the Iberian peninsula, were consciously and unconsciously preparing for how they would later deal with other heretics, "savages," and "barbarians" during the Age of Exploration that followed. Armed conflict, exploitation, deception, and brutality learned in the *Reconquista* were familiar methods. This was the layette prepared for the birth of the Renaissance. The rebirth of Western science and the Age of Discovery during this period ultimately spurred unprecedented European dominance. This historical convergence of social, ideological, and scientific events produced a fertile ground for the Renaissance birth of formal anti-Black scientific and biomedical racism.[141]

Race, Medicine, and Science during the Renaissance and Reformation

For a number of reasons, race emerged as a significant societal force shaping attitudes and events during the Renaissance in Europe. This contrasted with its lack of prominence in the ancient world and emerging importance in the Middle Ages. Europeans spread racialist thought throughout the world. Negative attitudes toward Blacks and other non-Whites affected various aspects of Renaissance life. These societal attitudes infiltrated the natural sciences and medicine; thus, the groundwork was laid for a new and distinct branch of *scientific racism*. A biological-determinist, anti-Black, hierarchical branch of racism based on the "new sciences" later dovetailed with and buttressed the classical Industrial Age concept of scientific racism that followed.

Beginning in late Middle Ages Europe, an unparalleled confluence of new and unprecedented circumstances arose between 1100 and 1400. Arabs, Arabists,* and the monks preserved, and often improved upon, the Hippocratic and Galenic medical and biological literature along with the Greco-Roman intellectual traditions in the preceding periods. An expectancy and excitement seemed to predict Western Europe's future: "Giorgio Vasari (1511–74), Florentine artist, architect, and man of letters, dubbed the period a *rinascita*, or rebirth, because of a common belief that the major force in its evolution was a return to the cultural priorities of ancient Rome and Greece."[142] However, the 350-year period from 1250 to 1600 was much more than a backward look at ancient Classical civilizations through a prism of their original writings, artistic masterpieces, architecture, and philosophic discourse.

The Renaissance was a much broader phenomenon. Some of the undergirding included, but was not limited to, new knowledge dissemination borne of the invention of the printing press and printing from movable type, which generated affordable books for the first time. It allowed the creation of a market-based money economy relying on trade. An economic explosion occurred linked to speculation and profits following the Crusades and the establishment of local industry throughout much of Western Europe. Meanwhile, the discovery of direct sea routes to the Americas, the Spice Islands, and India opened up new areas for exploration and European exploitation for trade and profits. Political stalemates early in the Renaissance between the Pope and the Holy Roman Emperor allowed for the existence and vitality, within political interstices of European power politics, of several prosperous city-states built upon international trade and commerce (e.g., Venice, Genoa). The shocking fall of Constantinople in 1453 changed the balance of political and religious power between Eastern and Western Europe and forced the migration of legions of Greek scholars into northern Italy and the rest of Western Europe. The religious Reformation and Counter-Reformation established a new baseline upon which individual freedom and republicanism would be defined in Western culture.

What happened to the concept of race in its relationship to Western biomedical sciences was also unprecedented. By 1700 the concept expanded beyond the boundaries of individual infusions of personal bias, condescension, and prejudice

---

*Arabists are contributors to the free and open Moslem intellectual tradition that included Jews, Egyptians, Chinese, Indians, and some Christians. They usually wrote in Arabic and for these reasons are sometimes referred to as Arabists.

against Black and other non-White peoples by physicians and scientists like Aristotle, Galen, and Avicenna to become a legitimate part of Western natural and biological science. As historian James Reed said of pre-twentieth-century scientific development:

> *The history of "scientific racism" before the 20th century is synonymous with the development of the modern scientific study of race. Scientific racism was not "pseudoscience" but an integral part of the intellectual world-view that nurtured the rise of modern biology and anthropology.*[143]

Racially prejudiced natural scientists, or scientists under the influence of commonly held social beliefs of their time taking cues from highly influential scientific forefathers like those mentioned earlier, were responsible for this phenomenon. Concomitantly, as the natural sciences increased in their social authority and influence, the data and viewpoint science produced became the new justification for racial hierarchies, White superiority, and the racial practices of the time.[144]

The Renaissance was marked by new modes of thinking and looking at the world. Instead of the blind-faith acceptance of Aristotelian-based teleology, Galenic dogma, and religious Scholasticism, the new Humanism encouraged Hippocratic-style approaches built upon open-minded observation, empiricism, and experimentation. A new age of science harkening back to the fundamental scientific values originally espoused by Classic Greek philosophers was in full swing by the fifteenth century. Although the first two centuries of the period were dominated by observation and empirical fact-gathering, by the sixteenth century some experimentation and quantification had begun. The Renaissance also marked the definite separation of the natural sciences from philosophy for the first time. Science and its present subdivisions, such as biology, chemistry, physics, and anthropology, would not emerge until after the eighteenth century. Ironically, the same emphasis on observation, detachment, and objectivity that had given people the possibility of freeing their minds of Biblical and historical sanctions, legend-myths, and ancient scientific dogma opened the way for pseudoscientific speculation to be used as "proof" of Black and non-Aryan racial inferiority. Moreover, this new approach was touted as being value-free, dispassionate, and objective—free of bias or personal subjectivity. Consequences of this emerging new breed of scientific racism flowered over the centuries into such phenomena as massive international systems of race-based chattel slavery; the genocidal near extermination of hundreds of North American, South American, and Caribbean Indian populations; and the slaughter of millions of European Jews in the Nazi Holocaust.[145]

The fifteenth-century Age of Exploration was emblematic of the European Renaissance. Utilizing new science-based instruments and methods of navigation pioneered by King Henry the Navigator's school at Sagras in Portugal, fifteenth-century Spain and Portugal dominated world sea exploration. The ulti-mate result was the discovery of sea routes to Africa, India, and the Spice Islands; circumnavigation of the globe; the discovery of North and South America; imple-mentation of exploitive commercial ties built upon militaristic coercion; a brutal new form of chattel slavery; and eventual political domination of African, New World, and Asian populations. Led by Portuguese and Spanish explorers, a perva-sive pattern of European exploitation of the native peoples of these various "lands of discovery" was rapidly established. Ensuing events, especially the Atlantic slave trade, would plunge Western European societies into unprecedented levels of corruption, wealth, greed, racism, and cruelty.[146]

Fifty to one hundred million black Africans were sacrificed to the slave trade, while between 10 and 20 million survived their transition to chattel slavery in the Western hemisphere. Western European medical participation in the Atlantic slave trade was heavy, with the British eventually making a surgeon a require-ment for slave ships. This represented a deeper level of Western biomedical and scientific involvement, as African patients' treatment became medically and ethi-cally "different" in Western physicians' eyes to accommodate the Atlantic slave trade. Despite medical participation, death rates from disease, poor sanitation, and brutality were enormous for the Black chattel slaves. The "different" status the Western medical profession conferred on Black Africans was borne out by the fact that whatever medical knowledge and practices made available during the period of Atlantic slavery were heavily focused on increasing the profitability of the trade instead of African American health improvement and the preservation of Black lives. The healthy, happy Black slave in English North America was a myth. Most Black slaves were neither happy nor healthy.[147] The primary reason slaves were treated, if and when they received any medical care at all, was to sustain their ability to perform as work units for profit in the slave labor force. If slaves died or were worked to death, they were replaced either through the Atlantic slave trade or through perpetuation of the work force by slave breeding after the Atlantic slave trade was abolished.[148]

Although the Renaissance had numerous positive effects on world culture, there were also regrettable occurrences. From a racial studies perspective many of these negative phenomena were directly or indirectly associated with the rise of science during the period. Negative social phenomena such as the slave trade, perceived White intellectual and biological superiority, and worldwide Euro-pean cultural intolerance and dominance seemed to be exacerbated by the rise of the "new science." Much of the scientific reawakening in the fifteenth and six-teenth centuries was concentrated in the fields of physics, astronomy, and mathe-matics based on the innovations of Nicolaus Copernicus (1473–1543), Galileo Galilei (1564–1642), and Tycho Brahe (1546–1601). These disciplines estab-lished the quantitative, numerical, and statistical standards by which other scien-tific disciplines such as biology and medicine were later judged. Scientific medical advances in these centuries, though at less mature levels than in these other disciplines, were led by Paracelsus (1493–1541), Ambroise Pare (1517?–1590), and Andreas Vesalius (1514–1564). Seventeenth-century advances, which were more mature scientifically, rested on the work of Galileo Galilei, René Descartes (1596–1650), and Francis Bacon (1561–1626). The work of all these men paved the way for Sir Isaac Newton (1642–1727), who is credited, somewhat overgenerously, with objectifying and quantifying the entire cosmos. Nevertheless, this reification of numerical methods and quantification was a major foundation upon which the legitimation of future racial pseudosciences such as anthropometry, craniometry, and eugenics rested. Seventeenth-century medical advance was led by men like William Harvey, Marcello Malphighi, Anton von Leeuwenhoek, Thomas Sydenham, and the obstetrical Chamberlains. Although most of these men had little to do with the origins of racial typology and the rise of racism in Western science, the few that did, such as Paracelcus, Malphighi, and von Leeuwenhoek, were of the first rank in their influence. Based on the scientific and cultural outcomes that followed, the effects were clearly devastating.[149]

From a biomedical perspective, the major scientific figures of the Renaissance were the "questioners," or iconoclasts who challenged the traditional Western biomedical dogma handed down to them from medical forefathers such as Aristotle, Hippocrates, and Galen. Some of these men were products of apprenticeship medical educations or rejected their own formal training out of hand if it inhibited their scientific quests. One early major medical figure in the Renaissance was Paracelsus. Born Theophrastus Bombastus von Hohenheim in 1493 near Zurich, Switzerland, he revolutionized Renaissance medicine by advancing prophetic theories and practices in drug therapy. He introduced mercury and iron into the pharmacopeia, earning him the title "Father of Pharmacology." By questioning and rejecting the ancients, he originated disease-specific inquiries and treatments in medicine emphasizing clinical rather than theoretical aspects. Paracelsus also conducted and reported pioneer studies in occupational diseases and public health. He was a prolific writer and has been highly praised by German medical historians; however, his recognition has been limited in that few of his works have been translated into other languages. One of the first books on the utilization of chemicals and metals as medications was his *The Triumphal Chariot of Antimony* (1604). Another of his works was the first book in the field of occupational medicine, titled *On Miners' Consumption* (1524).

Unfortunately, Paracelsus also espoused racist theories of separate creations, alleging that Africans, Asians, Indians, and other non-Aryan people of color could not be descendants of Adam and Eve. He theorized that they originated separately from inferior ancestors. The esteem with which Paracelsus is held in the history of science is rising. Whether this scientist's prejudiced racial attitudes will be considered a factor in the overall evaluation of his contribution remains to be seen. Due to his unpredictable and explosive personality and frequent and controversial behaviors, Paracelsus was not accepted within the scientific community of his time and is only belatedly recognized now. The impact of these rarely discussed views of Paracelsus on either scientific or social perspectives is a complicated question that deserves further study and future surveillance.[150]

The work of other biomedical giants in the early Renaissance has, so far, not been identified with the growth of scientific racism. They are briefly mentioned to lend some sense of the broad scientific world created that later shaped the future of modern medical science and health care. They serve as evidence that large blocks of Renaissance scientists were not preoccupied with race or racial differences. Niccolo Leoniceno (1428–1524), an early medical humanist, was noted for discovering and publishing botanical and medical errors in the works of Pliny, Hippocrates, and Galen. Ambrose Pare, a self-trained French Army surgeon born at Bourg Hersent near Laval, is credited with making surgery respectable in Western medical circles, challenging the surgical dogma passed down by Galen, Avicenna, and Albucasis. Perhaps his lack of formal training and his inability to read Latin insulated him from classical dogma, thus allowing him to focus on new and more productive thinking. His revolutionary techniques led to his becoming court surgeon for French kings and to his *The Method of Treatment for Wounds Caused by Firearms* (1545) and *A Universal Surgery* (1561). Mondino de Luzzi of the University of Bologna during the Late Middle Ages helped resurrect human dissection for teaching during the Renaissance with his *Anathomia*, written in 1316 and published in 1487. Although it contained a host of Galenical errors, his dissecting instruction book would not be retired until anatomy was redefined by Andreas Vesalius. When Vesalius published *De humani corporis fabrica* in 1543, scientific anatomy was established and Galenic anatomical dogma based on dissections of Barbary apes and pigs was abolished. With accurate, systematic, and artistic illustrations integrated with text, the *Fabrica* was praised as one of the greatest books, medical or not, ever published.

The century following the Renaissance, which some consider the "Age of Scientific Revolution," "The Age of Reason," and medical science's "Golden Age," was burdened with evidence of the growth of scientific racism marring the emerging and increasingly influential "new science." The sixteenth-century scientific explosion fueled advances in medicine and health care. By this period science was sophisticated enough by modern standards to make legitimate contributions to the corpus of racial thought. Classical definitions of scientific racism are usually built upon nineteenth-century English foundations borne of the Georgian Enclosures,* the Agricultural Revolution, and the Industrial Revolution — social circumstances discussed later. These phenomena were driven by

---

*The Georgian Enclosures refers to a series of Enclosure Laws passed by the English Parliament legally expelling peasants from what had been English common lands during the seventeenth and eighteenth centuries. The lands became the legal property of local manor lords. English Poor Laws were passed to provide relief to growing populations of landless small farmers and village artisans.

events that began in the seventeenth century. The British peasantry was driven into overcrowded, polluted, industrial centers clamoring for work that, because of inefficiencies in the political economies of the Industrial Age, was often nonexistent. Social pressures generated by these excess populations led to English Poor Laws and health-related relief programs. Criticism emanating from the first political economist, Thomas Robert Malthus (1766–1834)—based on rationales of overpopulation, overspending on the poor, and survival of the fittest—energized and organized the arguments leading to the classical version of scientific racism that arose during ensuing periods. Classical scientific racism, whose roots stretch back to the Age of Reason and Enlightenment, is considered a by-product of the Industrial Revolution. Science writer Allan Chase's definition of classical scientific racism in *The Legacy of Malthus: The Social Costs of the New Scientific Racism* serves best: "*scientific racism* . . . the creation and employment of a body of legitimately scientific, or patently pseudoscientific, data as rationales for the preservation of poverty, inequality of opportunity for upward mobility, and related regressive social arrangements."[151] Chase then mentions the branch of scientific racism whose origins we are tracing in this book. This is the branch of biologic-determinist, White superiority-promoting, anti-Black scientific racism whose origins antedate both modern science and the Industrial Age: "In the performance of these functions, scientific racism has often also institutionalized and lent scientific respectability to racist dogma and practices that were all far, far older than science itself."[152] This synthesis is analogous to the amalgamation of the Eurocentric cultural and psychological notions of Black filth, lasciviousness, savagery, and inferiority—the antithesis of civilization—antedating the Age of Exploration with the prejudices, degradation, and contempt associated with the scientific revolution, the Atlantic slave trade, and the institution of sixteenth- to nineteenth-century chattel slavery to form the peculiar U.S. notion of anti-Black racism. The conceptual frameworks reinforce each other, producing an amalgam that evolved into U.S. scientific racism. The predecessor branch of scientific racism was a unique response to an entirely different set of evolutionary circumstances and social pressures on the growth of Western science. Nevertheless, it left a permanent imprint on the U.S. notion of scientific racism.[153]

One societal pressure on the "new science" was the need for new rationales for social hierarchies in an enlightened age of individual worth, freedom, and democracy. For millennia, social hierarchies based on the divine right of kings, religious practices and beliefs, and maintenance of the social order had gone unquestioned in the West. Differences in wealth, power, and achievement based on birth and inheritance and other factors such as racism were expected and accepted. With the Renaissance spirit of inquiry, the Protestant Reformation, and the rebirth of democratic values, quiescent since the Classical Greek period, the justification of hierarchies based on ideologies grounded in progress, science, and change became the new norm. Travelers' tales of strange and different people from exotic lands and the so-called informed opinions of Renaissance physicians could only suggest racial and biological differences in mankind from a scientific standpoint. By the dawn of the Enlightenment in 1700, opinion leadership on such matters was transferred from social belief systems, scientific dogma, and religious orthodoxy to science and its quasi-priesthood—physicians and natural scientists. That science was reaffirming the unequal European social strata and racial hierarchies based on White superiority becomes comprehensible when one considers, as Lyons and Petrucelli state, "Three major influences from earlier centuries had to be reckoned with: Aristotelianism, Galenism, and Paracelsianism."[154] These major influences attended the birth of this vibrant new scientific age. It is strange and ironic that all three of these major figures, in founding the biomedical sciences, laid major foundations for the emergence of scientific racism, biologic hierarchies based on race, and biological determinism. Therefore, alongside the major strides in life sciences grew antecedents to pseudosciences, many with ancient lineages, such as physiognomy, anthropometry, and mysticism (alchemy, astrology, mesmerism, etc.). Instead of serving as self-correcting scientific systems that, given more facts, produce an ever-clearer picture of reality, pseudosciences, burdened by invalid assumptions and unverifiable hypotheses, perpetuate subjective belief systems, often with the trappings (numbers, statistics, tables, graphs) of real science. While reputable medical and scientific historians are justified in citing Aristotle, Galen, and Paracelsus as scientific giants, it is possible, in fact highly probable, that many were not aware of the negative contributions these icons made to the growth of scientific racism.[155]

It is significant that the series of scientific taxonomic efforts to categorize mankind on the basis of race began during the late seventeenth century. They are examples of what Wassermann, Haller, Stanton, and Jordan ably pointed out decades ago and Gould and Shipman reaffirmed more recently: Western scientists from the very beginnings of what can be considered the Age of Modern Science seemed to be almost morbidly fascinated by the subject of race.

Bacon and Descartes, while not physicians, influenced all of science with their theories and concepts. Their inductive* and quantitative approach and methodologies to empirical observations about the world sometimes led to erroneous and racialist conclusions. Lyons and Petrucelli pointed out that "Descartes' *Discourse on Method* in 1637 supported a generalization of the mathematical method and the development of a mechanistic picture of the world."[156] The uncritical promotion of inductive reasoning and unqualified near-worship of the scientific method led, inadvertently and almost inevitably, to the pervasiveness and success of many pseudoscientific racial theories. Resulting concepts, theories, and conclusions would later transcend time and have adverse effects on the image and health care of Blacks. Although good science has been a boon to

---

*The *inductive* method of science is based on the principle that the careful observation of many particular instances of a phenomenon leads to a pattern, a general law, or principle. While *deduction* follows a train of premises, *induction* depends on experience as the source of knowledge.

mankind, bad science has done grave harm to Blacks and most other non-White minorities.

Francis Bacon, a scientific seer who was not fully appreciated in his own time, promoted inductive reasoning and the scientific method, predicting that science would become the tool enabling man to control nature in the future. Dominance of these new views, in some important indirect ways, may have favored the formation of racialist thinking. For example, the mechanics of inductive reasoning, which emphasizes the inference of a specific law or causation from the observation and analysis of a particular instance or instances, easily justified reaching flawed, racialist conclusions. Induction is no sure-fire method of finding truth, as Milner notes: "One major problem is what is to be observed? If the scientist has no idea what he is looking for, he cannot know where to focus his attention or what facts to gather."[157] One example is misinterpreting the scientific and social implications of comparing the technical levels of European societies and those encountered in Africa and the New World. These societies were less developed in the industrial and technical sense. That they were also much less sophisticated than European countries in areas of foreign policy and diplomacy did not mean that they were necessarily inferior. Nevertheless, so-called objective observers repeatedly reached and recorded conclusions of inferiority. Europeans inferred that because African and Native American populations dressed in scanty costumes they were lascivious. The fact that American Indians often acted catatonic or committed suicide rather than submit to slavery was used as evidence that they were somehow biologically endowed with special, somehow inferior, "racial" temperaments. The simultaneous discovery of Black Africans and Great Apes, who had black coats and dark facial skin, in the same geographic areas on the coasts of Central and West Africa led to fallacious "scientific" associations between man and beast. There were even descriptions of alleged sexual intercourse between the two groups.[158]

Early efforts at hierarchical classification also prompted many scientific dead ends. Racial classifications based on obvious physical characteristics such as skin color and hair texture are glaring examples. Such differentiations turned out to be only superficial. Seemingly, the more that is discovered about the biology of the human species, the more closely related the races are to each other. Nevertheless, early attempts at racial classification based on appearance and geography reached wrong and tragic conclusions for many of the people involved.[159]

The mechanistic and quantitative approach also held the potential for flawed and dangerous "scientific" conclusions. Because naturalists could not explain most biological differences on any basis other than appearance or measuring body parts, they described and measured. When they tried reaching unsubstantiated scientific conclusions about these findings, they got into trouble. The efforts to relate mental capacity and personality and character traits to skin color or the size of a person's skull or the shape and location of bumps on the surface of his or her cranium are examples. Based on their acts and writings, Descartes and Bacon effectively reformed the philosophy of science and helped justify the generously funded infrastructures and societal authority science presently enjoys. However, they probably had no intention of providing through their proselytizing, nor could they have predicted, the liberties others would take with their valuable principles and philosophies to pervert science to support biased and often racialist views.[160] Many scientists are still attempting to relate complex matrixes of behavior such as intelligence and violence to skin color.[161] This is not new. Virtually all of the race-based conclusions reached by scientific giants like Benjamin Rush, Paul Broca, and Theodor Bilroth were either premature, based on mistaken sets of hypotheses, or simply racist.[162] Moreover, as Gould points out, whenever results are presented in numerical or statistical fashion, their power and immutability increases geometrically. That such presentations automatically have the panache of "objectivity" and lack of bias makes it more difficult to control their adverse scientific effects or social consequences. Herrnstein and Murray's *The Bell Curve* is a recent example.

However, this ideology, these processes and practices are being brought into question. Statements decrying race-based and racially biased research by scientific organizations such as the AAAS's—which stated that race is no longer a valid basis of human differentiation from a scientific viewpoint—is a first step toward openly addressing the problem. Other courses of action that may minimize scientific racism include, but are not limited to, the inclusion of African American and other disadvantaged ethnic American scientists in scientific societies, to make up for generations of *de facto*, if not official, exclusion policies; publishing and publicizing works that target scientific racism along with other perspectives that serve to counteract its effects; opening up American and international scientific societies to African Americans and other ethnic Americans; and ensuring that research focusing on the health and social needs of ethnic Americans is funded and supported by both public and private funding agencies. Such actions could go a long way toward counteracting the social biases and racial prejudices that, in actual practice, have always poisoned Western science.[163]

A major figure embodying the true scientific principles of the age and dominating seventeenth-century medical scientific advance was William Harvey (1578–1657). This Paduan-trained English physician's far-reaching physiological theories on human circulation served as mechanisms that helped launch the careers of two well-known contributors to the pseudoscientific notions of biological predetermination and Black inferiority—Marcello Malpighi and Anton van Leeuwenhoek. There is no evidence that Harvey shared pseudoscientific notions of biological predetermination or racial hierarchies. Questions on the continuity of the circulation raised by Harvey's classic book *Exercitatio Anatomica de Motu Cordis et Sanguinis in Animalbus* [*An Anatomical Treatise on the Movement of the Heart and Blood in Animals*] (1628) would be answered by the discoveries of Malpighi and van Leeuwenhoek.[164]

Malpighi (1628–1694), an Italian physician on the faculty of the renowned University of Bologna Medical School, earned the sobriquet "The Father of Histology." While systematizing the study of microscopic tissues, he documented microscopically the pulmonary capillary circulation. Of all his contributions to medical science, and there were many, this major discovery confirming Harvey's theories was his most important. Malpighi became one of the most highly respected physician-scientists of the day. Nevertheless, Malpighi's speculations on Black anatomical differences, black pigmentation,* and lesser intelligence in his research and writings and his promotion of the preformation theory became cornerstones of biological predetermination utilized by racial theorists for the next two centuries. Although Malpighi's career was not shaped by his racial investigations, his opinions and conceptualization regarding all biological matters were taken seriously—particularly within the scientific community—because of his prestige.

Harvey's theories were further verified by the 1688 findings of the pioneer Dutch microscopist Anton van Leeuwenhoek (1632–1723), who verified the peripheral capillary circulation in the extremities. This, again, corroborated Harvey's breakthrough physiological theories while placing this linen merchant from Delft in the pantheon of medical science. Later known as "The Father of Microscopy," van Leeuwenhoek was credited with the scientific discovery of spermatozoa, protozoa, and bacteria with his homemade equipment. So impressed was the scientific community with van Leeuwenhoek over the years that in 1680 he was made a member of the Royal Society in London—the most prestigious scientific society in the world. Unfortunately, this influential scientist also opened the door for speculation on Black inferiority.[165]

Another scientific "discovery" reported by pioneer Dutch microscopist Niklass Hartsocker (1656–1725), soon after van Leeuwenhoek's 1677 discovery of spermatozoa, exerted a major influence on scientific racism. When Hartsocker's *Essay de dioptrique* (1694) entered the natural science lexicon, it served as the pseudoscientific mechanism for most scientific racist and biologic predeterminist theoreticians for the next 200 years. The objects of Hartsocker's "discovery" were called "homunculi," or microscopic, preformed men that he allegedly found in spermatozoa. This "finding" led to one of the two major seventeenth-century theories on how embryos originated. The theory of *preformation* alleged that a miniature, fully formed individual resided in the sperm or egg and simply grew until it reached newborn size. That a woman's body contained miniature versions of her already fully formed offspring too small to see without the aid of microscopy became the most popular theory of embryo origin for at least the next 150 years. The opposing theory, *epigenesis*, hypothesized that an organism began as a primitive substance that evolved through a series of stages, gradually maturing and developing organs until the mature fetus formed. Preformation's assumption of biologically predetermined individuals, original members of a human race initially created by God, left little latitude for changing or altering any organism's biological potential.

This fit in neatly with the seventeenth century's mechanistic approach to

---

*Malpighi's name is eponymically associated with several of his major microscopic discoveries, including the renal corpuscles, the rete mucosum of the skin (the pigment layer), and the capillary nexus between the arteries and veins.

natural science and was later adopted by scientific racists as Social Darwinist explanations for permanent social hierarchies and inequalities and the inevitable and immutable inferiority of non-White races. Creating favorable living conditions or implementing social services or health programs perpetuating "inferior stock" wasted valuable resources. Malpighi and van Leeuwenhoek were staunch preformationists. In contrast, epigenesis, requiring a vital spirit to account for development, left open huge avenues for the environment to effect changes in the eventual biological outcome. Clearly, permanent Black chattel slavery, the lack of educational attainments and social refinements by slave and poor White populations, and the poverty of slave and peasant populations could be explained and rationalized with preformation theory.

Many scientific treatises, essays by learned scholars, and popular travelers' tales had openly referred to, or alluded to, Black and non-White inferiority by the seventeenth century. The first effort at racial classification possessing scientific rigor by the standards of the time was made by French physician and traveller François Bernier. His article "Nouvelle Division de la Terre, par les Differentes Especes ou Races d'Homme qui l'Habitent" ["The New Division of the Earth, by the Different Species of Races of Men Who Inhabit It"] was published in the Paris *Journal des Scavans* in 1684.[166] He attempted to classify people on the basis of skin color, hair texture, and appearance. However, even this first effort at human classification was disturbing, according to P. J. Marshall and Glyndwr Williams in *The Great Map of Mankind:* "[H]e expressed a common but potentially ominous belief when he allowed the American Indians to be the same species as Europeans, but not the African Negroes."[167] He also made derogatory comments about the Lapps. Such classifications undoubtedly affected the attitudes and opinions of other physicians and scientists studying these works. The next serious scientific efforts to classify mankind on the basis of race took place during the Enlightenment, sometimes referred to as the Age of Reason, which began in approximately 1700.[168]

Race, Medicine, and Science in the Age of Reason and Enlightenment

The Age of Reason and Enlightenment marked a rising tide of hierarchical thinking in all fields touched by natural philosophy. Medicine, anthropology, and the field that later became biology* were tainted by the pseudosciences. The new norms based on the hierarchical ranking of human groups spawned medical ethical conflicts on a clinical level, for all patients had a natural right to equal

---

*The term *biologie* was coined by the pioneer French evolutionist Jean-Baptiste Lamarck (1744–1829) in his book *Philisophie Zoologique* (1804) to refer to the study of plants and animals. It was quickly adopted in Europe.

treatment. Meanwhile, mesmerism, phrenology, and anthropometry, derogatory racial classification schemes, and "scientific proofs" and rationales of White superiority grew more popular in the scientific community. These theories and developments had lasting impacts on negative attitudes toward people of Black African lineage, especially as it was taught in academic institutions and medical schools.

This era's major effort at classifying mankind scientifically and biologically* occurred in the 1750s. Its creator, Swedish physician and naturalist Carl Linnaeus (1707–1778), was the "Father of Biological Classification." He named mankind *Homo sapiens*. Trained at Lund in medicine and botany, he received an M.D. degree in Holland (1735) and later became a professor of medicine and botany at Uppsala (1741). As Magnusson observed in the *Cambridge Biographical Dictionary*, "in his time he had a uniquely influential position in natural history."[169] Linnaeus's major contribution was binomial nomenclature of generic and specific names for plants and animals, which permitted hierarchical organization known as systematics. He and his students classified the known biological world of his time. Linnaeus published numerous naturalist classics, among them *Flora Lapponica* (1737), *Fundamenta Botanica* (1736), and *Critica Botanica* (1737), noted for its controversial "sexual system" of classification. Unlike other taxonomists of his time, Linnaeus added mankind to his scheme of classification.

Like Bernier earlier, Linnaeus relied heavily on racial appearances as the basis for his scientific classification of mankind. With progressive editions, over time, he added psychosocial characteristics—eventually categorizing Blacks as lascivious, inferior, and ape-like—to the world's premier book of scientific biologic classification, *Systema Naturae* (1735). As Marshall and Williams observed, "By the tenth edition of 1758 Linnaeus had reached a more elaborate classification in which the American Indian, but still more the African Negro, were viewed more negatively in comparison with the European."[170] Gould comments on Linnaeus's 1758 classification of man:

> *All leading scientists followed social conventions.* . . . *[I]n the first formal definition of human races in modern taxonomic terms, Linnaeus mixed character with anatomy* (Systema naturae, 1758). *Homo sapiens afer (the African black), he proclaimed, is "ruled by caprice"; Homo sapiens europaeus is "ruled by customs." Of African women, he wrote:* Feminis sine pudoris; mammae lactantes prolixae—*Women without shame, breasts lactate profusely. The men, he added, were indolent and anoint themselves with grease.*[171]

A classic and popular work, published in at least ten editions between 1735 and 1758, *Systema Naturae* dominated the field of biologic taxonomy throughout the

---

*Richard Bradley made a less sophisticated and a much less influential attempt at racial classification in A *Philosophical Account of the Works of Nature* (London, 1721).

eighteenth century.* The extent of the deleterious long-term effects of Linnaeus's offensive and racist classifications on Western science and society as a whole have not been fully spelled out.

Another dominant figure and colleague of Linneaus was the Comte Georges-Louis Leclerc de Buffon (1707–1788). Born of petty French aristocracy, Buffon studied law, medicine, botany, and mathematics at the universities of Dijonne and Angers. Between 1739 and 1788, while serving as director of the Jardin du Roi in Paris, the most prestigious scientific research institute in the world, he dominated eighteenth-century natural sciences. While in Paris he researched, compiled, and published the highly influential, comprehensive, 44-volume natural scientific treatise *Histoire Naturelle* (1749–1767). Eight supplementary volumes were published posthumously (1788–1804). If Linneaus was the scientific innovator, Buffon was the popularizer of the natural sciences throughout Europe. As Buffon groped for some type of evolutionary theory to tie together his thousands of observations in *Histoire Naturelle*, he made it clear he considered European Whites superior and Blacks, Native Americans, and other non-Whites inferior. Hugh Honour notes:

> In his multivolume Histoire naturelle *he set species and their varieties in a hierarchically ordered system with, not simply a man but a white man, at the summit. The people of Europe and western Asia—Caucasians of later categorization—were quite simply "the whitest and best-built men on Earth." Blacks he ranked at the bottom of the human scale as the ugliest of men, "as ugly as monkeys," he wrote, comparing them with pongos on the next step of the descending ladder.*[172]

He stated further that Negroes were "almost equally wild, and as ugly as the apes"[173] and alleged that orangutans were "ardent" for and copulated with Black women.[174] The impact of these derogatory and vile statements, published in highly regarded scientific documents, deserves further study. However, it is safe to say that for people of African descent, the racist outpourings of the two leading and most influential biological scientists of the eighteenth century were devastating.[175]

A lesser scientific figure compared to Linnaeus and Buffon, physician, surgeon, and anatomist Petrus Camper (1722–1789), in the process of pursuing artistic training, created, or resurrected,** an arbitrary system of physical measurements of the face and jaw called the "facial angle," which was utilized to categorize the races. When comparing the skull characteristics of antique Greek statues, his White ideal, with other races, Camper wrote:

Systema naturae may have gone through 12 editions during Linnaeus's lifetime. It was, obviously, a very popular book.
**The facial angle had actually been used as a criterion of beauty and intelligence as early as Aristotle. Greek gods got angles of 100 degrees, while other inferiors received lesser angles.

> When in addition to the skull of the Negro, I had procured one of a Cal-
> muck [or Mongolian] and had placed that of an ape contingent to them
> both, I observed that a line, drawn along the forehead and upper lip,
> indicated this difference in national physiognomy; and also pointed out
> the degree of similarity between a negroe and the ape. But sketching
> some of these features upon a horizonal plane, I obtained the lines
> which mark the countenance, with their different angles. When I made
> these lines to incline forwards, I obtained the face of an antique; back-
> wards, of a negroe; still more backwards, the lines which mark an ape, a
> dog, a snipe, &c.[176]

The White prototype was considered superior and most "beautiful." Camper's numerical measure of prognathism became a dominant manner of racial classification and hierarchy for two centuries. The more prognathic the specimen, the more animal-like and inferior. This work by an eighteenth-century biological scientist endured as a mainstream "objective" measure of non-Aryan inferiority until the downfall of Nazi Germany. Blacks, considered the most prognathic racial group, were considered the most inferior and most ugly. As Haller pointed out, "The facial angle was the most extensively elaborated and artlessly abused criterion for racial somatology."[177] This and other measurements created and promulgated by biomedical scientists of varying importance such as Louis Jean Daubenton (1716–1799) and Anders Adolph Retzius (1796–1860), creator of the cephalic index in 1840, were utilized as legitimate measures of racial difference for at least 142 years or until 1982. Had the Western scientific preoccupation with race been less intense, many of this last group of scientists would probably be forgotten today.

Efforts at racial classification and understanding human biology based on taxonomy (typology) by other influential scientists such as Johann Friedreich Blumenbach and Georges Cuvier (1769–1832), the "Father of Comparative Anatomy" and author of *Le Regne animal* (1817), followed. Of all of the racial taxonomy work done during the late eighteenth century, other than Linnaeus's, the work of Blumenbach had the most significant and permanent effect.

Johann Friedreich Blumenbach (1752–1840), "The Father of Anthropology," was a German anthropologist and professor of medicine. Born in Gotha, he studied at Jena and Gottingen, where he became an extraordinary professor of medicine in 1776. His lifelong interest in the study of racial differences resulted in the 1781 publication *On the Natural Varieties of Mankind*. It was a revolutionary work in the fields of anthropology and ethnology. While Bernier and Linnaeus based their classificatory systems primarily upon skin color, Blumenbach utilized a combination of skin color, hair texture and color, skull configuration and dimensions, and facial characteristics as the fundamental means for classifying the five varieties of man. His categories, which he labeled "varieties," consisted of Caucasian, Mongolian, American, Ethiopian, and Malay. His classification system dominated racial taxonomy into the twentieth century. He believed that the Georgians from the region of the Caucasus mountains (he invented the term "Caucasian") "to be the most beautiful race of men."[178] Appearance was not his only criterion; he theorized that the Caucasian was the basis from which the other races derived and was, by logical deduction, superior. As Blumenbach wrote in A *Manual of the Elements of Natural History* (1825):

> *The Caucasian must, on every physiological principle, be considered the primary or intermediate of these five principal Races. The two extremes into which it has deviated, are on the one hand the Mongolian, and the other the Ethiopian [African blacks].*[179]

The Mongolian and Ethiopian extremes were considered degenerative forms of the Caucasian ideal. A demonstration of the pervasiveness, persistence, and inappropriate validation of racial classification schemes in Western culture was Blumenbach's biographical sketch in a recent edition (1990) of the *Cambridge Biographical Dictionary*. It stated, "By his study of comparative skull measurements, he established a quantitative basis for racial classification."[180] Thus, the implication is that these "classifications," all predicated on scientifically invalid and arbitrary White, Aryan, European ideals, still possess some type of value.

Other lesser-known European and American naturalists of the late eighteenth century who were advocates of polygenesis and scientific promoters of Black inferiority included, but were not confined to, Christoph Meiners, the German philosophy professor at Gottingen who divided mankind into White and beautiful and Black and ugly; Frenchman Jean-Joseph Virey, who was a disciple of Meiners but who was particularly virulent relative to Blacks, whom he considered variants of apes; Englishman John Pinkerton, who even divided White Europeans into superior and inferior racial stocks; Scottish philosopher Lord Kames (1696–1782), who promoted separate origins for the races but was reluctant to rank them hierarchically; and Edward Long, who wrote a vitriolic, degrading, and widely read anti-Black history of Jamaica espousing racial differences and polygenesis. These opinion leaders may not have constituted the majority of learned men engaged in the monogenesis-polygenesis debate about the races, but they were important members of the intellectual elite who prepared the way for the idea of distinct races with inherently unequal capabilities that raged into the next century. Even the dominant monogenesis defenders, many of whom were still afraid to confront Biblical teachings, led by Linneaus, Buffon, and Blumenbach, believed that non-White racial types were degenerate forms of Caucasians. Black and non-White inferiority was a given. Under such circumstances, expecting European-dominated health systems to treat these various groups equally may be unrealistic. These physicians and scientists were representative of the period of racial typology, and their writings were studied by medical students and natural scientists of that time. Intellectuals of the era such as Thomas Jefferson were also strongly influenced by these theories. Attitudes about Blacks, acquired through such teachings and writings, had adverse social and medical-scientific impact on non-White populations throughout the world.[181]

Nineteenth-Century Race, Science, and Medicine

A plethora of natural scientists engaged in racial studies emerged in the nineteenth century. Although all of these scientists were not physicians, the major ones shifted the ground upon which the life sciences were based. Thus, as "race" grew in importance in scientific and medical-social senses, their contributions must be included. This was the period of racial typology. The most egalitarian racial scientists, called by Gould the "soft liners," assumed White racial superiority as a given or believed that non-Whites were deviants from an ideal European "norm." The more racist ones, the "hard liners," espoused Black and non-White animalistic and beast-like inferiority on biological, behavioral, and sexual grounds.

A prominent nineteenth-century attempt at racial classification was made by Georges Cuvier, a French anatomist credited as the father of paleontology, geology, and comparative anatomy. Cuvier was so influential by the turn of the nineteenth century that, as Berkowitz said, "His arrangement of animal species and higher groups in an order determined by anatomical principles and general relationships made his work in animal taxonomy the standard manual for most of the 19th century."[182] Born in Montbeliard, France, his love for, and expertise in, zoology led to his 1789 appointment as professor of natural history at the College de France and in 1795 as assistant professor of comparative anatomy at the Jardin des Plants at the Muséum d'Histoire Naturelle in Paris, then the leading scientific research institute in the world. During his tenure as director of the Muséum d'Histoire Naturelle (beginning in 1802), he wrote several influential books in natural science. Cuvier suggested a threefold division of the human race—Caucasian, Mongolian, and Negro. He referred to native Africans as "the most degraded of human races, whose form approaches that of the beast and whose intelligence is nowhere great enough to arrive at regular government."[183] Cuvier also theorized throughout his career that Whites were superior and Blacks were inferior, lascivious, and animal-like.[184]

Cuvier was only one of the three greatest nineteenth-century natural scientists to hold Blacks in low esteem. As Gould has pointed out, both Sir Charles Lyell, the founder of modern geology, and Charles Darwin, whose theory of evolution changed the scientific world, expressed anti-Black sentiments in their scientific writings. These men could be rightly considered the "big three" of Western science for the first two-thirds of the nineteenth century. For example, Lyell wrote "The brain of the Bushman . . . leads towards the brain of the Simiadae [monkeys]. This implies a connection between want of intelligence and structural assimilation. Each race of Man has its place, like the inferior animals."[185] Darwin, who is conventionally portrayed as an egalitarian liberal, alluded to a future when the gap between ape and human would increase by so-called intermediate forms such as Negroes, chimpanzees, and Hottentots dying off. In the *Descent of Man* (1871), he stated:

> At some future period . . . the civilised races of man will almost certainly exterminate, and replace, the savage races throughout the world. At the same time the anthropomorphous apes . . . will no doubt be exterminated. The break between man and his nearest allies will then be wider, for it will intervene between man in a more civilized state, as we may hope, even than the Caucasian, and some ape as low as a baboon, instead of as now between the negro or Australian and the gorilla.[186]

As Banton and Gould have made clear, virtually all of the eighteenth- and nineteenth-century naturalists and what we now categorize as biomedical scientists assumed Black racial inferiority based on biology, inheritance, or, at the very least, culture. A few "soft-liners" felt long-term programmatic education might enable Blacks to achieve White performance levels. However, even these felt that was aeons in the future and preferred racially separate development. The majority alleged that Black development was hopeless.[187]

Other nineteenth-century physician–natural scientists who attempted racial classification based on varying levels of Black inferiority included, but were not limited to, Charles White, author of *Account of the Regular Gradation in Man;* James Cowles Prichard, author of *Researches into the Physical History of Man;* Charles Hamilton Smith, author of *The Natural History of the Human Species;* and Robert Knox, author of *The Races of Men.* Although these men were not biomedical scientific giants of the stature of Darwin or Lyell, they were leading innovative researchers and biomedical scientists of their time. They taught at the great universities and medical schools throughout the Western world or determined what was being taught in those centers of learning. They published the scholarly literature on racial biology and anthropology dominating the scientific world of their day.

Charles White (1728–1813), from Manchester, England, was an eminent and highly regarded surgeon best known for his obstetrical work. His *Account of the Regular Gradation in Man* (1799) was a virulent, racist tract arguing that Blacks were a different species resembling apes in many ways. White, in his efforts to "raise apes and debase black humans . . . portrayed the simians as both slavers and sexual abusers,"[188] stating:

> They have been known to carry off negro-boys, girls, and even women, with a view of making them subservient to their wants as slaves, or as objects of brutal passion: and it has been asserted by some, that women have had offspring from such connections.[189]

Citing a physician-colleague, he alleged Blacks did not perceive pain like "real" humans:

> *They bear surgical operations much better than white people; and what*
> *would be the cause of insupportable pain to a white man, a negro would*
> *almost disregard. I have amputated the legs of many negroes, who have*
> *held the upper part of the limb themselves.*[190]

His opinions, which he did not consider racist, harked back to many features of the Great Chain of Being theory with Caucasians representing the apex of development.

Interestingly, White had been inspired by British physician and anthropologist John Hunter (1728–1793), one of the founders of modern scientific surgery. Hunter had been very impressed with the work of Dutch physician-anatomist Petrus Camper in his attempt around the 1780s to classify mankind objectively on the basis of bodily measurements. Camper's gradation of skulls from monkey to man had been especially intriguing. However, he was aware of both the scientific shortcomings of the work and the social implications of any work ranking other races above Negroes, a race whose relationship with European society was one characterized by subjugation, exploitation, and chattel slavery. English abolitionist James Ramsey reported after hearing Hunter lecture on "the gradation of skulls" at the Royal Academy "that the very doubt whether they might not be an inferior race, operated against the humane treatment of them; and God forbid, said he, that any vague conjecture of mine should be used to confirm the prejudice."[191] Thus, Ramsey was able to report that Hunter "drew no conclusion from the difference in them respecting African inferiority."[192] Physician-scientist John Hunter represents the highest ideals of both true science and moral principle. Although engaged in legitimate scientific investigations in ethnology and anthropology, work that could have fueled speculation injurious to Blacks, scientific integrity restrained him. Dr. Hunter would not write speculatively on these subjects.

James Cowles Prichard (1786–1848), an English physician and Edinburgh graduate who may have been the most respected ethnologist and writer on race in Europe during the first half of the nineteenth century, was not so careful. He argued for monogenesis and initially was a racial egalitarian, but he increasingly came to believe that Whites, especially of the Germanic varieties, were superior to all others. He authored *Researches into the Physical History of Man* (1813–1847), which expanded from one to five volumes by its 1836 edition. Another British physician who was the epitome of the racial typology movement was Charles Hamilton Smith (1776–1859). A disciple of Cuvier, Smith hypothesized three races: "the wooly-haired or Negro; beardless or Mongolian; and bearded or Caucasian."[193] The Negro's lowly place was due to his small and developmentally arrested brain, Smith explained in *The Natural History of the Human Species* (1848). He presaged the theories that led to the founding of the discipline known as *race relations* by referring to "the deep rooted hatred of the Caucasian races towards the typical Negro."[194] Thus, "natural" disdain, aversion, and bigoted feelings among Whites toward Blacks became, for the first time, "scientific" factors. Smith also disseminated his racial views through scientific lectures to lay and medical audiences.

Robert Knox (1791–1862) was an English physician and a determined propagandist for racial typology. He lectured extensively in medical schools, placing racial studies prominently in the curriculum, where he ranked the races hierarchically with Blacks on the bottom. He authored *The Races of Men* (1850 and 1862). The effect of this racial typology movement on scientific and lay opinion in Europe intensified because nineteenth-century biological science simultaneously emphasized morphology and the stability of "pure types." This hardening of the notion of biological hierarchies and biased racial attitudes disguised in the legitimacy of science led Banton and Harwood to label the nineteenth-century phenomenon as the "peak" for "this science of race."[195]

The first major American scientific work on racial differences was published in 1787. The Reverend Dr. Samuel Stanhope Smith, president of the College of New Jersey (later renamed Princeton University) and an eminent minister and gentleman scientist of that era, released *An Essay on the Causes of the Variety of Complexion and Figure in the Human Species.* This tract espousing monogenesis defended a Scriptural perspective on racial typology and conceded Black/White differences, but "hoped that American blacks, in a climate more suited to Caucasian temperaments, would soon turn white," according to Gould.[196] Smith went so far as to say that black skin color was actually a "giant freckle."[197] The few scientific defenders of Black and non-White people were classified as degenerationists.* By the time the second, enlarged edition of Smith's *Essay* appeared in 1810, it had become the center of a scientific firestorm. Attacks arose from Northern and Southern biomedical scientists—most of whom were also physicians.

Although there is anecdotal evidence that Smith's monogenesis-based theories on racial differences, which also conceded that Blacks were members of the family of man, were already under fire in the late eighteenth century, attacks surfaced publicly in 1809 from within the medical profession. John Augustine Smith, a prominent New York physician and medical school professor at the College of Physicians and Surgeons of the University of New York, fired the first volley in his medical school lectures. Fresh from postgraduate medical training in a Europe teeming with proliferating racialist theories based on the latest anthropometric, anthropological, and Biblical data, he returned to espouse his personal racialist synthesis. Citing authorities such as Petrus Camper, Georges Cuvier, and Charles White, his "scientific" theories were grounded in Black racial inferiority and separate origin—which challenged Biblical doctrine. He would eventu-

---

*Degenerationists believed that human races are a product of degeneration from Eden's perfection. Races declined to differing degrees—Whites the least and Blacks the most.

ally become the president of the College of Physicians and Surgeons of the University of New York and, later, William and Mary University.

Another of Dr. Samuel Stanhope Smith's volatile and persistent critics was a well-known North Carolina–born physician named Charles Caldwell (1772–1853). He received his medical training at the prestigious University of Pennsylvania School of Medicine. After a tour of duty on the university's faculty, he began lecturing vigorously and frequently throughout the United States in 1811, espousing separate origins of the races and Black, animal-like, inferiority. He became strongly allied with the phrenology movement, which was highly influential in the early nineteenth century. Direct contact with this movement, which had strong racialist overtones, occurred in 1821 when Caldwell visited Paris to purchase books and apparatus for the new medical school he was establishing at Transylvania University in Kentucky. He met Franz Joseph Gall, the founder of phrenology, and Kaspar Spurzheim, Gall's disciple, while attending their lectures. These lectures and intellectual exchanges permanently converted him to their "science." After returning to the United States, he placed phrenology in the curriculum of Transylvania's medical school and traveled widely delivering lectures on race and phrenology, becoming America's best known phrenologist by 1830.[198] His book, *Thoughts on the Original Unity of the Human Race,* a work on racial differences and phrenology, was published that same year. The work questioned Biblical chronology, and doubted that Blacks and Whites could have become so different in less than 2,000 years. He speculated that Blacks were closely related to apes. A highly motivated Caldwell continued what was tantamount to a national racialist campaign while simultaneously founding two Southern medical schools before his career ended.[199]

As Horsman and Gould have observed, the growing controversy around Black slavery triggered by the Revolutionary and Federalist periods highlighted the importance of the scientific arguments on race. By the 1830s active African colonization and abolition movements led to much more aggressive and vigorous defenses of slavery by Southerners. Throughout the Black experience in English North America beginning in 1619, an increasing sociocultural assumption of Black biological racial inferiority emerged. Buttressed by scientific movements of the eighteenth and nineteenth centuries, the entire community, both scientific and lay, had another powerful rationale leading to an inevitable devaluation and trivialization of Black life and health. Based on the evidence, commercial considerations were unable to countervail such basic cultural attitudes and behaviors. Black longevity and birth rates declined during the economic boom-period of the Antebellum South, reiterating that the image of "the contented, well-cared-for Black slave" was largely a myth.* These developments did not bode well for Black experiences or their future in the English North American health system.[200]

---

*The "Gold Standards" of public health including life-span, mortality rates, and infant mortality rates, which deteriorated among Blacks during the Antebellum Period, are also indicators of the quality of life of a given population.

Racial studies during the era of racial typology, which encompassed the entire nineteenth century, were dominated by Americans from the 1830s to the Civil War. In many respects this was a natural extension of the early steps in the scientific method as efforts at taxonomy matured and the process of analysis and quantification began. Throughout this period virtually all of the major efforts regarding mankind focused on classifying the human family according to race. Easily observed, measurable, and quantifiable features such as skin color, hair texture, cephalic indexes, cranial indexes, cranial volumes, body part measurements and dimensions, illness profiles, and detailed descriptions were the dominant parameters utilized. Moreover, the efforts of scientists such as Adolphe Quetelet in Europe and Samuel George Morton in the United States in the early part of the century to quantify racial differences based on bodily measurements and dimensions further extended the power and authority of racial studies in increasingly number-conscious nineteenth-century scientific and lay communities. Although figures such as James Augustine Smith and Charles Caldwell laid the foundations, internationally respected U.S. biomedical physician-scientists such as Morton, Louis Agassiz, Josiah Clark Nott, and Samuel Cartwright helped put the "American school" of anthropology on the map.[201]

Roots of the "American school" of polygeny and anthropology can be traced back to the physiognomy movement of the eighteenth century. This movement poisoned the conception of race within the biomedical and newly emerging behavioral and psychosocial sciences. It devalued and marginalized patients of African descent within the health and sciences subculture responsible for delivering their health care. Physiognomy, the theory that facial or body features could determine one's character or mental capacity, had been promoted in the preceding century by Swiss mystic and physician Johann Kaspar Lavater (1741–1801). However, he failed to elevate this notion, which utilized Classical Greek physical features as the "ideal," to a science. Physician scholars such as Petrus Camper, Johann Blumenbach, Franz Josef Gall (1758–1828), and Kaspar Spurzheim (1776–1832) had extended physiognomy to create the pseudosciences of phrenology, and later, craniometry, a branch of anthropometry. These disciplines were temporarily elevated to the status of "science" but lost credibility over time as legitimate scientific evidence against their validity mounted. Anthropometry, the study of human body measurements especially on a comparative basis, was popularized as serious science by Belgian statistician, sociologist, and astronomer Lambert Adolphe Jacque Quetelet (1796–1874) in the 1830s. Physical body measurements, such as those used in craniometry, were utilized to statistically develop a theoretical model he called the "average man" (*l'homme moyen*). Quetelet attempted to create a social physics based on evaluations and comparisons of discrete versions of his average man. White Europeans were his standard, and much of the work based on his efforts would be utilized to categorize groups of men hierarchically. The physical parameters and culture-based behaviors were weighted such that Blacks and other non-Whites were usually placed on the bottom. The various relations compared included physical, social, and moral parameters. It was considered the "IQ" test of the age and did not lose its hold on the U.S. scientific community's imagination until well into the twentieth century. Quetelet's work was so influential that it was resurrected at the time of the American Civil War as the basis for racial studies of Black and White Union soldiers.

Samuel George Morton (1799–1851) was an internationally famous faculty member of the University of Pennsylvania Medical School. From a patrician background, he also served as the president of the Academy of Science. After earning a second medical degree from Edinburgh in 1823 (his first was at the University of Pennsylvania, 1820), he studied in Paris where it is thought that he interacted with, and was influenced by, the great French physicians: the statistically based clinical researcher, Pierre Louis, and the founder of phrenology, Franz Josef Gall. Morton returned to the University of Pennsylvania where he taught medical students at the Philadelphia Hospital, Pennsylvania College, and the Philadelphia Alms-House Hospital. Articles, lectures, and textbooks later produced by Morton and used in medical presentations were riddled with racist text, assertions, and illustrations (e.g., *Crania Americana, Crania Aegyptica*). His quantitative work greatly strengthened the so-called scientific legitimacy of sociobiology, White superiority, and non-White inferiority.

By 1830 Morton's efforts in ethnology, craniology, phrenology, and statistics were more than an abstract interest and avocation to a zealous taxonomist. As Gould noted: "He had a hypotheses to test: that a ranking of races could be established objectively by physical characteristics of the brain, particularly by its size."[202] Between the 1820s and his death in 1851 he collected more than 1,000 human skulls of a wide variety of racial and ethnic groups, many of which he utilized for his studies. Through his skull collection, nicknamed in scientific circles "the American Golgotha," he graded the races hierarchically based on "inherent intelligence" and cultural potential he related to elaborate skull volume and cranial measurements. Thereby, Morton won worldwide respect as the world's empiricist and data gatherer on racial typology and ethnology questions. Gould later found that because of his probable unconscious biases he had distorted much of his "objective" data, thus rendering it useless from a scientific standpoint. Based on this flawed data, Morton alleged that Whites were superior, Indians intermediate, and Blacks inferior. After *Crania Americana* was published in 1839 he became the world's leading nineteenth-century empiricist of polygenesis and White racial superiority and the father of American physical anthropology. *Crania Americana* was considered the world's primary ethnological-scientific reference "documenting" Indian, Black, and non-White inferiority. His later *Crania Aegyptica* (1844) extended his work in racial science. Although a smaller volume, it was the product of more mature research. *Crania Aegyptica*'s anthropological allegations included, but were not confined to, evidence that the Black African physiognomy or mentality had not improved for over 3,400 years, since their time in ancient Egypt; proof that Black Africans were slaves and servants in ancient Egypt, reaffirming their nineteenth-century position in the social hierarchy; indications that the anthropological evidence significantly set back the date of Creation, refuting Archbishop Usher's date of 4004 BC; and "documentation" that the ancient Egyptians, then thought of as the originators of Western civilization, were definitely not Black but were a blend of several branches of the human family, including Caucasians, Semitics, and Austral-Egyptians. *Crania Aegyptica* evidenced the new attitudes and events of the early nineteenth-century United States that channeled ethnological research into the service of racial hegemony. The new focus of the "American school" emphasized Black inferiority and the immutability of racial types, viewed race in biological-deterministic terms, and alleged that Blacks could not have been the founders of civilization. Morton and his colleagues collaborated and proselytized these views throughout their careers.[203]

If Morton was the empiricist of the polygenic school, Louis Agassiz (1807–1873) was its theoretician.* A highly regarded Swiss naturalist, physician, and student of Cuvier of Paris, Agassiz migrated to America in the 1840s where he became the most highly respected biologist of his generation. Although he cloaked his theories of separate human races in scientific terms, his bias was grounded in gut racism. As Horseman and Gould reveal in his letters recounting his first contact with African Americans:

> *It was in Philadelphia that I first found myself in prolonged contact with negroes; all the domestics in my hotel were men of color. I can scarcely express to you the painful impression that I received, especially since the feeling that they inspired in me is contrary to all our ideas about the confraternity of the human type [genre] and the unique origin of our species. . . . Nevertheless, I experienced pity at the sight of this degraded and degenerate race, and their lot inspired compassion in me in thinking that they are really men. Nonetheless, it is impossible for me to repress the feeling that they are not of the same blood as us. In seeing their black faces with their thick lips and grimacing teeth, the wool on their head, their bent knees, their elongated hands, their large curved nails, and especially the livid color of the palm of their hands, I could not take my eyes off their face in order to tell them to stay far away. And when they advanced that hideous hand towards my plate in order to serve me, I wished I were able to depart in order to eat a piece of bread elsewhere. . . . What unhappiness for the white race—to have tied their existence so closely with that of negroes in certain countries! God preserve us from such contact.[204]*

---

*See Agassiz L. The diversity of origin of the human races. *Christian Examiner* 1850; 49:110–145; Gould SJ. *The Mismeasure of Man*. New York: W. W. Norton and Company, pp. 42–50. Restored, original letters in Harvard's Houghton Library; and fraudulent versions of his letters/papers cleansed of derogatory racial content in Agassiz EC. *Louis Agassiz: His Life and Correspondence*. Boston: Houghton Mifflin, 1895.

Secure as head of the Museum of Comparative Zoology at Harvard (1847–1873), he soon found "scientific evidence" to support his beliefs. He would publish papers and monographs and engage in research "documenting" Black inferiority throughout his career.

Other members of the "American school" of anthropology, which remained internationally influential until Darwin's theory of evolution swept the field in 1859, included Dr. Josiah Clark Nott, Dr. Samuel Cartwright, archaeologist Ephraim G. Squier, and Egyptologist-lecturer George R. Gliddon. Josiah Clark Nott (1804–1873) was a University of Pennsylvania, European-trained physician and anthropologist. One of the South's leading surgeons, he became famous as a defender of polygenesis, slavery, and Black inferiority. Samuel Adolphus Cartwright (1793–1863) was another Southerner trained at the University of Pennsylvania who became a prominent physician. Residing in Natchez, Mississippi, and New Orleans, Louisiana, and often affiliated with academic institutions, Cartwright published and spoke extensively on Negro biological difference, inferiority, and suitability for slavery. George Gliddon (1809–1857) and Ephraim G. Squier (1821–1888), primarily followers of Morton and Nott, collaborated with all these men, publishing books (*Types of Mankind*, 1853; *Indigenous Races*, 1856) and papers and giving lectures on their scientific racist theories throughout the middle of the nineteenth century.[205]

Less constrained by scientific considerations than Morton, some of these men wanted to codify, publicize, and inject these pseudoscientific racial findings into the public policy debates raging in the United States on Black slavery and the future of Native Americans. Their work carried the devaluation and marginalization of Blacks as full-fledged human beings and patients beyond the confines of the biomedical and scientific subculture into the realms of society and politics. Even though the evolutionary aspects of the "American school" of anthropology and its world leadership in ethnology and evolutionary biology were undermined by Darwin's theory of evolution after 1859, influences of the movement lingered.

Perhaps the most prominent evidence of the influence occurred when the U.S. Sanitary Commission, serving the Union Army, employed modifications of Quetelet's old methodology, seeking to "quantify" racial differences anthropometrically during the Civil War. (See Table 1.2.) These data were utilized to rank the races hierarchically until the mid-twentieth century. Thus, this numerical and statistical approach to racial typology and ranking, through the efforts of men like Samuel George Morton, was lent further scientific legitimacy, influence, and force—although the basic scientific premises to which the numerical methods were applied proved incorrect. Another important area of influence wielded by this new anthropological and ethnological information was the pre–Civil War defense of Black slavery. Pro-slavery supporters utilized these findings as part of their projection of slavery as a "positive good." After the war scientific racism was utilized to "prove" Black inferiority, justifying segregation, Jim Crow laws, and hierarchical Social Darwinism. It therefore had the effect of increasing the deci-

Table 1.2 An Ethnographical Table Showing Autopsy Results on White and Negro Brains

ETHNOGRAPHICAL TABLE,
Derived from 405 Autopsies of White and Negro Brains. Made under the direction of Surgeon Ira Russell, 11th Massachusetts Volunteers.

Number of Autopsies.	Grade of Colour.	Average weight of brain.	Maximum weight of Brain.	Minimum weight of Brain.	Brains, 60 ounces and over.	Brains, 55 and under 60 ounces.	Brains, 50 and under 55 ounces.	Brains, 45 and under 50 ounces.	Brains, 40 and under 45 ounces.	Brains, 35 and under 40 ounces.	Brains less than 35 ounces.
		oz.	oz.	oz.							
24	White.	52.06	64	44¼	1	4	11	7	1	. . .	. . .
25	¾"	49.05	61	40	1	. . .	10	12	2	. . .	. . .
47	½"	47.07	57	37¾	. . .	2	13	19	12	1	. . .
51	¼"	46.54	59	38½	. . .	2	10	22	11	6	. . .
95	⅛"	46.16	57	34½	. . .	1	15	50	21	7	1
22	¹⁄₁₆"	45.18	50½	40	. . .	. . .	3	10	9	. . .	. . .
141	Black.	46.96	56	35¾	. . .	5	42	51	38	3	. . .
405	. . .	. . .	. . .	. . .	2	14	104	171	94	17	1
Autopsies of Clendenning, Sims, Reid, and Tiedemann. 278	Whites, collated from various sources.	49½	65	34	7	28	99	97	39	7	1

From a study appearing in an 1869 Anthropological Review comparing the brain weight of White and Negro soldiers authorized by the United States Sanitary Commission during the Civil War. Such pseudoscientific comparisons were used by scientific racists to justify racial discrimination against Blacks well into the twentieth century.

Source: Sanford B. Hunt, "The Negro as a Soldier," *Anthropological Review* (1869). Courtesy of National Library of Medicine.

sion making and public policy authority of racial science on previously political and social issues and subjects such as social and class inequality, racial discrimination, and Black chattel slavery.[206]

The great scientific strides in biology unleashed by Darwin's theory of evolution germinated the next stage of scientific racism and facilitated the future dominance of statistical methodology following the Civil War. Utilizing virtually any set of observations ranging from the litters resulting from hog breeding to the intelligence of Africans according to travelers' accounts, Francis Galton (1822–1911), a partially trained physician and gentleman scientist, believed he could create measurements and discern scientific truths. In the process of applying his methodology to convince the world that the rich and powerful were endowed with superior abilities by heredity (*Hereditary Genius*, 1869), Galton became the apostle of quantification. He applied statistical correlation to his heredity studies, laid the foundation for biometric research, and extended the boundaries of his work to generate the science of eugenics (the science of breeding the "best"). As Chase observed in *The Legacy of Malthus: The Social Costs of the New Scientific Racism*, "He reduced such 'data' to elaborate statistics that were taken seriously as 'science' for over a century, and which proved to Galton and his followers that there is an inborn or hereditary difference of at least three magnitudes of intelligence between white people and black people."[207] Galton's disciples Karl Person and Cyril Burt continued his statistical distortions on psychological and intelligence testing data, grading groups of human beings, in actuality, on the basis of race and class, well into the twentieth century.

The "scientific" discovery of immutable hereditary gifts confirmed philosopher Herbert Spencer's (1820–1903) beliefs. He and his disciples, such as William Graham Sumner (1840–1910) of Yale, combined statistical and demographic data on so-called inferior groups—such as immigrants, Native Americans, and Blacks—and applied Darwin's theories to them. Spencer's "survival-of-the-fittest" formulation explained the social order and justified the cruel aspects of *laissez-faire* capitalism. According to these biological deterministic and social Darwinistic theories, the poor and "unfit" were "eliminated" by the inexorable laws of evolution. William Graham Sumner, who besides being a university professor of political and social science was an Episcopal rector, warned Blacks and the poor that "a man may curse his fate because he is born of an inferior race," but God would not pay the slightest heed to such "imprecations."[208] Seemingly, science confirmed not only racial but also class, ethnic, and societal prejudices and distinctions. These ominous nonbiological nineteenth-century antecedents of the sociocultural period of racial thought did not thwart the course of mainstream science in the twentieth century.[209]

The Social Sciences and Twentieth-Century Race, Science, and Medicine

The work of Darwin and Mendel had shifted the scientific terrain of evolutionary biology by the late nineteenth and early twentieth centuries. Their work, Darwin's theory of evolution and Mendel's breakthrough explanatory mechanisms of genetic transmission, profoundly affected all the related disciplines, including but not limited to biology, ethnology, geology, paleontology, archaeology, chemistry, botany, and anthropology. This included the fields constituting the life sciences and the discipline Banton later called "racial thought." Nevertheless, neither the U.S. scientific nor life sciences subcultures—the milieu where Blacks were forced to seek medical care—addressed or corrected the degradation, devaluation, and marginalization Black patients had undergone, and were experiencing, as a result of scientific racism. The correction of history-based health deficits in such a medical-social environment seemed to be an unrealistic goal.

Darwin's theory of evolution forced natural scientists to openly confront and reconcile the immense time periods required for biological evolutionary changes to occur. Moreover, it corroborated "millions of years" time estimates cropping up in geological, archaeological, and paleontological studies. Much to his chagrin, Darwin also indirectly brought Creationism theories into question concerning chronology and questions of change and dynamism. However, as Gould and others have pointed out, evolution did not preclude the hierarchical ranking of the races. It simply changed the basic assumptions and mechanisms in which White superiority and non-White inferiority were framed. In fact, it encouraged the new pseudoscience of eugenics and legitimized Spencer's harsh and authoritarian social theories—Social Darwinism. Even though Darwin succumbed to racial hierarchical thinking before he died, the synthesis of evolutionary thinking with the new disciplines of genetics and natural history* would revolutionize both the human life sciences and racial thought.

A new level of legitimate scientific progress in genetics began with the work of Austrian monk Gregor Mendel and August Weismann. It continued with European genetic pioneers Dutchman Hugo de Vries, the German Carl Correns, and the Austrian Erich Tschermak and was combined with the twentieth-century work of British geneticists Ronald A. Fisher and J. B. S. Haldane and American workers Sewall Wright, Thomas Hunt Morgan, and Hermann Mueller. By the 1940s, the synthesis and reconciliation of evolutionary biology with Darwin's work was finally completed through the efforts of Julian Huxley, Theodosius Dobzhansky, George Gaylord Simpson, and Ernst Mayr. Their work emphasized the dynamic, diverse, and evolutionary aspects of heredity and race.

However, the application of numerical and statistical methods that had altered the profile of racial studies in the early nineteenth century would extend and expand the influence of accomplishments in the fields of population and molecular genetics. Even the new biological definitions of race based on genes were dynamic and unfixed, emanating from the new sciences of genetics, biochemistry, and, later, molecular biology. Efforts to preserve static, hierarchical, racial typology–based classifications and human evolutionary hypotheses by scientists such as Earnest Hooton, William H. Sheldon, and Carlton Coon failed

---

*This broadly inclusive field of study included zoology and botany, paleontology and comparative anatomy, inheritance and variation, geographic distribution, and ecological adaptation.

and were ultimately rejected. Scholarly, though backward-looking, books such as Hooton's *Ape, Men and Morons* (1937), Sheldon's *The Varieties of Temperament: A Psychology of Constitutional Differences* (1942), and Coon's *The Origin of Races* (1963) and *The Living Races of Man* (1965) could not stem the late twentieth-century tide against scientific and anti-Black racism. Shipman covers this contemporary story in greater detail than is warranted here in *The Evolution of Racism* (1994).

Change and dynamism, for the first time, were rendered acceptable in biological circles by Darwin's theory of evolution. The biology of races became a matter of studying diversities within — as well as among — groups. Thus, the natural scientific studies of *organic* evolution, to borrow Outlaw's term, focus on changes in the gene pool of a group or groups. This objectivity and accuracy borne of the "new synthesis" between laboratory research in genetics and field work in physical anthropology and biology to produce modern evolutionary biology eventually led to the overthrow of the White superiority and biological predetermination theories that had for so long influenced the discipline of racial thought. Although static typological theories were dismissed as being unscientific or unsubstantiated, their lingering impact on society at all levels, including medicine and health care delivery, persists today.[210]

Added to these developments was a new emphasis on the social science of race, that is, understanding the social implications and outcomes of groups sharing certain distinctive biological features. The social sciences of anthropology, sociology, psychology, and ethology matured and contributed significantly. Thus, the twentieth century heralded the beginning of the sociocultural period of race. In response to challenges by modern biological, social, political, and behavioral scientists of the previous century, many old biological and typological-based concepts of race were first disproved and, later, dismantled. Debates with the social and behavioral scientists greatly enriched the field of racial thought.

Through the integration of ecological concepts and analysis along with disciplined survey and demographic-based research performed in the field, social scientists such as W. E. B. Du Bois, Robert E. Park, Lloyd Warner, and Hortense Powdermaker shifted the attention of racial studies to physical differences as signs of membership in competing groups, which call forth conscious and unconscious behaviors. Such behaviors translated into power relationships, social customs, class and caste structures, and institutional structures and functions that were, ultimately, driven by race. John Dollard, a psychologist, applied the new European psychoanalytic methods defining a Freudian theory of racial relations. He formulated psychoanalytic methodologies and introduced them to racial studies. Analysis of the social system as a machine with social, sexual, economic, and political components, all of which were influenced by race, was a hallmark of the sociocultural period of race. An excellent overview of the early development and accomplishments of this latter period is presented in Gunnar Myrdal's *An American Dilemma.* Other contributions to the field of racial thought by scientists such as Melville Herskovits, E. Franklin Frazier, Christopher Jencks, Andrew Hacker, William Julius Wilson, James H. Jones, and Ronald Takaki constitute a cross-section of much of the subsequent body of this work.

The twentieth-century focus of racial thought had shifted to the sociocultural and psychological impact of possessing certain biological features such as dark skin color or kinky hair on individuals and groups. Such investigations and concepts fall under the category of racial studies Outlaw refers to as *superorganic* evolution. These studies focus on changes in the "behavior repertoire" or the sociocultural development of the individuals or groups in question. Moreover, as Outlaw remarked about extending the boundaries of the inquiry, "[I]t became possible at least to work at synthesizing insights drawn from both natural science (genetics, biochemistry) and social science (anthropology, sociology, psychology, ethology) for a fuller understanding of . . . races."[211] These developments highlight the fact that in postmodern, late capitalist, global society, studying groups of persons strictly on the basis of their shared genetic homogeneity has become a scientific anachronism, as evidenced by the fact that the American Association for the Advancement of Science (AAAS) stated clearly at their 1995 conference: "Biologically . . . race is no longer a valid scientific distinction."[212]

Despite scientific racism's tragic World War II outcome resulting in the Jewish Holocaust, new waves of biological determinism based on the misuse of evolutionary biology, ethology,* and race reemerged between the 1960s and 1980s. As Barker notes in "Biology and the New Racism" about the lineage of the movement, "There are strong lines of continuity, both personal and doctrinal, between the ethologists and the prewar eugenicists."[213] One branch of this movement surfaced publicly as a series of facile books applying scientific animal behavior theories directly to humans. Books such as Konrad Lorenz's *On Aggression* (1966), Robert Ardrey's *The Territorial Imperative* (1966), Desmond Morris's *The Naked Ape* (1967), and Lionel Tiger and Robin Fox's *The Imperial Animal* (1970) captured the imaginations of both the lay and scientific communities. What had begun as pre–World War II scientific efforts at understanding animal behavior became a superficial "pop ethology" projection of humanity as aggressive, incorrigible, territorial killers. Because of its superficiality, the scientific influence of this branch of the biological determinist movement waned within a decade.

The other branch of this biological determinist movement had to be taken more seriously. Building on Darwin's landmark study of animal behavior, *The Expression of Emotions in Man and Animals* (1872), exploring how animal and human behavior evolved—complemented by a resurgent IQ testing ideology—a coterie of well-trained biological and behavioral scientists headquartered at prestigious U.S. and European universities launched a new wave of scientific racism. In essence, this movement posited that Linnaeus's and Darwin's well-established acknowledgment that species *Homo sapiens* were animals implied that mankind's

---

Ethology is the study of animal behavior.

specific patterns of behavior and social arrangements were biologically predetermined by their genes. Therefore, the ethology and sociobiological* movements articulate their aims of cultural, national, and ethnic exclusion and discrimination in terms of the concept of *instinct* elaborated in biological and genetic terms. Sociobiologists under the leadership of Harvard entomologist Edward O. Wilson in 1975, building upon the 1940s and 1950s scientific work of men such as Earl Wendel Count and some of the less distasteful work of Konrad Lorenz, intended to "codify sociobiology into a branch of evolutionary biology."[214] Attribution of complex human behaviors such as criminality, homosexuality, and racism to genes purportedly rendered them inevitable, heritable, nonjudgmental, and virtually uncorrectable. Moreover, these theories justified the status quo in the U.S. social order. People were in their present positions because of *natural* evolutionary mechanisms at work.

As Goldberg notes in the *Anatomy of Racism*, "The scientific sophistication that this new racism furnishes has served to modernize the terms of racist exclusion generated by Enlightenment anthropology, nineteenth-century cranial and eugenic measurements, and twentieth-century intelligence testing."[215] However, the new movement founders on flawed methodology characterized by oversimplification and reification inherent in its strict reductionist approach to complex social, educational, and behavioral problems. Ultimately, sociobiologists were unable to prove their elaborate and circuitous hypotheses and theories. Moreover, as Goldberg noted, "[T]hese presumptions are unwarranted in terms of the very Darwinian outlook the new racism claims to represent."[216] This scientifically flawed neo-Darwinian evolutionary outlook, like other predecessor scientific racist schemes, exculpates and perpetuates flawed social hierarchies and racial conflict and discrimination. After much acrimonious scientific debate and scrutiny, sociobiology fell out of scientific favor by the late 1980s. Nevertheless, IQ and "criminal gene" studies continue to be defended by a cadre of scientists. The race and class aspects of these scientific inquiries continue to generate controversy. Hotly debated efforts to "prove" the biological and genetic basis of homosexuality also continue.[217]

Clearly, the dominant sociocultural and scientific definitions and implications of race have changed drastically since the eighteenth century. So much has been done and so much change has occurred, that today's intellectual landscape in health-related areas is totally different. Therefore, an examination of the modern construct of race has been undertaken; what follows is an investigation of the contemporary interface between "race" and U.S. society. The goal is to lend per-

---

Sociobiology is the systematic study of the biological basis of all social behavior. Largely through genetic mechanisms, these biologists and behavioralists offer biological explanations for such human cultural manifestations as aggression, competition, entrepreneurship, criminality, homosexuality, dominance, slavery, territoriality, tribalism, religion, ethics, warfare, genocide, cooperation, conformity, indoctrinability, and spite (this list is incomplete).

spective and understanding to the sometimes incomprehensible racial conundrum of "cultural pluralism," "reverse discrimination," and the racial politics and polarization we face in the U.S. today, and to relate this to racism in medicine and the health delivery system.

Race, Class, Ethnic Politics, and Health Care

> *The country's image of the Negro, which hasn't very much to do with the Negro, has never failed to reflect, with a kind of frightening accuracy, the state of mind of the country.*
>
> JAMES BALDWIN, *THE PRICE OF THE TICKET*

To understand the relationship between the concept of race and the racial inequities and inequalities in health status, health care outcome, and other determinants of the quality of life in the United States, one must understand that this state of affairs is directly linked to the greater problem of race in U.S. and Western society. As far as race is concerned, the Reverend Jesse Jackson often says, "There is a mean mood in America." As the title of this section suggests, race in the United States has recently assumed an amorphous and complicated new form. Terms like "racism" and "discrimination" now have unsure meanings to many people—even African Americans. Racial discrimination no longer has the strong moral and ethical overtones it once had. Anti-racist measures such as anti-discrimination rules designed to protect disadvantaged minority groups such as Blacks and Native Americans, victims of centuries of invidious racial discrimination, are now used to protect Whites. The subjects of race and racism have seemingly become more complicated, but less discussed. Offering Blacks or other disadvantaged ethnic Americans an opportunity to participate in the mainstream of American life through admission of qualified applicants to professional or graduate school is now being viewed by Whites as being socially detrimental. Some citizens, both White and Black, allege that admission of qualified Blacks to professional schools through affirmative action programs is somehow injurious to African Americans. Although scholarly investigations and political events indicate that race remains a hot-button issue, it often lies hidden behind a consolidating veil of irrationality. Many Whites and "the system" itself openly attempt to make race a nonissue, as if overt and covert anti-Black racial discrimination no longer exist in the United States. These signs and symptoms indicate that efforts toward understanding and ameliorating problems caused by race are critically needed.

As the postmodern, late capitalist era advances, it is important to acknowledge that the issue of race has moved into spheres dominated by politics and cultural imagery instead of national morality or ethics reflecting seriously held American creeds and values. Conciliation seems elusive, and hostility levels are rising.

Some principal reasons this transformation in the racial climate has taken place include, but are not limited to, the new psychological profile race has assumed within White America's consciousness in a new and dehumanizing cultural environment. This increasingly prevalent psyche is a by-product of a postindustrial, increasingly technological, manipulative economic state. Through combined effects of the political-economic system, mass media, and cultural traditions, many White Americans have come to look upon racism as no longer being a problem—but a past sin. The U.S. political economy since World War II has allowed most European Americans to relocate to placid and relatively safe suburbs escaping many of the pressing inner-city, socioeconomic status, and urban problems in the process. The mass media, projecting and reinforcing U.S. cultural icons of equal opportunity, rugged individualism, and the classless society, promote the myth of the "American dream" in an increasingly class-bound, race-bound society. Not only are U.S. class problems ignored, but their relationship to racial inequality is also increasingly denied and unappreciated. These phenomena have bred both geographical and psychological isolation between the races. Andrew Hacker's book *Two Nations: Black and White, Separate, Hostile, Unequal* captures the situation both in its title and content. The old cliché "out of sight, out of mind" increasingly applies to America's racial divide.

Behavioral scientists have always contended this modern industrialized market (capitalist) environment breeds bureaucratic inhumanity and exists largely outside the psychological realm. The inability of both Black and White Americans to comprehend the class problems plaguing U.S. society, as they are bombarded with the myth of a classless society, intensifies the economic and social distance between the races. Structural inequalities between races and classes, such as unequal schools, inadequate health care facilities, *de facto* segregation, insufficient environmental and social services, institutionalized economic disparities, and lack of political representation as a result of the transformation of the U.S. economy, are problems social scientists such as William Julius Wilson and Jonathan Kozol have articulated. They are problems with which many White Americans and some members of the new Black middle-class refuse to come to terms.[218]

Other major reasons for the transformation of the U.S. racial state is the historical rearticulation* of race as both scientific and intellectual concepts over the past 60 years. Unexpectedly limited and sometimes unfulfilled promises of the 1960s and 1970s Civil Rights Movement in America have also exacerbated the process. As many of the racial barriers before the 1960s were transformed into institutional and class impediments after legal segregation was outlawed—a response to a Civil Rights Movement largely based on Black middle-class desires instead of structured and enforced public policies—the actual status or treatment of the majority of Blacks did not substantively change. The class-structured limi-

---

Rearticulation is the process of redefinition of political interests and identities through a process of recombination of familiar ideas and values in hitherto unrecognized ways.

tations on correcting economic inequalities in a competitive, capitalist, technical society went unaddressed and thus uncorrected.* Martin Luther King, Jr., and Malcolm X, the two Black leaders who began addressing the core problem of race-based economic inequality, were murdered. Only the small upwardly mobile African American middle-class and a small percentage of poor Blacks benefited from the limited equal opportunity and affirmative action programs, while the status of the Black working class and impoverished majority deteriorated. These contradictory and confusing changes have also been strongly exaggerated by resurgent, but superficial, ethnic and cultural diversity movements.

Sociologists such as Stephen Steinberg reject prevailing views and projections that traditional cultural values and ethnic traits are major determinants of the economic destiny of ethnic and racial groups in America. He views the current emphasis on cultural diversity and ethnic purity as a publicity-oriented diversion avoiding the more fundamental race and class issues that actually determine the economic performance of different racial and ethnic groups in the United States. This is more evidence that the psychological mechanisms of racism have moved away from the dominative forms toward aversive and metaracist models.

While these psychological changes are of pivotal importance, the progressive dehumanization of U.S. society, an environmental phenomenon occurring beyond the limits of psychology, is generating a fertile garden in which American racism flourishes. As Joel Kovel observed about the anti-human environment:

> *The racist sentiment which pervades the life of virtually all white Americans is . . . not the only obstacle to . . . racial justice. Equally important as a general psychological factor is the general apathy and remoteness, the nonspecific coldness that prevails in our time. . . . [W]e do not care for one another; we can be momentarily aroused to compassion, fear, or even rage, but as a rule we soon slip back into the comfortable torpor that typifies our life.[219]*

Cultural dehumanization is not new in the United States. For the racism involved with slavery to work, dehumanization, the psychological transformation of human beings into "things," had to take place. That dehumanization, concentrated on the Black slaves, was more focused. The new form of dehumanization is more diffuse, described as "more rationalized . . . the omnipresent manipulation of taste, thought, style, and wants in the interest of stimulating demand and rationalizing activity . . . with the aim of controlling and maintaining the material productivity of our society."[220] Both subtle and pervasive, other aspects of the new dehumanization process are described as follows:

---

*Neighborhoods, schools, and institutions, remained *de facto* segregated. Blacks continued to experience financial, institutional, and workplace discrimination and remained poor.

> *People experience it, although often unconsciously, as a kind of general falseness, a bogus and synthetic quality that seems to permeate every aspect of life. It is crushing, squeezing and suffocation, a dry, cold force dressed in the guise of good cheer and objectivity; it is the concern of image over substance and for technique over truth, and it exists everywhere — in supermarkets, among politicians, on television shows.*[221]

The generalizability of this mind-numbing, virtual "living lie" environment represented by its increased capacity for dissemination through mass media makes it more dangerous:

> *What we contend with today is cultural falsification: systematized, reasonable, pervasive mendacity, dished up with all the resources of electronic technology and used as a regulator of social activity. It is presented as an objective necessity and seems to be accepted with blind acquiescence. . . . [I]t represents the cutting edge of all the antihuman forces in Western culture.*[222]

Anti-human to the core, in this new environment morals are numbed and aggression and violence proliferate. This helps explain why the limits and the definitions of the arguments on race relative to all aspects of Black life in America, including health care, have become much less "human." Instead, they have become more economically based, technocratic, and sociopolitical in nature, such that even children are being publicly victimized by politicians and policy makers.[223] The utility of the technique of falsification in the interests of consumerism and productivity on the human level is that it automatically creates alienation, increasing remoteness, and distances people from each other. All of these dehumanizing processes facilitate racist processes.[224]

These dehumanizing phenomena, along with the new definitions and construct of race (sociocultural construct), render dominative or aversive forms of racism less necessary in the production of European American class dominance and racially disparate outcomes between African Americans and Whites in the United States. Institutional, economic, and technocratic means mediate the new racism, usually with a deadly efficiency. With the new dominance of the metaracist mechanism — racism carried out through technocratic or economic means in its many guises — it is easier to explain and understand the "disconnect" we are presently experiencing in the health system wherein deep, race-based health disparities in virtually all disease states and health services are downplayed, if not ignored. There is no medical-ethical or medical-social outrage here, even from a legitimate public health perspective — except the largely sublimated rage of African Americans. In lieu of the ongoing systematic and rational scientific dismantling of the biological or genetic explanatory hypotheses for these health differences, there is virtually no appropriate response from any aspect or component of the health system.

Why and how the concept of race was rearticulated in the middle of the twentieth century, along with its contemporary configuration, deserves investigation. The plasticity and shifting of ground undergirding the concept of race generates many mysteries clouding contemporary events and impedes comprehension, and thus communication, across the racial divide. The changes are so rapid that scholars in the field, civil rights leaders, and politicians of all races seem baffled and confused. The public, who confront real race problems daily, seems just as, if not more, confused. Many of the polemics and inconsistencies noted here are rendered clearer and placed in a "presentist" context against the background of the earlier intellectual rearticulation of race as a sociopolitical concept that evolved during the 1930s. Such a historical investigation also serves as a paradigm for analyzing the present rearticulation of race.[225]

The major modern scholarly studies on race in the United States were triggered by the ideological and sociopolitical struggles surrounding the New Deal — the anti-dictatorial, anti-colonial, anti-capitalist, and anti-racial struggles that reached their peaks during the 1930s. In the era between the wars, spurred by the Great Depression, "emancipatory projects" focusing on race, gender, and class broke out across areas of the world dominated by Western culture (e.g., French Indochina, Germany). Many of these emancipatory events had racial overtones or involved Black, Jewish, previously marginalized, or non-White people. Women's suffrage, the early phases of the Russian Revolution, the Weimar Republic, the League of Nations, the Marcus Garvey movement, and the New Deal are examples. However, there were also a series of repressive and fascist events taking place in post-revolutionary Russia, Italy, Germany, Africa, and in Asia and the Pacific Rim. In addition, Europe, especially during periods of economic downturn and destabilization, was inundated by recurrent waves of anti-Semitism. During the 1920s *critical theory** studies, largely triggered by anti-Jewish discrimination and persecution and focusing on racial prejudice and social domination, emanated from social scientists such as Max Horkheimer (1895–1973) and Herbert Marcuse (1898–1979) at the Institute for Social Research in Frankfurt, Germany. Their work laid new groundwork with practical applications for understanding the new social dynamics and definitions of race and its relationship to social domination.

Especially troubling was the mounting evidence that many of the anti-racial, anti-colonial, anti-dictatorial struggles were failing. The rise of totalitarian and fascist regimes in Russia (1917), Italy (1922), Japan (1925), and Germany

---

Critical theory in general is any social theory that is at the same time explanatory, normative, practical, and self-reflexive. It was first developed by Max Horkheimer describing the Frankfurt School's (1923–present) revision of Marxism. It is now applied to a wider critical theoretical approach to areas such as feminism, racism, and liberation philosophy.

(1932) was even more disturbing. So troubling were these failures to some members of the social science community that they sought methods of studying and understanding the social dynamics and mechanisms causing these "freedom" movements to fail. Concern was also mounted initially in Europe, and later in America, about the interaction between race and the authoritarian personality on emancipatory movements in society at large. Was racial prejudice adversely affecting areas such as economics, education, health, and social welfare? A group of German social scientists responded to the challenge. "Critical theory" is the name that Max Horkheimer, an early director of the Institute of Social Research,

> gave to what he projected as the appropriate character and agenda for theoretical work directed at understanding—and contributing to the transformation of—social formations that, in various ways, blocked concrete realizations of increased human freedom.[226]

Thus, critical theory emanated from a 1920s European social scientific institute (also known as the Frankfurt School) founded to critically analyze Marxist socialism and to study anti-Semitism and the rise of fascism. Devising science-based methods, which built upon their original studies, to combat these negative social forces was also envisioned.

After being forced to move to the United States by 1935 due to Hitler's rise to power, the Institute of Social Research's original focus on anti-Semitism became a more diffuse interest in prejudice in general, especially as it related to authority and authoritarianism. Therefore, by the early 1940s with the onset of World War II and the beginning of the Jewish Holocaust, the promise evoked by the early twentieth-century intellectual and socially based "emancipatory projects" of men such as Gunnar Myrdal, Franz Boas, and Ashley Montagu had "foundered on the crucible of 'race,'"[227] according to Outlaw. Based on Hitler's and Mussolini's racial agenda for Jews and U.S. policy regarding people of African descent, W. E. B. Du Bois's prediction that "the problem of the 20th century is the problem of the color line" had come true figuratively and literally. These anti-democratic forces had irretrievably damaged and distorted twentieth-century Western social development and promise to continue to be a dominant factor in twenty-first-century Western cultural life.

As a result of the rekindled interest in the U.S. race problem triggered by the Great Depression, the Carnegie Corporation funded an extensive 1937 study of the U.S. race problem under the supervision of Swedish social scientist Gunnar Myrdal. His project's collaborations with the Institute of Social Research the University of California at Berkeley's Psychology Department, and the American Jewish Committee's Department of Scientific Research resulted in a major transformation in U.S. racial thought. This process also facilitated the transfer of the U.S. race problem into the less emotionally charged, technocratically supervised, political sphere as batteries of specific anti-racial public policy and political reform recommendations were made.

The results of this basic rethinking and the policy recommendations on racial issues crafted by the social and behavioral science communities were artic-ulated and displayed best in the books born of two major racial studies released as World War II ended. We have previously alluded to Myrdal's *An American Dilemma: The Negro Problem and Modern Democracy* (1944). The other was Adorno et al.'s *The Authoritarian Personality* (1950). The ongoing major empiri-cal studies of the bases and dynamics of prejudice on all levels, including the individual, group, institutions, and communities, defined and clarified the psy-chological origins and mechanisms of *social discrimination*. The more Horkheimer studied racial and religious hatreds, the more he believed that scien-tists were "imbued with the conviction that the sincere and systematic scientific elucidation of a phenomenon of such great historical meaning can contribute directly to the amelioration of the cultural atmosphere in which hatred breeds."[228] The dramatic need for research in the fields of racism, fascism, and anti-Semitism in Western culture revealed by World War II and its racial and political consequences—such as the Holocaust and the African American demand for first-class citizenship—were unanticipated at the inception of the major empirical studies of prejudice and racism. By the end of the war promoters of a critical theory on race were joined by the international United Nations move-ment and internationally respected scholars at the United Nations Educational, Scientific and Cultural Organization (UNESCO), who reaffirmed the assump-tion that enlightenment on race would eventually lead to the emancipation of oppressed groups of all kinds. This changed paradigm was viewed by progressive thinkers as a mechanism for fueling emancipation for Blacks and other oppressed groups throughout the world.[229]

Not only were the theoretical frameworks of how race worked in Western soci-ety changing, but historical events such as World War II also countervailed more than three decades of fascism by extending certain branches of the emancipatory process into the 1960s and 1970s. Virtually all agree that the end of World War II largely dismantled the fascist movements, prepared the way for the Civil Rights Era and the liberation of non-White colonial countries in Africa and Asia, and led to the women's liberation and environmental movements in America. These devel-opments altered the way race was viewed in America; thus, it led the way for legal desegregation of U.S. society at large and the health system in particular. For exam-ple, while changing the legal arrangements such as hospital desegregation and overthrowing discriminatory aspects of the Hill-Burton Act,* civil rights reforms had the effect of allowing individuals of color to negotiate both the health system and society differently. Nevertheless, levels of institutional racism have persisted

---

*This was the $1.3 trillion government-funded program lasting from 1946 to 1974 to erect and upgrade the private hospital infrastructure in the Southern United States after World War II. It

such that it negatively affects the majority of African Americans in both the U.S. society at large and the health delivery system.[230]

These persistent, authoritarian, and invidious racialist phenomena have had antithetical effects on the future of liberalizing Western cultural events. Although some incidents laid the groundwork for democratic and anti-dictatorial movements throughout the developing world and Europe, there have been more examples of dictatorships and repressive governmental regimes worldwide following the late 1980s economic collapse of socialist states in Russia and Eastern Europe. The late-1980s fall of the Eastern Bloc after decades of a post–World War II Cold War is part of the positive continuum of the often countervailing emancipatory trends. On the down side, there have been potentially dangerous readings of recurrent failures and compromises surrounding the issues of freedom and race in the United States — and in the free world at large. In the United States this has become especially relevant, as the "New Right," led initially by the presidential administrations of Ronald Reagan and George Bush and presently by the conservative Republican Congress, has taken charge. Buttressed by a fundamentalist Christian political movement, this right wing ideology has become popular enough in the Congress to successfully reframe issues of racial justice and discrimination, often held to be synonymous with civil rights in the United States, away from the high moral ground connected with democratic ideals and the American creed into technocratically dominated political and public policy areas.

This mood has had more than an exclusively domestic impact. Internationally, the World Bank has been allowed to cast the economic progress of the developing world into reverse gear by imposing Draconian economic policies based on the manipulation of the international debt structure. Many impoverished nations are being forced to pay back loans to rich Western nations that grew wealthy while colonizing them in lieu of feeding their starving populations. As these technocratically framed, but hostile, international policies continue, African, Asian, and South American nations, all with long economic histories of colonial exploitation by the United States and Western Europe, may never be allowed to enter the mainstream world economy.

This process has also included detaching race from its historical moorings in the United States and submerging racial debates in the confusion and obscurity created by confounding terminology, disingenuous political and legalistic debates, and mind-numbing euphemisms. Issues directly involving both overt and covert racism are increasingly relegated to areas of discourse such as art, culture, and African studies instead of political science, public or health policy, and economics. A gutting of progressive and functional social programs, such as Head Start and school lunch programs, along with the stripping away of foreign aid

---

promoted government-funded, legally sanctioned, segregated health facilities until legal battles resulted in anti-discrimination provisions in 1964.

accompanied by signs of a numbing new isolationism, are also trends related to and reflecting authoritarianism and intolerance. Although these conceptional and ideological changes originated largely independent of the health delivery system, they have profoundly affected America's health institutions and the environment in which health policy is framed in this country.[231]

During this decades-long multifactorial process of reframing racism into predominantly political and cultural diversity issues — divesting it of its serious societal implications, ethical overtones, psychological mediations, and historical memory for the general public — in intellectual circles race itself has also become reconceptualized, in part, as "ethnicity." *Ethnicity* is a concept extending the view that differences in people are a function of sociology and culture rather than biology. Michael Banton, a specialist in race relations, noted the retreat of racial arguments from the parapet of biology in *The Idea of Race:*

> *In a matter of years, Western culture has come a long way from propagating racism as a doctrine that a man's behavior is determined by stable inherited characteristics deriving from separate racial stocks having distinct attributes and usually considered to stand to one another in relations of superiority and inferiority.*[232]

Reasons as to why eighteenth- and nineteenth-century biological concepts of race receded as the major scientific focus and influence in racial thought have been discussed. New racial theorists from fields as varied as evolutionary biology and the behavioral sciences had facilitated such conclusions by drastically shifting racial assumptions, arguments, and basic definitions. Investigators and scientific opinion leaders in group relations and social dynamics such as Ashley Montagu and Daniel Levinson had already homogenized the old concept of prejudice directed at racial groups into a new and expanded version of Robert Park's "ethnocentrism":

> *Prejudice is commonly regarded as a feeling of dislike against a specific group; ethnocentrism refers to a relatively consistent frame of mind concerning "aliens" generally. . . . [E]thnocentrism refers to group relations generally; it had to do not only with numerous groups toward which the individual has hostile opinions and attitudes but, equally important, with groups toward which he is positively disposed. A theory of ethnocentrism offers a starting point for the understanding of the psychological aspect of group relations.* [emphasis in original][233]

Informed by the past abuses the term *race* had experienced, many investigators, such as Julian Huxley, Ashley Montagu, and the committee formulating the UNESCO Statement on Race (1950), suggested the term was no longer valid. Although it was suggested that the term *race* was no longer legitimate, other translations, or versions, of the term continue to affect attitudes toward certain groups in society at large and in the health delivery system. Institute of Social Research investigator Daniel Levinson, seeking greater understanding of the modern psychosocial dynamic of racism, realized that *ethnocentrism* was a larger gathering concept for the more diffuse and subtle racist phenomena they were observing in their studies. This further justified the shift from *race* to *ethnic group*, when referring to the various groups of people being studied. As Levinson explained:

> [A]*part from the arbitrariness of the organic basis of classification, the greatest dangers of the race concept lie in its hereditarian psychological implications and in its misapplication to cultures. Psychologically, the race theory implies, whether or not this is always made explicit, that people of a given race (e.g., skin color) are also very similar psychologically because they have a common hereditary family tree. . . . [F]urthermore, the term race is often applied to groups which are not races at all in the technical sense. . . . [T]here is no adequate term, other than "ethnic," by which to describe cultures (that is, systems of social ways, institutions, traditions, language, and so forth) which are not nations. . . . [F]rom the point of view of sociology, cultural anthropology, and social psychology, the important concepts are not race and heredity but social forms and individual personalities. To the extent that relative uniformities in psychological characteristics are found within any cultural grouping, these uniformities must be explained primarily in terms of social organization rather than "racial heredity."*[234]

Well into the late capitalist-postmodern era an assimilationist school of progressive thinkers predicted that the socially divisive aspects of ethnicity would disappear in a social-cultural "melting pot" of ethnic assimilation. Although these new categories were both useful and appropriate for analytic purposes, the expected "smooth sailing" on the racial front did not occur. More recent investigators such as Steinberg, Outlaw, Hacker, Kovel, Simone, Farley and Allen, Zweigenhaft and Domhoff, Massey and Denton, and Feagin and Spikes have added caveats to this optimistic prediction. Their reservation is that as far as the African American experience is concerned, race remains a separate and overarching concept relative to class,* language, culture, or other variables. This postmodern-late capitalist reconceptualization rooted in the recent racial realities moves far beyond the now classical and narrow 1960s and 1970s Black Nationalist defense of race being more important than *class* in understanding "the Negro question." As Steinberg noted, relating race to the experiences of other immigrant and ethnic groups in the United States:

---

*Hereafter the simplified notion of class will be used: the socioeconomic, material, and cultural conditions in which people live.

Although the prejudice against immigrants was greater than is gener-
ally realized, it still was not as virulent, as pervasive, or as enduring as
that experienced by racial minorities; nor was it given official sanction.
But the qualitative differences are even more important. Immigrants
were disparaged for their cultural peculiarities, and the implied mean-
ing was, "You will become like us whether you want to or not." When it
came to racial minorities, however, the unspoken dictum was, "No mat-
ter how much like us you are, you will remain apart." Thus, at the same
time the nation pursued a policy aimed at the rapid assimilation of
recent arrivals from Europe, it segregated the racial minorities who, by
virtue of their much longer history in American society, had already
come to share much of the dominant culture.[235]

The "forever remaining apart" phenomenon is playing itself out in the 1980s, 1990s, and early twenty-first century as evidenced by recently transplanted Asians surpassing Blacks economically and educationally in the United States. This continues to happen despite survey research evidence that continues to reaffirm Myrdal's finding that African American attitudes and values are more "American" than virtually any of the later-arriving ethnic groups. It is especially disturbing and also has many parallels in the health system: Other ethnic American groups—many of whom are recent immigrants to this country—already experience superior health indicators compared to African Americans. Nevertheless, despite the ominous directions of race in the United States, the perceived force of the race issue on postmodern U.S. society has been vitiated in normal discourse and, therefore, is consistently underestimated. This may explain why some investigators who had predicted the U.S. system's potential and predisposing affinity for accepting a fascist system of social control found such a development to be unnecessary by the mid-1980s. There was no organized liberal-progressive left wing to be controlled or conquered, and the race issue has been "buried alive." Thus, reactions to social inequities such as the inequalities and invidious racial discrimination in the health system were never made important health policy issues; in fact, they were hardly acknowledged or discussed. All of these internally pacified, metaracist developments are relevant as one views the most recent sociopolitical construction of race in the United States and its effects on the health system.[236]

The reservations about the purely ethnic analysis applied to race have proved to be important. After observing that the projections by some scholars that the socially divisive aspects of ethnicity would disappear in a social-cultural melting pot of ethnic assimilation did not occur, especially with the physically identifiable non-European ethnic groups, a more conservative pluralistic school turned the concept on its head. They described and encouraged the maintenance of ethnic identity as a liberating mechanism—which it clearly has not turned out to be.

This turned into an example of the metaracist flexibility to invert a potentially racist phenomenon into a so-called "anti-racist device." As was clear from the U.S. experience, the realities and result of cultural pluralism and maintenance of ethnic identity often had cross-cutting and conflicting results if the protagonists were non-White or racially identifiable:

> In actuality, the native cultures of Indians and blacks were ruthlessly stamped out, though paradoxically, the extreme segregation of these groups allowed for an evolution of distinctive ethnic sub-cultures built upon vestiges of their original cultures. In comparison immigrant minorities had greater freedom to promote their special identities, which they did in the communities that developed around ethnic populations. Nevertheless, given their position at or near the bottom of the class system, and dependent economically on the surrounding society, immigrants were compelled to relinquish much of their European heritage in order to achieve their aspiration of social and economic mobility. . . . [I]n short, American society provided only a weak structural basis for ethnic preservation.[237]

Since resegregation was occurring anyway as a result of this new wave of cultural pluralism, conservative theoreticians, within the framework of metaracism, disingenuously adjusted their theories to fit the new circumstance. However, it was clear that *ethnic pluralism* and *cultural diversity* taken to extremes could be a double-edged sword. Therefore, ethnic pluralism, racial pride, and, some would contend, cultural pluralism, with their "Balkanizing" tendencies, had the potential to rip the American social fabric apart.

One disingenuous strategy put forward to prevent this from happening was restricting their application to "private" matters. Reassurances were provided alleging that any wide-ranging adverse social consequences of this movement toward ethnic pluralism, or cultural diversity, would be modulated by sacredly held principles of the American creed and the emerging body politic based on *radical individualism*. Individuals in society would advance "without regard to race, creed, color, or national origin" based on demonstrated achievement and merit. In lieu of covert and overt racial discrimination in employment, education, housing, economic development, and social interaction, the system would be forced into the false mold of a "colorblind society."

Some European Americans, believing they were not being promoted rapidly enough because of the few Blacks or Hispanics hired, alleged that they were victims of racial discrimination—thus, *reverse discrimination*. This is another working example of metaracism, wherein an anti-racist measure is inverted and utilized for racist purposes. Not only is a racist outcome obscured, but the inverted mechanism is also legitimized in the process.[238]

Anyone questioning these basic principles of the body politic in America during the postmodern period has been politically and intellectually marginalized. This paradigm has largely served the political agenda of the New Right as a cover for the sometimes explicit, but always programmatic, domination of African American and other disadvantaged peoples. Systematic inattention to the dramatic and history-based health needs of the African American population has been one of the results. The 1978 Allan Bakke case, whereby a European American won a Supreme Court case alleging he had been discriminated against on the basis of race because Blacks had been admitted to medical school, is one of the landmark reverse discrimination cases. This major case emanating from the University of California at Davis turned back the clock on disadvantaged minority participation in the cognitive professions. As a result of this decision, many affirmative action mechanisms for admitting qualified Blacks to medical school were attenuated or ended. The direct effects on the U.S. medical profession may perpetuate a historical tradition. African Americans constituted 2.6 percent of the U.S. medical profession in 1910 when they constituted approximately 10 percent of the population; in 1995 they represented between 2.8 and 3.4 percent of the medical profession when they constituted nearly 13 percent of the U.S. population.[239] (See Table 1.3.) It is significant that the health system, relative to the Bakke case, was in the vanguard of the racial retrenchment away from justice and equity taking place in American society.[240]

The question is whether the political agenda that evolved around race, as a result of the tumultuous and sometimes violent protests of the early 1960s and urban riots and uprisings of the late 1960s and 1970s Civil Rights Movement, has achieved racial justice. The African American population seemed placated after the Civil Rights Era by the enactment of liberal and anti-racist policies in the wake of the 1964 Civil Rights Act, Voting Rights Acts and programs, and Housing and Employment Acts. The right to vote, something other Americans achieved as a birthright, and legal access to public accommodations did virtually nothing to correct race- and class-based economic inequalities. Contingent on an assumption of continued U.S. economic growth, these policies were to create "an epoch in which 'race' as such was to be obliterated as a mark of distinction, black and white together becoming increasingly absorbed in a gray, consumerist society watched over by a technocratic state projecting its violence outward, through nuclear weapons if necessary."[241] This would deflect, and largely divert, the White psychological energy generated toward the "Others" outward, instead of directly onto Black and other identifiable minority groups. With all of these contradictory and negative events clouding the U.S. racial picture as we enter the twenty-first century, close scrutiny of the result of the 1960s civil rights emancipatory effort is warranted.

Table 1.3   African American Physician Numerical Estimates

African American Physician Numerical Estimates
Table. Total, Number, Percentages African American Physicians, 1990

	Total Physicians	Black Physicians	Percent Black Physicians
U.S. Census Data	562 350	21 538	3.8%
G King, R Bendel study	562 350	16 282	2.8%
JS Todd/AMA	562 350	19 000	3.4%

In response to census data inaccuracies, the King-Bendel study documented a lower number of African American physicians than had been previously projected. The AMA concurs with the overestimation, submitting a compromise figure on the true numbers.

Sources:
U.S. Bureau of Census
The AMA Physician Masterfile
National Medical Association Masterfile of Black Physicians (NMAMBP)

Cited References:
Adapted from reference 33 and US Department of Health and Human Services. Bureau of *Health Professions Factbook—Health Personnel United States, Detailed Occupation and Years of School Completed by Age for the Civilian Labor Force by Sex, Race, and Spanish Origin: 1980.* Supplementary Report PC80-51-8. Population data derived from US Bureau of the Census Public Information Office Release CB91-100 and US Bureau of the Census Current Population Reports Special Studies Series P-23 No. 80.
King G, Bendel R. A statistical model estimating the number of African American physicians in the United States. *J Natl Med Assoc* 1995; 87:264-272.
Todd JS. Letters to the editor: African American physicians. *J Natl Med Assoc* 1996; 88:69.

Evaluative Benchmarks of Black Progress

Evaluative benchmarks that would indicate whether the goal of the colorblind society virtually everyone espouses and reifies has been—or is being—achieved are not encouraging. They include, but are not limited to:

- The economic gap between Blacks and Whites—according to the new cadre of social scientists, this major indicator of racial injustice and discrimination is wider than ever.
- Major improvements toward Black/White equalization in health and quality of life indicators have failed to take place, and in many areas Blacks are worse off than they were a few decades ago.
- Black/White race relations seem to be deteriorating and indicators are that complex new factors are thwarting the

nation's initial efforts at racial desegregation and equal opportunity for all racial and ethnic groups—this, accompanied by a rightward drift of the political apparatus since the 1980s, predicts a guarded future for African Americans.

- Hard-won Black political gains, especially as a function of municipal governments and the Congressional Black Caucus, are not yielding the expected positive results and are presently under assault.[242]

The first, and probably most important, major evaluative benchmark measuring social equity in postmodern–late capitalist America is economic status. As Kovel states in *White Racism:* "The most striking indication that a profoundly racist structure continues in America is the level of economic inequality between whites and blacks."[243] Confirming this impression is David H. Swinton, a Harvard-trained economist and expert on African Americans in the U.S. economic system, who said in 1993:

> *The past 12 years have been a period of no progress towards achieving the long-sought-after goal of economic parity for African Americans. To be sure, some African Americans have advanced. However, the central tendency for the group as a whole has been stagnation or retrogression in absolute status and increased disparities in relative status.*[244]

Blacks, since they began receiving wages following emancipation in the United States, have always received less in wages than Whites in both relative and absolute terms. Recent experience predicts little change in that status. This becomes especially important in a market-driven, for-profit-dominated, capitalist health delivery system—the delivery mechanism the political representatives of the American majority continue to endorse. Based on recent and projected future experience, employment status and income levels have, and will continue to have, a tremendous impact on the ability to gain access to comprehensive health services in the United States. As long as insurance principles, especially experience rating,* guide the U.S. health system, Black and poor people will be at a disadvantage (they are both sicker and poorer). Health care will continue to be distributed based on class considerations and the ability to pay rather than on medical needs.

Between 1940 and 1970 the income between Blacks and Whites converged, as indicated by the fact that the median income of Black men as a percentage of that of Whites increased from 41 percent in 1939 to 58 percent in 1969. However,

---

*Individuals or groups are charged insurance premiums proportional to their expected level of utilization.

since the mid-1970s the income of Black men has fallen faster than that of White men, leading to larger racial differences. This divergent trend in incomes has increased since the 1980s. For Black women the income results have been mixed, with some indications of their incomes reaching parity with White women by 1970. However, as White women entered the labor market in increasing numbers, often demanding wages and promotions equal to those of White males, the pay gap between White and Black women has again increased in recent years.

Racial comparisons of family incomes have not fared any better. Between 1970 and 1990, the Black family income, in constant dollars, hardly changed, going from $21,151 to $21,423; White family income rose from $34,481 to $36,915, an increase of 7.05 percent. Translating this to relative terms, Black incomes dropped from $613 to $580 for each $1,000 received by Whites. Although there was a 46 percent increase in the proportion of Black households with incomes over $50,000 between 1970 and 1990 compared to a 35 percent rise for Whites, indicating a measurable increase in the Black middle class, the true wealth differentials remained alarmingly disparate. Middle-class White families have household assets at least 11 times those of Black families, depending on how it is calculated, a difference that is much larger than that reflected by income. As Edward N. Wolff noted in *Top Heavy: A Study of the Increasing Inequality of Wealth in America*, a 1995 Twentieth Century Fund Report: "In 1983, the median white family had eleven times the wealth of the median non-white family. By 1989 this ratio had grown to twenty."[245] Whites also hold more professional degrees, are employed overwhelmingly in the private sector, and can more often derive the social benefits from mothers being at home with children because of sufficient income of single wage earners. As Ellis Cose noted in a 1999 *Newsweek* report, though there were slight improvements in education, health, and economics fueled by the booming economy: "blacks remain a race apart in America."[246]

The racial employment picture is even more alarming. Recent Black unemployment data are daunting. Since access to health care in the United States is for the most part directly related to employment status, this has profound implications for the nation's most unemployed, poorest, and sickest population. Black unemployment, another major economic indicator, has remained at double-digit levels since 1974, reaching almost 20 percent in 1983. It has remained in double digits,* at more than twice the White rate, since 1976, with the Black/White gap increasing throughout the 1980s. As Reynolds Farley and Walter Allen pointed out about the lack of racial convergence in employment since the post–World War II era:

> In some important manner, the increasing educational attainment
> of blacks, the more liberal racial attitudes of whites, and civil rights

---

*The Black unemployment rate in 1995 was 10.4 percent compared to 4.9 percent for Whites, according to the U.S. Bureau of Labor Statistics.

legislation have failed to narrow the significant gaps in employment and unemployment. Indeed, the evidence . . . convincingly demonstrates that racial disparities in employment are growing larger among young women and among men at all ages except the oldest. If present trends continue, blacks will fall further behind whites in terms of employment.[247]

Regarding economic status in the 1990s, Swinton states: "In terms of relative inequality, that is, the position of African-Americans in comparison to the position of white Americans, the degree of inequality increased somewhat since the 1980s. Blacks have lost ground."[248] The maintenance of economic inequality has emerged as one of the principle mediators of postmodern–late capitalist racism.

Assessment of the characteristics of the Black middle class reveals its fragility. These include, but are not limited to:

- Most Black families classified as middle class are based on both parents working.
- Black middle-class families are heavily employed in the public rather than private sector.
- Middle-class Blacks do not have levels of training or credentials equivalent to their White counterparts.
- Middle-class Blacks have a net worth one-third or less of White middle-class families.
- Black middle-class members, including college graduates, are less likely to be employed, have much higher risks of being laid off, and are fired much more often than their White counterparts.

The economic and social progress represented by the highly touted, but fragile, Black middle class has not grown to more than 20 to 31 percent, depending upon criteria and the sources utilized, of the African American population. In lieu of these limited gains, this progress has been offset by substantial growth of the Black economically disadvantaged. Since the lion's share of the new Black middle class is employed by governmental and public agencies, which are in the midst of Draconian cutbacks by "less government" zealots, maintaining these levels of middle-class incomes seems unlikely.

These economic forces have also divided Black America, creating "a more prosperous stratum whose fortunes become increasingly identified with the white population, and a growing mass of paupers, increasingly defined as useless and without stake in the future of their society,"[249] as Kovel observed. Economic and geographic divisions vitiate African American communities politically and socioculturally just as they do for other groups. Potential political power is fragmented, and further deterioration is encouraged because of the absence of a middle-class base.

Moreover, the liberal and progressive focus on Great Society, anti-discrimination, and affirmative action programs has failed to relate the economic fate of poor minorities to the dramatic changes and functionings of the postmodern–late capitalist U.S. economy. Since 1970, William Julius Wilson observes that this "has resulted in sharp increases in joblessness, poverty, female-headed families, and welfare dependency"[250] in inner-city minority neighborhoods. This has allowed conservative forces to disingenuously focus on the "culture of poverty" and "underclass" formation as explanations instead of the political economy for what has been a series of reactive rather than proactive social phenomena in the nation's racially segregated inner cities. Most of these behaviors are natural and expected results of inferior educational and training opportunities, living in dangerous and crime-ridden environments, and the paucity of good jobs. This public policy failure to achieve economic equity between the races and classes predicts dire consequences in a market-based health care system. If high incomes and costly insurance plans are necessary to access the best the U.S. health system has to offer, the prognosis of America's sickest and poorest populations appears grim. If the public funding and policy necessary to restructure the health system's structure and financing are undercut, poor health outcome for Black and other disadvantaged groups is preordained.[251]

Another major evaluative indicator that the racially disparate order in the United States remains intact and weighted against African Americans is that major improvements toward equalization in health and other quality-of-life indicators between the Black and White populations have failed to take place. Some of these indicators have deteriorated over recent years. As in the past, over the last three decades Blacks in the United States have not developed the power to influence or affect public health policy or public policy in general. Virtually none of the "gold standards" measuring the quality of life and the health of the Black and White populations are the same. The stagnant or retrogressing indicators include mortality, longevity, and infant mortality figures along with demographic and economic indicators.[252] Black life expectancy, in contrast to the rest of the U.S. population (the United States only ranks 23rd overall in longevity as of 1995), has not improved since 1984. In fact, between 1984 and 1989 Black life expectancy actually declined for both sexes for the first time in this century and was projected to return to 1984 levels by 1994 (official figures are always three years behind). By 1996 there was a 6.6 year Black/White disparity in life expectancy—5 percent more than the 1980 figure (6.3 years). The National Center for Health Statistics projected that Black male life expectancy would continue its decline until the year 2000.[253] (See Table 1.4.) The major factors causing this racial divergence in life span as of 1996 are cardiac disease and cancer. These illnesses, accounting for 55 percent of all deaths, are improving for all other segments of the population largely due to improved medical interventions and treatments. Unfortunately, African Americans displayed stable or widening racial disparities according to age-adjusted death rates for both illnesses, demonstrating that on a relative basis Blacks are not benefiting (in some instances, actually falling farther behind) from mainstream health improvements. Simultaneously, Black mortality rates remain 1.5 times higher than White rates. African American infant mortality rates remain at least two times the White rates, while Black maternal death rates are three to four times as high as White rates. Blacks are differentially and adversely impacted by HIV infection and deaths and experience homicide rates and deaths due to violence at rates many times higher than Whites. The most distressing fact is that one could assess hundreds of health status, outcome, and utilization measures having nothing to do with AIDS, violence, or drug abuse and could document racial disparities of the same magnitude. Moreover, this is a nearly four-centuries-old continuum.

Nevertheless, as the authors of this book and other public health investigators such as M. Alfred Haynes, William Darity, and D. S. Greenberg have noted repeatedly, specific measures to improve Black health do not rank high on the nation's public policy or health policy agendas. Moreover, the health toll imposed on Blacks by the brutal consequences of their relationship with the economic system based on their differential unemployment status is immense. This is especially relevant when the *New York Times* reported about the health/employment relationship in the United States that "each one per cent rise in the unemployment rate is accompanied by a 2% increase in the mortality rate, a 5–6% increase in homicides, a 5% increase in imprisonment, a 3–4% increase in first admissions to mental hospitals, and about a 5% increase in infant mortality."[254]

The toll such grim economic, health, and environmental factors takes on families is immense. African American families are no exception. Joblessness and poverty contribute to the increased incidence of crime. These are well-known sociological principles. Well-crafted and fact-based arguments utilizing these

Table 1.4 Male Life Expectancy, According to Race

Year	Male Life Expectancy (Age at Death)	
	Black	White
1970	60.0	68.0
1980	63.8	70.7
1990	64.5	67.7
1995	66.6	73.4
2000	66.5	73.9

Although there have been some improvements since 1970, with a decline between 1984 (65.3) and 1990 (64.5), the National Center for Health Statistics projects Black male life expectancy to decline again by the year 2000.

Source: National Center for Health Statistics

principles augmented by statistical databases by social scientists such as William Julius Wilson and Andrew Hacker have more weight than the forceful, and sometimes well-intended, arguments by conservative scholars that attribute these problems to the social values of a ghetto underclass. Most of the analyses of Black crime, joblessness, and illegitimacy, both liberal and conservative, are oversimplifications failing to grasp the complexities and realities of inner-city, urban existence in the contemporary United States. Nevertheless, pursuit of the underlying causes of these inner-city social dislocations and the dangerous and pathological environments created thereby should not be deflected. Wilson and others allege that they are largely reflections, and indeed products, of fundamental changes in the nation's economy. As Nicholas Lemann notes in *The Promised Land: The Great Black Migration and How It Changed America*, they also mirror a generation of failed public policies relative to major areas of U.S. life such as employment, economic development, housing, welfare, public health and health care, and public education. Lemann contends the American political and public policy systems failed to address or correct the changes wrought by the great Black migration from the rural South to the cities. This, and not flaws inherent in the people themselves, has led to central city deterioration and the growth of a permanent, dependent, socioeconomically disadvantaged class. Due to these circumstances and shortfalls, individuals and families caught in the midst of urban inner-city life have often succumbed to circumstances that have perpetuated their own degraded status. Columbia sociologist Herbert Gans refers to many of these behaviors as *poverty-related* effects in his recent book, *The War Against the Poor: The Underclass and Antipoverty Policy*. Current figures measuring some of the effects are staggering: Almost two-thirds of Black children are born out of wedlock; more than one-half of Black families are headed by women; in over half of these households the women have never been married; and among African American women in their mid- to late-30s, less than one-half have intact marriages. Inner-city neighborhoods have become toxic crime- and drug-ridden danger zones. Since 1950, violence, crime, and drug abuse have become epidemic in urban Black neighborhoods. Moreover, this has been exacerbated by the fact that they are differentially utilized as sites for toxic wastes such as lead, mercury, arsenic, and steroids—known carcinogens and toxins with known harmful effects on childhood mental development. Exact relationships between these toxic and poisoned environments on Black health and behavioral problems are unclear. Although partially responsible for, and victim to, the overall crisis in Black America, African Americans do not presently possess the economic or political power within their own communities to prevent such exploitation of their communities or reverse all of these trends and benchmarks of social disorganization and racial injustice without outside help.[255]

Adam Walinsky cited a study on Black men in the District of Columbia, ages 18–34, in *The Atlantic Monthly*. The findings were as follows:

> *On any given day in 1991, 15 percent of the men were in prison, 21 per-*
> *cent were on probation or parole, and six percent were being sought by*
> *the police or were on bond awaiting trial. The total ... involved with*
> *the criminal-justice system was 42 percent. . . . 70 percent of black men*
> *in the District of Columbia would be arrested before the age of thirty-*
> *five. . . . 85 percent would be arrested at some point in their lives.*[256]

This distressing situation is also reflected in U.S. prison statistics. Between 1970 and 1986 the Black prison population increased from 35.8% to 45.3% of the total. By 1992 Blacks made up 51% of the U.S. prison population. It is well known that prison populations do not receive high-quality health care services. This country compares only with South Africa and the former USSR when it comes to crime and incarceration rates. The United States, with more than 1.8 million people behind bars, now "imprisons more people than any other country in the world — perhaps half a million more than Communist China."[257] California holds more inmates in its jails and prisons than France, Great Britain, Germany, Japan, Singapore, and the Netherlands combined. As one scholar stated about the deteriorating African American condition relative to crime and environment:

> *[I]t indicates the real object of contemporary racism: the workless black*
> *underclass, created by structural economic injustice, cut off from their*
> *bourgeoisiefied fellows, and set adrift among family disorganization,*
> *wretched educational opportunities, dwindling public services of all*
> *kinds and decaying urban enclaves. That these circumstances would lead*
> *to a marked rise in criminalization is inevitable. . . . [T]his becomes the*
> *signifier of their role in the racist order . . . [A]bout a third of the black*
> *population are becoming not simply invisible, but outlawed.*[258]

The reaction to the fundamental changes in the modern industrial American economy is the bifurcation of the labor force into highly technical, information-based, economically renumerative employment and low-skilled, minimum wage, service employment. The old blue-collar, urban workforce Blacks depended upon in the past has been either dismantled, transferred to the suburbs, or moved overseas. Corporate America has determined that low-skill jobs can be more cheaply performed overseas in underdeveloped countries. Neither the complex racial nor class dimensions of these phenomena are being addressed. Therefore, the excess uneducated and undereducated are banished to the work force trash heap. African Americans trapped in inner-city enclaves of poor education, virtually no job training, and pathological welfare-based subcultures are disproportionate victims of this political economy dynamic. Instead of full-employment, inner-city economic development, childcare, and job training, the most prominent public policy solutions have recently turned to victim blaming and incarceration. The overwhelming majority of these political and policy decisions are made by privileged White males. Institutions such as banks, real estate agencies, public and private schools, the health system, and the criminal justice system, which were originally structured on the basis of race and class, continue to function basically as they always have. Institutional discrimination goes unquestioned and largely unaddressed. The adverse quality-of-life health effects of these threatening economic and social environments and developments are exacerbated by the collapsing inner-city health infrastructures many African Americans depend upon, such as city hospitals, community health centers, and public clinics. They are either being closed or fiscally starved.[259]

More than 40 years after the *Brown v. Board of Education* public school desegregation ruling by the Supreme Court and 30 years after passage of the Civil Rights Act, the state of affairs of Black/White race relations is not favorable. Evidence of this abounds based on Black/White survey and opinion poll results, the largely ineffective results of the 1960s desegregation efforts (e.g., in housing, public schools, private sector workplace), and the right-wing takeover of the political apparatus since the 1980s. The stubborn persistence, if not worsening, of the race-based health status and outcome disparities are but one piece of the puzzle. Virtually everyone agrees that the signs of improved race relations—the outlawing of legal segregation of public accommodations; *de jure* desegregation of public schools; and rules and programs outlawing discrimination in the workplace, in housing, or on the training site—are superficial. All were projected as being good for the country. Many factors, however, have been effective in maintaining segregation, White racial privilege, and European American economic dominance. They include:

- Resistance of the European American population to racial equality and integration through White flight to the suburbs, maintaining residential segregation
- Erection of alternative private education systems while continuing to dominate and restructure public education
- Defunding and abandonment of the public health care sector while expanding the power and influence of the private health sector
- Manipulation of the mass media to perpetuate a consumer-oriented, myth-producing (the American dream, land of opportunity, etc.), conservative society
- Concession and surrender of political and public accommodations rights to African Americans that cost the system nothing while maintaining a stranglehold on the U.S. political economy
- The resurrection of a strong political right wing through conservative political action committees (PACs), think tanks, and the Republican party

- Political and legal activism through administrative, electoral, and legal maneuvers favoring maintenance of the racial hierarchy

For one-fourth of African Americans, economic, educational, and social progress has been considerable, even though it has failed to meet Black middle-class expectations. Although middle-income Blacks are able to educate their children to levels almost equivalent to well-to-do Whites, they are not thriving equitably on economic, professional, or social levels. Their concerns, articulated by social critics and social scientists such as West, Cose, Pinkney, Swinton, Feagin and Spikes, and Massey and Denton, indicate that much of the racial progress is less than profound and probably results more from lower levels of White repression and withdrawal of interest than from fundamental change.

Thus, there is a state of racial "quiet" rather than racial "peace." The dichotomy in racial opinion became prominent by 1980 when a Gallup poll showed that 68% of Whites felt that Blacks now had equal standing and 75% held that there had been steady improvement in the quality of life for African Americans. However, only 44% of Blacks felt their lives had improved and 25% believed they were worse off than 10 years earlier. This divergence in opinion has not changed. Louis Harris and National Opinion Research Center surveys performed during the late 1980s, not to mention news media surveys in the 1990s, have continued to display stark contrasts between rosy images of race relations painted by White Americans and the disillusionment based on reality among Blacks. As Kovel said, "Such a radical gap in perception suggests that the racist structure of American society persists, and that the 'ease and pleasantness' of racial relations is more a matter of superficiality than of a real harmonization."[260] Moreover, a post–Los Angeles riot survey conducted by UCLA's Center for the Study of Urban Poverty in 1992 shockingly revealed that Blacks with household incomes over $50,000 felt more alienated from American society than any subgroup in their sample. This alarming Black middle-class alienation is no isolated incident. It reflects their increasing perception that the present "quiet" hovering over U.S. race relations does not represent true peace—representing form rather than substance, rhetoric rather than reality. However, the short recapitulation of some post–Civil Rights Era indicators that have helped shape the racial profile of postmodern–late capitalist America makes the emergence of these attitudes understandable.[261]

Soon after the Civil Rights Movement achieved its greatest successes, including the outlawing of public school discrimination, passage of the 1964 Civil Rights Act, passage of the Voting Rights Act, and a variety of equal opportunity programs in employment, housing, and education, it was systematically attacked by conservative, sometimes racist, Whites. Resistance to social change such as that embodied in the Civil Rights Movement could have been expected from conservatives, who since the days of Edmund Burke have tended to uphold hierarchies, defend social distinctions, and perpetuate inequalities in the name of stability. As Anthony

O'Hear states, "The conservative tendency will always be to defend the tolerable and even the tolerably bad against what he fears will be immeasurably worse."[262] For most conservative Whites in the United States, segregation and discrimination based on race, the status quo for nearly four centuries, meet these criteria. The conservative approach to political and social questions as outlined by Burke, and containing lines of thought dating back to Hobbes and Aristotle, is empirical rather than rationalistic, cautiously skeptical rather than dogmatic, and often seeks to preserve the status quo. Conservatism advises against wholesale revolution or the overthrow of existing institutions, as many of the civil rights changes such as *Brown vs. Board of Education*, federal court decisions, and new civil rights laws and programs were viewed. Much of this activity is interpreted as undermining the decentralization, pluralism, and maximum amounts of individual and social autonomy so loved by conservatives. Thus, many conservatives were often placed in the midst of overt racists with both groups openly resisting desegregation and, often, equal opportunity laws and programs. A review of a few examples of these attacks follows:

- The South systematically, and more or less successfully, resisted court ordered integration of public schools for more than 20 years after the 1954 Supreme Court desegregation ruling.
- Civil Rights Enforcement Chief Leon Panetta was fired by President Richard Nixon at the beginning of Nixon's second term—one alleged reason being overvigorous enforcement of civil rights laws.
- Government-sponsored attacks on court-ordered busing to end school desegregation was led by the Department of Justice under several attorneys general, including John Mitchell and Assistant Attorney General for Civil Rights William Bradford Reynolds.
- After the courts forced Southern schools to accommodate somewhat to integration laws, communities over the entire nation, led by Boston, illegally resisted court-ordered busing for public school desegregation by local interposition, nullification, community campaigns, and the opening of "segregationist academies."
- President Reagan declared open war on affirmative action, including open attacks on Executive Order 11246* and government-sponsored social welfare programs that differentially benefited disadvantaged minorities and women.

---

*This was the executive order issued by President Lyndon Johnson on September 24, 1965, ordering affirmative action programs based on race in areas like employment and education to be implemented by the Department of Labor. Gender would be added later due to pressure by feminist lobby groups.

- The Rehnquist Court struck down minority set-aside plans and restricted the reach of anti-discrimination laws through rulings handed down in 1989.
- Despite the reservations of many in the African American community (and with the support of others), Clarence Thomas replaced Justice Thurgood Marshall as the only African American on the U.S. Supreme Court in October, 1991, and has since voted against cases positively affecting African American interests virtually 100% of the time.[263]
- A strong national movement to end affirmative action is gaining momentum and was being articulated and politicized by ex–California Governor Pete Wilson, who led in dismantling much of that state's affirmative action programs since 1995.

Events such as these explain why much of the civil rights effort is viewed as having failed in many ways by many African Americans—even those constituting the much-publicized middle class. Other reasons for these attitudes include, but are not limited to, the fact that 40 years after the Supreme Court outlawed segregated schools, most Black children continue to attend one-race schools; as the United States dismantles its public school system, educationally many Blacks are worse off today than they were three decades ago; the Black/White economic gap has not only persisted, but has in many instances intensified; the civil rights promise of Black equality of opportunity has benefited a small middle-class Black minority who were positioned to capitalize on the complex education- and training-based opportunities; and newfound Black political power has not translated into improved well-being for the majority of the African American community.

These disappointments and perceived "broken promises" also affected the "health care–civil rights movement" that started in the 1960s. African Americans, the only group forced to view health care as a civil rights issue, made significant advancements during the Civil Rights Era. Although health care attracted little attention at the time, the promise of future health care advances seemed brighter with the community health center movement, passage of Titles XVIII and XIX, and hospital desegregation rulings in the courts. Hospitals and health facilities were *de jure* and *de facto* racially segregated over the entire South and *de facto* segregated throughout most of the North before the 1960s. The federal courts ruled in 1963 that "separate but equal" was unconstitutional in health care delivery when it involved public funds (in this case Hill-Burton funding) in *Simkins v. Moses Cone*, a suit filed by a group of Black physicians and dentists in Greensboro, North Carolina, against Moses Cone Hospital. Passage of the Civil Rights Act of 1964 and the Medicare and Medicaid programs, enacted in 1965 as Titles XVIII and XIX of the Social Security Act, had much greater potential to end racial segregation in the health system. However, between 1975 and 1980 it became clear that the race-based health status and outcome disparities would persist and that little would be done by national health policy makers or the health system to remedy them.[264]

Nevertheless, the intent of this mass of Health Education and Welfare (HEW) legislation, Title VI of the Civil Rights Act, and health programs targeting the poor was not to be served. Health system desegregation efforts did not integrate or equalize the system from race and class perspectives for many reasons. Discriminatory barriers, which were actually complex matrixes of history- and culture-based race and class practices and problems at institutional, health policy, and medical-social levels, were not adequately or appropriately addressed. This explains why as public health care sector funding levels declined in both relative and absolute terms during the Reagan-Bush era, hard-won African American health progress ground to a halt. Fundamental structural changes toward a unitary health system failed to occur. Race and class segregation continued and differentials in the quality of care between the upper and lower tiers of the system persisted, if not worsened. Some reasons for the failures include, but were not limited to:

- Narrow and timid interpretation of HEW anti-discrimination regulations toward hospitals and health facilities, such as demanding minority "admissions" only and not forcing complete desegregation of the facility (e.g., segregated rooms, wards, and hospital staffs continued in many facilities)
- HEW failure to enforce, or cursory enforcement of, their own anti-discrimination laws
- Hospital resistance by finding loopholes in the law, such as declaring themselves "sole providers" in an area or as "emergency facilities" only or simply signing compliance paperwork and continuing to segregate
- Failure of HEW or Congress to deal with racial segregation in private physician's offices or health facilities
- Failure of the Office of Civil Rights (OCR), formed by HEW to investigate and enforce compliance, to effectively investigate or prosecute delinquent institutions
- The notorious and well-known HEW failure to punish proven violators of anti-discrimination regulations or laws
- The gradual and progressive defunding of the OCR apparatus by the Congress, which added to its administrative nonfunctioning

Therefore, as in many other areas of American life, at least one-half of African American and other disadvantaged minority patients continued to receive lower quality health care in facilities that are *de facto* segregated based on race, class, and geographic location. On a day-to-day basis one continues to see underfunded, lower quality, segregated health care delivered in the nation's cities around the nexus of race and ethnicity.

One need only visit some of the surviving large public facilities scattered throughout the United States, such as Kings County Hospital Center in Brooklyn, Cook County Hospital in Chicago, Boston Medical Center (the merged entity between Boston City Hospital and Boston University in Boston), Grady Hospital in Atlanta, or King-Drew Medical Center in Los Angeles, where over 90 percent of the clients are African American, Latino, other people of color, or poor Whites, to see failed desegregation and absence of unitary health system policies in action. Moreover, other real and perceived barriers currently being erected by White America block virtually all areas of racial progress, and this pattern is intensifying. Examples abound. Black poverty levels until very recently have been the same as they were in the 1960s. Nationally, the Harvard Project on School Desegregation showed that the 1991–1992 school year was the most segregated (segregation refers to African American children attending predominantly minority Black [50–100% minority] schools) since 1968, with 66% of African American children attending segregated schools. This trend continued through 1999. Blatant racial discrimination remains an everyday occurrence in the United States for virtually all African Americans, including within the health system. Segregation in housing as well as in the health delivery system is as prevalent as ever and may be growing. In such a hostile race relations environment, therefore, the persistence of the race-based health status, outcome, and services utilization disparities perpetuated by a tiered and unequal health delivery system structured for nearly four centuries on the basis of race and class becomes much more comprehensible.[265]

Any analysis of race relations must recall that, as Kovel and others have stated, "[R]acism . . . is the tendency of a society to degrade and do violence to people on the basis of race, and by whatever mediations may exist for this purpose."[266] The dominant new form of racism pervading this current era of race relations, metaracism, is no less violent; it simply represents a shift in character. Moreover, this character shift in postmodern–late capitalist American racism is much more detached and technocratic, much less emotion-laden, usually impersonal, increasingly systematic, often clothed and projected favorably by the culture-consciousness media industries, often presented as anti-racism, often projected in a friendly manner (a form of Bertram Gross's "friendly fascism"), often confounded by traditional American values, and often clothed in the quantitative language of objectivity and science. As racism is clothed in a more technocratic framework and integrated into accepted modes of capitalist interactive behavior, Simone observed the following about racism's new anti-human and deceitful character in the corporate world:

> *Contemporary administrative and corporate forms seek to bury differ-*
> *ence. They are ready to proclaim that only exemplary and optimum per-*
> *formance or competence now matters, regardless of sex or ethnicity,*

deftly ignoring that such competence must be nurtured. In this omission, we return to a state where competence is a matter of biological endowment even though we're supposedly not talking this language anymore.[267]

The New York Times and others have recently observed that the U.S. health system is rapidly transforming itself into a corporate-dominated managed care system. Gordon MacLeod, Professor of Health Services Administration at the University of Pittsburgh School of Medicine, tracked this phenomenon:

The 20th century in the United States witnessed the transformation of society from rural to urban, from an individual orientation to institutional domination, from an agricultural to a manufacturing economy, and from self-employment to employee status in increasingly larger corporations. During the same time period, medical practice made the transition from generalist to specialist, from solo to group insurance, and from a predominantly cottage industry to increasing emphasis on the corporate management of medical care.[268]

This corporate transformation has been described by Peter Drucker:

During the last fifty years, society in every developed country has become a society of institutions. Every major social task, whether economic performance or health care, education or the protection of the environment, the pursuit of new knowledge or defense, is today being entrusted to big organizations, designed for perpetuity and managed by their own managements.[269]

Drucker further warns that "on the performance of these institutions, the performance of modern society—if not the survival of each individual—increasingly depends."[270] The health care implications of these changing relationships should concern every citizen. Inclusion of the racial aspect of the corporate takeover of health care becomes increasingly relevant to African Americans. Corporate characteristics, inherent in their legal enactments for the transaction of business, render them more rational and distant. *Barron's Law Dictionary* defines *corporation* as "an association of shareholders" or "an artificial person . . . having a legal entity separate and distinct from the individuals who compose it." These traits render postmodern–late capitalist racism associated with corporations more "cold" and anti-human in nature. However, the older "hot" forms of racism that energized Western race relations for centuries still exist. For example, the generalized American resistance to, and eventual defeat of, busing for school desegregation represents the older forms of White aversive racism. The Rodney King incident in 1991, wherein a crowd of Los Angeles police officers (although only 4 of the 25 policemen were eventually charged and tried) brutally and publicly beat an African American traffic violator in front of a video camera, reveals the persistence of authoritarianism in the American character and of lingering violent forms of dominative racism. After all the officers were acquitted, a major urban race riot ensued. The policemen were finally tried and convicted for violating King's civil rights. The acquittals followed by riots that finally forced federal action in the King incident are emblematic of the mixed reactions of regional, predominantly White, metropolitan populations to the phenomena surrounding the politics of control among large, minority, inner-city populations.

This is even more tense and volatile in majority-minority cities in which the actions of encircling White populations are mediated by fears of race-based poverty and social disorganization. How these urban areas continue to be controlled by White power structures does not resonate as racism. However, Kovel reminds us, "The fact that it is mediated by fear of poverty and social disorganization instead of the traditional signals of racism does not make the reaction any less racist; it only means that racism keeps changing its face."[271] The Justice Department's enforcement of the Civil Rights Act of 1964 to protect White employees against discrimination in hiring is an example of the new "upside-down" race relations. President Reagan, under the banner of egalitarianism, attempted to give schools with openly discriminatory admissions policies tax-exempt status. These are examples of the fact that today's racism can be cloaked by anti-racism. Another example of these "upside-down" racist mechanisms is the closure since 1965 of virtually all of the approximately 200 Black hospitals in the name of integration, economic efficiency, and other positive technocratic reasons. This rendered African Americans completely dependent on the White health institutions that traditionally had rejected and mistreated them for decades and which are still under virtually lily-White management and administration. Black acceptance in professional sports with the preservation of White hierarchies in the front office and ownership levels is another example of a more subtle form of racism that evokes less emotion in Blacks, including the players. They function as the physically working menials while White males, almost exclusively, supervise and administer the multi-million-dollar industry. Although they remain stereotyped and discriminated against, Blacks have been projected by the culture and communication industries as sports heroes. These African American males are then expected to play out stereotypical, sometimes derogatory, roles in advertisements and sales promotions for these new foundries of media-promoted metaracism. These new cerebral, media-slick mediators of racism in no way decrease the levels of violence inflicted on Blacks, nor are such mediators less repressive.

The outmigration of White populations to racially segregated suburbs is a continuum of aversive racism that is centuries old and shows no signs of abating. Despite the 1968 Fair Housing Act, which banned racial discrimination in the sale and rental of housing, African Americans of all classes continue to be channelled into segregated housing. Through the collusion of banks, real estate agencies, insurance companies, and lending institutions a new form of white-collar racism continues. This geographic segregation has a great deal to do with determining the quantity and quality of health care institutions and facilities that are conveniently available to African American populations. Therefore, African Americans are getting signals that they may have to wait generations for the abatement of residential segregation in order to obtain justice and equity in vital necessities such as health care and education. It is abundantly clear that new forms of subtle, technocratic, media-oriented racism define modern race relations.

Of all the signs and symptoms of the declining fortunes of African Americans, one of the few evaluative beacons of progress virtually everyone agrees on is the gains in Black political power. The first manifestations of this political success resulted from two phenomena. The first was the passage of the Voting Rights Act in 1965 and the increasing concentration of African Americans in the nation's urban areas. Moreover, the rise of Black leaders such as Martin Luther King, Jr., and Malcolm X also raised political awareness and spawned a generation of national and regional African American political and community leaders. Due to political memory and sociopolitical and class realities, most Black political activity has been confined to the Democratic Party after the Franklin Roosevelt era. The 1967 election of Mayor Richard Hatcher in predominantly Black Gary, Indiana, notwithstanding, the first African American elected to govern a truly major city in the United States was Carl Stokes in Cleveland, Ohio, that same year. Stokes accomplished this with a Democratic coalition of a bloc of White voters and a solid African American electoral minority. Tom Bradley was elected mayor of Los Angeles six years later when the city was less than 20% Black. Since then Chicago, New York, Newark, Baltimore, Atlanta, and Washington, D.C., to name a few of the more than 200 cities, have all had Black mayors. Interestingly, of the 26 major cities with Black mayors as of 1992, only nine had majority Black populations. However, many have hypothesized that these were Pyrrhic victories in that virtually all of these cities were in the throes of infrastructure collapse and were turned over to Blacks only after they became "ungovernable."

These new strides in political power have not usually translated into improved quality or functioning of the health systems in African American–controlled jurisdictions. The monolithic nature of the health system seems, at times, impervious to political forces or change. For example, Atlanta, Georgia, a city strongly influenced by African American politicians such as Maynard Jackson and Andrew Young for more than two decades, with a predominantly Black city hospital, continued until recently to "red-line" the predominantly Black Morehouse School of Medicine in support of Emory University's control of the medical and professional training that takes place at Grady Hospital. Emory graduates few, if any, physicians that serve Atlanta's Black community after their training phase is over. Nevertheless, Morehouse, which trains predominantly African American physicians, many of whom serve Atlanta's Black community, is grudgingly being allowed participation in training activities involving their own people. There was until recently a similar situation in Nashville, Tennessee, in which the Vanderbilt University Medical School successfully undermined predominantly Black Meharry Medical College's full participation in training programs at Nashville General Hospital from 1893 until the early 1990s. Vanderbilt continues to block Meharry's participation in the staffing or training programs involving the federally funded Nashville VA Hospital and the publicly financed Children's Hospital. In 1998 Vanderbilt subsequently moved back in to assume control over the new city hospital Meharry virtually donated to Nashville. Of course, Blacks never exercised the political clout in Nashville that Atlanta Blacks have wielded.

Nevertheless, African American political representation, although far from proportional, has made impressive gains. It represents one of the few bright spots in the wake of the Civil Rights Movement of the 1960s. Despite Black voter turnouts never equalling the 58% of the 1968 presidential election, there are now at least 8,000 Black elected officials. Almost two-thirds of them hail from predominantly Black jurisdictions. However, there are disturbing recent events that wreck the African American political success story. The Congressional Black Caucus (CBC), after flexing its newfound muscle in the 103rd Congress and growing from 26 to 40 members, including Carol Mosely-Braun (D-Ill.),* the first African American senator since Edward Brooke in the 1970s, was virtually stripped of power by the Republican takeover of both houses of Congress in 1994. This has great potential for undermining the CBC's health care efforts as we enter the twenty-first century. Moreover, over the last several years African Americans have lost mayoral seats in some of the largest cities in the country, including Chicago, Philadelphia, Los Angeles, and New York City. This political distress is compounded by the fact that the Democratic Party is increasingly distancing itself from its 20% Black support—which, paradoxically, is hurting the party politically.

The latest blow to the correction of Black political underrepresentation, especially in the U.S. Congress, is the 1995 Supreme Court ruling outlawing certain methods involved in the creation of minority-dominated Congressional districts. Although White politicians have gerrymandered political boundaries for over a century to negate Black political power, efforts to correct this history-based inequity regarding African American political representation have been declared illegal. How much racism was tainting the political process in the United States by 1995 is hard to measure, but if the upcoming battles over affirmative action and the Republican agenda for dismantling the "welfare state" are examples, the color line remains a big factor in American politics. Whether African Americans will find new and creative ways to participate in the political process is one of the major questions that must be answered as we enter the twenty-first century.

From a health policy perspective, election of the 103rd Congress and the prospect of national health reform geared toward a more egalitarian system engendered the most hopeful period for African Americans in decades. The CBC and the Summit '93 Health Coalition, a consortium of more than 155

---

*She was defeated in the 1996 elections.

minority and progressive organizations supporting egalitarian health reform, placed health care on minority America's national agendas. The CBC was in the process of establishing a public policy foundation that was to have a health care policy component. However, the 1994 electoral landslide by Republicans essentially put these plans on hold for the foreseeable future. Rejection of health reform by the 103rd Congress, followed by removal of health reform from the political agenda by the 104th Congress, was just as significant in a negative direction.[272]

Whites are largely detached from African Americans both geographically and psychologically. This is also reflective of a new racism that is largely structural and institutional and requires virtually no psychological mediation to exercise its racist result. The cold and heartless efficiency of this postmodern–late capitalist system is enhanced and compounded by the cultural effects of the dehumanized and anti-human cultural environment. Moreover, the new racism is protean in nature and can be clothed in anti-racist rhetoric or long-held American values such as self-reliance, individual achievement, meritocracy, personal responsibility, and individual autonomy.

This brief survey of contemporary race relations indicates that anti-Black racism and racial discrimination are vibrant, if not burgeoning, forces in contemporary American life. Neither painting the old race-based quality-of-life disparities with new political and ethnic faces nor deceptively dressing them in traditional, albeit victim-blaming, costumes composed of traditional American values changes their ugly faces. Expecting the health delivery system to remain immune to these forces is unreasonable.[273]

Strategies to Overcome a Dream Deferred: Race, Justice, and Equity in Health Care As We Enter the Twenty-first Century

Based on the evidence, the African American Civil Rights Movement, along with the Chicano and Black Power movements of the 1950s through 1970s, failed to transform the U.S. racial state. Official endorsement of *de jure* apartheid ended. However, *de facto* racial segregation is still prominent for the majority of African Americans. Deep inequalities in quality-of-life measures such as socioeconomic status, major health parameters, educational attainment, housing, and environment remain. Possibilities of hope for future progress for African Americans in the United States are contingent upon justice and equity in education, employment, housing, health care, the criminal justice system, and the living environment. Despite current domestic shortfalls in these areas, Ali Mazrui, one of the eminent scholars on Black Africa, contends that both Africans and the Black Diaspora look to African Americans for an improved worldwide African future:

> From a political point of view, Black America especially is Africa's most
> important external human resource, precisely because it constitutes a

> *large concentration of people of African ancestry lodged in the most*
> *powerful nation in the world, and certainly a nation with immense*
> *capacity to do Africa harm or good. A re-Africanisation of Black Ameri-*
> *can allegiance and sympathies could help to re-orient American foreign*
> *policy towards Africa, and transform it in the direction of greater sensi-*
> *tivity and sympathy with African aspirations and values.*[274]

This and other developments are concrete evidence that improvements in these areas of deficiency in the African American freedom movement warrant our attention and efforts in the future.

The shortfalls in race relations pointed out here occurred despite the previous 60 years of critical theory development. The progressive development and matura-tion of critical theory included the incorporation of more comprehensive and sen-sitive definitions of the concepts required to study modern conformations of race such as prejudice, ethnic groups, and ethnocentrism; the creation of new objec-tive tools to study race such as the Bogardus Social Distance Scale; access to and guidance from comparative data from statistically significant and accurate, peri-odic, serial surveys studying the various racial and ethnic groups; the inclusion of the results of massive, longitudinal, prospective, statistically analyzed, psychologi-cal and behavioral cohort data sets; and an extensive potpourri of social scientific investigations focusing on the unique U.S. racial environment in the North and South around the time of World War II. Although the corpus of racial studies and analyses had become more sophisticated and the tools available to public policy makers more diverse and efficacious as a result of these developments, the hoped-for eradication and amelioration of racism and the race problem did not occur.

As the various social and intellectual forces reshape the race problem into a confusing and often obscure political and public policy amalgam of concepts and euphemisms, debating the use of terms such as *interest groups, class warfare, illegal aliens, welfare dependency, the underclass, inner-city poor, ethnic friction, nationality, cultural identity,* and *cultural pluralism,* the basic power relationship between Blacks and Whites has not changed enough to enable full-fledged Black participation and first-class citizenship for African Americans at this juncture. White racial dominance mediated through economic, political, and, more recently, social forces not only became entrenched and internalized through dif-ferent mechanisms, but is assuming an ugly face as well. As Sniderman and Piazza in their analyses of the National Election Study (NES), the General Social Survey (GSS), and the Race and Politics (RAP) Survey, all conducted in 1986, have observed, White Americans no longer feel restrained or obligated to be polite about their negative attitudes about Blacks, nor do they feel compelled to mask their feelings of impatience or intolerance regarding African Americans. Negative racial stereotyping, strongly perpetuated by the culture-conscious media corporate infrastructures, is still very prevalent. Although the concept of race has been transformed by mechanisms of metaracism to such an extent that its racist signals are more complex and hard to read, abundant evidence of White racial dominance is still in place. The postmodern–late capitalist politics of race has become complex and obscure enough that students such as Sniderman and Piazza have divided their political survey studies on race into easier-to-discern components such as the social welfare agenda, the equal treatment agenda, and the race-conscious agenda. How do we interpret this grim picture from a racial perspective in a society purportedly constructively engaged in a civil rights struggle toward equity and eventual equality among the races?[275]

With all these confusing forces, what is the racial reality in the United States? Kovel's original psycho-historical analysis seems to be borne out by the cascade of events 25 years after he proposed the original hypothesis. His updated contention bears repeating:

> [R]acism is a category of Western civilization, and Western civilization is saturated, not merely with racism—that is obvious enough—but with the elementary gesture out of which racism is constructed: splitting the world in the course of domination. It follows that:
> - racism antecedes the notion of race, indeed, it generates the races;
> - racism supersedes the psychology of prejudice, indeed, it creates that psychology for its purposes;
> - racism evolves historically, and may be expected to appear in different phases in different epochs and locales;
> - racism cannot be legislated out of existence, since what is put into law always serves to legitimate the system which generates racism and is defined by it.[276]

This broad construct of modern racism is one of the few that adequately explains the complex, sometimes baffling, racial phenomena that occur today. Michael Omi and Howard Winant's notion of *racial formation* also appears useful as an explanatory hypothesis of postmodern–late capitalist racism. Their construction, *racial formation*, is a sociohistorical notion created to displace race as a fixed, concrete, and objective "something." With this in mind, Omi and Winant suggest that race should be understood as

> an unstable and "decentered" complex of social meanings constantly being transformed by political struggle. . . . [T]he crucial task . . . is to suggest how the widely disparate circumstances of individual and group racial identities, and of the racial institutions and social practices with which these identities are intertwined, are formed and transformed over time. This takes place . . . through political contestation over racial meanings. [emphasis in the original][277]

Their argument is centered on the notion that race is built upon a foundation that is both historical and social and that it changes secondary to social struggle. Projection of race as a "mere *illusion . . .* which an ideal non-racist social order would eliminate"[278] renders racial problems less concrete. Such a conception is hopeful and suggests that the present complex and seemingly intransigent U.S. race problem is a candidate for replacement by racial formation. This validates Outlaw's conclusion that " '[r]ace,' in a racial state, is thereby irreducibly political."[279] For those focused on the applicability of utilizing racial theory in the formulation or shaping of future health policy, such an approach appears potentially useful.[280]

These constructs, one psychohistorical, as laid out by Kovel, and the other sociohistorical and ultimately political, according to Omi, Winant, and Outlaw, are promising for public health and medical-social utility in the future. These hypotheses are based on the historical construct of race, thus preserving the sociohistorical constructivist (socially formed) dimensions of race. By placing this matrix of social, cultural, psychological, historical, scientific, behavioral, ethical, and biological concepts in perspective and into coherent and understandable relationships and systems, these paradigms should lend understanding and perspective to the race problem in modern America. These principles should be applicable to the modern market-capitalist U.S. health system. They should also become tools for, and make contributions to, the analytical process for generating hypotheses leading to solutions for the health system's race and class problems. It is also significant that the social and political nature of some of these concepts makes their integration into the political process a real possibility.

Another useful paradigm that serves our purpose as reluctant historians of racism in the health system, while adding social and historical richness to the inquiry, is well articulated by George Fredrickson in his 1987 introduction to the reprint edition of his classic *The Black Image in the White Mind:*

> [T]*he most useful approach for the historian of racism is to study the interaction between culture — preexisting beliefs, values, and attitudes — and social structure, defined as the stratification of classes based on relationship to the market or the means of production.*[281]

Fredrickson's history-based connections between culture and class-based social structure and their direct relationships with economic markets and means of production are strikingly prescient. Many students of race, including Eric Williams, Du Bois, and Manning Marable have posited the comfortable relationship between market capitalism and racial and social injustice. This relationship, which fostered chattel slavery, colonial exploitation, social hierarchies, and even genocide as far as people of color were concerned, was a major reason these scholars leaned toward socialist conceptions of a world order. The lessons learned from these scholars' experiences and writings are especially germane as the health system transforms into a purely economic market. This transformation was predicted by

managed care experts like Kongstvedt, Drucker, and other contemporary authorities in the *New York Times,* while race- and class-based medical and medical-social
needs seemingly go unheeded. Is one corollary of this transformation of the U.S.
health system into a competitive market a prediction of race and class conflict in
the health system's future? Nevertheless, Fredrickson's recognition that race awareness and racism are products of a complex interplay between culture and society
reaffirms Lévi-Strauss's classic contention that statements about race are statements
about culture, and vice versa. Or as Fanon pointed out, "Racism is never a super-
added element discovered by chance in the course of investigation of the cultural
data of a group. The social constellation, the cultural whole, are deeply modified
by the existence of racism."[282] These paradigms interface easily with the sociohistorical, and ultimately political, construct of Omi and Winant while buttress-
ing the psychohistorical hypotheses of Kovel. Thus, despite the postmodern
pretense that racism is no longer a major problem, objective evaluation of concrete economic, educational, legal, political, and health care outcomes and
masses of survey research involving African Americans reveals that racism and its
manifestations are alive and well in the United States. This, of course, includes
the health system. Insights gained as a result of this inquiry, along with the over-
powering weight of the evidence, demonstrate that the failure to come to grips
with this reality can be interpreted as another manifestation of postmodern–late
capitalist American metaracism. Clearly, the persistent health disparities being
experienced by African Americans are, in part, a result of this overarching racial
dynamic. Nevertheless, we must be mindful that this racial-cultural interplay is so
complex that it defies monocausal explanations. In that the immense U.S. health
care system involves a distinct culture and immense social, institutional, and
political infrastructures, Lévi-Strauss, Fanon, and Fredrickson's analyses are relevant and lend understanding and perspective to any investigation of these entities. Additionally, the theories and paradigms about modern racism articulated by
Outlaw, Omi and Winant, Kovel, and Fredrickson should be incorporated into
any new critical theory on race.[283]

Virtually all agree that U.S. sociopolitical and economic systems have been
dominated by European Protestant White males. All other resident subgroups
have been consigned some form of "Other" status. Nevertheless, as has been reit-
erated by many noted scholars, the interplay, especially in its negative dimensions, between U.S. race relations (including Native Americans, Hispanics,
Asians, and Blacks) and the "Other" dynamic has been energized and symbolized by the ongoing, nearly four-century-old Black/White relationship.

Only the Native American experience approaches the African American one
in negativity and dehumanization. Native Americans probably lost eight million
souls in the process of White domination of North America; people of African
descent lost at least 50 million in the slave trade alone.[284] The chronology of the
African American ordeal in the U.S. has been 246 years, or a little more than
eight generations, of chattel slavery, followed by 100 years, almost three and one-
half generations, of legal segregation and discrimination, and one generation of

legal but not actual equality. Moreover, the relationship has been characterized by its brutishness, brutality, violence, overt and covert invidious discrimination, and sexual depravity (e.g., a high incidence of miscegenation and the frequent imposition of castration as official punishments during slavery and as unofficial events during lynchings after slavery). For no other group has the White dominance been so brutal and devastating. Perhaps for these reasons classic reconceptualizations and rearticulations of Western civilization's old race problem into "ethnicity," "ethnocentrism," or "cultural-societal interaction" have foundered on the rocky shores of racism in the United States.

There is no intention here to get bogged down in the specialist details of the intellectual debates about race over class (Black nationalist), class over race (classical Marxism), or ethnic group over race, but only to utilize concepts from them to understand the dynamic of racism as it affects the health system in postmodern America. Therefore, Terry's model in which *power relations, problem definition, resource distribution,* and *standard setting* are regarded as the basic mechanisms for maintaining White/Anglo dominance within the society at large, including the health system, a model also crystallized by Kovel in somewhat different terms, has been vindicated. Recent events in the United States, Great Britain, France, unified Germany, Bosnia-Hergozovina (the former Yugoslavia) and Kosovo, where racial and ethnic conflicts have occurred, reflect a new wave of dangerous racist thinking throughout the West and the failures of recent conservative political strategy, either locally or internationally, to counteract and ameliorate it. The 1992 Los Angeles riots, along with a rash of "blackface incidents" at Northeastern universities and some of the nation's leading medical schools during the 1990s, are evidence of the highest degree of Black/White racial polarization in recent U.S. memory.[285]

Both Kovel and Omi and Winant's racial paradigms emphasize learning as essential to the formation of a new critical theory. This new synthesis of theoretical work directed at understanding and transforming the social formations that have blocked the concrete realizations of increased human freedom, especially as far as race and racism were concerned, would integrate and incorporate new bodies of knowledge and discourse. New operative mechanisms of racism, contemporary psychological paradigms of race and racism, recent data accumulated by utilizing up-to-date analytic instruments, and new models and hypotheses surrounding race would be included. Such new knowledge incorporated into a new critical theory could be essential if improving the Black/White relationship in the United States is to be accomplished efficiently. If analyses and examination of problematic racial-ethnic relationships threatening to tear apart the fabric of the American nation are not carried out, it could have profoundly negative consequences. Moreover, bridging the Black/White racial divide would go a long way toward transforming the U.S. founders' ideals into social reality. Application of these findings could lead to fact-based explanatory hypotheses, formulations of creative solutions, and implementations of socioculturally sensitive and relevant corrective actions toward solving the nation's race-based social problems. Medical-social applications could also eventually result in a fair and equitable health system.

Moreover, these major contemporary models help explain the complex con-
volutions the racial struggle is undergoing, as race is being rearticulated in the
United States today. Kovel's linkages of White racism to the psychological roots of
Western "human nature" and imperial domination are rational and interesting,
but they go beyond the scope or reach of our study. Similarly, Outlaw's recommendation that Omi and Winant's reconstruction of a new critical theory of race
be juxtaposed and intermingled with Black Nationalist racial theories is appreciated as a plea for future scholarly challenges and endeavors for specialists in the
field. These are areas that should dominate forthcoming scholarship in the discipline of racial thought, but have limited utility here. For the authors of this book,
who are striving to place the relationship between race and the U.S. health care
system in a clear and analytical light, the outline of a new critical theory of race
suggested by the work of Outlaw, Marcuse, the Frankfurt School, Omi and
Winant, and Kovel is sufficient. However, we submit this chapter as a notice of
warning. As Devisse, Mollat, and Courtes related in *The Image of the Black in
Western Art:* "[T]his . . . is a beginning, a groundbreaking, an invitation to look
further, to be curious: it is not the soft pillow on which the hasty certitudes of hur-
ried civilizations too often fall asleep."[286] Much remains to be examined and clarified about the relationship between race, biology, medicine, and health care.

As has been stated by Sniderman and Piazza and Simone, there has been a disappearance of the race problem's moral or ethical squint in the United States. New
models of race relations are needed that will protect vulnerable minority populations as these conflicts are addressed and resolved in the future. This is especially
relevant regarding changes in the health system where life, death, and well-being
are at stake. Dangerous times seem to be ahead for U.S. race relations. The African
American future in the U.S. health system appears no less dangerous. Therefore, if
attempting to formulate a new critical theory of race is a good thing, and we feel it
is, amalgamating elements of these efforts represents a good, and useful, beginning.
Lucius Outlaw, who in many ways has intellectually overseen the racial thought
aspect of this inquiry, points out the advantages of a new critical theory, stating:

> [W]e would have at our disposal the prospects of an understanding of
> race in keeping with the original promises of critical theory: enlighten-
> ment leading to emancipation. Social learning regarding "race," steered
> by critical social thought, might help us to move beyond racism, without
> reductionism, to pluralist socialist democracy.[287]

If such an outcome could be anticipated for the present racially divided and
inequitable U.S. health delivery system, then our labors and efforts to explore the
topic of race have been worthwhile. Recent events indicate Du Bois's prediction
that "the problem of the twentieth century is the problem of the color line" has
been borne out and will plague Western culture well into the twenty-first century.
There is no better evidence of this than the U.S. health care system, and there is
no better cause deserving of our efforts at amelioration.[288]

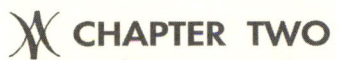 CHAPTER TWO

Race, Medicine, and Society: From Prehistoric to English Colonial Times

Since prehistoric times medicine has been a major human endeavor. Healing and administering health care have always held special places in the sphere of human interactions and have possessed inordinate, even quasi-magical and mystical powers in both primitive and civilized societies. Our investigation delves into how, why, and when race and racialist dogma, or their precursors, were first injected into the life sciences. Other major concerns are the origins of America's individualistic and hierarchical approaches to health, healing, and health care. How these medical-social principles and practices, which have always been factor-loaded against African Americans, became entrenched in U.S. medical and health care systems is a critical question. These same principles and practices became encumbered with quasi-religious ideological and moral overtones with the potential to justify proscription, exploitation, and even condemnation of particular patient groups. These evolutionary trends in the health system's subculture, having roots and precursors stretching back to Mesopotamian, Egyptian, and Greco-Roman times, have led to profound race and class problems plaguing the contemporary U.S. health system.

Ancient Western Medicine and Health Care: Race and Class Considerations in Predecessor Health Systems

Western medical science, and health care as we know it, can be traced to the valleys of two great river systems. Both areas were located on the pre-African land mass of the supercontinent Pangaea 130 million years ago. The civilizations girding these river systems trace their origins mythically before 6000 BC and in writing from at least 4000 BC. One culture producing early medical practices and documents originated in the southwest Asian region known as Mesopotamia, which literally means "between the rivers." The two rivers, the Tigris and the Euphrates, have their headwaters in the mountains of Asia Minor and flow into the Persian Gulf. We know the region today as Iraq and Kuwait. The other early civilization originated along the banks and the delta of the Nile River in northeastern Africa at approximately the same time.[1]

The prehistoric origins of Western medicine and health care from these two regions reflect medicine's religious and magical overtones. The Egyptian and Mesopotamian models were only two examples of what has been called "archaic medicine" by Temkin and others. Other examples of ancient medical systems having archaic characteristics are the ancient Chinese, Indian, Central American, South American, and most recently, some sub-Saharan African medical systems. Ancient medical systems lacking these characteristics are categorized as primitive. Although both categories shared religion and magic as distinct features, there were several characteristics that distinguished archaic medicine from primitive medicine. Some of these distinguishing characteristics included empiricism, systemization, and practical organization in contradistinction to primitive medicine; archaic medicine recorded its experiences and cases for the future utilization and growth of the profession and, because of its germination in heavily populated relatively urban areas, incorporated some public health measures into its corpus of knowledge and practice.

Early physicians in these Western medical traditions were also priests. This was analogous to the European health system in the early Christian era. Only in Greek times were successful attempts made to sever these ancient and seemingly cyclical relationships between religion and medicine. However, the difficulty in severing these relationships is evidenced by Greek medicine's dominance (500 BC to AD 500) of temple complexes functioning as religious-oriented spas, sanitariums, and hospitals. The fall of the Roman empire and the spread of barbarism over Europe would drive medieval Western medicine back into the arms of the Church.[2]

The first documented Mesopotamian records of a formal medical profession and codified medical treatments date back to approximately 3000 BC. Some of this medical and medical-legal information is included in the Code of Hammurabi dating from around 1700 BC. Although just as ancient, Mesopotamian medicine seems less codified, more mystical and less rationalistic, and less systematized than its Egyptian counterpart. Several major sources indicate that although surgery was performed in Babylonia, it was much less prominent, less documented, or professionally focused upon than it was in ancient Egypt.

There were also definite evidences of a class hierarchy in both the Mesopotamian and Egyptian systems regarding the receipt of health services. Traditions espousing the tiering of health care and health services are important progenitors to America's health system. Even if the hierarchical delivery and organization of health care and services were not encouraged, their establishment is still significant. These status-based health policies were especially prominent in Mesopotamia, where slaves received less treatment, from less trained and less prestigious practitioners, at lower fee scales.[3] Though class was a prominent social force in the delivery of health services in both ancient systems, disparities in this regard did not seem to be racially motivated.

Mesopotamian medicine was based on an assumption of divine punishment leading to illness as a mark of sin. This spiritual approach to disease from a scientific standpoint seemingly handicapped the region's medical attempts at rationality, scientific objectivity, and surgical advances. Physicians were, therefore, heavily dependent on divination and priestly functions to practice. Mesopotamian physicians seemingly were trained primarily in schools located alongside religious temples, although in Nippur and some other locations in Sumer there is archaeological evidence that suggests that there may have been specialized institutions functioning as medical schools.

Although there is evidence of minor surgery, Mesopotamian medicine focused on demonological and divine approaches to medical disorders. However, some of the preoccupations with these fear concepts resulted in strict hygiene practices when a person was ill. Quarantine, isolation of the sick, and merging social disability with the "sick role" are legacies of Mesopotamian medicine passed along to us through Hebrew and Greek medical traditions. The inclusion of hyoscyamus, opium, and belladonna in its pharmacopeia are thoroughly contemporary. Other drugs such as hellebore and mandrake were also known in Mesopotamia. Although heavily bound by harsh and punitive forensic limits of malpractice, Mesopotamian physicians leave no evidence of ethical traditions for treating all patients equally or equitably.[4]

Around 6000 BC a complex, highly technical, multiracial civilization flourished in northeastern Africa along the 4,000-mile length of the Nile River. By 3000 BC this civilization, along with ancient Mesopotamia, had perfected the use of paper, ink, pens, and the writing skills necessary to record its experience. By the third millennium the Egyptians had transcended primitive levels in medicine as they had in agriculture, technology, science, architecture, and art. The impact of Egyptian medical traditions on Western medicine is incalculable. Although Greeks have been credited with founding Western medicine until recently, authorities such as Thorwald have suggested otherwise:

Many decades were to pass before this unrealistic view was corrected
and it was recognized that a body of medical experience and knowledge
had existed long before the Greeks; that the Greeks had, in fact—with
"the vitality of bastards," as a modern medical historian expressed it—
absorbed everything they could from older sources.[5]

Egypt provided Western medicine with a tradition of trained physician-specialists; an extensive medical armamentarium of diagnostic maneuvers, medications, and medical and surgical treatments; a rich corpus of scientific medical data and textbooks; and an untapped tradition of medical-social responsibility and obligation leading to the provision of most health services to all members of society in an equitable and ethical manner. They also left a legacy of cognitive elitism and professional secrecy—health professions' traditions whose effects may be adversely impacting Western and U.S. medicine today.[6]

Like all ancient medical traditions, the Egyptian tradition was strongly religious; the earliest physicians had priestly functions. Physicians were well thought of in Egyptian society and were trained at schools affiliated with religious temples. Imhotep was the chief physician of Pharaoh Zoser around 2980 BC and was a major founder of Egyptian medicine. According to Sir William Osler, he was "the first figure of a physician to stand out clearly from the mists of antiquity."[7] He was also an architect, priest, and scribe. Imhotep was later deified and his teachings and philosophies came to dominate Egyptian medicine for the next 2,500 years. As early as 2500 BC, Egyptian medicine was divided into specialties—with physicians focusing on care of the eyes, the abdomen, or the anus, for example. The first identifiable dental physician, Hesi-Re, Chief of the Court College of Physicians, suggested the high standing of tooth specialists, as noted in documents at Saqqara (c. 3000 BC). However, specialization may not have been indicative of the medical advancement it would later become but may have been Egyptian physicians' mechanism for not having to master the massive corpus of Egyptian medical knowledge. During that 2,500 years of medical dominance, Egyptian physicians and medical schools were considered the state of the art throughout the Mediterranean basin. Homer, as early as 1000 BC, noted that Egyptians were the finest physicians, and Herodotus, in the fifth century BC, reaffirmed that opinion.[8]

Egyptian physicians treated both medical and surgical conditions, including, but not limited to, infections such as tuberculosis; diseases resulting from water and food contamination; parasitic infections; diseases of the eyes such as night blindness, cataracts, and trachoma; atherosclerosis; women's diseases; pneumonia; appendicitis; arthritis and gout; kidney and bladder stones; cirrhosis of the liver; hernias; and certain tumors such as those of the ovaries and bones. There is evidence that diagnoses were made based on histories given by patients and by complex examinations including probings of body parts and study of sputum, feces, and other body fluids and products. Diseases were treated with a wide range of agents, including the use of purging and enemas and a vast number of medicinal plants, herbs, minerals, metals, and other agents with the effects of narcotics and antibiotics.[9]

After training, physicians became members of a hierarchical structure. Both the standards of training and practice were set by the Pharaoh's physician, who was at the top of the hierarchy. Beneath him were palace physicians, lesser chief physicians (or inspectors of physicians), and a lower order of physicians who comprised the majority of practicing physicians. Evidence that the Egyptians were considered leaders of ancient healing arts is that their schools attracted physicians from Western Europe, Greece, Asia, and Asia Minor to study medicine until well into the Roman era. The Greeks displaced them from this pinnacle after successfully co-opting, often plagiarizing, and incorporating Egyptian medical knowledge and techniques.[10]

The Egyptians preserved their achievements through a series of religious and emperico-rational medical documents. Egyptian physicians wrote medical textbooks as early as 4000 BC. These texts constitute the most comprehensive and systematic ancient corpus of medical knowledge in Western culture. The best-known products of this scholarship are the *Edwin Smith* (1600 BC) and *Ebers papyri* (1550 BC). The former is largely surgical in content, while the latter is a more encyclopedic, medically oriented document. Both refer to a formal medical tradition dating from at least 2500 BC. There are several other lesser-known Egyptian medical papyri. For example, the *Kahun* gynecological papyrus, compiled around 1900 BC, dealt with subjects such as contraception, determination of the sex of the child during pregnancy, infertility, premature labor, amenorrhea (absence of menses), dysmenorrhea (painful menses), venereal diseases, and inflammations of external and internal genitalia. Upon close examination, a high level of medical sophistication is observed from diagnostic, prognostic, and therapeutic standpoints. Some of the more recent papyri, such as the *Hearst Papyrus* (1500 BC), the great *Berlin Papyrus* (1300 BC), the *London Papyrus* (1350 BC), and the lesser Berlin papyrus *(Westcar)*, are largely restricted to prescriptions and contain much more magical content. Such evidence implies that ancient Egyptian medicine deteriorated with the occurrence of foreign incursions and Greek dominance. Nevertheless, many hypothesize and maintain that Western medicine would not attain these levels of complexity and expertise again until the nineteenth and twentieth centuries.[11]

Unlike the Mesopotamian medical traditions, Egyptians were surgically oriented and reset fractures, treated wounds, and trephined the skull. There is not much evidence of formal hospitals per se; Egyptian physicians, however, made house calls, had officially assigned duty stations at temples, and were formally assigned to military units. Thus, whatever surgery was performed seemingly took place at these sites. Most Egyptian medical treatises seem to involve solitary practitioners attending patients. The "medical team" concept of assistants like nurses and therapists may not have occurred until the Greeks implemented it later in the Asclepiad temple complexes. Moreover, there are suggestions that these surgical traditions, along with circumcision and Caesarean section births, were transmitted by way of Upper (Southern) Egypt from sub-Saharan Africa.[12] The Egyptians also contributed a variety of therapeutic principles, including wound dressings, application of antiseptic and antibiotic powders, therapeutic and medicinal enemas, and a pharmacy of more than 1,000 agents. Egyptian physicians usually compounded their own medicines. Some included opium, prescribed for pain and infant colic; belladonna alkaloids for gastrointestinal problems; sedatives; and castor oil for various applications. Some of these pharmacologic principles and therapeutic agents are utilized today.[13]

Egyptian medical-social attitudes toward health care and health services delivery were, in some ways, more advanced than our own. They provided medical services to virtually all of the population despite class, race, or social status through an organized system of state-salaried physicians. This provision of medical services to the masses included public health services. Egyptian physicians conducted sanitation inspections and designed public health programs based on their findings. Thus, many Egyptian homes contained bathroom facilities, and waste disposal was planned and organized to prevent pollution of the Nile and other rivers. Cities were kept clean and homes generally were sanitary. Doctors were formally assigned as temple physicians, which made medical care available for virtually the entire population. Citizens were encouraged to visit these facilities. Some physicians were specifically assigned to care for slave or worker populations. Others were assigned for duty with military units. Egyptian physicians charged with the care of slave and peasant populations enacted strict sanitation, hygiene, and quarantine measures that influenced Hebrew and Greek medicine in later periods. Race was not an important matter in the Egyptian health system. The racial aspects of the Egyptian medical contribution seem more a matter of modern rather than ancient concern, epitomized by the current academic debate surrounding the racial identity of ancient Egyptians—including Imhotep, the "father" of Western medicine. Paradoxically, the way Egyptian and sub-Saharan medical traditions are perceived, projected, and conceived of in the context of Western culture is symptomatic of the West's racial health dilemma. The shift away from the tradition of projecting Eurocentric particularity in the achievements and progress of the life sciences toward a pluralistic, inclusive, nonhierarchical perspective regarding contributions and participation is important. Such an approach demands cultural equality and respect that could favorably influence the U.S. medical and health subcultures.[14]

Until very recently Egyptians, traditionally viewed as major contributors to Western civilization, were projected by Egyptologists, archaeologists, and historians as White. Contemporary investigations by intellectuals such as Cheikh Anta Diop, George G. M. James, Ivan Van Sertima, St. Clair Drake, Basil Davidson, Molefi Kete Asante, Charles Finch, and Martin Bernal have refuted this scholarly misrepresentation, which has distorted Western history since the nineteenth century.[15] As early as the 1920s scholars like J. A. Rogers and W. Montague Cobb had maintained that Imhotep—like many other Western icons—was Black, based on studies of primary sources.[16] Such efforts were ignored, discredited, or marginalized by mainstream scholars. With the maturation of a cadre of Afrocentric* and unbiased White scholars, the historical and cultural distortions produced by the co-option of Egyptian civilization by White Europeans and trivialization of the contribution of Black sub-Saharan Africans has begun to be corrected. Briefly stated, evidence shows that many of the ancient Egyptians in the highest positions were Black; that ancient Black populations were not closely related to the Arab groups that occupy Egypt presently; that ancient Egypt was more closely linked with Black sub-Saharan Africa than previously suspected; and that Black sub-Saharan Africans possessed highly sophisticated cultures and were not the primitive barbarians they have been depicted as for the past two centuries.[17]

Having said this, it can now be credibly stated that some contemporary scholars of medical history present compelling evidence that a substantial portion of Egyptian medical knowledge and practices originated in the then-fertile Saharan and sub-Saharan areas. Knowledge transfer to Egypt began during prehistoric times. A mounting body of evidence demonstrates that the traditional African practitioner of ancient times had formidable medical and surgical skills and contributed a great deal to ancient Egyptian medicine.

Although slavery was a given in the ancient world, there seemed to be little concern with race in ancient societies before Hellenic civilization. Contrary to popular belief, ancient contributions to early medicine and health care are surprisingly multicultural, and they emanated from many racial and ethnic groups. Major contributions to Western life sciences came from the Egyptian, Mesopotamian, and Hebrew medical traditions. Moreover, interaction with southern African cultures such as Punt or far Eastern cultures such as Indonesia or China makes their inclusion as participants in Western medical progress likely. There is sketchy travel evidence and relatively strong, though indirect, pharmaceutical evidence that some contact with these distant neighbors was made by Egypt and Mesopotamia. Not only did there seem to be a wide variety of medical and technical input from all of these civilizations, but health services delivery also varied from a relatively equitable and open Egyptian system to more elite-oriented and socially rigid examples from Mesopotamia. This open, multicultural atmosphere of professional and technical exchange would change with the passage of the medical torch to ancient Greece.[18]

There is much of interest from a medical-social perspective contained in the ancient medical experience of the West. For the first time in history, ancient Egypt wrestled with defining medical attendance and health services as a social good. Although primarily motivated by maintaining the workforce and developing

---

Afrocentricity is a scholarly movement that seeks to discover African agency in every situation without advancing African particularity as universal.

disease-prevention strategies, Egyptians defined health services as a universal right worthy of state subsidy. They provided medical care and health services for slaves and free men alike. Egyptian physicians also monitored and supervised remarkably satisfactory sanitation and hygiene conditions throughout the kingdom. Despite the view that keeping workmen and slaves healthy was in the ruling class's self-interest, the concept was an advanced one. Additionally, the Egyptian medical profession did portray themselves as a highly moral class who cared for all members of Egyptian society, from nobility to slaves. These were progressive medical-social concepts. Although Western European countries have implemented unitary health delivery systems dating back to the turn of the century, the polemic still rages in the United States today. Only the Republic of South Africa* and the United States continue to maintain stratified and unequal health systems based on race and class among the developed countries.[19]

A less communitarian approach to health care coexisted north of Egypt. The Mesopotamian medical experience includes Sumer, Akkadia, and Babylon. All of the various groups that dominated the region adopted and shared a common culture — including medicine and health care. Their approach to medicine and health delivery demonstrates that the hierarchical and unequal delivery of medical care also has ancient antecedents. The lower classes and slaves in their systems received virtually no health care, and little or no provision was made to supply it. The relationship between medicine and society was a meaner one than Egypt's,** reflecting the "eye for an eye, tooth for a tooth" philosophy transmitted to us through the Old Testament traditions nascent in the area. The monarchies and medical professions in that region of the ancient world obviously reconciled the disparate health delivery their systems provided on both the practical and ethical levels. Moreover, the sanitation and hygiene conditions of the civilizations occupying the fertile crescent were inferior to Egypt's.[20] Whether Egypt's African origins and that continent's strong tendencies toward collective living, generalized sharing of responsibilities, and aversion to individual ownership of vital resources has anything to do with these divergent patterns in health delivery and professional ethics poses interesting departures for future investigation.[21]

Ancient Greece: Establishing Western Science and Hierarchies

The Greek story is a pivotal one for several reasons. Greek civilization was a major contributor to Western culture and life sciences. The Greeks brought change. Most of these contributions were positive, and shaped the practices and

---

*The Republic of South Africa is making hesitant first steps toward a more just and equitable health system. Reform seems slow and a unitary system seems to be in the distant future.
**In some instances Mesopotamian doctors were punished by their hands being cut off if their patients died.

mores of Western civilization that we share today. The glowing imagery of Greek medicine portrayed by Sigerist, Nuland, and Lyons and Petrucelli is true but incomplete.[22] From the perspective of people of color, the Greek contribution was flawed, for it was tainted with certain aspects of both the biological and socio-cultural concepts of race and racism that continue to plague our civilization. Greek, and later European, ethnocentrism led to the deemphasis and often exclusion of contributions made by predecessor civilizations like the Egyptians. The Greeks can thus be portrayed with more complexity, as both heroes and villains. They elevated Western culture to new levels while planting the seeds of, if not actually initiating, some basic flaws relative to Western concepts of race, ethnicity, and class. Because of these dichotomies and tensions, examination of the Greek contribution to medicine and health care from an African American perspective is revealing, interesting, and challenging.

Greek philosophers introduced the reliance upon, and popularization of, the concepts of empiricism, objectivity, and logic. Under the influence of philosopher-scientists such as Thales (640?–546 BC), Anaximander (fl. c. 560 BC), Anaximenes (fl. c. 546 BC), and Pythagoras (fl. c. 530 BC), the Greek approach to the world deemphasized the mystical, magical, and superstitious—replacing them with the concrete and the natural. Medicine was no exception. These founding principles have shaped many facets of Western learning and have served as the foundation of the modern scientific method and the basis for much social progress.

Greeks were the dominant force in Western medicine from approximately 500 BC until AD 500. Until very recently, everyone was taught that Western medicine and health care started with ancient Greece during its golden age, around the fifth century BC. Upon closer examination, this turns out to be an oversimplification and, sometimes, a distortion of the facts. Such a wary appraisal of the conventional view of exclusively Greek medical beginnings seems appropriate in light of the evidence of the direct Greek medical borrowings from Mesopotamian and, especially, Egyptian medical traditions.[23] It seems that this cultural "kidnapping" had been successfully completed by the time of Alexander the Great in the fourth century BC. His installation of Ptolemy as Egypt's Pharaoh and establishment of Alexandria as the fount of Western knowledge and training served to further obscure and confuse the Egyptian contribution. By the time of the Roman Empire the myth of Greek pretensions as the sole originators of Western civilization, science, and medicine was formidable. The Romans, being a highly pragmatic people, both adopted and despised the Greeks' scholarly pretensions. Some of the most gifted Greek physicians and teachers were held as Roman slaves. As Diop, Bernal, Davidson, and Van Sertima have documented recently, it would require nineteenth-century European scholars to complete the process of reifying the Greeks and ablating the Africans' Egyptian contribution.[24]

By the time of the Classical Period of Greek civilization (ca. 500 BC), Greek cultural predispositions toward ethnocentricity, intolerance, and detachment began to distort and mar their more obvious gifts to Western civilization. The economic dependence of Greek civilization on the institution of slavery added another dimension to their negative cultural influence. The result was that such prominent Greek philosophers as Plato and Aristotle, often considered the philosophical fathers of modern science and medicine, began arbitrarily assigning slaves of all races a lesser status within the human family; they speculated that slaves were inherently inferior and less intelligent. There is also evidence that they injected and added some specific color prejudice toward Blacks and Asians.[25] This hierarchical ranking of the family of mankind based on slave status and color was something new. Chattel slavery was as old as civilization itself, and virtually all ancient civilizations and racial groups participated in the institution. Moreover, the majority of evidence suggests that before the period of Greek prominence in the Mediterranean basin, slaves were considered biologically and intellectually equal to all other people, and race was inconsequential.[26] There is no evidence that this did not apply to the medical arena.

The Greeks incorporated Imhotep along with the corpus of Egyptian medicine into their Asclepiad medical tradition. This was later grafted onto the Hippocratic medical and ethical traditions that linger today. Recent scholarship has documented that much of what was previously credited to Greek civilization is of African origin. Not just the spiritual impact of Egyptian medicine, as some scholars have projected, but also the emperico-rational and scientific approach to diseases and illnesses are medical legacies not wholly belonging to the Greeks. Both the Egyptians and Mesopotamians contributed heavily.

After beginning as itinerate, haphazardly trained, synthetic adherents of Mycenian, Cretan, Egyptian, and Asian medical traditions, Greek physicians began to change and establish a distinct identity by the sixth century BC. Pre-Socratic philosophers like Pythagoras, in a quest for harmony, explored medicine in great detail. Spawned by a litter of Greek medical schools at Croton, where Pythagoras dwelt; in Sicily; in Cyrene; in Asia Minor and the Archipelago at Rhodes; and in Cnidus and Cos, Hippocrates (460–370 BC) emerged as the "ideal" physician. He was a contemporary of Plato, a semi-legendary practitioner who travelled widely in Egypt and the Levant performing medical miracles for that time. Facts about him are few. We do know that he lived during the fifth century BC, that he was a famous practitioner and teacher of medicine, that he was born at Cos, and that he was a physician member of the Asclepiad cult. Most of his immortality is derived from his writings, called the Hippocratic Corpus, a huge collection of medical monographs, textbooks, manuals, speeches, extracts, and notes. His corpus, which originates from a variety of sources and authors, establishes that Greek medicine had become "a highly developed healing art which had succeeded in ridding itself of the magical and religious elements that still clung to ancient oriental medicine, and that it was guided by observation and experiment."[27] After the establishment of the Greek school of medicine at Alexandria, which collected and disseminated Hippocrates' corpus, his fame outstripped other legendary Greek physicians such as Praxagoras and Chrysippus.

This established him as the virtual deity of Western medicine. This tradition continues today.

During this "Golden Age," Greek physicians contributed many valuable principles to medicine — the most important being the detachment of disease and illness from superstition and religion. The empirical, objective approach to medicine would mature into the medical facet of the scientific method. By the time of the dominance of the cults and "schools" of medicine (actually, associations of philosophers, medical teachers, practitioners, and students) at Cnidos and Cos in the fifth century BC, Hippocratic physicians approached both diseases and sick patients as "natural" phenomena. They applied the principles of hypotheses, meticulous observation, and empiricism to their patients and their disease processes. This approach existed beside, and often complemented, the religious spa-like approach to illness perpetuated by the more ancient Asclepiad temple complexes.

These temple complexes have origins extending back to the Homeric healing god Asclepias as early as 1200 BC. They were variegated groupings of buildings that occupied grounds located in airy, wooded areas preferably near bodies of water. There were 200 to 300 Asclepiad temple complexes throughout the Classical Hellenic world. Sited on these park-like grounds were tablets, memorials, and benches containing gifts and testimonials to the miraculous cures effected at the Asclepian, as the complexes were called. The buildings usually consisted of a temple of Asclepias, which contained an altar, precious representations (often gold and ivory statues) of the god, and areas for the pilgrims to pray and sometimes convalesce; an *abaton* where the ill were placed to sleep, receive medications and treatments, and be visited by the god (represented by a priest-physician) and his attendants; a *tholos*, which was a round building usually containing purifying water from a pool or bubbling spring; entertainment buildings such as theaters, stadia, and gymnasiums; and often inns and temporary housing for visiting patrons. Healthy Greeks, who were as preoccupied with health as contemporary Americans, attended these Asclepia in numbers as great, if not greater, than the ill.

The Greek contribution was extremely positive relative to the establishment of Western medicine at the professional, didactic, and therapeutic levels. However, its medical-social contributions to health care cannot be viewed so favorably. Many authorities have noted that the Greeks institutionalized arrogance, social distancing, professional self-interest, class exclusivity, and cult-like behavior as acceptable norms within the medical profession; established a professionally focused, highly individualistic, societally irrelevant, paternalistic, materialistic, amoral medical ethic; laid the groundwork for the biomedical sciences to become involved in the hierarchical ranking of humanity; established a scientific climate of intolerance toward deviation from Western Classical physical norms; began the process of couching racist ideology in pseudoscientific guise; and encouraged a professional approach toward health delivery and health services reflecting Greek society's slavery and its medical profession's self-serving and weak social covenant. Close scrutiny of the Hippocratic Oath and corpus by medical ethicists reveal these characteristics. The public perception and trust in the medical profession's lofty ideals, dogged commitment to patients, and rigorous ethical codes are often misguided, or, at the very least, misunderstood.

Medical ethicists have pointed out that the Hippocratic Oath is a highly individualistic contract between independent agents, demonstrating little bonding, commitment, or concern with social well-being. Much like a religious order, physicians swear to maintain "trade secrets," vow to cover up for each other's mistakes or deficiencies, and pledge to preferentially channel the educational process to each other's children. The medical profession has done an excellent public relations job in the utilization of this relatively selfish, elitist, and autocratic oath.

Much of this ideology is reflected in how the Greeks delivered and distributed health services. Members of the Greek medical profession traveled widely in pursuit of fees from patients. Trained professionals had little concern for the poor, slaves, or lower classes. Both Plato and Aristotle described the hierarchy of Greek physicians and the different ways they practiced on different classes of people. As M. I. Finley stated about Plato's description of Greek medicine:

> There were actually two sorts of doctors . . . the free and their slave assistants, and "in most cases" it was the latter who treated slaves. That the slave's fees were substantially less is a further implication from the way Plato develops the difference between the two "kinds" of medical practice.[28]

The less fortunate got less sophisticated, less scientific care. Most fully trained physicians worked on a strictly fee-for-service basis and courted upper-class patients.[29]

In contrast, the Asclepiad cult's tradition provided some "charity" services for the poor. By the Classical Period, the Asclepiad temple complexes were manned predominantly by priests. Much self-congratulation and adulation centered around and was focused upon providing these eleemosynary services. Fee-for-service practice was also encouraged in the Asclepians for the majority of attendees. This is what allowed them to "write off" small amounts for the poor. All in all, slaves, the poor, or the lower classes received little medical attention in ancient Greece.

These practices established a precedent of "walling off" the poor and disadvantaged from health services as the norm for Western medicine. It also served to institutionalize the medical profession as an upper-class vocation from the professional, patient, and health services perspective. Obtaining health care was certainly a "privilege" from a Greek perspective. This allowed the Greek medical profession to rationalize the inequitable delivery of health services based on the highly individualistic characteristics of the Hippocratic ethical tradition.[30]

Whether these traits, which still linger in the American medical profession, are part of this continuum is debatable. Many still defend the individualistic ethical concerns of the U.S. profession based on Hippocratic traditions. American allusions to the worthiness of idealizing Classical civilization pervade everything from the nation's art museums and academic traditions to its institutional architecture. Evidence that the idealization of ancient Greek civilization has not always been put to good use in the United States was its application as a defense of the antebellum South's slave-based plantation system in the nineteenth century.

Moreover, Greek attitudes toward hierarchies, typologies, and categories spilled over into their medical science. Greek physicians Herophilus (c. 300 BC) and Erasistratus (c. 260 BC) of Alexandria were possibly the first Western physicians reputed to use prisoners for vivisection at a time when that practice was banned universally.[31] As Celsus (fl. 14–37), the Roman scholar-historian, wrote of their experimentation on the defenseless:

> *Herophilos and Erasistratos . . . laid open men whilst alive—criminals received out of prison from the kings—and whilst these were still breathing, observed parts which beforehand nature had concealed, their position, colour, shape, size, arrangement, hardness, softness, smoothness, relation, process and depressions of each, and whether any part is inserted or is received into another.*[32]

The overutilization of the poor, defenseless, and disenfranchised for medical experimentation and demonstration purposes had begun in Western medicine. Slaves and criminals were especially convenient subgroups for these purposes. However, most ancient pagan religions served to limit these professional activities. Later, the teachings and doctrines of the Christian church, with its prohibitions on dissection and murder, would inhibit the medical profession in this regard. Physicians would be attacked and mobbed for human dissection, experimentation, and suspected grave-robbing until the nineteenth century in Europe. Later, African American slaves, who were routinely exploited for such purposes, would benefit from far less societal or religious protection.[33]

Roman Medicine: Legions, Slaves, and Public Health

Roman medicine is an enigma. Historians ask why the most sophisticated civilization of the ancient world was so backward medically. As Harvard physician-historian Guido Majno observed about Roman medicine, "Hippocrates passed away; Alexandria sprang up, Greek medicine discovered the laboratory. And all this time the Romans had no physicians at all."[34] Pliny may have answered questions surrounding this shocking revelation in very commonsense terms. He offered a six-word explanation about this mystery: *"non rem antiqui damnabant, sed artem;* 'it was not medicine itself that the forefathers condemned, but medicine as a profession . . . chiefly because they refused to pay fees to profiteers in order to save their own lives.'"[35] Thus, Majno alleges that "for six hundred years the frugal Romans carried on with folk remedies. Surely there was no reason to pay for *those.*"[36] Even if that does not answer the major questions regarding the health status, outcomes, and care received by Black and disadvantaged Romans, a primary focus of this inquiry, it says a great deal about the Roman character and attitudes about health care.[37]

Only when a plague struck in 293 BC and the Romans sent an emergency envoy to Epidauros, the famed Greek healing center, did their medical isolation end. Whatever the charm was that the Greeks sent (reputedly it was Asclepios in the form of a snake), it worked. For unknown reasons, the plague abated. Nevertheless, it was not until 219 BC that the first Greek physician, Archagathus, immigrated to Rome and established a successful medical practice. These are the incredible and unlikely legends surrounding the birth of scientific Roman medicine. Pliny's first-century account corroborates Majno's impressions, stating: "The Roman people for more than six hundred years were not without medical art but were without physicians."[38] However, the Roman reception to the learned, but limited, ancient medicine remained lukewarm throughout the time of the empire. Because of the limited efficacy of ancient medicine, though the Greek version was the best, the Romans were never convinced that medicine was a legitimate profession worthy of the costly expenditures associated with its administration. This helps explain why throughout Roman history, medicine remained a profession dominated by foreigners—the Greeks, Egyptians, and the Jews—most of whom were probably slaves. The pragmatic and cynical character of the Romans again remained consistent.[39]

It is not rash to say that Roman medicine was in many ways a Greek afterthought. The Greeks truly dominated Roman medicine in both word and deed, and the Romans never became jealous of their dependency upon, and lack of participation in, what they considered an unwholesome and somewhat unworthy profession. As Guthrie reiterates in *A History of Medicine:*

> *Measured in terms of the diagnosis and treatment of disease the Roman contribution was negligible, because . . . medical practice was in the hands of the Greeks. . . . [W]hile Rome, apart from Greek aid, contributed little to the advance of scientific medicine, she set a great example to the world by the inauguration of a system of public hygiene which in some aspects has never been excelled.*[40]

The latter three quarters of the Roman period from 250 BC to AD 600 served as one of the major transitional periods between ancient Greek medical innovation and the European Renaissance. Arabic medical dominance during the early

Middle Ages served as the other. Therefore, scientifically, the period can be looked upon as one of consolidation instead of innovation in many fields—and medicine was no exception. It was consistent with the pragmatism and sobriety of the Roman character to emphasize military medicine and public health.

Because of epidemics and the growing awareness of their practitioners' shortcomings, foreign physicians were summoned and encouraged to settle in Rome after 250 BC. With the arrival of Greek physicians such as Archagathos in 219 BC, Asclepiad and Hippocratic traditions began to dominate Roman medicine. With the Roman conquest of the Greeks, this transformation was completed on the intellectual and practical levels.[41]

However, the lowly status of the physician in Roman society still hung like a cloud over the profession. The tradition of consigning the role of physicians to slaves persisted, with Greek slave-physicians being preferred over other ethnic physicians. The strong academic inclinations and standing of the Greeks continued their tradition as tutors and teachers. Paradoxically, the Romans came to depend on physicians, although in many ways they despised them. Ambivalent feelings were counteracted by incessant wars, which had created a Roman market for competent, efficient physicians and surgeons. Greek physicians performed so well and acquired such exalted reputations that by the time of Julius Caesar they were being granted honorary Roman citizenship for their services, especially if they worked as military physicians.[42]

Rome became the capital of the world, and medical success during that time was largely defined there. Influential Greek physicians such as Asclepiades (first century BC), Thessalus of Tralles, and Soranus of Ephesus during the second century AD migrated to practice in Rome. Although challenged by schools of medical theory and practice such as the Dogmatists, Methodists, and the Empiricists, the Hippocratic school would come to dominate because of the efforts and writings of Soranus and the last demigod of Greek medicine, Galen of Pergamum (AD 129 to c. AD 199).

Galen was the dominant figure in Roman medicine. He was an amalgamator and synthesizer of the major currents of Greek philosophy, medicine, surgery, and therapeutics. Early in his career he added some anatomical and scientific discoveries to the Greek corpus through experimentation, but later in his life he transformed into one of the most dogmatic scientists of recorded history. Although his anti-Black prejudices and contributions to scientific racism were alluded to in Chapter 1, his medical scope was encyclopedic and he recorded virtually everything he touched. His massive written legacy would be preserved by passing through Oriental Christian and Arab cultures, helping elevate him into a medical deity in the process. Galen's humoral theories, anatomical treatises, and physiological explanations remained unquestioned until the Italian physician-anatomist Vesalius in 1543 and English physician-physiologist Harvey in 1628 disproved some of his work. Thus, he and his Arab promulgators truly dominated Western medicine for an unprecedented 45 generations.

Though somewhat backward scientifically and therapeutically had it not been for the infusion of Greek physicians and medical practices into their system, Roman medicine broke new ground from a public health standpoint. As Guthrie has noted: "Although the Romans were content to leave the practice of medicine and surgery to the Greeks, they were not slow to realize the value of organization of medical teaching and of medical services for the poor and for the army and navy."[43] This is a reflection of the Romans' singular and brilliant organizational and administrative talents. Seemingly, they viewed medicine and health care delivery as weapons of public and diplomatic policy. During the period of Roman dominance the following public health triumphs occurred: the marshes surrounding Rome responsible for endemic malaria and other diseases were drained; the Cloaca Maxima, or main sewer, was constructed by the sixth century BC; after the third century aqueducts were built supplying Rome with copious amounts of fresh water; Roman houses were provided with plumbing and sanitation; and magnificent public baths were available with dressing rooms, hot and cold baths, gymnasia, and swimming pools. Such public health feats and programs would not be approached in the West again until the nineteenth century. It must be remembered that most physicians in Rome were foreigners and slaves. Although the overwhelming majority of physicians in the empire were denied high social status, or even freedom for that matter, they were essential cogs in the system. For example, under the reign of Emperor Vespasian (AD 69–79) teachers of medicine were provided at public expense. This measure was probably implemented to ensure an adequate supply of physicians for Roman military and public service. Guthrie observes that in the Roman army's fighting services, "medical men were part of the establishment, and although they ranked only as noncommissioned officers, they were exempt from taxation and from combatant duty."[44] There were both legionary and cohort surgeons working as a team, and each ship of the line had an assigned surgeon. Early in the empire's history, public physicians, or *archiatri*, were hired to attend the poor. Though the quality and pay of these providers varied, they were distributed to towns and districts according to the population. Another Roman innovation with public health implications was their establishment of hospitals. The legend of the first civilian hospital established in Rome involves the same plague or pestilence described earlier, which struck the city in 293 BC. The legend is that the emergency mission that was dispatched from Epidaurus sent a ship armed with a sacred serpent entrusted with healing. The ship landed on the island of St. Bartholomew in the Tiber River. Rome survived the plague, and the hospital that was built there survived to become a hospital for slaves and the poor. In a subsequent period, an emigrant monk from the site, Rahere, was sent to and founded St. Bartholomew Hospital in London in AD 1123. By the first and second centuries AD, there are creditable records of well-developed private and public hospitals, nursing homes, and military hospitals established at various strategic points throughout the empire.[45]

Despite these strikingly modern features, the overall Roman system perpetuated the hierarchical approach to medical care initiated by the Greeks and Mesopotamians. The few academically trained Roman physicians, virtually all of whom were of Greek nationality, focused their attention on caring for rich or upper-class patients. This was expected in a system where, as Bullough points out, there "was a lack of any legal regulations for either the training or qualifications of medical teachers or practitioners."[46] Thus, Galen's vitriolic outbursts about this situation were seemingly grounded in fact. There was a chronic shortage of well-trained physicians for the empire's growing needs. Indirect evidence supporting this impression is that:

> *Caesar, for example, during the famine of 46 BC ordered the expulsion of foreigners from Rome but specifically exempted physicians and teachers. . . . Even slave physicians received special privileges. The Emperor Augustus granted physicians immunity from taxes and other burdens, and these privileges were renewed or confirmed by the Emperor Vespasian and later codified by the Emperor Hadrian.*[47]

Seemingly, as noted earlier, even military physicians were well treated. One result of this situation was that on the rare occasions disadvantaged people in Rome received medical care or services, slave physicians or assistants were retained by physicians, institutions, or governments to provide medical services to them.[48] Moreover, the Greek attitudes of slave inferiority were perpetuated if not intensified during Roman times. As historians and classicists such as Sir Moses Finley, Jean Devisse, and St. Clair Drake observed about the deteriorating racial relations affecting the Roman empire by the early Christian era:

> *[T]he color symbolism of Ethiopian bodies arose in the cultural context that produced the fundamentally racist ideas of Julian the Apostate* and Galen the physician—a multiethnic Roman Empire that was bringing people of different racial groups into contact on a scale never before seen, thus exacerbating ethnic and class tensions.*[49]

Galen exacerbated these already escalating race and class tensions by passing along his negative racial attitudes toward Blacks in his medical writings. He

> *mentions ten specific attributes of the Black man, which are all found in him and in no other; frizzy hair, thin eyebrows, broad nostrils, thick lips,*

---

*Julian the Apostate was the fourth-century AD Roman emperor in Constantinople who, although raised as a Christian, tried to reinstate paganism as the state religion. He also wanted to implement racial discrimination and segregation, arguing that the wide range of physical differences among men was not consistent with the theory of a common ancestor.

> *pointed teeth, smelly skin, Black eyes, furrowed hands and feet, a long*
> *penis and great merriment. Galen says that merriment dominates the*
> *Black man because of his defective brain, whence also the weakness of*
> *his intelligence.*[50]

Although Roman medicine seemed not to be preoccupied or dominated by racism, there is evidence that Galen's attitudes influenced medical teachings in the Byzantine, Arab, and Medieval Christian worlds.[51] Since Galen and his Arab protegés dominated Western medical teachings for 45 generations, logic dictates that these prejudicial racial attitudes have had a negative impact on the Western scientific medicine that followed. How much effect these ideologies, writings, and practices had on the later pseudoscientific biological justification and rationale for racism in Western culture is still being studied.[52] These negative racial attitudes within the life sciences had to affect the health status expectations regarding Blacks, the efforts exerted to ensure equal health service delivery to Blacks, and the professional and policy responses to the poor health status of patients of Black African descent. Results of these phenomena were devastating to Black people.[53]

Another set of forces descended on the Roman health and medical-social worlds. The rise of Christianity paralleled the Roman era. This was especially so during the Empire's latter centuries. Christianity's medical effects were largely confined to the medical-social and ethical spheres. Although there probably were Christian physicians, their number and prominence were relatively small, and they probably exerted minimal effects on medicine professionally, or upon health services delivery.

Christian doctrine brought into question the dominant hierarchical approach to health care delivery. The new religion advocated care and compassion for the poor and disadvantaged. This conflicted with Roman social practices. Although Christianity was burdened with the old Canaan and Ham legends (which ascribed incestuous and other negative characteristics to the dark-skinned son of Noah), it did promote an egalitarian social ethic. Religion's contribution to the Black inferiority myth would become more prominent and important during later periods.[54]

Further Roman contributions to medicine or health care would be cut short by the military dissolution of the Roman Empire after the sixth century AD.

The Middle Ages

The Middle Ages are conveniently looked upon as the period from the fall of the Roman Empire (some date this as early as AD 476, when the final Caesar, Romulus Augustulus, was deposed by invaders) to the beginning of the Renaissance (often dated as 1453, when Constantinople fell to the Turks). After the Greco-

Roman military collapse starting in the fourth century AD, the Roman Empire gradually dissolved. So-called barbarian invasions swept over Italy and most of Europe, with Rome finally being sacked by the Visigoths and Vandals in AD 410 and AD 455, respectively. These Caucasian northern tribesmen, including the Lombards, Franks, Goths, Saxons, and Burgundians, were the ancestors of most of the present European population. Uneducated and unsophisticated for the time, they sometimes crippled or destroyed the previous social, legal, political, and educational infrastructures. However, just as often they adopted and incorporated much of the sophisticated Roman culture into those they established. Their destructiveness and negative effect have been overemphasized by historians, for the replacement of the decayed remnants of the Roman Empire had been eminent since before AD 300.[55]

Christianity had been on the rise in Rome since the days of Peter and Paul around AD 67. Evidence of the power of this largely unrecorded social movement, heavily adopted by the poor and underprivileged, led to an edict of toleration of Christian worship in the Empire by AD 312. Constantine (AD 274–337), the Roman Emperor, would be baptized a Christian 24 years later, and Christianity would later become the official state religion. The rise of the Christian Church during the dissolution and splitting of the Empire during the fourth century led to Church domination of the political vacuum left after the Empire's collapse on the Italian peninsula. The Eastern Roman Empire headquartered in Constantinople since AD 395 charted its own history until 1453. In Western Europe, Christian conversion of Germanic invaders led to an Age of Faith, or a domination of the supernatural over the natural world in men's minds. Led by philosophers such as St. Augustine, this mute acceptance of inevitability, fatalism, and substitution of faith for reason by the converted Germanic Christians led to the characterization of this epoch as the "Dark Ages." Illiteracy, serfdom, and feudalism dominated Italy, the old seat of the Roman Empire, and most of Europe by the eighth century.[56]

Such a dominance and submission to religion stagnated the mode of thinking that usually resulted in medical progress. Dissection was strictly outlawed until the late thirteenth century, and experimentation was frowned upon by the Church. Aggressive interventions such as surgery into divinely determined illnesses were circumscribed, and questioning supernatural explanations of diseases or illnesses was considered heretical. The result was a return to religious medicine. It became more magical and mystical instead of scientific, and declined in social and scientific influence.

In Europe medical practice came to be dominated by clerics in the early Middle Ages. The period between AD 500 and AD 1130 can be considered the age of monastic medicine. This occurred because Christian monks felt that healing and health care represented an extension of their moral obligations to assist the poor and disadvantaged. Beginning with St. Benedict, healing and health care were adopted by the monks. Thus, the earliest European hospitals and craft-like medical schools were located in monasteries or near churches. Moreover, the monks being the sole, secure repository of literacy, copied and preserved the available medical manuscripts, textbooks, and literature. This also served to supplement their database to function as practitioners. The dominant sources they preserved included medical forefathers such as Aristotle, Galen, Rhazes, Avicenna, and Hippocrates. There is no evidence at this time that the monks added to or compounded the net effect of this racist material as they translated, copied, and preserved the classical and Moslem medical corpuses.

The monastic-dominated period of Medieval medicine lasted until the twelfth century. Because of doctrinal considerations the Church began pressuring monks to dissolve their medical missions and functions. When the Council of Clermont in 1130 forbade monks to practice medicine, considering the profession too disruptive for an orderly life in monastic sequestration, the age of monastic medicine began to be terminated officially. This divorce of medicine from the clergy was further accentuated by the Council of Tours in 1163, which effectively took surgery out of the hands of church-based physicians by forbidding clergy to perform surgery. This divorce between medicine and surgery in Europe would not be healed for centuries.

As these repressive measures changed the profile of European medicine, taking medical teaching out of the cloisters, mature Arabic medical traditions emerged. Moreover, scholastic-based monastic medicine had been ideal for classroom, not clinical, teaching. These forces increased the move toward a more secular-based university system of medical education in Western Europe. Medical schools affiliated with the new network of European medieval universities at places such as Salerno (c. ninth century) in southern Italy, Montpellier (c. ninth century) in France, and Bologna (c. thirteenth century) in northern Italy arose to fill the breach. They not only produced practitioners but also helped professionalize medicine.

Christian doctrinal and sectarian battles at Constantinople led to medical sects like the Nestorians being expelled to Asia in AD 431. A group of Christian sectarians who were driven out of the Byzantine Empire, the Nestorians relocated and translated Greek authors into Semitic languages such as Syriac or Hebrew, and later Arabic. By the tenth century, the Arabs, grounded with this classical Greek background, had developed and innovated their own classical medical literature. Christian sectarians had translated all the classical Greek medical writings into Arabic at Damascus by AD 707, Cairo by AD 874, and Baghdad by AD 918.

The Christian sectarians also assisted in establishing medical schools and hospitals and prospered at places such as Edessa by AD 489. They eventually established a medical school and hospital at Jundi Shapur in Persia. Jundi Shapur was the dominant intellectual crossroads of Asia during this period, and the Nestorians flourished under royal patronage. When the city fell to the Arabs in AD 636, the university was not only preserved but also adopted by the Moslem conquerors. It became the Moslem empire's principal medical training center. This medical center became one of the major bibliographic trunklines preserving and later transferring Hellenic and Galenic medical knowledge. During the next six centuries, this scientific medical knowledge would reach the West. The interaction between Arab and European medicine at cities such as Salerno, Montpellier, Toledo, and Cordoba allowed the vital transfers of knowledge to European medicine.[57]

The late Middle Ages would mark the beginning of a joint clerical and secular-based hospital movement that spread all over Europe. Some early examples were the Hotel-Dieu of Lyon, France (c. 542); the Hotel-Dieu of Paris (c. 652); and the Santa Maria della Scala in Siena, Italy (c. 898).[58] These facilities, largely controlled by university-trained professional physicians, facilitated the dissemination of medical treatments to a large base of the population. They also involved the European medical profession and their patrons in the health of their communities and provided a base for professional advancement on technical and therapeutic levels. The stage was gradually set for medicine to become a true profession. Moreover, this process and pattern of early legitimization and acceptance of medicine into the mainstream of university training in Europe would profoundly affect observed differences between the European and American professions. In contrast, the American profession would remain a somewhat powerless, craft-like profession with little cultural authority until the late nineteenth century. Only after worship of the new science became integral to a new American ethos would a window of opportunity for accrual of medical power and authority present itself in the nineteenth century. Furthermore, the U.S. profession would remain largely detached from the university system until then. These dynamics help explain American medicine's fears regarding untrained practitioners and the monumental sectarian wars that raged within the profession until the twentieth century. Moreover, American medicine's future development would be shaped largely by professional self-interest instead of within a framework of providing a service and medical social good, as required by the royal, clerical, and aristocratic patrons of the university-trained European physicians and their institutional and educational systems. Thus, the origins of the U.S. medical profession's detachment and social insensitivity, if not irresponsibility, becomes more comprehensible and understandable.

Meanwhile, access to medical care declined for the average citizen in Western Europe. This was most striking during the early Middle Ages. Not until the Renaissance would availability and access to medical care approach Roman levels. The number of secular practitioners declined. During the early Middle Ages the relatively rare clerical practitioners functioned strictly within the confines of their religious institutions. Moreover, they were preoccupied with metaphysical and deontological aspects of medicine instead of patient care. Only the rational and scientific medical approaches of the Arabists (who embraced all components of the tradition, including Nestorian Christians, Persians, Jews, Orientals, and

Arabs) incorporating the classical Greco-Roman preservations and their contemporary contributions in therapeutics and clinical medicine counteracted these trends. Not until the rise of the university-based medical schools and the community hospitals in the thirteenth and fourteenth centuries would these trends begin to change in Western Europe.

Who received appropriate medical care and how often was socially determined. Whether a patient was well treated from a medical, technical, or social standpoint when he or she interacted with the health system was, and continues to be, largely determined by the physician. These facts reveal the early linkages between the societal and professional effects of racism as a dominative sociocultural construct affecting health services delivery. Currently there is a growing scholarship about negative European attitudes toward Blacks during the Middle Ages. With the dissolution of the Roman Empire it is clear that with the exception of the Iberian peninsula, European interaction with Black Africa declined. As Jean Devisse, one of the modern scholars studying racism during this period, states in *The Image of Blacks in Western Art*:

> *Particularly between the sixth and the eleventh century the Occident fashioned an entire imagery based on prejudice and errors which "cultivated" minds substituted, century after century, for objective thinking about Africa and Blacks. This situation sprang primarily from lack of knowledge which was sustained by the absence of physical contact between Africa and Europe.*[59]

Moreover, until 1453 the European demand for chattel labor had largely been satiated by trade with the East, which supplied slaves of Slavic or Asian lineage. There is some visual representational, literary, and documentary evidence in this new field of inquiry that this period of racial isolation tended to intensify negative Black images as anti-ethical and contrary to purity and chastity; undermine positive mythical Black images, such as the noble Ethiopian, the noble king (i.e., the Black wise man), and Prester John; and, allow the Christian curse mythology of Canaan and Ham to become crystallized in the public mind and institutionalized. Little-known today is the fact that Blacks have not always been considered inferior as a group. Not until the concept of racial inferiority was buttressed by the authority of Western science after the fifteenth century was Black biological and racial inferiority a universally accepted Western cultural assumption.[60]

When we pick up the European thread of racial history after widespread use of the printing press in the fifteenth and sixteenth centuries, Europe had already developed prejudicial racial attitudes toward Blacks.[61] History has also yielded evidence that despite medical ethical oaths or lofty, professional public images, physicians—American or otherwise—treat patients on medical-social and professional levels in ways that mirror the dominant social norms. Medical writings, professional conduct, and the clinical treatment of African Americans during slavery and during the apogee of pseudoscientific racist belief during the late nineteenth and early twentieth centuries by the White American medical profession serve as examples.[62]

Although racial biases and negative stereotypes toward Blacks were contained in Greek, Roman, and Arabic medical literature and writings, their effect on the minuscule amount of Black patient care or health delivery that must have been rendered by White physicians to Black patients in Europe (excluding the Iberian peninsula) during this period is impossible to measure. However, the inclusion of racial material with this bias, especially Galen's, in the academic corpus of the profession certainly laid a foundation for future problems at all levels of the biomedical sciences. If this body of literature guided and informed the future progress in fields like clinical medicine, anatomy, biology, physiology, pharmacy, surgery, public health, health services, and medical ethics, the roots of the medical-cultural and racial problems affecting these fields today becomes comprehensible. Being educated by these writings would logically affect future physicians like Carl Linnaeus, Petrus Camper, and Benjamin Rush—men whose racial biases would mar a great deal of what they did from a contemporary perspective. Moreover, the effect that opinion and pronouncements from these disciplines have had on the general society's rationalizations and justifications for racism is incalculable. Galen and the scientific community began and perpetuated a tradition of helping make Western culture's racial prejudices "legitimate."[63]

The Arabic Legacy of Race and Slavery

During the first 500 years of the Christian era (AD 500–1000), barbarian invasions of the West, recurrent pestilences and disasters, and the zealous anti-Hellenism of the Christian Church destroyed many of the Greek and Roman writings that formed the basis of Western civilization. The loss to medicine was substantial. During this lull in Western dominance, Muhammad (570–632) founded the Islamic religion. Over the next century, Islam swept through the Near and Middle East into Africa, Spain, and southern France. This religious-based revolutionary dispersion of Moslem culture spurred the founding of three dynastic caliphates: the Abbasids (750–1258) in Persian Baghdad, the Umayyads (756–1031) in the Spanish West headquartered at Cordova, and the Fatimids (909–1171) based at Egyptian Cairo.

Beginning with works by early scholars like Stanley Lane-Poole and later research by Bernard Lewis and Ronald Sanders, we discover that the Iberian social climate was quite different from the rest of Europe from a racial perspective. Black/White contact was not only frequent but was sometimes adversarial and marked by violence. In fact, this area served as the embattled interface between African-Moslem and European-Christian cultures between 711 and 1492. Moreover, these wars of the *Reconquista* by the White, European Christians against the dominant rulers—the Black African Moors—planted many of the seeds of European color prejudice and racism that later guided European relationships with non-White peoples. Significantly, this provided a training ground in racial antagonism and dominance toward people of color for the Spanish and Portuguese— who later led the Age of Exploration. The depiction of Black Moors as villains and the recurrent waves of intolerance, inquisition, and expulsion of Moors and Jews that have marked Spanish history are celebrated and well known today.* These connections explain Sanders's reference to the "Iberian germ of racism" as a major theme in his *Lost Tribes and Promised Lands: The Origins of American Racism*.[64]

Internally, the openness and tolerance characterizing early Black Moorish rule, which transmitted the brightest cultural light to Europe in the Middle Ages, would erode Moslem power. The slave trade, polygamous family structures, and an erosion of discipline and morals among the ruling Umayyad elite led to the dynasty's end in AD 1031. As George O. Cox states in *African Empires and Civilizations*:

> This penetration [of the Black race by the Caucasian] *was facilitated not alone by the dominant position of the African race, but also by its tendency to polygamy . . . on the one hand, a violent penetration of the conquered people by the polygamous invader, through their womenfolk; and on the other, the attraction exerted by the Saracen women . . . upon men of the defeated race.*[65]

This undermining process was augmented by a burgeoning slave trade. As Chandler points out, "This slave trade changed the racial mix in Al-Andulus. The use of European women as concubines gradually lightened the complexion of Moorish Spain."[66] The societal effects of these complex processes tended to institutionalize color prejudice against dark-skinned Blacks, mark them as a predominantly slave class in Iberian culture, and lay the foundation for the racism that would later undergird the Atlantic slave trade.[67]

Between the eighth and twelfth centuries, Western knowledge and intellectual traditions were rescued, preserved, and perpetuated by Arab Moslem cultures. Increasingly, the major contribution to medicine by the Arabs is now being acknowledged. They made miraculous academic, therapeutic, and pharmacological contributions to Western medicine, but some unfortunate medical-social ones. Arab preservation of Classical medical texts by masters such as Aristotle, Galen, and Hippocrates provided the fundamental medical traditions required for continuity, progress, and survival. The almost reverent adoption of the Galenic and Hellenic medical texts containing their racist typology and stereo-

---

*Celebrations of Christian-Spanish conquest of the dark Moslem Moors and expulsion or conversion of the Jews from the Iberian peninsula are reenacted today in both Spain and New World countries with Iberian roots.

types, combined with the social dynamic taking place on the Iberian peninsula, had adverse effects on Moslem medical practices. Thus, Moslem physicians, including Avicenna, added their own anti-Black prejudices, which had been incorporated into Arabic society, to the racial biases they inherited from Roman physicians such as Galen. Although not preoccupied with racist ideology and considerations, Moslem medical practices were marred by the institutional effects of slavery and racism. Slaves received less medical care and attention, and blackness accentuated this discrimination.[68]

Based on a Moslem cultural tradition of respect—even worship—of knowledge, Arab possessors of a relatively backward indigenous medical tradition attended medical schools at Alexandria and throughout the Levant and quickly caught up and surpassed their European, Egyptian, Jewish, and Asian teachers. Between the eighth and fifteenth centuries, the Arabs made remarkable and irreplaceable contributions to medical progress. Between the ninth and thirteenth centuries they were emblematic of scientific medicine, totally dominating the Western profession.

Physicians such as Rhazes (d. 925), Isaac Judaeus (850–950), Haly Abbas (fl. tenth century), and Avicenna (d. 1037) in the Eastern Caliphate, and Averroes (d. 1198), Avenzoar (1091?–1162), Miamonides (1135–1204), and Albucasis (d. after 1009) in the Western Caliphate led Western medicine for 400 years and influenced it for another 1,500 years. Moreover, there was a great deal of interaction between the Moslem and Christian professions. This interaction took three primary forms. The first was through the translation of the Classical and Arabic medical treatises, textbooks, and documents by the monks in monasteries scattered throughout Western Europe; the second, through transmission of the Arabic and Classical medical traditions through medical school faculty activity and clinical teaching during the late Middle Ages, especially when those physicians were of Jewish, Arab, or Nestorian Christian backgrounds; and the third, through the direct transmission of Classical and Eastern medical traditions through Constantine the African (1010–1087) and his activities enhancing and expanding the Salernitan medical school's database with the largest transfusion of Classical and Eastern data up to that time. Some of the effects Arabic medicine had on Western medicine are still manifested today.

As was noted previously, Plato, Aristotle, and Galen—pillars of the Classical Greek medical tradition—transmitted prejudicial, and some clearly racist, material in the corpus of their works. Some of these serve as the foundations of Western medicine. Initially collected and preserved at Alexandria and later incorporated in the sometimes encyclopedic medical works of Moslem physicians such as Rhazes (author of the *Almansor*) and Avicenna (author of the *Canon*), these medical-social views were transfused into Western medicine. Moreover, unfortunate racially biased attitudes toward Black people grew in Moslem culture throughout the same period. Undoubtedly, these racist developments affected the Moslem institutions of slavery throughout the period of the Middle Ages, the social and political systems with regard to race in Moslem society, and health care as reflected in the deprecatory view Moslem physicians had toward Black people. Again, in the aggregate, this conundrum of events was, and continues to be, devastating for Black people.[69]

The Scientific and Medical Renaissance: Inauspicious Racial and Medical-Social Roots

The Renaissance can be viewed as that transition period between Medieval and modern times that took place between the fourteenth and sixteenth centuries. It was marked by a humanistic* revival of classical influence. This resulted in a flowering of the arts and literature and the beginnings of modern science. The Renaissance is said to have begun in Italy in the 1300s, as symbolized by the paintings of Giotto and Masaccio, sculptures of Pisano and Donnatello, architecture of Brunelleschi, and the writings of Petrarch and Dante. The emergence of modern science was similarly associated with the works and writings of Nicolaus Copernicus (1473–1543), Tycho Brahe (1546–1601), and Galileo Galilei (1564–1642).

This was the epoch in which science emerged as an entity distinguishable from other branches of philosophy. Until the Renaissance, for example, scholars who focused on the material world of the solar system, plants, mineral and organic substances, and animals were referred to as natural philosophers. Other contributors to knowledge of the physical world were identified with the realm of magic and alchemy. The artisans and craftsmen who built the machines, structures, and devices required by increasingly complex civilizations were a third influence altering man's relationship to the material world. By the end of the Renaissance, after much interaction and cross-pollination from these three realms, their descendants would be called scientists.

Aristotle and the Greeks had brought reason, rationality, and objectivity to science—a method of dispassionate observation. Most influenced by these antecedents were astronomer-mathematicians such as Copernicus, Galileo, and Kepler, who added quantification and numbers to the study of natural phenomena. Much of the scientific reawakening in the fifteenth and sixteenth centuries was concentrated in physics, astronomy, and mathematics. After the end of the Renaissance, with the publication of Sir Isaac Newton's *Principia* in 1687, the disciplines of mathematics, physics, optics, astronomy, and motion had been synthesized into a coordinated system of scientific inquiry built upon previous observation and experimentation, which provided the foundation for further research.

Humanism is the notion that humans are the measure of all things and that the fulfillment of each individual's potential is the goal of civilization.

A series of scientific instrumentation and measuring tools had also evolved. Although these men's work and craftsmanship focused largely on astronomy, mathematics, and physics, their ideas influenced the activities in all fields of science.[70] Even though medical treatments remained largely ineffective, scientific discoveries and progress were also being made in medicine and biology.

Many important events that occurred in the pre-Renaissance period prepared the field for the emergence of scientific medicine. Not only had there been an increase in medical activity between 1050 and 1225, but medical schools also became centers of medical practice in Europe. These schools were supplied with classical medical data of Egyptian, African, Mesopotamian, Hebrew, Oriental, and Greco-Roman origin that were preserved and transmitted through Arabic and pre-Renaissance medical schools and training facilities like Jundi Shapur (fifth- and sixth-century Persia), Cordoba (eighth- to tenth-century Spain), and Salerno (tenth-century Italy). European medical schools affiliated with universities opened at Bologna (early thirteenth century), Montpellier (twelfth century), Paris (thirteenth century), and Padua (thirteenth century). The study of medicine joined theology and the law as highly respected European academic courses of study. In contrast with American academic medicine, which would not become institutionally affiliated with universities until the nineteenth century, medical studies would remain highly respected components of European academic life.[71]

Built upon this foundation, Western medicine flourished during the Renaissance. For the first time medical forefathers such as Plato, Aristotle, and Galen would be questioned and their theories refuted and discarded based upon more objective, scientific information. The ultimate effects of their pseudoscientific, culture-based, biological deterministic, sometimes racist, material on Western medical development and practices remains virtually unevaluated. Scholars such as Stephen Jay Gould, James H. Jones, Allan Chase, Allen M. Brandt, and Stephen Thomas have recognized the importance of this field of inquiry in light of the subsequent misuse of science to validate racial and class-based social prejudices and discriminatory practices.[72]

Renaissance medical forefathers such as German physician Theophrastus Bombastus von Hohenheim, or Paracelsus (1493–1541), originated disease-specific inquiries and treatments and pioneered public health and occupational medicine besides. Paracelsus, considered the "Father of Pharmacology" for his advances in chemical therapeutics, introduced therapies such as mercurials for syphilis and iron for various ailments. However, Paracelsus also espoused a racist view of separate creations for Africans and other peoples of color whom he felt originated from different and inferior ancestors.[73] With the June 1543 publication of Vesalius's (1514–1564) *De humani corporis fabrica libri septem,* Galen's 1,400-year-old anatomical mistakes were corrected scientifically for the first time. Another graduate of the University of Padua's medical school, William Harvey (1578–1657), placed physiology on a scientific basis with his 1628 publication,

Exercitatio anatomica de Motu Cordis et Sanguinis in animalibus [*On the Movement of the Heart and Blood in Animals*].

The scientific method and experimentation, which revolutionized medical and biological progress as shown by this tiny sample of examples, was also augmented by the fact that anatomical dissection became accepted by clerics and the general populace for medical training in the thirteenth century and became commonplace throughout Western Europe by the fifteenth. Although Catholic Church policies shifted away from the study and practice of medicine around the thirteenth century, the medical profession was supported by both the church and the aristocracy in the building of hospitals and financial provision of health care. The passing of the torch of medical advance to Western Europe by the time of the Renaissance by this confluence of scientific and social circumstances becomes comprehensible.[74]

From a medical-social perspective, the fourteenth to sixteenth centuries represented increasing contact between European societies and Africans through the evolution and development of the Atlantic, and to a lesser extent the Mediterranean, slave trade. The rise of the Ottoman Empire (late thirteenth to early twentieth centuries), especially after the 1453 Moslem Turkish conquest of Constantinople, blocked the brisk Mediterranean slave trade in Slavs from the Balkan, Persian Gulf, and Black Sea areas, rerouting the trade toward the African continent. Black slavery subsequently spread to Sicily, Italy, and the Iberian peninsula. The growth and dominance of capitalism and the Age of Exploration, along with the Protestant Reformation, resulted in economic benefits and cultural traits that plunged Western European societies into unprecedented depths of corruption, wealth, greed, racism, and cruelty. Slavery, along with these major social developments, altered the medical ethical landscape and the delivery of health care to people of Black African descent.[75]

Increased levels of prejudice bred of isolation, the transmission and perpetuation of ancient racial prejudices, religious legends and myths, and stereotypes generated during the Middle Ages created environments favorable to the development of many of the social and medical-social race-based problems of today. Of the three Medieval Black/White racial interface points noted by Scobie—"in Spain from Morocco-Sudan; from and in Italy through Sicily, Tunis and Cyrenaica; and through Jerusalem from the lands of the Nile (Egypt, Ethiopia and Sudan)"[76]—the former came to dominate with the growth of the Atlantic slave trade.[77]

The same Christians who led and came to dominate the world during the Age of Exploration completed the 800-year-long reconquest of the Iberian peninsula with Ferdinand and Isabella's capture of Grenada in 1492. This represented the overthrow of a Moorish Moslem population by a White Christian one. The Spanish and Portuguese Christians transferred their attention and methods of dealing with non-White peoples outward and turned the Atlantic slave trade into big business. The Spanish and Portuguese hostile and aggressive brand of race relations and practices regarding non-White peoples, which had developed during the *Reconquista*, accompanied them on their voyages and is detailed by Stannard and Sanders.[78] By far the most important event affecting race relations in Western culture was the Atlantic slave trade. For Black Africa, this became the turning point shaping its history. Although Iberian colonial and slave-based medical systems were organized and relatively advanced technically, prejudicial and hierarchical race- and class-based attitudes affected how they functioned.[79]

Black Health before and during the Slave Trade: Beginnings of a Health Deficit Legacy

Black Africa sacrificed 40 to 100 million souls to the slave trade; 15 to 25 million survived to enrich the Western hemisphere. Descendants of this importation survive as the African American population of the United States; Black, mulatto, and hybrid populations in the Caribbean; and Black, mulatto, and mixed African-European-Indian populations of central and South America. Scholars such as Savitt, Kiple, and Sheridan have begun the process of probing the detailed relationships between health events and the nefarious institution of chattel slavery. Although the work remains fragmentary, discernible, fact-based patterns based on this experience have emerged.[80]

Ransford and others have documented that the African continent was, and remains, a peculiar health environment. With the exception of the North African coastal regions and the Nile basin, this huge continent was relatively isolated from other populated areas of the world. The interchange that did occur with this land mass over three times the size of the United States was confined to a few caravan routes, commercial sailing ports, and immensely long trails in the interior connecting village markets.

Until the nineteenth century this huge continent was virtually an outline on most cartographers' maps. Because of its lack of deep bays or gulfs and lack of navigable rivers (most contained sand bars and rapids blocking their mouths) and the fact that most of the continent is on a high plateau beginning only a few miles inland at most points, it remained remarkably impenetrable. Moreover, as early as the sixteenth century Europeans recognized the lethality of Africa's mysterious fevers and diseases, about which we will discover more later. The presence of heavy mangrove swamps immediately beyond the seaboard exacerbated this geographic isolation and provided excellent breeding grounds for insects and other purveyors of pestilential diseases. Until Europeans conquered Africa's geography and diseases in the nineteenth century it remained the "Dark Continent."

Thus, the African continent seemed inaccessible and invisible to European explorers. On a human level, completely foreign civilizations strongly laced with animism and magic seemed incomprehensible, crude, and worthless to the new visitors from a cultural standpoint. Moreover, African civilizations seemed technologically backward to warlike Europeans armed with muskets, cannons, and military science. All of this was exacerbated by the "strange" and foreign physical appearance and dress of the Black Africans to European eyes. Human interaction and interchange were further stunted by the fact that the African continent was sparsely populated. However, this kept endemic diseases localized and was automatic prophylaxis against epidemics.

For Africa the health environment has always been a major factor. As Ransford has reported, "[T]he great mass of Africa, that part lying within the tropics, has carried a more grievous burden of disease than any other area in the world, and it very largely determined the history of this vast region."[81] Of the three major regions of the continent, Black Africa stretches from about 15 degrees north to the Cape of Good Hope. It dominates more than three-fourths of the continent. It is drastically different from the Mediterranean littoral and the high Ethiopian plateau climatically, politically, and culturally and has been so throughout recorded history. Much of the interior is shielded from penetration by muddy swamps reinforced by tropical forests and thick walls of vegetation constituting a hot, steamy coastal plain. This largely tropical environment has always served as an excellent breeding ground for the insect and parasitic transmitters of malaria, sleeping sickness, yellow fever, bilharzia, hook worm disease, filariasis, and river blindness. Adding to the mysteriousness of this aspect of the "Dark Continent" was the fact that these diseases were largely beyond the purview of European and Arabic medicine. Moreover, the Black Africans seemed to exhibit some specific immunities* to this lexicon of ailments.[82]

Despite these cursory European impressions borne of limited and casual contact with the interior of the continent and its peoples, African longevity was very short and infant mortality was extremely high. Health factors were major determinants producing results as varied as low population densities, high fertility rates, and cultural practices such as polygamy and extended families. Africans developed very specialized immunities to their local diseases. The delicate epidemiologic balance was also preserved by the geographic isolation between villages and tribes, precluding epidemics or the spread of unfamiliar diseases among already high-risk populations. The exploding Atlantic slave trade during the sixteenth century, which disrupted this isolation, had devastating health effects on Black Africa.

The effects of the Atlantic slave trade on the African continent itself are usually downplayed or ignored. Current estimates of slave mortality and the number of Africans displaced by the forced diaspora of slavery are serious underestimates based on naval lists and port registers.[83] The sizeable toll exacted by events on the African continent (some estimate mortality in Africa as high as 50 percent) and after arrival in the New World (some estimates are as high as 30 percent in the

---

*A *specific immunity* is a state of altered responsiveness to a specific substance acquired through immunization or natural infection.

first year after arrival) are not included. The toll on the African continent's peoples, their societies, and their economic potential is recently being considered. As Davidson and Mazrui have observed, Africa lost millions of vital skilled workers, reproductive-age women, and children—people in their prime years. As huge numbers of Blacks became necessary to supply the triangular trade between Europe, Africa, and the New World colonies, the slave trade became much more systematized. Moreover, the slave wars, round-ups, and marches from the interior to the coast inflicted high death tolls. An expanding commercial enterprise required deeper and more circuitous penetrations into the African interior, larger numbers and longer journeys traveled by slave coffles, and larger, more dense, concentrations of slaves in storage pens, slave castles, and on ships, elevated the death rate from slavery to at least 50 percent before they even left Africa. Europeans also imported new diseases such as tuberculosis, syphilis, smallpox, and measles. Moreover, the process itself—generating artificial "slave wars," rounding up the captive slaves, and marching slave coffles from the interior to the African coast—spread and intermingled local African diseases to large populations of nonimmune Africans. (See Figure 2.1.) Thus, epidemics and the spread of local diseases occurred among the African captives in transit. From their network of slave castles and trading posts along the West African coasts, the Portuguese and Spanish, and later English, Dutch, and French, comingled the various tribal groups in slave barracoons, storage ships, and castles. This added to the devastating death toll. The Atlantic slave trade was an epidemiologic nightmare for an African continent already burdened with excessive disease. This may account for the eighteenth- and nineteenth-century accounts of the depopulation of large tracts of the African continent. Thus, as African scholar Basil Davidson has repeatedly pointed out, sociologically and epidemiologically, the coming of the Europeans in the fifteenth and sixteenth centuries was the worst thing to happen to Black Africa.[84]

Although physicians of that time could do little to lessen disease mortality and morbidity, medical support for the Atlantic slave trade was quite advanced and well organized during the sixteenth and early seventeenth centuries when Spain and Portugal dominated. As Sheridan observed, comparing British slave ports with Spanish-run ports early in the era of the Atlantic trade, English "ports lagged far behind Cartegena and other Spanish ports where slaves and slaving vessels underwent thorough health inspections,"[85] and at Spanish slave embarkation points and slave markets "instead of being quartered in the towns of Spanish America, new slaves were kept on outlying farms and restored to health before they were sold."[86] Unfortunately, by the end of the seventeenth century when the Dutch, British, and French became the major slavers, many of these health practices were abandoned. Although the British felt that medical support was vital to the successful support of the slave trade, financial rather than health care concerns dominated the beginnings of a pathological White doctor–Black patient relationship in Anglo Saxon–dominated Western cultures. (See Figure 2.2.) As

Figure 2.1 Exposure to New Diseases Devastated Slaves

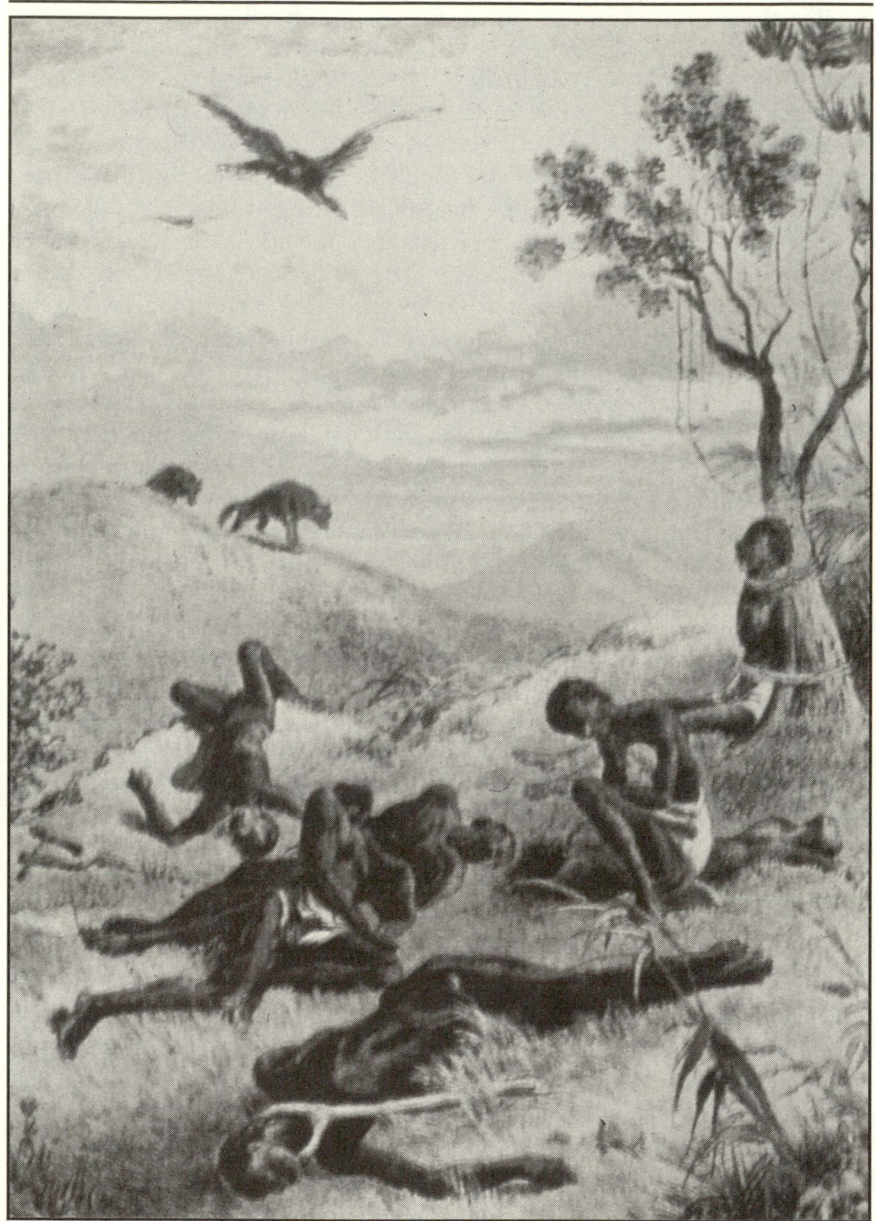

The native African population, already demonstrating the lowest population density and heaviest disease burden of any continent, previously lived in relatively isolated pockets from the general population. The slave trade with its mobilization and interaction with strange disease-bearing populations had even more devastating health effects on the African.

Sheridan noted, "Surgeons in the Guinea trade were motivated primarily by economic gain and secondarily by humanitarian concerns."[87] By the eighteenth century, slave ship surgeons were considered so indispensable to the successful passage of slaves to the New World, they were frequently the second-highest paid employees on board, surpassed only by the captain.[88]

The indigenous medical practices and practitioners encountered in Africa were largely of a traditional type, strongly based in rituals and magic. Though some of the African therapeutics and surgeries were effective, they were largely empiric rather than scientific. Besides their magical charms, amulets, and fetishes, highly respected medicine men had a broad-based pharmacopoeia for medical conditions. Both ancient and modern accounts of these African practitioners skillfully performing Caesarean sections and surgical amputations are documented. The tradition of African medicine men, root doctors, and midwives survived the cultural ablation Whites incorporated into Black slave indoctrination, and descendants of these practitioners practiced their crafts in the New World. From many accounts neither African Americans, South American Africans, nor Caribbean Africans fully accepted White Western-trained physicians unless they were

Figure 2.2　The Medical Examination before Embarkation

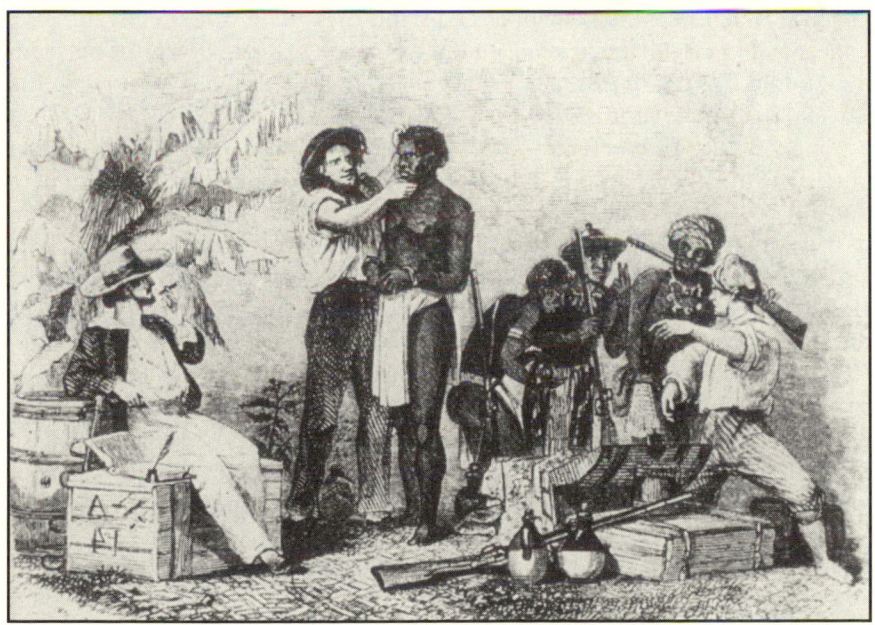

Medical examination was a vital part of slave trade. A healthy-looking slave was more likely to survive the notorious "middle-passage" and brought more money on the auction block. Slave ship surgeons became a requirement in the British trade. The examination usually took place in either the barracoon, on the ship, or in the slave fort.

coerced. Thus, traditional slave healers, herbalists, and midwives were eventually incorporated into a *slave health subsystem* alongside the planters, their wives, and the overseers. Formally trained physicians were not called in for most ailments and then only as a last resort. Thus, traditional Black healers often became the American slave's sole available medical treatment. Traditional root doctors, herbalists, and voodoo practitioners continue to have a quiet and persistent presence in African American communities today.[89]

Transportation of slaves from Africa to the Americas had profound health effects. This may have been the most massive epidemiologic catastrophe for the various involved populations (i.e., Amerindians and Black Africans) in world history. Only the Black Plague of the fourteenth and sixteenth centuries and the influenza epidemic of the early twentieth century had comparable historical impact epidemiologically. Both African and American populations' epidemiologic isolation was traumatically ended. The slave trade transported malaria and yellow fever to the New World. Both of these diseases devastated the Amerindians, probably being more responsible for their extinction in many areas than the notorious Spanish *Leyenda Negra*—the Black Legend atrocities. Added to their already tremendous indigenous disease and death toll, African mortality during the Middle Passage was between 20 and 50 percent. Another third of the slaves died during the first months in the Americas.[90]

The net effect of the tremendous mortality present in Africa before the slave trade, combined with the huge death toll secondary to the trade itself along with the Middle Passage, means that a "slave health deficit" actually began with the Atlantic slave trade even before Blacks' arrival in the North American English colonies. Blacks were certainly "different" types of patients for the European physicians heavily engaged in the slave trade. When not cast as lower animals, they still were not considered equals of the same caliber, or worthy of the same consideration, as their regular White European patients.

After the exploration of this background, the story of Black health in the United States shifts to the North American English colonies after the arrival of slaves in 1619. Although Blacks such as Esteban had been members of the earliest sixteenth-century Spanish exploring parties and expeditions, colonization was not the primary thrust of these efforts. No permanent institutions resulted. English and Dutch colonial settlements of the early seventeenth century, by contrast, were intended to be permanent from the beginning. Before long, a Black African presence in English North America in the form of slavery became prominent.[91]

✕ PART II

Race, Medicine, and Health in the North American Colonies and the Early U.S. Republic

Black Health in the North American English Colonies, 1619–1730

A Background with Iberian Roots

A little more than 500 years ago, there were no European settlers in the vast lands that now constitute North America. To understand the Black health experience in English North America from 1619 to 1730, a brief digression into New World history is necessary. The tragic story of the eradication of Native American populations throughout the Western hemisphere provides a cultural foundation for exploring the European response to non-White people. An examination of Spanish, Portuguese, English, and French medical practices will place slave health status and outcomes in context.

Following Christopher Columbus's 1492 landfall in the Caribbean archipelago, Spanish colonization quickly spread throughout Central, North, and South America. The Spanish colonizers emphasized conquest of the native lands and peoples. Their goal was to claim discovered lands for the crown and to acquire riches through mining for precious stones and metals and trade, not to establish permanent agriculture-based family farms and settlements. Acquisition of slave manpower for commercial interests was rationalized and given official Catholic Church sanction, as was the conversion of "heathen" Native Americans to Christianity. The colonizers' empire grew to include most of the Caribbean islands, Florida, New Mexico, Mexico, Central America, and South America. In North America exploration parties established a few temporary settlements. Subsequent demands for manual, primarily slave, labor generated by plantation agriculture, mining for precious metals, and the erection of new factories, towns, and institutions ensured intercontinental racial interaction and disease exposure that had profound, often unexpected, health effects.

Although North American settlement by Europeans began with Spanish conquests in 1519–1521 in Mexico, the first permanent colonial outpost in what later became the United States was in Saint Augustine, Florida, in 1565. Iberian health care policies and practices transported from Europe were fairly well organized and sophisticated for the period. As Guenter B. Risse notes in *Medicine in the New World*, "The regulation of medical practice in New Spain followed closely along the lines established in the mother country."[1] This included the establishment of medical regulating committees composed of trained physicians, auditors, magistrates, judges, and law enforcement agents called *protomedicatos* by the Spaniards, as well as hospital openings, including the first North American general hospital by Hernando Cortes in 1521—the Hospital de la Concepcion de Nuestra Señora in Mexico City—and the first North American medical school in 1578, the Royal and Pontifical University of Mexico located in Mexico City.[2]

The Spaniards soon realized that their dream of a new route to the Orient had not been attained. However, some of the new lands possessed significant mineral deposits and agricultural potential. If the colonies were to succeed financially, these resources had to be exploited. As menial work was anathema within Iberian culture, a work force for mining, farming, and building had to be mobilized. The huge indigenous non-White Amerindian population was initially chosen for this role as slave laborers. Health policies ensuring native survival based upon a slave system were indicated. An extensive system of hospitals affiliated with Spanish missions grew to approximately 128 institutions for Indians and slaves by the seventeenth century. These hospitals not only provided illness care for Amerindian and Black populations, but were also designated as centers for evangelization and religious conversion while ensuring the survival and increase of these populations for utilization as slave labor.[3]

Through a combination of Spanish brutality and massacres, the transmission of European diseases against which the Amerindians had virtually no resistance, and a policy of working slaves to death, the Amerindian populations were virtually eliminated over the entire Western hemisphere where the Spanish had landed. Within 50 years of Spanish arrival, native Amerindian populations had been eradicated at genocidal levels totaling hundreds of millions in Hispaniola, Florida, Cuba, Mexico, Central America, and Peru. Although the Spanish empire grew by leaps and bounds, these developments signaled the failure of one phase of the nascent colonial slave system. It also marked the failure of a progressive, slave-based, Iberian health policy.[4]

Under Spanish policies it became apparent that Amerindians could not meet the colonial demand for slaves. Aside from the huge mortality rate, Amerindian work habits were chaotic, Amerindians seemed unable to meet the physical demands of slave labor, and they often ran away and resisted forced labor. These circumstances were exacerbated by the fact that the Spanish were cruel taskmasters who often forced natives into slavery through kidnapping, murder, and brutalization.

Amerindians were also incredibly susceptible to diseases such as yellow fever, smallpox, influenza, and malaria. Despite Spanish medical efforts, which were highly organized for that period, the native inhabitants died in droves. It is evident that Spanish medical efforts were modulated by racial superiority feelings harbored by Spanish physicians. Scholar David Stannard has documented racial antipathy by the Spaniards in his work *American Holocaust.* Such feelings were reflected by the highly regarded sixteenth-century Spanish physician Diego Alvarez Chanca, who stated that the Amerindians' "degradation [was] greater than that of any beast in the world"[5] and concluded that the natives were barbarous and unintelligent.[6]

Driven by misgivings about the failed work force strategy and the inhumane and sometimes barbaric treatment and eradication of the Amerindian population, Spanish policies regarding the administration of the colonies changed through a campaign led by Dominican friar Bartolome de las Casas in 1540. The designation as slaves was transferred away from Amerindians to Black African populations by 1572. The policy proposals of las Casas went further than protecting the Amerindian population. He aggressively worked to assign Blacks to permanent chattel slavery. As Isabelle August noted in A *Pictorial History of the Slave Trade,* "Bishop Las Casas . . . proposed to Ximenes, a cardinal and regent of Spain, that a systematic importation of blacks be organized."[7] This policy was condoned by both the state and the Catholic Church. These policy changes, combined with the proven success of Black plantation slavery in Saõ Taome, Fernando Po, and other locations, set a trend that persisted into the nineteenth century. By the time the English and the Dutch entered the colonial competition and the slave trade in the seventeenth century, the success of the Iberian approaches to slavery were evident. The lessons learned from favoring Black African slavery and colonial mercantilism were not lost on Spain and Portugal's English, French, Dutch, and Danish colonial competitors.[8]

The North American English Colonies

Initially, North American exploration and settlement were dominated by the Spanish and Portuguese and later by the French, whose approach to imperial expansion focused on trade and economic exploitation, not necessarily on the establishment of permanent agricultural-based colonies. Their activities in North America were, therefore, largely confined to coastal port facilities and strategically located inland trading posts and mining sites. Life was usually isolated, male-dominated, and rustic with long forays into wilderness areas where living

accommodations and relations with Native Americans were uncertain and sometimes dangerous. Moreover, these explorers' commitments to colonies often were
not lifelong, nor did they usually involve the importation of European women or
children. In societies dominated by hunting, exploration, trading, and animal
trapping, health care considerations and provisions tended to be minimal.

Instead of establishing multiple trading posts along the coasts and rivers as
the Spanish and French had done, the English and Dutch struggled to establish
permanent settlements at Jamestown (1607), Plymouth (1620), New Netherlands (1624), and New Sweden (1638). These late sixteenth- and early seventeenth-century efforts by the English and Dutch settlers established permanent
colonies to claim and cultivate the land. Their permanence was reinforced by the
fact that these early settlers had migrated to the Americas in search of religious
freedom, economic opportunities, and, for many, new beginnings. Some of these
New World settlers could be characterized as religious zealots and others who did
not fare well in a Europe fractured by the Protestant Reformation and counter-
Reformation; as miscreants, debtors, misfits, prostitutes, and prisoners often
rounded up by colonial corporations to supplement sparse European populations
in the colonies; and, as those dissatisfied with European class hierarchies, traditional feudal political systems, and the lack of economic and upward mobility.

For an increasing percentage of Europeans, the post-Jamestown Colonial
Era involved extreme hardship in a dangerous environment and barely hanging
on in a strange land. Months-long hunting and exploring parties in uncharted
forests where life depended on rugged individualism, wilderness skills, and intimate bartering relationships with Amerindians became less important for the
Europeans' existence. Nevertheless, life in these newer colonial areas was characterized by solitude, deprivation, and hardships in harsh environments. Moreover,
these agricultural settlements were often surrounded by lukewarm to hostile
Native Americans who variably shared their survival skills with the Europeans.
This necessitated delicate and sensitive diplomacy with Indians for these early
settlements' very survival. Maintaining agricultural sufficiency in lieu of labor
and capital shortages, and political and military integrity despite episodes of
Native American hostility or aggression, were requisite for continued existence.
Scant attention or resources remained to devote to health, sanitation, or medical
considerations.

Provision of basic human needs was the dominant preoccupation in the earliest settlements. Food was provided by planting and harvesting meager crops.
Nutrition was often inadequate, and several colonies suffered casualties from
starvation. Provisions were supplemented by hunting, trading, and selling cash
crops such as tobacco, which could be sold to England. Shelter was crude and
often inadequate, especially in the beginning. Sanitation was crude and dangerous. Thus, the colonists' health status was often poor, and they frequently died
from overexposure, malnutrition, typhoid fever, dysentery, influenza, and other

epidemic diseases. These factors helped to account for their poor health status and the slow development of a health care infrastructure.

This "third generation"* of Europeans in North America faced the challenges of claiming the new lands, clearing the lands, and creating an agricultural work force. After short adjustment periods in colonies such as Jamestown, Plymouth, and New Amsterdam, Amerindian displacement and Black chattel slavery became the chosen methods to achieve these goals.

As it became clear that cash crops for export based on a plantation economy would be vital to the colonies, labor became a major concern. Clearly, European colonists were not numerous enough to compete internationally as "work units" in the mass production agricultural machines represented by plantations. Alternatives to sole reliance on institutionally based chattel slavery were attempted initially. Indentured servants supplied much of the early labor in the colonies. But as profitable crops such as tobacco, rice, and sugar cane were identified, this system proved to be inadequate for several reasons. Indentured servitude was a temporary status, often lasting less than 10 years, and most indentured servants were European. Thus, after serving out their indenture, they became citizens in the community who could become influential—even family members.** Such factors created problems when brutal, dangerous, long-term gang work became necessary. Moreover, escaped European workers were difficult to identify. These problems resulted in economic inefficiency.

One of the most momentous events to occur during the formative stages of English North America was the introduction of Black slavery. As John Rolfe, the liberalizer of the Anglo-Indian relationship by his marriage to Pocahontas, wrote in his journal in 1619: "About the last of August came in a dutch man of warre that sold us twenty Negars [*sic*]."[9] His matter-of-fact entry reflected a Black/White relationship in English North America that paralleled the one initiated more than 70 years earlier by Bartolome de las Casas in the Spanish colonies. By the end of the seventeenth century, Black chattel slavery as the basis of a plantation economy was a system that was tried, tested, and true.

Cash-crop, plantation-based economies fed by commodities such as indigo, rice, tobacco, and sugar cane dictated a plantation system. Such a system's dependency on gang labor virtually ensured some method of slavery. Early North American attempts to adapt Amerindians to a slave system were undermined by

---

*The "first" European group exploring North America was the Norsemen between 986 and 1024; the "second" group, the Spaniards, beginning in 1492. Although Englishman John Cabot discovered mainland North America in his 1497 landing at Labrador, the English did not pursue that breakthrough for almost a century.

**Freed White indentured servants could, and did, marry White colonists, becoming members of many early American families. This almost never applied to Black indentured servants in the early Colonial Period.

the fact that, compared to other peoples enslaved and exploited by Europeans throughout the world, they did not perform well at gang labor, tended to grieve and sulk in captivity, and commonly escaped. Their morbidity and mortality rates were high, and recapturing these slaves created diplomatic and political problems with surrounding Amerindian populations. These developments, along with the secondary economic shortfalls, generated pressures favoring permanent Black chattel slavery. Although it would take 40 years to clearly define Black chattel slavery socially and an additional 30 years to carve out its legal status in the North American colonies relative to White indentured servants, the economic, social, and ideological advantages of such a system for European interests determined the eventual outcome. As early as 1705 the "difference" in treatment meted out to Blacks had been codified into law in Virginia, the "model" colony. A. Leon Higginbotham (*In the Matter of Color: Race and the American Legal Process: The Colonial Period*) noted that the House of Burgesses passed direct provisions codifying the obligations masters owed White servants:

> In addition to the prohibition against publicly whipping a naked white Christian servant, masters were admonished to "find and provide for their servants wholesome and competent diet, clothing and lodging, by the discretion of the county court." Church wardens were authorized to provide for servants who become so sick or lame that "he or she cannot be sold for such value . . . as shall satisfy the fees and other incident charges accrued."[10]

With regard to the care and maintenance of Black slaves:

> In contrast to the detailed delineation of duties owed a servant by the master, the statute was silent as to any obligations owed to the slave by the master. Masters were apparently allowed to feed, clothe, and nurse their slaves in whatever manner they saw fit.[11]

The health care implications of such laws help explain the inferior health status, outcome, and services with regard to African Americans. The fact that slave masters had no official environmental or health provisions to live up to had profound and far-reaching health care implications.[12] Thus, a new social and, by extension, medical ethical landscape was created—anticipating the "blind spot" James Jones hypothesized that White physicians had regarding Black patients in the United States centuries later during his investigation of the Tuskegee experiment.[13] Degraded racial status was beginning to be reinforced by the legal system, and the pathological relationship between Blacks and the White medical profession—whose roots preceded Black arrival on North American shores—was to become greatly distorted by the implementation of Black chattel slavery in the North American English colonies. This aspect of the social and legal deterioration of African American status in the North American colonies grew out of a form of indentured servitude into a singularly brutal form of chattel slavery (mutilation, castration, and burning alive were almost exclusively punishments for Blacks).

Black Africans hailing from sophisticated agricultural and craft-based cultures and backgrounds in Africa worked well within New World plantation systems. They also seemed to be stronger, hardier, and more resistant to several dreaded diseases, such as malaria and yellow fever, than were the Amerindians. This was especially important in a crude and physically hostile environment in which little medical care was available. Moreover, unlike the Amerindians and European indentured servants, Black slaves had no contiguous political or cultural allies. Thus, when they escaped, Black slaves not only were easier to track and identify, but they also had fewer sympathetic co-conspirators or easily accessible refuge sites.

The scientific and religious environments of the time promulgated the institutionalization of Black slavery. They provided traditional justifications and rationalizations within Western culture, allowing such status to be transferred onto this "different" and somehow "inferior" Black race of people. The Biblical Canaan and Ham myths were well known to Europeans by the seventeenth century. There is also evidence that myth- and culture-based anti-Black attitudes had intensified during the Middle Ages within northern Europe, as evidenced in the writings of several prominent intellectuals, physicians, and artists of the period.[14] Moreover, the scientific advance that had been reawakened during the Renaissance was strongly influenced by Great Chain of Being theories, which emphasized the progression from simple to more complex and advanced beings (with the Greek ideal as the ultimate biological model). The natural sciences, yet to separate from the general discipline of philosophy, were in the taxonomic stages of development. Such developments led, almost naturally, to the scientific flaws of reification (attributing concrete, quantifiable status to abstract concepts) and hierarchical ranking. Each of these developments helped reinforce social and cultural beliefs that "proved" that Black Africans and other non-Whites were separate and unequal beings compared to White Europeans.

Primitive circumstances, sparse populations, and the absence of formal hospitals and clinics dictated that sick colonists were cared for at home during the early Colonial Period. For these reasons, North America was slow to develop hospitals for the delivery of health care. In the few communities large and urban enough to afford them, the first institutions that systematically provided inpatient health care to the public were the almshouses and poorhouses. Private hospitals and dispensaries used by the general population did not appear in America until the eighteenth century. From the beginning, institution-based health care would have strong relationships to class distinctions and stewardship for the poor. Blacks, relegated to the lowest classes or chattel slavery status by the end of the early Colonial Period, intermittently had access to these facilities.[15]

Black Slave Health: Effects of the Diaspora

In terms of health, Black slaves entered the North American European colonies, to use a metaphor, in a deficit situation. Much of this health disadvantage was related to the Atlantic slave trade and its epidemiologic disruption of exposure to diseases indigenous to the African environment, was augmented by the slaves' vulnerability to diseases foreign to the African continent, and was compounded by the stresses and trauma of the trade itself.[16] This deficit consisted of mortality rates associated with the experiences on the African continent due to "slave wars," round-ups, and marches from the interior of the African continent to the coast; storage experiences at slave castles and posts; Middle Passage deaths due to sanitation, contagion, and exposure conditions; disease epidemics and maltreatment during the enslavement process; and deaths caused by the "breaking-in" period after arrival in the New World. Another important factor created by the slave trade, a legacy lingering over the U.S. health system today, is the effect of slavery on the medical profession in America. Often unmentioned are the implications of the pathologic relationship between White physicians and Black patients established during the Atlantic slave trade. The expectation of poor health status and outcome became the "norm" for Black and poor patients in the United States as far as White physicians were concerned. This centuries-old expectation was articulated by a White Harvard physician-activist as late as the 1960s:

> [C]ertain forms of medical and psychiatric illness are so widespread as to seem "normal"; they are everybody's lot. . . . I no longer notice with surprise the terribly rotted teeth, the poor hearing, the eye-sight too long neglected, and hence hopelessly impaired. . . . I often find myself taking for granted the occurrence of parasitic diseases. Rat bites no longer seem rare and awful; rodents are everywhere, in the halls and in the apartments as well as in the littered alleys. Finally, there are to be found in the poor a host of diseases, deficiencies and developmental disorders that even medical students in pursuit of variety and experience rarely see. They are illnesses and erosions of the body that go with poor diet. They are the neurological disorders brought on by untreated or poorly treated injuries or diseases. They are the serious congenital and metabolic flaws—in us they are quickly spotted and treated—that have been allowed unimpeded existence or growth.[17]

It is doubtful that the expectation and acceptance of poor Black health status and outcome—exacerbated by the pattern of nihilism and inattention to high medical or ethical standards regarding the system's race and class problems exhibited by organized medicine today—would be as problematic without the slavery experience.[18]

Examining the origins of conservative estimates of the 50 percent overall mortality rate of the entire Atlantic slave trade is important. More realistic calculations posited by authorities such as W. B. Blanton estimate that "not one in ten survived the capture, coffle, barracoon, middle-passage and seasoning."[19] Documentation of Black morbidity and mortality from the slave trade in the interior portions of the African continent is sparse and largely dependent on slave and travelers' accounts. Middle Passage mortality, the most documented phase of the Atlantic slave trade, is based on port registrations and shipping manifests. "Breaking-in" period morbidity and mortality rates, less organized and largely under private aegis, are also virtually undocumented.

For most Africans, the slave experience provided their first contact with the Western medical profession. While on the African coast, most slaves underwent a physical examination and evaluation by a slave ship surgeon, who helped determine which slaves were purchased and their dispensation while both on the coast and during the voyage. Ominously, these physicians suspended their normal medical ethical relationships with this new category of "patients." Based on the numerous written accounts left by slave ship surgeons themselves, they quickly adopted practices that contributed to the dehumanizing process and conformed to the sociocultural ideology of Black inferiority. Though unable to successfully treat many diseases during that era, valuable slave ship surgeons were often the highest paid persons on the ship after the captain.

African populations that had been geographically isolated for millennia brought certain diseases to the coast with them. Yaws, sleeping sickness, hookworm disease, and sickle cell disease were rare and virtually unknown among non-African populations. Based on peculiar susceptibilities, this exchange of diseases on the coast took a heavy toll on all groups involved in the slave trade.

The most devastating phase of the Atlantic slave trade was the Middle Passage. Sanitation conditions were horrible aboard slave ships; the slaves were crowded below on shallow decks with inadequate sanitation provisions. The chattel were shackled and stacked like spoons on shelves. Besides being overcrowded they had to lie and sleep in their own waste. Slaves attempted suicide by jumping overboard or attempting starvation. Horrible sanitation conditions encouraged disease outbreaks, the effects of which were compounded by monotonous and nutritionally inadequate shipboard diets.

Diseases encountered during the Middle Passage included dysentery, diarrhea, ophthalmia, malaria, scurvy, worms, yaws, and typhoid fever. Epidemics of smallpox, yellow fever, and measles occasionally broke out. As Sheridan noted in *Doctors and Slaves*, "Slaves also suffered from friction sores, ulcers, and injuries and wounds resulting from accidents, fights, and whippings."[20] By far the greatest killer disease during the Middle Passage was the bloody flux: amoebic dysentery. The overall mortality from this traumatic, disease-ridden, transoceanic experience was around 15–20 percent, sometimes climbing to 50–80 percent. (See Table 3.1.) Mortality rates were directly related to a length of voyage greater than the average 42–50 days. (See Table 3.2.) If slaves survived this ordeal, they encountered disease-ridden ports awaiting their day of sale.[21] Although slave ship surgeons were well paid, they were technically ill equipped to successfully treat most of these illnesses. Their most valuable medical contribution would have been their insistence on adequate sanitation, good nutrition, and implementation of preventive disease measures on board ship. Preventive medicine standards did exist in the seventeenth century, as Blanton points out:

> [T]here did exist some wholesome ideas about the causation and prevention of disease. One sees this in the current disapproval of poor food, crowded quarters, foul ships, marshy land, stagnant drinking water, and in the recognition of contagion and the need of quarantine.[22]

Had the doctor–patient relationship been normal and more wholesome, perhaps records of such activity by physicians involved in the Atlantic slave trade would have survived rather than the abundant records documenting indifference, avarice, and complicity contributing to poor health.

Black slaves arrived in the Americas less healthy than usual populations. By 1619 this had been a fact for more than a century. On a relative basis, the medical care rendered in the Atlantic slave trade in the sixteenth century during the Spanish and Portuguese dominance of the trade may have been superior— although few ancestors of African Americans would have benefited from that experience.*

Another critical period was the *breaking-in period*. This period lasted from six months to three years after arrival in the Americas. Medically, the breaking-in period was one of increased risk for the slaves, including the shock of adjusting to a new disease environment, new climatic conditions, and a strange indigenous population. The stress of being torn away from home and familiar environments combined with the American program of deculturation (e.g., drums for communication were outlawed, speaking African dialects was forbidden, and African religions were outlawed) in the English colonies compounded the situation. The overall result was a 30–50 percent mortality rate for newly arrived slaves. Diseases involved were endemic, such as tuberculosis, pneumonia, and cold injuries. Moreover, the newly arrived slaves seemed to be more prone to epidemic diseases such as plague, influenza, typhoid fever, and yellow fever.[23]

---

*Most Spanish and Portuguese slaves were transported to Caribbean, Mexican, Central American, or South American destinations.

Table 3.1   Loss of Slaves in Transit Sustained by the Slave Traders
             of Nantes, 1715–75

Period	Mortality from Disease (%)	Mortality from All Causes (%)
1715–19	12.2	19.1
1720–24*	19.1	22.4
1725–31	13.5	13.5
1732–36	18.4	18.4
1737–41	19.4	19.6
1742–45	11.1	16.8
1746–50	10.8	11.5
1751–55	15.8	15.8
1756–63	5.9	7.9
1764–68	13.2	13.2
1769–73	14.2	14.8
1774–75	5.3	8.6
Mean, 1715–55	14.5	·16.2

Nantes was a major French slaving port. This table records their losses during the Middle Passage between 1715 and 1775. Their mean mortality of 16.2 percent from all causes closely approximates the estimates of the Committee of the Lord's Privy Council on the African Slave Trade of the British Parliament relative to the British slave trade.
*No shipping returned to Nantes in 1725–26.

Source: Martin, *L'Ere des negriers,* pp. 15 ff. and graph.

Table 3.2   Loss of Slaves in Transit Related to Length of Voyage,
             1817–43*

Length of Voyage in Days	Destination Brazil	All Destinations
10–19	—	7.9 (1)
20–29	5.1 (31)†	4.8 (47)
30–39	6.0 (60)	5.9 (83)
40–49	8.3 (19)	8.5 (25)
50–60	13.7 (18)	13.1 (21)
61 or more	25.9 (20)	22.0 (29)
All voyages in sample	9.7 (148)	9.0 (206)

This table documents the positive correlation between rising mortality rates and increasing lengths of transit to the New World.
*In percent of slaves lost during voyage.
†Numbers in parentheses indicate number of ships in sample.

Origin of a Race- and Class-Based Health System

This background is a prerequisite to a largely untold story. It provides a beginning to a medical-social profile of Black health in America that is a grim continuum of poor outcomes, indifference or exploitation by an elite White medical profession, neglect, active scientific racism, and occasional gut racism. Such a perspective is obviously related to the poor health status and outcomes experienced by African Americans for nearly 400 years. How closely remote and recent historical and evolutionary events are related to present health system performance and how they have affected Black health from America's colonial beginnings to the present can be seen in the explanatory hypotheses forwarded by researchers Todd Savitt, Herbert Morais, Montague Cobb, and Edward Beardsley. As Paul Starr eloquently stated in *The Social Transformation of American Medicine*, "[T]here is . . . no necessary and invariant relation to social structure of a function such as caring for the sick. Social structure is the outcome of historical processes."[24] It is necessary to understand the evolution of the structure of the race- and class-based health delivery system in the United States, in order to understand the current "structural arrangement." According to Starr: "To understand a given structural arrangement . . . one has to identify the ways in which people acted, pursuing their interests and ideals under definite conditions, to bring that structure into existence."[25] Investigating and revealing these relationships, events, and actions represents a significant part of this treatise. This represents an extension of the intellectual revision taking place in the social sciences, medical history, public health, and U.S. history itself.

As has been explained, the early health system in the North American colonies was primitive. From the beginning, treatment for different racial groups was separate. It was segregated on the basis of class and increasingly on the basis of race. For middle- and upper-class Whites, most health care was rendered in the home. Hospitals, organized institutions in Europe by this time, were largely absent and were feared by the general population (both Black and White). Compared to the Iberian colonial health system, very little organized medical activity, including hospitals, quarantine facilities, and publicly determined health care, was present for poor citizens or slaves. Beriberi and scurvy were diseases reflecting common dietary deficiencies in the colonies. Malaria, plague, smallpox, measles, and the flux (bloody diarrheal disease) were common. Because of primitive sanitation conditions, typhoid fever was a prominent problem. Most mortality in the colonies, which was very high for the period, was due to these causes.[26]

Between 1641 (Massachusetts) and 1750 (Georgia) slavery was legalized in 10 states. As Black reality became locked into the social and legal paradigm of chattel slavery in the North American colonies, the Black health experience came to be almost totally dominated and shaped by that institution. The health system's response was total. Whites were maintained in a separate system of care and institutions physically and ideologically and eventually were legally segregated from Blacks. Thus, by the end of North America's early Colonial Period, Black health could be equated with slave health. This would have profound future implications. As Stanley M. Elkins pointed out in *Slavery: A Problem in American Institutional and Intellectual Life*:

> *How a person thinks about Negro slavery historically makes a great deal of difference here and now; it tends to locate him morally in relation to a whole range of very immediate political, social, and philosophical issues which in some way refer back to slavery.*[27]

Until recently, very little scholarship has directly related slavery's institutional effects on Black health. Although Black slave health data are sketchy, a definite pattern of poor Black health outcome survives. African American health would be shaped directly by slavery for the first 246 years of their experience in North America and indirectly by its sequelae to the present day.

As levels of social organization increased in North American colonies and the profile of a health system became discernible and then more institutionalized, the influence of the separateness would increase. There are abundant examples of race and class stratification and its effects on the American health delivery system. As early as the late seventeenth century this "difference" was incorporated into law. By 1717 in South Carolina, a White servant could complain to a justice of the peace if his or her master did not provide a "competent diet, clothing and lodging, and . . . [did] not exceed the bounds of moderation in correcting them beyond the merit of their offenses."[28] The effects of overwork, maltreatment, and deficient health services and environments were taking a toll by the early Colonial Period. Black health disparities were already discernible, and the deplorable state of the nation's few public hospitals and health services available to African Americans was obvious.[29]

In contrast to Western Europe, hospitals were only grudgingly accepted by White Americans as sources of medical care until the late nineteenth century. There were few private hospitals before then. As early as the eighteenth century colonial cities were forced to open almshouse, pesthouse, and poorhouse hospitals. Institutions such as Charity Hospital in New Orleans, founded in 1737, and Bellevue in New York City, founded in 1735, are well-known eighteenth-century examples of the nation's public hospitals that were opened to provide some care for the city's "worthy" and "unworthy" poor.* Many of these institutions were heavily populated by Blacks, both slave and free.

---

*The "worthy" poor were impoverished people whose circumstance was considered no fault of their own: citizens such as elderly working men or widows who were sick with no families; orphans; or the noncriminal insane. In America the receipt of charity health services included a strong moral

For the tiny minority of African Americans fortunate enough to live in Northern communities with White advocates, where their admission to hospitals was even considered, class and caste considerations were compounded by racial ones. Racial segregation and discrimination remained the rule in hospitals until the twentieth century. As Charles Rosenberg noted in *The Care of Strangers:*

> *Class was not the only social relationship that reenacted itself within the hospital. . . . Black patients continued to occupy the least desirable locations in non-segregated hospitals; in some cases they remained in older wings when new wings . . . were constructed. In others, they were shunted into basements or attics.*[30]

At the New York Hospital, one of America's oldest hospitals, "Private white patients would hardly patronize an institution in which they might be expected to share rooms (or even floors) with blacks."[31]

Most colonists in the North American English colonies had little access to formal medical care. Primitive conditions and the absence of trained physicians were determining factors. Thus, most early colonists diagnosed and treated themselves. These medical-social circumstances combined with a frontier ethos to breed a distrust for physicians and formal health care. These factors retarded the development of a trained, respected physician class with designated authority and responsibility in health matters.[32]

In most communities, hospital facilities were not provided for Blacks. Many accounts exist of African American incarceration in jails, quarantine facilities, and poorhouses for illnesses. When they were available, public almshouse hospitals were racially segregated and usually overcrowded. Long waiting lists for admission for Blacks was the rule.

As chattel slavery became institutionalized, a *slave health subsystem* evolved that would attempt to serve the Black population's health needs for the next 246 years. Composed of slave midwives, root doctors, and spiritual healers strongly imbedded in African healing traditions, Blacks treated and attended the majority of Black illnesses. Planters, their overseers, and their wives participated in the provision of care in this health subsystem. This arrangement was reinforced by the trust and acceptance of these Black healers by the slaves. During the early Colonial Period physicians were seldom involved in the care of Black patients for various social and economic reasons.

---

component. The "unworthy" poor were impoverished people in need of health services whose circumstance was considered morally reprehensible: victims of venereal diseases, unwed mothers, alcoholics, and young unemployed men are examples. Many charity hospitals required a letter of character from an influential citizen for admission.

There were few physicians in the North American English colonies. The prevailing ethos of democratic ideals and staunch republicanism did not promote the granting of social authority or privileges to any professional group. Not only did this create an atmosphere of self-reliance in American patients, but it also bred a strain of distrust toward any elite profession. This lack of professional status would dog American medicine into the twentieth century. It would also serve to isolate them from meeting the medical-social needs of the American public, White or Black.[33]

Another barrier to equitable health treatment and policy for African Americans by the seventeenth century was the growing input by the medical profession itself into the pseudoscientific corpus of racial inferiority. Publicly held beliefs about the separateness and inferiority of Black people—buttressed by science—precluded appropriate medical care or health policy. Physicians were just as vulnerable as laymen were to this growing ideology. Moreover, when members of the medical profession made racial inferiority pronouncements, it seemed to create more impact in a society just starting to acknowledge the authority of natural sciences.[34]

An Embryonic Healing Profession

The first English physician to land on the American continent was probably Henry Kenton, who arrived in 1603. Of the few doctors that were available, the overwhelming majority were apprentice trained. This created a hierarchy within the profession: a tiny elite class (constituting less than 10 percent of the profession) of cosmopolitan European-trained physicians practiced in cities agitating for professionalization, and a larger group of practitioners varied from self-trained conjurer-healers to apprentice-trained physicians who often resisted formal regulation. In contrast to the situation in Europe, the medical profession was not connected with the colony's underdeveloped university system, nor was the occupation granted the high prestige or authority of a cognitive profession. Many American physicians were very self-conscious of their lowly status and made scattered and frantic efforts to organize medical societies, create licensing laws, and improvise professional standards. Insecure in their own status, American physicians were intolerant of practitioners who deviated in any way—professionally, racially, or along gender lines. Moreover, it bred a defensive "us vs. them" posture that would characterize the American profession for the next 250 years. The paucity of trained physicians, the crude state of the higher education system in the colonies, and American character traits of self-reliance and distrust of elites and intellectuals were all barriers to medical professionalization.[35]

From an African American perspective, there were barriers to high-quality medical care between themselves and the White medical profession from the beginning. Not only was the relationship between Western medicine and Black Africans distorted by the exigencies and perpetuation of chattel slavery and the Atlantic slave trade, but the growing influence of the social and pseudo-scientific stigmata of racial inferiority further complicated the picture. As Basil Davidson points out in *The African Slave Trade*, the trade was socially, economically, culturally, politically, and demographically devastating to Black Africans. He also noted that "[i]t produced among Europeans the mentality of race superiority that helped to hasten colonial conquest and still lingers like a poison in our midst."[36] Naturally, such attitudes were devastating to patients of African descent. Moreover, the medical profession concentrated its efforts on the well-to-do. This pattern, which was also prominent in Europe, had the effect of eliminating or negating the importance of Blacks from a medical standpoint. Moreover, as Black social and legal status deteriorated toward legalized, permanent, chattel slavery, this further isolated African Americans from routine medical-social interactions. Medical institutions and facilities were often not provided for Blacks. When they were, they were inferior or segregated, often both. Furthermore, good health—which was considered an inherently worthy social good by the majority society—was driven almost exclusively by economic self-interests with regard to Blacks, who were in essence considered to be forms of livestock or chattel. Moreover, the impression that slaves were well treated from a property perspective is not borne out, either by the documentary evidence of slave owner records or by data on Black health status and outcome.[37]

A Black Healing Tradition

During the early Colonial Period in English North America there were virtually no apprentice or institutionally trained Black physicians. The single recorded exception seems to be Lucas Santomee, a Dutch-trained physician who practiced in New Amsterdam during the 1660s. (See Figure 3.1.) Seemingly, Santomee was successful and a property owner. He was discovered by Black historian J. A. Rogers, who shared his find and collaborated with noted medical historian W. Montague Cobb in the 1930s. There were, as has been mentioned earlier, many African American medical practitioners. This can be viewed as a continuation of ancient African medical traditions and was the healing method with which slaves were most comfortable. These healers could be described as slave midwives, root doctors, spiritual healers, conjurers, or "kitchen physicks." They were the hands-on medical work force that staffed the slave health subsystem and provided the medical care and attention most Blacks received. Begun during the early Colonial Period, this informal system became more elaborate, consistent, and specialized over the subsequent 200 years before the Civil War.

However, the restriction of participation by Blacks exclusively in the slave health subsystem would not be permanent. As free Black populations grew along-

Figure 3.1   Blacks Receiving Training in Eighteenth-Century Europe

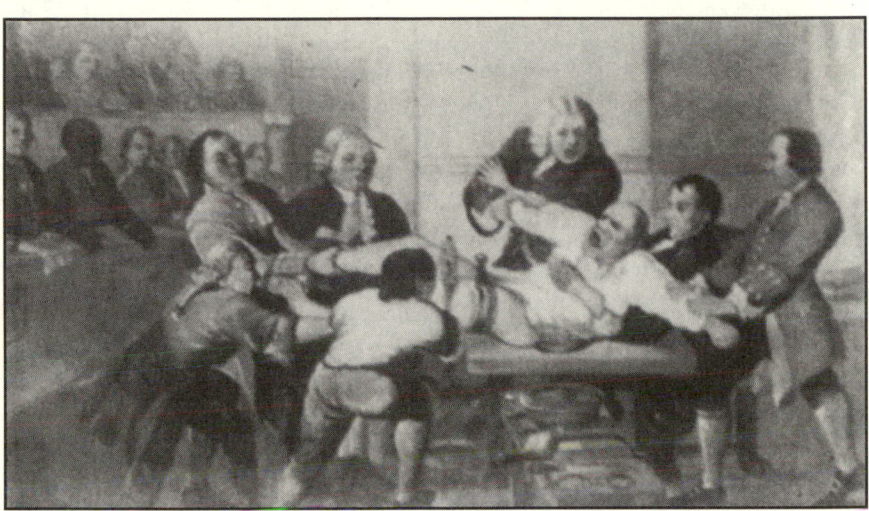

This eighteenth-century watercolor depicting a medical demonstration in England is from the collection at the Royal College of Surgeons. Though exaggerated, the absence of antisepsis and anesthesia in this limb amputation is clear, but most shocking is the Black medical student in the audience (seated in the amphitheater on the left). It documents a Black presence in the European medical educational system as early as the 1700s. Suddenly Lucas Santomee, the first trained African American physician who appeared less than a century earlier, does not seem to be such an anomaly.

side the slave population, African Americans continued to strive to become trained and recognized members of the healing professions. They would be amazingly successful, considering the odds and barriers set against them. As early as the eighteenth century Black efforts to participate as full-fledged health providers would bear fruit.[38]

The Black health experience in the early Colonial Period of the North American colonies was one of nascency compounded by hardship. At the time of African arrival in 1619 the colonies were a crude and threatening health environment for all. The Amerindian population was probably much healthier until their contact with Europeans and Africans. Their mortality was predominantly from infectious diseases. Colonists and their slaves were also vulnerable to nutritional deficiencies such as pellagra (niacin deficiency), riboflavin deficiency, scurvy (vitamin C or ascorbic acid deficiency), beriberi (thiamine deficiency), and general starvation. Overexposure to the weather often translated into health problems such as pneumonia, frostbite, and heat injuries. Western medicine had little therapy available to counteract these poor health outcomes.

By the seventeenth and eighteenth centuries the corpus of Western medical knowledge already contained a core of racial inferiority, anti-Black, biological determinist information. This negative health environment was compounded by the distorted relationship already established between European-trained White physicians and Black slaves beginning with the Atlantic slave trade. The expectation of a normal medical outcome or the expenditure of maximum medical efforts and resources on Black slaves were, at best, wishful thinking. There was almost an expectation reinforced by a self-fulfilling prophecy that Blacks were, and would always be, sicker. These medical-social and health cultural trends continue today and are reflected in the attitudes, expectations, and responses by the medical establishment and general public to poor Black health status in the United States. This may be the most important and damaging African American health legacy from the Colonial Period.[39]

Black Health in the Republican Era, 1731–1812

The rugged and threatening natural environment of the sixteenth and seventeenth centuries made a compelling case for improving the health system in the eighteenth and nineteenth centuries. During the 1500s the North American continent was colonized by Spanish, French, Dutch, and English explorers. Multiple trading posts were established along the coastlines and rivers. By the late 1600s some European settlements had spread inland. Most Spanish and Portuguese efforts focused on exploration, land claims, and get-rich-quick schemes. Seventeenth-century life in North America was characterized by European colonists surviving precariously in dangerous environments, scratching out an existence in strange lands. Health systems were crude and sparse and were operated with a limited supply of physicians.

From a European perspective, these lands seemed sparsely populated and empty. Spaniards had already depopulated large tracts of the Atlantic coast during the previous century of contact with Native Americans through disease transmission and displacement via military and vicarious violence. During the seventeenth century, the English, Swedes, and Dutch had struggled to establish permanent settlements at Jamestown (1607), Plymouth (1620), New Netherlands (1624), and New Sweden (1638). Health conditions were horrible; in fact, half of the Mayflower's passengers died within three months of their arrival. But despite the high mortality rates caused by contagions and epidemics in these nuclear settlements, the original colonies grew.[1]

After the early eighteenth-century beginning of the Republican Era, the North American English colonies had expanded to thirteen with the founding of Georgia in 1733. The late eighteenth century was an era of spectacular growth in both population and wealth. Energized by the Great Awakening (1734–1738), a religious revivalist movement, and reaffirmed by the earlier Puritan notion that America was to be a "city on a hill," a special place of God's work, the colonies stood in sharp contrast to what was regarded as corrupt and irreligious England. From a population of 250,000 in 1700, the mainland colonies south of Canada grew to 2.25 million by 1775 and 5.3 million by 1800.[2]

From the beginning, America's medical system had unique tendencies. Medical practices were strongly influenced by religion, as Ackernecht noted in *A Short History of Medicine:*

> As a rule the only educated men in the struggling young colonies were the clergy, as had been true in medieval Europe and in the early stages of civilization in many parts of the world. It is therefore not surprising that the practice of medicine was largely carried on by clergy.[3]

Men like Samuel Fuller, Cotton Mather, and Thomas Thatcher, author of the first American medical publication in 1677, were theologians as well as physicians. Nevertheless, it was social standing and wealth, not health conditions, that determined the availability of medical care.[4]

Expansion of the colonies over the Appalachian highlands into the Ohio Valley triggered a French military response by 1749. Establishment of a string of forts was the first measure taken to arrest the English incursions into French territories, resulting in the French and Indian Wars (Seven Years' War) between 1754 and 1763. This long series of conflicts exaggerated the French tendency to rely on their military for medical support. Thus, French military surgeons were the common health caregivers to French colonists and Native Americans. Following the French defeat, Britain took over much of France's colonial empire along with Spanish Florida. The English superimposed their less organized approach to health care matters on the "systems" encountered in captured territories.

Relieved of the French threat from Canada, Americans gained new confidence. With no contiguous hostile power, the need for British military protection now seemed more imagined than real. Besides, with the new series of British taxes and regulations the colonists came to feel that English military garrisons were designed to control—not protect—them. Moreover, myriad new parliamentary taxation schemes were designed to raise revenues to pay for military occupation of the colonies. Thus, the British Parliament seemed to want it both ways; they wanted additional control of the colonies while making the colonists pay for it. Increasingly, the American colonies agitated for more independence from England and resisted increasingly repressive British taxation. While the agitation for severing political and economic ties with Great Britain gained momentum, the colonial health system became more dependent upon and more and more imitative of the English system. However, there were dramatic differences necessitated by the progressive institutionalization of Black chattel slavery. It required the erection of a dual and truncated, unequal, and racially segregated health system.[5]

As the pre-Revolutionary War institutionalization and expansion of the slave system proceeded during the 1680s to 1710, "It saw, now under the conditions of comparative prosperity, the full emergence of the plantation as the basic unit of capitalist agriculture."[6] Starting as a numerically insignificant, prohibitively expensive labor system available only to the very affluent, Black slaves became a mass market agricultural work force for a massive plantation system. Slave prices declined and the volume of the slave trade increased. Black slaves became inhuman "work units" producing commodities from large agricultural machines (plantations). The provision of health services to Blacks, who constituted one-fifth of the American population in a massive and separate labor system built upon chattel slavery, became a major factor in the health care system from personnel, logistical, and health policy perspectives. As a result, a large and relatively complex slave health subsystem matured during this period.[7]

Early colonial advancements eventually led to the Revolutionary War between 1775 and 1781 and to the colonies liberating themselves from Great Britain. The new United States formally dominated the eastern third of the North American continent after the signing of the Treaty of Paris in 1783. Through generous arrangements with England and the other European powers, the republic occupied the continent from Canada south to Florida and from the eastern seaboard to the Mississippi River. During this turbulent period, the nation's first voluntary hospitals (1752) and medical schools (1765) were founded. They opened on the bases of racial exclusion and segregation.[8]

Due to climatic and other factors, not to mention a growing cultural predisposition, slavery flourished most profitably in the agriculture-based South. The ideal of the eighteenth-century European farmer was to acquire a small farm to support his family. For Americans the agricultural ideal was a commercial enterprise to produce staple cash crops for export. This commercial attitude based on laissez-faire capitalism dovetailed with the ideological and philosophical foundations upon which the Republic was grounded. For example, many large plantations would not spare land to grow nonstaple crops or livestock but were forced to import provisions for both master and slaves. These large plantations grew to function as virtual self-contained societies and economic units. One consequence of this development was that the plantations often developed their own health systems complete with independent pharmacies, clinics, and hospitals.[9]

Significantly, by the early nineteenth century the South had become the world's only slave-holding system that developed a positive defense for slavery (alleging that the institution was a positive, social good). Some of the justification for this position, as we have explored, came from the realms of biomedical science.[10] It seemed a natural development from science's assignment of Black and non-White people to immutable, permanent, biology-based inferiority. The debate on constitutionally allowing slavery in a democracy where "all men are created equal" was shuffled to the background by the tides of commerce and capitalism buttressed by burgeoning market and industrial revolutions. The introduction of Eli Whitney's cotton gin (1793)—which reinvigorated plantation slavery and the cotton economy—and the development of steam boats and steam engines symbolized this technological transformation.[11]

As a consequence of the Napoleonic wars in Europe, the Haitian slave rebellion in Santo Domingo, and a French military defeat inflicted by Toussaint L'Ouverture in 1801, Napoleon sold Louisiana to President Thomas Jefferson in 1803. The Haitians' military resourcefulness and a yellow fever epidemic defeated a French military expeditionary force of 33,000, commanded by Napoleon's brother-in-law General Leclerc, sent to recapture Haiti.[12] As Ransford wrote in *Bid the Sickness Cease:*

> [Y]ellow fever killed twenty-nine thousand of the soldiers and only a sickly remnant of the expeditionary force returned to Europe. Thereafter, Napoleon abandoned his ambitions in the New World, selling the state of Louisiana and the surrounding country to the infant American republic.[13]

The Louisiana Purchase represented another great expansion of the United States, literally doubling the size of the American republic.

From the republic's beginnings, Black chattel slavery, growing at its fastest rate between 1780 and 1810, created a rift between the northern and southern states. Both the politics and the processes of institutionalizing a separate sociopolitical and economic system for one in five Americans had profound effects. The health system was no exception. Revolutionary and libertarian rhetoric notwithstanding, a separate and inferior quality of life for one group of Americans had to be made legal, profitable, acceptable, and insulated from being dismantled or outlawed in the future. As a consequence, slavery became a major, contentious agenda item for every session of the Continental (1774–1777) and Confederation Congresses (1777, 1781–1787). Measures to placate Southern representatives, such as the "three-fifths clause," surfaced in the Confederation Congress as early as 1783. Finally, at the Federal Convention in 1787, the "three-fifths compromise" between the North and South was enacted. The compromise decreed that the slave population would be counted for proportional representation purposes as three-fifths of "other persons." This provision, along with assurances of delays in governmental interference with the slave trade—first until 1800 and then until 1808—remained a part of the nation's "Great Compromise" regarding slavery. Despite the convention's efforts to skirt the slavery issue by not mentioning it or slaves by name in the Declaration of Independence,

Constitution, or Bill of Rights and by adopting a fugitive-slave clause borrowed from the Northwest Ordinance of 1787, the issue would not go away. The North-South conflict over slavery would not be reconciled until the cataclysm of the Civil War.[14]

Seeds of a Multitiered, Unequal Health System

The Republican Era's new affluence and sophistication translated into drastic changes in health and the health system in the colonies. Large urban populations developed and, despite somewhat meager improvements in sanitation, nutrition, and the environment, the health status of some White Americans improved. Mortality and morbidity data in some areas came to approximate, if not surpass, that of Western Europe. Nevertheless, the rudimentary health system adversely affected an early nineteenth-century America entering what Wilson Smillie refers to as the "The Period of Great Epidemics":[15]

> The country . . . was young and poor, with a considerable amount of ill-ness. Polluted water supplies, unsanitary means of sewage disposal, unhygienic methods of food preparation and transportation, and the lack of any control over mosquitoes, flies, and other insect vectors exposed many people to illness. Among the rural and poor urban inhab-itants, malnutrition, poor housing, and exposure to weather grossly intensified the harsh effects of the more general factors. Illness was thus a major part of the lives of Americans, and major epidemics as well as persistent endemic diseases were characteristic of the period.[16]

With few exceptions, advances in health status have been attributed to improved environmental factors rather than to breakthroughs in medical care. Although the medical profession became more skilled at the observation, description, and prognostication of disease processes, therapeutically it offered little.

Hospital development in America, although progress was later and slower, mirrored the classical stages outlined by Henry Sigerist, who observed that the rise of hospital care in medieval Europe was a side effect of incarceration in jails and poorhouses, that there was a thirteenth-century second stage of hospital development when identifiable medical institutions focused their care on the indigent and dependent sick, and that the nineteenth century marked the devel-opment and evolution of the modern European hospital.[17] American develop-ment was slower and overlaid with a heavy emphasis on class distinctions and morality, with race always lurking as an extra factor (see Figure 4.1). Details con-cerning the opening of the nation's first almshouse hospitals at Philadelphia in 1732, New York in 1734, Charleston in 1736, and New Orleans in 1737 are cov-ered elsewhere, but Harry Dowling in *City Hospitals* made this observation

Figure 4.1   A Moral and Physical Thermometer Governing Health Care

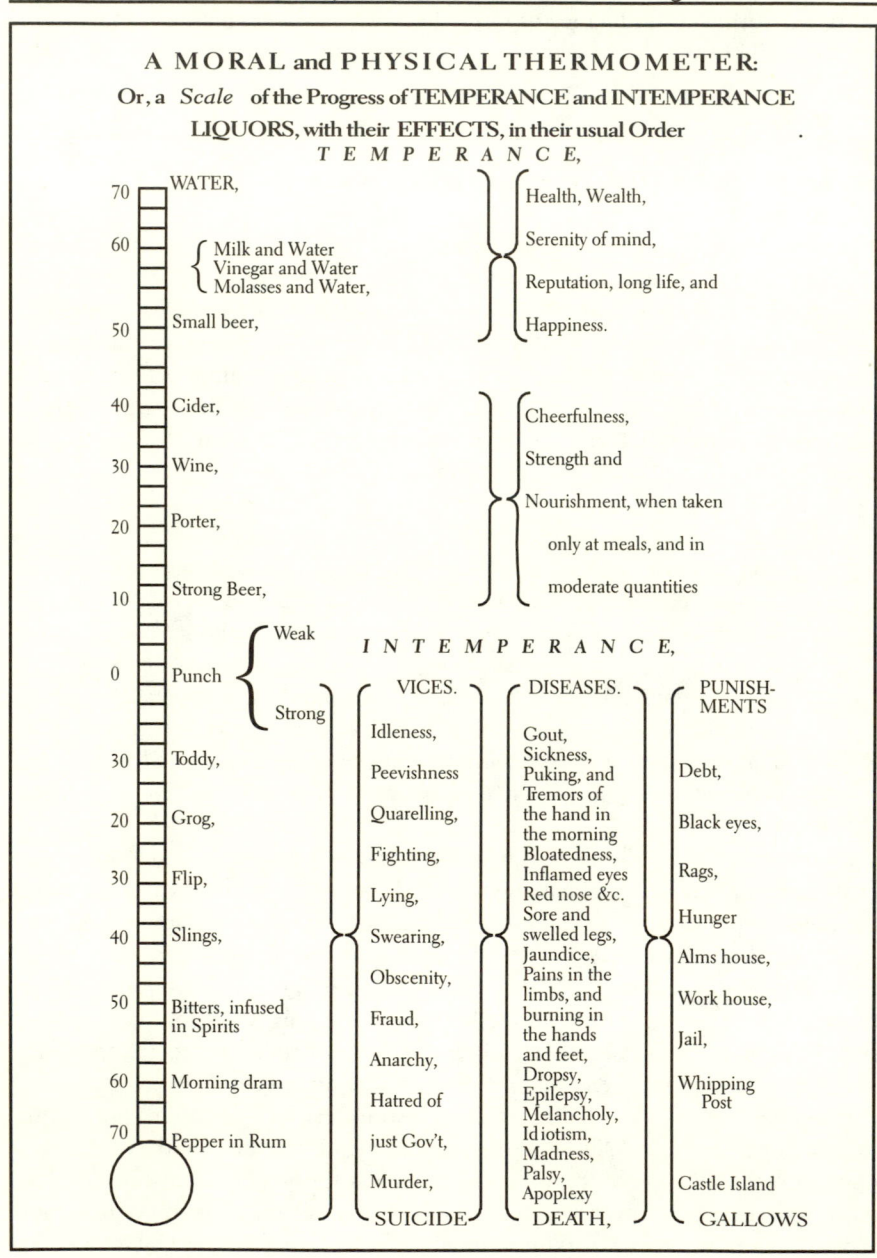

The early American health care system had a strong class, moral, and racist overlay. This document objectifies attitudes prevalent in a health system that condemned patients for intemperance, behavioral problems, and contracting "certain" diseases (i.e., madness, epilepsy, melancholy).

regarding early public health facilities: "[A] prison atmosphere was present also in the iron cages for psychiatric patients and whipping posts for slaves sent by their owners to be punished."[18] The different status and treatment of these special categories of patients in the early health system was clear. It is also comprehensible why most working-, middle-, and upper-class Americans received their health care at home, refusing to consider utilizing such hospitals. Acceptance of hospital care by mainstream White Americans would not occur until the nineteenth century after evidence of advances in medical science and surgery was clearly discernible and the character of the institutions had changed. Thus, the bulk of the earliest hospital care rendered in this country affected socially marginal populations. Nevertheless, it was even worse for Blacks, whose patient status did not protect them from the abuses of slavery or racial discrimination when they were admitted to these institutions.

The eighteenth century's increasing urbanization and population concentration in cities—especially in the Northeast—created growing populations of urban poor who were dependent and homeless. Having little formal social support, their needs during illnesses required institutions to provide domiciliary and medical support. Many communities were forced to establish tax-supported poorhouses and almshouses that provided *de facto* hospital care. According to Novotny and Smith, many of these institutions served as workhouses and houses of correction "where wardens were often permitted to fetter or shackle, moderately whip, and even starve inmates."[19] These inadequate facilities also provided whatever quarantine provisions existed in a community. In urban areas that were large enough, separate pesthouses for isolation were provided. They were sometimes located outside the town or placed on the most isolated area of the almshouse-hospital's campus. Maternity wards for unwed mothers and orphanages were often contiguous. All of these facilities were provided under the stewardship of community leaders and local governments for the "worthy" and "unworthy" poor. In many areas, where racial segregation laws allowed, these institutions were heavily populated by Blacks, both slave and free. For many of these institutions, Bellevue in New York City being a prime example, separation of the hospital from these other functions of poorhouse care would not occur until the nineteenth and twentieth centuries.[20]

Staffing of these facilities varied. As Rosenberg points out, a superintendent or warden usually supervised the facility. Some jurisdictions formally hired a physician to provide medical services. There were often informal arrangements with a number of physicians in the community. Professional staff positions at almshouse hospitals in cities with medical school teaching activity—such as Philadelphia, Boston, or New York—were highly prized. Many of these physicians were European-trained and had experienced the value and role of clinical training on that more medically sophisticated continent. Moreover, such appointments allowed these medically elite physicians to specialize, concentrate on teaching, and conduct experiments and research. These physicians pushed for the establishment of the nation's first medical schools, formal credentialing and licensing of all physicians, and strong medical professional organizations. In other, nonacademic settings, such appointments were training grounds for personally improving medical skills, or simply became a professional burden and community responsibility assumed by the medical community.[21]

From such a firmament arose the colony's first medical schools. Physicians such as William Shippen, Sr., John Morgan, and Benjamin Rush—who were European-trained and closely tied to the Friends Almshouse of Philadelphia—became founding fathers of the College of Pennsylvania (later the University of Pennsylvania) medical school in 1765. This was America's first medical school. Another hospital founder, Samuel Bard (founder of New York Hospital in 1771), established the medical department of King's College in New York City, the nation's second medical school, in 1768. Medical schools immediately began to rotate their trainees through these institutions as the value of clinical training in the medical education process grew. The elite medical leaders among American physicians, most of whom trained at either Leiden or Edinburgh during the eighteenth century and Paris during the early nineteenth century, patterned American medical curricula on these European models. Despite attempts to professionalize the medical profession and to have committees and boards of academically trained physicians granted legal authority through regulation and restrictive licensing laws, colonial physicians were frustrated in their efforts until the late nineteenth century. Moreover, none of these efforts increased access to medical care for the average American. Medical care continued to be expensive and available almost exclusively to the rich. Blacks and the poor, who were viewed as lesser beings whose only "real" medical value was as "training material," were of little health policy concern relative to improving community standards and perceptions regarding quality of care and decent facilities.[22]

Race, Medicine, and Health Care: Reassessing the Late Eighteenth and Early Nineteenth Centuries

As medical science and health systems developed in English North America during the eighteenth century, pseudoscientific theories of biological determinism and racial inferiority began to replace old travelers' tales and Biblical justifications for Black racial inferiority and White racial superiority in Western scientific culture. Until the middle third of the nineteenth century, most of these theories emanated from Europe. The growing influence of this racially biased scientific racism had detrimental biomedical, health policy, and medical-social effects on non-White people worldwide. It was especially devastating in a new republic increasingly committed to racial slavery.

Many precursors of the pervasive scientific racism of the 1700s and 1800s emerged during the Renaissance.* Examining these precursors lends perspective to emerging eighteenth- and nineteenth-century scientific and medical attitudes toward Blacks. During the Renaissance, European physician–natural scientists such as Andreas Vesalius (1514–1564) and William Harvey (1578–1657) pioneered significant advances in biology and medicine. However, other scientific luminaries such as Paracelsus (1490–1541) and Marcello Malpighi (1628–1694) lent their names to racial inferiority speculations that helped establish Blacks in scientific and popular minds as separate, subhuman beings.[23]

Spurred by the scientific advance of the Enlightenment in fields like astronomy, physics, and mathematics, natural scientists concentrating in life sciences found themselves at a disadvantage. The epistemological terrain of biology was different from these other disciplines. As Gossett in *Race: The History of an Idea in America* noted:

> The attempt to explain the universe in terms of natural laws had made possible the development of the sciences of physics and chemistry, but not that of biology. . . . [T]he result was that biology remained a subject generally outside the mechanistic propositions which were applied in physics and chemistry.[24]

Life scientists were also on explosive and dangerous ground with reference to the religious and social implications of their work, as Winthrop Jordan wrote in *White over Black: American Attitudes Toward the Negro, 1550–1812*. To Jordan the plight of natural scientists was both complicated and "unfortunate. . . . [W]hen natural philosophers set about arranging animals and man, they found their materials inherently less easy to manage than the steadily orbiting planets and their findings more liable to unleash disturbing religious and social questions."[25]

Another example of the complicated social environment confronting physician-scientists and their efforts to objectify biological variations and racial typology was the effect of the valuable scientific contribution of physician Edward Tyson. Between the fifteenth and eighteenth centuries there was a growing and pernicious European perception that of all mankind, Blacks were most closely related to, if not variants of, apes. The European tradition to which Winthrop Jordan refers in his research can be traced back to the published medieval bestiaries and travel legends and accounts describing monsters and beasts inhabiting distant and unknown lands. As Landau notes in the *In the Age of Mankind*, similar legends and myths mark the early reference works in evolutionary science and

---

*Recall that several of scientific racism's precursors, such as the "Great Chain of Being" theory and the theory that facial angle correlates with intelligence and sterling character, date back to Greco-Roman times.

biology.[26] When the great apes were serendipitously encountered on the West African coasts between the Dark Ages and the fifteenth century at the same time most Europeans were "discovering" Black Africans, the derogatory associations made between apes and dark men were devastating. In 1699 Tyson performed the first detailed and scientific dissection of a chimpanzee (referred to in that era as an "orang-outang"). It has been described as a masterpiece of critical scientific investigation. Objective information regarding the comparative anatomy of great apes relative to human beings at that time should have been both welcome and positive from a scientific perspective. Scientists and writers that followed Tyson instead misused his work. However, as Jordan noted in *White over Black*, "Tyson's conclusions did nothing to weaken the vigorous tradition which linked the Negro with the ape."[27] Therefore, many cited Tyson's work as more "scientific proof" of Black separateness and inferiority. In the complex and stereotypical eighteenth-century environment in which Tyson's scientific work appeared, it could be misrepresented and misconstrued to reinforce traditional and popular racial attitudes and beliefs.[28]

The first recorded formal scientific effort at racial classification had been performed by French physician François Bernier in 1684. Bernier's methodology was revolutionary for that time. Based on his wide travels, Bernier broke ranks with others regarding human differences, stating, "The geographers up until this point have divided the world only according to the different countries or regions."[29] His travels suggested that a classification based upon the color and physical types of people was needed. Winthrop Jordan notes that Bernier's article in a Paris journal predicted future scientific efforts, observing that he "relied more upon color than anything else in chopping mankind into four (or possibly . . . five or six) categories, the Europeans, Africans, Orientals, Lapps . . . and perhaps American Indians and Hottentots."[30] Also during English North America's Republican Era, "Linnaeus . . . first . . . transformed the game into a science"[31] with his landmark effort *Systema naturae*.[32]

After the 1735 release of *Systema naturae*, the definitive book establishing binomial nomenclature as the standard in biological classification, Swedish physician-scientist Carl von Linnaeus earned his sobriquet the "Father of Biological Classification." His book dominated the field of biological taxonomy for over a century. However, *Systema naturae* designated Africans as "phlegmatic, . . . crafty, indolent, negligent, . . . governed by caprice,"[33] and "mulled over the possibility that the Hottentots were not men but apes, though he rejected the idea."[34] It has been documented that Thomas Jefferson, who was fond of viewing himself as a gentleman scientist, read *Systema naturae* as part of his background for his writings—alleging Native American and Black inferiority in his 1786 *Notes on the State of Virginia*.[35] These activities, led by the world's leading physician-scientists, were devastating for Blacks. Such developments could not avoid affecting the basic components of America's embryonic health system. Attitudes and practices spurred by such pseudoscientific knowledge bases distorted the health profession, health delivery institutions, and medical education infrastructure for centuries to come.[36]

Imprecision in the life sciences during the Age of Reason and Enlighten-ment generated another set of problems. One consequence of the confusion and disarray plaguing the biomedical sciences was the emergence of approaches and methodologies from indefinite, even mystical, sources. Previous contributions from mystical scientists like Paracelcus and the alchemists to Renaissance medi-cine had set ambiguous precedents. Physiognomy was one of these marginal pseudoscientific eighteenth-century developments. One of the early influential sources of physiognomy, the theory that facial or body features could determine one's character or mental capacity, was Swiss mystic and physician Johann Kas-par Lavater (1741–1801), known as the "Father of Physiognomy." Lavater attempted to elevate physiognomy to a science. To codify the theories he had col-laborated on in Zurich with clerics such as Fuseli during the 1760s, he published the richly illustrated *Physiognomische Fragmente* between 1775 and 1778. The ideal standards delineated in the book, indeed in all of Lavater's work, were based on Caucasian, often Greek, models. This automatically disadvantaged non-White peoples or people who deviated from these models physically, creating a false impression of their ugliness, deviousness, and inferiority. Physician scholars active during English North America's Republican Era, such as Camper (1722–1789), Blumenbach (1752–1840), Gall (1758–1828), and Spurzheim (1776–1832), men we will speak more of later, extended physiognomy to create the pseudosciences of phrenology and, later, craniometry. Within a 50-year period these so-called objective pseudosciences, rich with numbers, tables, and calculations, were misused by biological determinists and became the founda-tion stones to define and support influential White racial superiority and Black inferiority theories until well into the twentieth century.[37]

Another major effort directed at biological racial classification occurred in 1781. University of Gottingen professor of medicine Johann Friedreich Blumen-bach, in the second edition of *On the Natural Variety of Mankind* (1781), expounded on a mature racial classification of the human family. As Haller remarked about Blumenbach's then-landmark classification of mankind in *Out-casts from Evolution*, "His division into Caucasian, Mongolian, American, Ethiopian, and Malayan races, with the added Linnaean descriptive peculiari-ties, became the subsequent basis of most nineteenth-century anthropometrical studies."[38] While Bernier and Linnaeus had based their classification systems upon skin color, "Blumenbach considered a combination of color, hair, skull, and facial characteristics as fundamental means for classifying the five varieties of man."[39] He felt the "Caucasian"* Georgian "to be the most beautiful race of men."[40] Appearance was not his only criteria, for he theorized the Caucasian was the basis from which the others derived. As Haller notes about Blumenbach's cri-teria of skull shape, "[H]e argued that the Mongolian and Ethiopian were

---

Caucasian was a term Blumenbach originated referring to Mount Caucasus. This mountain's southern slope had been the home of the Georgians.

extreme degenerations from the original. . . . [H]e relegated the two other races, American and Malayan, to transitional phases of only minor importance."[41] After relegating non-Whites to "degenerate" forms of the Caucasian "ideal," Blumenbach's scheme dominated racial anthropology and typology for most of the next century.

Another dominant eighteenth-century European natural scientist and physician, Comte de George-Louis Leclerc Buffon (1707–1788), author of *Histoire Naturelle* (52 volumes, 1749–1804), was considered the leading scientist and one of the great minds of his day. *Histoire Naturelle* included virtually all the known facts of natural science, including allegations that Negroes were as wild and ugly as apes—even consorting sexually with them.[42] In academic circles *Histoire Naturelle* was the most comprehensive treatise on nature up to that time and was considered the only academic document rivaling Diderot's 35-volume *Encyclopedia* (1751–1772).[43]

Petrus Camper (1722–1789) was a Dutch surgeon and anatomist born in Leiden. His work in anatomy, racial anthropology, and art had profoundly negative medical-social effects on Blacks that have lasted nearly two centuries. A professor at Franeker (1749–1761), Amsterdam (1761–1763), and Groningen (1763–1773), he wrote a series of works on human and comparative anatomy during the Republican Era.* Camper was an accomplished artist whose work evolved from an artistic perspective, overemphasizing physical appearance that in many ways paralleled Lavater. Both proselytized a Classical Greek ideal. In 1786 Camper resurrected the facial angle (the angle formed by two intersecting lines—one drawn horizontally from the ears to the nostrils, the other a line formed by the shape of the face from the forehead to the front teeth), a measure dating from the time of Aristotle to indicate intelligence and to compare humans and lower animals. Horsman states, "At 70 degrees was the Negro, usually illustrated in later works as just above the orangutan or ape; at the apex was 'the Grecian antique' with an angle of 100 degrees."[44] Thus, Negroes were the most *Prognathous* race, which was unfavorable—Caucasians the most *Orthognathous*, a favorable determination. Camper's work, complemented by that of Lavater and Blumenbach, helped ensure that comparisons of the skull, face, and head would figure prominently in later nineteenth- and twentieth-century racial classifications. Some of the measurements Camper pioneered were used to "document" Black inferiority during the Civil War. Arguments citing Dr. Camper as a scientific reference alleging Black inferiority were noted in medical textbooks and journals and in the U.S. Congress's debate against passage of the Fifteenth Amendment after the Civil War.[45] Such is the role that science has played in the nation's sociopolitical affairs.[46]

---

*Art books sold in U.S. bookstores in the 1980s still utilized Camper's methodology and some of the eighteenth- and nineteenth-century scientific racist racial classifications. Camper is known today for his anatomical research involving Camper's angle, chiasm, fascia, ligament, and line.

Georges Cuvier (1769–1832) was a legend in his own time. A French anatomist credited as the "Father of Paleontology and Comparative Anatomy," his influence went far beyond that, for he virtually dictated policy on zoological matters to the entire world from his headquarters at the Jardin des Plante in Paris during the formative years of this nation. He was the most influential naturalist in the late eighteenth and early nineteenth centuries. Moreover, his work went beyond lower animals to include scientific study and speculation on human beings.

The French Revolution seemingly had little adverse effect on Cuvier's career, for he survived and prospered through Napoleon's government and the new republic. His love for zoology led to his 1789 appointment as professor of natural history at the College de France and in 1795 as assistant professor of comparative anatomy at the Museum of Natural History in Paris. By 1802 he was the director of the Jardin de Plante, where he wrote several influential books in natural science. Some of his important works were: *Lecons d anatomie comparee* (1801–1805), *L'Anatomie de mollusques* (1816), *Les Ossements fossiles des quadrupedes* (1812), *Histoire naturelle de poissons* (1828–1849), and *Le Regne animal distribue d'apres son organisation* (1817).

Cuvier was interested in racial matters. His research on this subject matter seemingly highlighted some of the weaknesses in his personality. Stocking, Gould, and others have revealed that he demonstrated ruthlessness and insensitivity toward less fortunate and less sophisticated people if they were members of groups he was studying. Human beings, to Cuvier, were "subjects of scientific study" who lost their humanity in the process. His interest in Black people led to his theorizing, lecturing about, and publishing that Blacks were unintelligent, inferior, lascivious, and animal-like. An account of Cuvier's pursuit of Saartjie Baartman, a Black South African Khoi-San woman called the "Hottentot Venus," across Britain and continental Europe to test his theories on racial differences follows. After "studying" her and dissecting her body at autopsy, he published his "scientific findings"—distorting them to "document monkey-like" racial differences that conformed to his personal European-based prejudices. This scientific giant was cited universally as a scientific authority "documenting" Black inferiority for more than a century.[47]

Another major late Republican Era contributor to the scientific racist, Black inferiority myth was an English surgeon practicing in Manchester, Charles White (1728–1813), a physician-naturalist best known in medical circles for his work in obstetrics, where he promoted absolute cleanliness during obstetrical delivery. In 1795 White presented his polygenist theories on human classification to the Literary and Philosophical Society of Manchester. It was the last scientific defense of the Great Chain of Being theory. Much of White's argument was a lengthy catalog of the particular ways in which he believed Blacks more closely resembled the ape than the European. He published his findings in 1799 as *The Regular Gradation of Man, and in Different Animals and Vegetables*. As Stephen Jay Gould noted, "[H]is conventional ranking of human groups with European whites on top

The "Hottentot Venus" and Nineteenth-Century Racial Science

As the curtain rose on the nineteenth century, science was coming of age and was increasingly asked to explain natural phenomena such as differences in the races of man and how they ranked. Naturalist Baron Georges Leopold Cuvier (1769–1832), world-renowned Director of the Jardin des Plante in Paris acknowledged as Father of Paleontology and Comparative Anatomy, felt qualified to answer these questions. Already an international figure in natural science, he influenced worldwide scientific biological thought for the next century. His conceptual framework on racial thought persists as scientific debates over biological racial differences rage today.

Another protagonist in this tragedy is Saartjie Baartman. A woman who could be viewed as a beautiful female specimen, she represents the epitome of scientific and media exploitation, with racism as a major subplot in this drama. Saartjie was a member of the Kung tribe of Bushmen who reside in South Africa; they are now designated as the Khoi-San people. In the nineteenth century they were commonly known as "Hottentots" and were considered one of the lowest forms of humanity from a "scientific" perspective. Women of the Kung tribe are characterized by steatopygous (large fat accumulation) buttocks and prominent labia minora (the smaller or inner lips of the vagina). Saartjie, considered as beautiful as the Venus de Milo by her own people and prominently possessing both these traits, was misled, exploited, and prominently displayed as "proof" of racial inferiority throughout Europe. This calamity was orchestrated with the full complicity of the nineteenth-century scientific community.

Atypical or deformed humans were displayed as objects of amusement during the nineteenth century. P. T. Barnum's rise to fame and the "elephant man" debacle are examples. Scientists contributed to this trend. Although Saartjie did not fit this mold, Europeans considered her a "curiosity" in that her body habitus was inconsistent with European ethnocentric standards of physical beauty. After being misled by Europeans who promised Baartman wealth and fame on the stage, she was transported to Europe during the early 1800s and displayed like an animal throughout Great Britain and the continent until her death in Paris in 1815. Curiosity seekers patted, poked, and viewed her body, buttocks, and private parts, which were considered ugly, lascivious, and outrageous. Saartjie's most prominent feature, her buttocks, created a sensation triggering scandalous European reactions.

After being alerted to Saartjie, European natural scientists made matters worse. Cuvier utilized the "Hottentot Venus," as *his* prototype of a separate, subhuman species. He was determined to prove that Hottentots and people of African descent were inferior scientifically. Cuvier had students and colleagues in Paris study Saartjie, often when she was unaware and without her permission; he also commissioned scientific reports such as the one written by eminent zoologist Geoffroy Saint-Hilaire (1772–1844), which alleged her racial inferiority and kinship to apes; and, in the end, he displayed her corpse and body parts in the Museum of Natural History in Paris as an inferior "scientific" curiosity. Upon hearing of her illness Cuvier publicly stalked her as a scientific specimen and ultimately performed her autopsy. Although never obtaining the scientific evidence of her inferiority, Cuvier continued to opine and write of her inferiority and lasciviousness. He obsessively associated her physical peculiarities and Africanoid features, such as flat nose, high cheekbones, and kinky hair—characteristics having nothing to do with biological or genetic superiority—with apes. The ultimate abominable exploitation occurred after her death when Cuvier and his colleagues mutilated her body (cutting out her vagina and storing it in a specimen jar for display) and mummified her corpse and body parts, placing them, along with her skeleton, on display in museums where they remained for more than a century. Baartman supposedly represented the ultimate example of a biologically inferior, subhuman race of mankind.

Long after Cuvier's racist concepts had been scientifically disproven, Saartjie's mummified body, brain, vagina, skull, and skeleton remained on display in Paris at the Musée de l'Homme until at least the 1980s. Subsequently, the features Cuvier had listed as "proof" of Saartjie's inferiority and kinship to apes—such as her steatopygia, "monstrously large" lips, flat nose, kinky hair, and prominent labia—have been suggested by some contemporary scientists as signs of advanced biological development based on the anthropological concept of paedomorphosis* when compared to features such as thin lips, long straight hair, and general body hairiness in other human groups. Saartjie's mental quickness, mastery of several languages, and excellent coordination, noted by many observers, were ignored. The public display of her body as an example of biological racial inferiority and, later, of biological ethnic differences (from modern scientific and genetic standpoints these differences are considered trivial) was finally taken down at the Musee de l'Homme by 1985. As of 1989 her body and body parts remained stored in the museum. They may serve new purposes as case material for documenting and debunking an unfortunate period of Western scientific racism and reassessing the cultural roots of arbitrary and ethnocentric standards of physical beauty by which women of African descent are judged today.

Interestingly, playwright Suzan-Lori Parks's 1996 off-Broadway musical comedy *Venus* is based on this tragic tale of scientific exploitation. Although not named specifically, Baron Cuvier is referred to as "the Baron." Moreover, according to Parks, his interests in Saartjie, whose Christian name (she was christened in 1811) was Sarah, may have been much more personal and prurient than the scientific accounts reveal. Perhaps this excellent musical may serve as a vehicle for opening dialogue on Western science's persistent problems with social and scientific racism in the future.

---

*Humans have evolved by a general slowing down of developmental rates, leaving our adult bodies quite similar in many respects to juvenile, not adult, forms of our primate ancestors—an evolutionary result called *paedomorphosis*, or "child-shaping." Khoi-San people are now considered the most paedomorphic of human groups—thus, the least simian and most human of all *Homo Sapiens*.

Notes

Campbell J. *Historical Atlas of World Mythology*. Vol. 1. *The Way of the Animal Powers*. Part 1. *Mythologies of the Primitive Hunters and Gatherers*. New York: Harper and Row, 1988, 40–42, 90–101, 100.

Gould S J. *The Mismeasure of Man*. New York: W.W. Norton and Company, 1981, 56, 85–86.

Gould S J. The Hottentot Venus. In *The Flamingo's Smile: Reflections in Natural History*. New York: W. W. Norton and Company, 1985, 291–305.

Honour H. *The Image of the Black in Western Art*. Part IV. *From the American Revolution to World War I*. 2. *Black Models and White Myths*. Cambridge: Menil Foundation, Inc., distributed by Harvard University Press, 1989, 52–55.

Milner R. *The Encyclopedia of Evolution: Humanity's Search for Its Origins*. New York: Facts on File, Inc., 1990, 24–26, 33–34, 41–42, 104–105, 125, 190–191, 201, 379–382.

Parks S-L. *Venus*, the program of the Joseph Papp Public Theater, May, Volume 2, Issue 7, New York, 1996.

Ransford O. *Bid the Sickness Cease: Disease in the History of Black Africa*. London: John Murray Publishers Ltd., 1983, 14–15.

Samuels A. Black beauty's new face. *Newsweek*, November 24, 1997, 68.

Stocking GW. French anthropology in 1800. In Stocking GW. *Race, Culture, and Evolution: Essays in the History of Anthropology*. Chicago: The University of Chicago Press, 1982, 13–41.

Winchell A. *Preadamites; or A Demonstration of the Existence of Men Before Adam; together with A Study of their Condition, Antiquity, Racial Affinities, and Progressive Dispersion over the Earth*. Chicago: S.C. Griggs and Company, 1880, 53–55, 72.

and African blacks on the bottom certainly reinforced the prejudices of his comfortable Caucasian contemporaries."[48] Before and during the process of debasing Blacks, White makes a disclaimer attributing his racially derogatory findings to objective and scientific facts, as opposed to any personal biases. He then debases Orientals and Blacks, ranking both as inferior and close to lower animals, having stronger body odor, being lascivious beasts, and being insensitive to pain. Resorting to devices ranging from fact falsification to artificially unifying unrelated groups of animals and concepts, and finally appealing to aesthetic criteria, White could neither prop up the static Chain of Being that he hypothesized nor fill in the gaps or explain the copious variations in nature that his own data revealed.[49]

From the North American English colonies themselves arose another influential voice on racial classification during the Republican Era. The colony's most famous physician, medical educator, signer of the Declaration of Independence, and anti-slavery activist Dr. Benjamin Rush (1745–1813), sent curiously mixed messages regarding his attitudes toward African Americans. Although he was an avid anti-slavery activist, Rush nevertheless displayed basic scientific racist and anti-Black views and assumptions in some of his statements and writings. Inadvertently, he contributed to the corpus of negative biological determinism and scientific racism against African Americans. Accounts reveal that Rush convened a special meeting of the American Philosophical Society on July 14, 1792, to report his theory that "the Black Color (as it is called) of the Negroes is derived from the LEPROSY."[50] He hypothesized that the disease was congenital and implied that it appeared in mild form in most Blacks. Disease was allegedly responsible for the African Americans' appearance (large lips, flat nose, and woolly hair); black and smelly skin; morbid insensitivity to pain; and "notorious" sexuality and venereal desires. For those agreeing with Rush's hypothesis, Henry Moss, a man who collected fees in taverns for displaying himself as a Negro in the process of changing colors, seemed to be undergoing a spontaneous "cure." This reflected the intense scientific and public interest in the origins and changes associated with skin color during this period. It was probably the well-known pigmentary disorder vitiligo.* Despite almost schizoid admonitions against racial separation and discrimination, possible contagion demanded that Dr. Rush prescribe strict isolation and segregation until either a cure or spontaneous regression of the "disease" occurred. Though he was condescending, contradictory, and paternalistic in modern terms, Rush represented the best of the eighteenth-century White medical profession as far as Blacks were concerned. Much of the distorted view of Blacks that Rush shared with other American physicians was shaped by the so-called science of the day. Racist scientific events and personages shaped the beginnings of the distorted, often pathological, medical-social environment that African Americans have contended with and endured in the health system in America.[51]

Although the scientific validity of these derogatory (for non-White people) eighteenth- and early nineteenth-century pseudoscientific racial theories and classifications was refuted over time, they were still highly influential. These ideas and concepts polluted everything in U.S. society from medicine and health policy to politics and public policy. Moreover, there is documentary evidence that when physicians expressed these beliefs, it increased not only their social power and authority but also the credibility and acceptance of the derogatory beliefs themselves. This body of information and data was read by and influenced powerful men such as Thomas Jefferson, John M. Daniel of the *Richmond Examiner*, and Mississippi Senator Jefferson Davis (who later became president of the Confederacy) and exerted a pernicious influence on virtually every aspect of American life. These early efforts, by authoritative eighteenth- and early nineteenth-century scientists who helped shape the contours of the life sciences of the Republican Era, did not bode well for the treatment of non-White peoples in the emerging biomedical sciences. Authorities who were active during this era in the United States were quoted in biomedical, political, and intellectual circles, and their theories were viewed as "proof" of Black inferiority well into the twentieth century.[52]

A "Slave Health Deficit" Institutionalized: 1731–1812

The Republican Era is important in many ways from a health perspective. It is the first historical period wherein America had a clearly defined health system with contours, functions, and institutions—the descendants of which are recognizable

---

Vitiligo is the appearance of white patches on black skin due to the loss of pigment without other trophic changes.

today. The nation's first medical schools were opened, the first private hospitals were established, and the medical profession organized and made halting steps toward legal recognition. It was also the first period in which some cities and towns collected morbidity and mortality data that anyone with a public health background could evaluate and appreciate. Even before U.S. independence, academicians recognized the problems faced by the new American medical schools as they struggled to keep up with increasingly demanding scientific curriculums streaming overseas from Europe. Health delivery and educational institutions became active in promulgating the system's race and class differences in health status and outcome, which continue to plague us today. By the end of this period, for the first time, the health system could reasonably be held culpable for some of the differential race- and class-based outcomes.

The maturation and eventual independence of English North America meant that the apron strings from Britain were cut. Moreover, Black health status and outcome could no longer be attributed to lingering effects of the African environment, the Atlantic slave trade, or primitive frontier conditions of New World colonies. Furthermore, by 1730 Black chattel slavery was a pervasive and prominent American institution that was shaping the health system for African Americans. Despite Republican Era rhetoric of "freedom and justice for all," slavery grew as a malignancy on the new democracy that would not be excised until the Civil War almost a century later.

Within this sociopolitical and economic environment, certain factors defined the contours of "difference" that African Americans have historically experienced in the health system:

1. African Americans have always suffered different and worse health status and outcomes, initially manifesting as a slave health deficit.
2. Blacks have from the outset been victim to different, weak, and ineffective health policies and logistics from facility, resource allocation, and expectation perspectives.
3. American society has always viewed Blacks as different from biological and physiological perspectives, providing rationales for the contented, well-cared-for slave myth as justifications for poor Black health, Black/White health disparities, social performance, and outcomes and as rationalizations for racial segregation, White control, and exploitation.
4. African American health providers have traditionally been treated differently, being systematically excluded from or discriminated against within the mainstreams of professional training or health delivery.
5. Until very recently, White physicians have found it socially and politically expedient to view Black patients as different (e.g., citing genetic, constitutional, or biological differences)—thus justifying and rationalizing poor Black health status, outcomes, and expectations.[53]

Although the government began rudimentary census taking in 1790, 1850 was the first year the U.S. Bureau of the Census surveyed and tabulated deaths by disease and race. It was the only official national census taken before the Civil War. Although the data were collected in only a few states, they are as complete as any available before 1933, when the entire United States was included in the Death Registration Area (DRA) for the first time. Bureau of Census data reliability is further compromised relative to African Americans, as most authorities feel that data collected on Blacks are less accurate. Adult, child, and infant mortality data on Blacks before this time came from plantation records on slaves and from records collected by local governmental authorities. These rates were determined by factors such as quality of available medical care, income, nutritional status, environmental quality (e.g., including sanitation conditions, water quality, and air quality), and cultural habits.

The "gold standards" of health status and outcomes from a public health perspective are measures of longevity and mortality and the infant mortality rate (IMR). Douglas C. Ewbank, who published a groundbreaking 1988 study in *The Milbank Quarterly* of mortality trends of American Blacks between 1800 and 1940 compared to mortality trends of American Whites, stated:

> *Throughout the period studied, blacks had substantially higher mortality rates than whites living in the same area. Although the amount of excessive mortality among blacks differed from place to place and period to period, we did not find a single area or time when black mortality rates were close to those of whites.*[54]

His conclusions and results must be seriously considered, as Ewbank utilized modern analytical methods, analyzed old and previously forgotten virgin census data, reanalyzed previous data utilizing modern methodology, and utilized U.S. government health data banks, which are the finest in the world.[55] In 1970 Jitsuichi Masouka reported on Bureau of Census comparative health data for slave and free populations and the small amounts of less reliable, cruder information available for the 1731–1812 period. Masouka indicated that "due to the incomplete reporting of Negro deaths"[56] it was not clear if Black mortality was higher than White mortality.[57] However, Masouka conceded that Baltimore's annual recorded mortality rates compiled before the Civil War—which date back as early as 1812—record only one year before 1830, specifically 1821, in which the Black mortality rate was lower than that for Whites. Reuter observed that in Northern cities where statistical data on mortality was more adequate, "[T]he mortality rate of the Negroes was always higher than that of whites."[58] Although Robert Fogel notes almost a century-long decline in slave mortality beginning around 1700, "[I]t came to a halt during the 1810s or 1820s and then began to rise."[59] Nevertheless, Richard Sutch summarizes the overall situation, succinctly noting, "[T]he most conservative estimate gives white males five more years of life expectancy at birth than male slaves."[60] Until the late nineteenth century Black male life span was approximately 30 to 32 years and life span for Black females was approximately 34 years in most areas, while White longevity climbed to 50 years or more. Clearly, based on the available evidence, if mortality is a "gold standard" of health status and outcome, Black slaves fared much worse than did Whites.

Many experts feel that infant mortality rates and childhood mortality are more sensitive measures of the standard of living and of the slave health experience than are most other indicators. They certainly reflect the same factors that adult mortality figures represent, such as quality of available medical care, income, nutritional status, environmental quality (e.g., including sanitation conditions, water quality, and air quality), and cultural habits. As Ewbank stated about African American childhood mortality, "It is clear that during all periods studied mortality rates were substantially higher for blacks than for whites."[61] Moreover, Fogel noted that fetal and infant death rates, perinatal mortality rates, and childhood death rates also are indicative of other factors, such as the work patterns of pregnant slave women, nursing practices relative to slave infants, and nutritional supplementation for pregnant slaves. Slave babies, probably disproportionately less than 5.5 pounds at birth, were predisposed to diseases such as diarrhea, dysentery, whooping cough, respiratory diseases, and worms. This could account for the fact that early childhood mortality rates for slaves were at least twice as high as the level experienced by white infants and children in the United States. These low birth weight figures may also be related to the high rates of spontaneous abortions, stillbirths, and "mysterious" deaths (Savitt feels some of these might be undiagnosed instances of sudden infant death syndrome [SIDS]) recorded for slaves. There is also strong evidence that malnutrition and undernutrition in early childhood and preadolescence strongly predicted increased overall Black mortality. All of these indicators of the "slave health deficit" were identifiable as early as America's Republican Era. These deficits have constituted a major measure of Black/White "difference" in equality of opportunity and quality of life in the United States since the beginnings of our country.[62]

Because of the paucity of numerical and statistical data collected between 1731 and 1812, our descriptive epidemiology-based analysis of Black health resumes in the Jacksonian Period, for which more information is available. We now shift to more readily available qualitative, descriptive, and clinical information concerning the health of the slaves during late the eighteenth and early nineteenth centuries. Much of this information focuses on how the health of African Americans in slavery was affected by living and work conditions. A survey and overview of the major disease areas impacting slave health during the Republican Era is covered.

High mortality rates for Black slaves were associated with dysentery, typhoid fever, cholera, hepatitis, and worms. Most of these diseases, as Savitt, Kiple, and others have pointed out, were related to the terrible sanitation conditions in most slave quarters. Latrines and sewer disposal systems were rare in eighteenth-century America. Although a few urban slaves living in metropolitan centers such as New Orleans had access to sanitary waste disposal facilities, they were virtually unknown in most slave domiciles. Another condition adding to the risk of gastrointestinal disease transmission was the absence of provisions for adequate hand, dish, or utensil washing. Life in well-defined areas known as "the quarters" was worsened by slave utilization of water supplies contaminated by their own wastes. These risks were compounded by some plantations' use of "night soil" (human feces) and compost heaps for fertilizer. Thus, any larvae or parasites infecting a slave's alimentary tract were disseminated to the entire slave quarter through careless handling of wastes, contaminated produce, and runoff into wells or water tables. Such poor sanitation conditions led to flies in "the quarter" transmitting bacterial infections such as *Vibrio* (cholera), *Salmonella* (typhoid fever and food poisoning), and *Shigella* (bacillary dysentery); viral infections such as viral hepatitis; and protozoal infections caused by *Entameba histolytica* (amoebic dysentery) through feces-to-food transmission. High population density on some larger plantations, where morbidity and mortality was always greater, exacerbated the spread of enteric diseases.

Although there were exceptions, most slave quarters were filthy, allowing huge pest and parasitic infestations and promoting diseases associated with poor hygiene at the personal (few opportunities for baths, hair washing, and haircuts) and environmental (unclean beds, unwashed clothes) levels. Impetigo (a skin disease characterized by infection, pus, and ulcers) was a problem, especially in slave children. Rats killed infants in the slave quarters regularly and transmitted diseases carried by fleas (e.g., the bubonic plague, murine typhus, and dog tapeworm). Worm infestations of various types were rife. Ascariasis (large roundworms often passed in stools) caused malnutrition and chronic anemia. Tapeworms compromised already marginal slave nutritional status and occasionally caused intestinal obstruction. Murine typhus (caused by *Rickettsia mooseri*) and scrub typhus (caused by *Rickettsia prowazeki*), transmitted by body lice and rat fleas, often swept through the slave quarters. Yaws, a deforming, tumor-producing, weeping ulcerative disease of the skin, thrived because slaves often couldn't bathe. Being unable to change clothes for months at a time made this bad situation worse.[63]

Other killers of African American slave populations were ailments attacking the respiratory system. The slaves experienced higher death rates from respiratory diseases than other populations because of their historical lack of exposure to chest diseases such as tuberculosis and pneumonia combined with their seemingly lower tolerance of cold environments. Cold, drafty, sometimes underground, crowded living quarters, compounded by poor ventilation, worsened already deplorable conditions. Tuberculosis death rates were high in the slave quarters due to close proximity, air droplet transmission, and compromised resistance due to poor nutrition and clothing. Diphtheria took a heavy toll among slave children, and pleurisy was ubiquitous in the slave quarters during the fall months. Influenza was a major and periodic problem that often became a killer when slaves had lowered resistance because of other factors. Streptococcal infections in all forms ravaged the slaves. Streptococcal-related pharyngo-tonsillitis, rheumatic fever, and erysipelas were scourges during the pre-antibiotic era.

Pneumonia, often precipitated by upper respiratory infections, took a major toll on slave populations.

Though relatively high in calories, the slave diet led to many nutritional deficiencies. Poor nutrition led to decreased resistance to most major diseases. For slaves, pork was "King of the Table." The bases or staples of the slave diet were 1/2 pound of pork and 1–1 1/2 pounds of corn (usually cornmeal). Although most authorities felt this diet provided between 4,000 and 6,000 calories, such levels were required for the long hours of heavy work demanded of a field slave. However, this pork and corn diet, even when supplemented with molasses, sweet potatoes, cabbage, collard greens, turnips, and turnip greens, did not provide adequate amounts of niacin and tryptophan to prevent pellagra (caused by niacin deficiency). There is evidence that slaves suffered with this disease, described in some accounts as "black tongue." Riboflavin deficiency might have been the cause of the "sore mouth" often reported by slaves. The *slave diet* also failed to provide adequate calcium or vitamin A unless there was heavy supplementation with milk, bright orange sweet potatoes, or cow peas, which were seldom provided to the slaves in large amounts. Vitamin A deficiency accounted for the frequent reports of "sore eyes" noted by Postell. Due to the method of storing, curing, and preparing slave rations of pork and corn, the slaves may have suffered from a spectrum of thiamine deficiency leading to dirt/clay-eating (geophagia) or to full-blown beriberi. The more severe form, the wet type of beriberi, was mislabelled "Cachexia Africana" by many Southern physicians busy creating a lexicon of new diseases peculiar to Black slaves. This serious variety of beriberi was sometimes complicated by hypochromic anemia and hookworms. Clinically the victims exhibited a perverse craving for clay, and, as Sutch elaborated, "extreme sluggishness, great edema, pallor (particularly of the mucous membranes), great susceptibility to cold, diminished secretions, blood thin and watery, of a livid purple hue."[64] The eventual outcome was death. The unembellished slave diet was thus far from ideal considering the stresses under which they lived, and it also predisposed them to many other illnesses.[65]

Slaves were able to survive this dietary stress by supplementing the basic slave diet with green vegetables from their personal gardens, fish from lakes and streams, and greens and game acquired from hunting and scavenging. Some masters provided these items when crop harvest was bountiful. When red meat and fish were not added, anemia, protein malnutrition, and lassitude resulted. Valuable calories and iron were added by molasses, which the slaves thought only added flavor and good taste. This entire dietary spectrum, even when nutritionally sufficient, was high in cholesterol and triglycerides, predisposing the slaves to coronary artery disease and heart attacks, strokes, and complications from vascular blockage.[66]

Diseases associated with animal exposures, although not foreign to Whites, were prevalent with slave populations. Many slaves were compelled to work with animals as they engaged in daily agricultural pursuits. Moreover, animals were the sole means of transportation at the time. Thus, slaves had a significant incidence of brucellosis (undulant fever or Malta fever), a disease of pigs, goats, and cattle. Clinically, this disease presented as an intermittent fever; therefore, it was probably often confused with malaria and other similar fevers. Humans were infected through several routes, with direct contact with skin wounds being the most common. The incidence of brucellosis rose during hog-killing or beef-butchering times. Leptospirosis (also called mud fever) was also a disease acquired from domestic animals. *Leptospira* organisms were transmitted oropharyngeally, through abraded skin or wounds on the body. Contact with organisms also took place in swamps, muddy pastures, and rice paddies where domestic animals such as pigs or cattle had urinated. Clinically, the disease presented as chills and fever accompanied by a headache as the organism invaded the bloodstream and spinal fluid. Muscle pain was also common. Anthrax, a disease of pigs, cattle, sheep, and other domestic animals, remains a threat to both man and animals, especially in developing countries. The animals ingest the bacterium in their food. Humans handling the animals' hair, hide, or infected meat develop skin pustules, fever, vomiting, general malaise, and diarrhea. Depending upon the spread pattern, some slaves died of meningitis and septicemia.

Black slaves, who may have had distinctive patterns of disease predisposition, were probably at somewhat increased risk for thermal injuries due to cold. They were frequently exposed because of inadequate heating, the absence of shoes, and a lack of clothing. Although they may have been at slightly decreased risk of heat injury, African Americans were not immune. For example, Savitt quotes the record left by Hill Carter of the Shirley Plantation in 1825 about slave responses to heat: "Hottest day ever felt—men gave out and some fainted."[67] Subsequent scientific evidence has suggested that Blacks may be slightly more resistant to heat injury (e.g., heat exhaustion and heatstroke) than Whites and may be somewhat more prone to cold injuries such as frostbite. Because Black slaves performed long hours of outdoor work in all seasons in different parts of the country, their risk for thermal injury, especially in winter, is clear. Little was known of preventive hydration and prophylactic salt administration (considered of questionable value) in the eighteenth century; thus, the slaves' risk of heat injury would have been high in summer months. Numerous accounts document the inadequacy of clothing provided to slaves. The absence of adequate footwear or being forced to wear poorly made footwear were especially prominent problems, exacerbated by the fact that manufacturing resources in the South were inadequate and slave clothing and shoes had to be ordered from as far away as New York or New England.[68] Such practices substantially increased the risk of cold injury.

Venereal diseases were a problem with poor populations throughout the colonies. The slave population was no exception. The institution of slavery, which encouraged casual sexual activity to increase fertility and lessen restrictions caused by close family ties, was an incubator for gonorrhea, syphilis, and other sexually transmitted diseases. Moreover, treatment for sexually transmitted diseases for the most part was relatively ineffective, lengthy, and costly. Toxic treatments with heavy metals such as mercury were the cornerstone of therapy. High rates of gonorrhea caused much suffering and disability among both males and females and was probably a major cause of female sterility. Syphilis became epidemic in slave populations, and congenital syphilis was not uncommon.[69]

Miscegenation involving masters and overseers and slave women exacerbated an already bad situation. Encouragement of pregnancy was one of the distinguishing characteristics of English North American slavery. By the mid-eighteenth century, Black slave populations increased dramatically. Legal closure of the Atlantic slave trade by the British Parliament in 1807 and the United States Congress in 1808 increased the necessity of the internal or domestic slave trade. Slave breeding became profitable and necessary to perpetuate the institution of slavery. Thus, casual fornication was encouraged, if not forced. The older, upper South states such as Virginia became slave exporters to new slave states in the west and lower South. As slavery became big business, the domestic slave trade transformed into a massive infrastructure. This increase in slave populations was the opposite of the slave system in the Caribbean and Central and South America, where annual slave importation was necessary to sustain slave populations. All of these developments had a tremendous impact on the health system.[70]

The beginnings of the Industrial Revolution during this historical period meant that more slaves were involved in industrial work. Hiring slaves out for industrial work was common in the ensuing decades. Five percent of the total slave population worked in Southern industries during the Antebellum Period. The practice of "hiring out" also meant that slaves often worked in strange and unfamiliar environments under the supervision of masters who had no vested interest in maintaining them. Diseases such as tobacco lung and silicosis, forms of chronic lung disease with progressive respiratory insufficiency and respiratory failure, emerged and became more common. Victims became increasingly disabled pulmonary cripples, eventuating in death. Lead toxicity from foundry work was reported with progressive mental deterioration and nervous system involvement. Accidental injuries were also a real risk to slaves, who often labored in dangerous workplaces. As Todd Savitt notes in *Science and Medicine in the Old South*, "Farm accidents . . . took their toll on slaves. Falls, overturned carts, runaway wagons, drownings, limbs caught in farm machines, kicks from animals, and cuts from axes or scythe blades were the commonest types."[71]

Throughout the U.S. slavery experience, childhood mortality was extremely high. Infant and childhood mortality were directly responsible for a significant proportion of excess slave deaths and for statistically shortening slave life spans. Birth was usually attended by untrained Black midwives, which increased the risks for deaths from obstetrical complications and birth injuries. Black prematurity and stillbirth rates were at least twice as high as those for other populations. Improper handling of the umbilical cord led to a high incidence of neonatal tetanus, a uniformly fatal disease at that time.[72]

Even if the infant survived the neonatal period (the first 28 days of life), mortality rates for children in the slave quarter were still very high. Poor sanitation conditions in the slave quarters led to infections and infestations with ascariasis (roundworms), hookworms acquired by walking in infected soil, tapeworms acquired through ingesting infected meat, and typhoid fever and hepatitis through poor sanitation and oropharyngeal transmission. Diarrhea and dysentery were common killers of children in the slave quarters. Smallpox vaccinations were seldom carried out by penny-pinching masters. Therefore, Black children commonly succumbed to smallpox. SIDS was a relatively common problem in slave populations and was often attributed to the mother "laying over" her young or being suspected of foul play.

High maternal and infant death rates reflected multiple obstetrical system deficiencies. As was noted earlier, deliveries by poorly trained midwives often resulted in bad outcomes for both mother and child. Although there is ambiguity expressed among medical historians specializing in slavery, slave women's unfortunate outcomes relative to infant mortality, perinatal mortality, and maternal mortality testify that they were not overly pampered while pregnant. More than 90 percent of slave deliveries were attended by such midwives, and physicians were only called in when serious complications arose. Pregnancy outcome was also compromised by poor slave nutrition and massive overwork for slave women. Slave women received insufficient rest while pregnant and nursing. They worked virtually until they went into labor and returned to the fields two to three days after delivery. It was observed that slave infants "are suckled hurriedly, whilst the mother is overheated."[73] A lack of prenatal care, inadequate rest, and insufficient diets led to pregnancy complications, anemias, and small babies. Intergenerational dietary deficiencies may have predisposed slave women to contracted pelvises and abnormal labors and, eventually, to maternal deaths.[74]

Female diseases and gynecological disorders worked special hardships on slave populations. Women slaves often had to work while enduring severe abdominal or pelvic pain. Such conditions were relatively common and sometimes interfered with work. Frequent childbearing compounded by heavy work and lifting made genital prolapse (the "falling out" of the womb and bladder from the vagina) relatively common among slave women. Vaginal discharges and infections were also common, although cancer seemed to be relatively rare— probably due to short slave life span. These conditions may have influenced already high miscarriage and stillbirth rates. Infertility could often pose serious problems for younger slave women, who could be sold off or punished for failing to become pregnant.[75]

Another factor that changed the profile of slave illnesses was the reign of terror that swept over the slave South beginning in the Republican Era. An unfortunate fact of history is that whenever Whites perceived a threat of Negro rebellion or violence in Western Hemisphere slave systems, punishments meted out to Blacks increased exponentially. Slavery specialist Eugene Genovese noted, "As early as 1522 the slaves of Hispaniola rose in what was probably the first black slave revolt in the New World."[76] Responses to reports of slave rebellion such as those that occurred on the *Clare* in 1729 and the *Dolphin* in 1732 were vigorous in English North America. The reports that had the most impact were those of rebellions in the Caribbean, such as the ones that occurred in the Virgin Islands and Jamaica in the 1730s. Especially terrifying were domestic incidents of slave resistance. In English North America, African and Native Americans invaded Hartford, Connecticut, as early as 1657. As Katz observed in *Breaking the Chains*, "The eighteenth century . . . gave birth to slave uprisings from New York to Georgia."[77] In 1712 New York slaves rose to wound and kill more than a score of Whites, and recurrent riots occurred there in 1740 and 1741. McManus notes in *A History of Negro Slavery in New York* that as a result of the 1741 riot, "Altogether, fourteen slaves had been burned at the stake, eighteen hanged, and seventy-two deported from the province."[78] Whether the purported slave uprisings in 1741 in New York were real or simply based on White hysteria is debatable. Nevertheless, the adverse outcomes for Blacks remained basically the same. Three slave uprisings rocked South Carolina in 1739, the last being the Stono Rebellion where slaves seized a warehouse full of arms and ammunition, marched in military formation, and killed about 30 Whites. There were incidents in Hackensack, New Jersey (1741); Maryland (1766); and Virginia (1781), where Blacks were punished for arson. Black punishments in the United States, especially in the eighteenth and early nineteenth centuries, often went to ghoulish extremes, including, as Woods notes in *Black Majority: Negroes in Colonial South Carolina from 1670 through the Stono Rebellion*, "castration, nose-splitting, and chopping off such extremities as ears, hands, or toes."[79] (Some of the unusual psychosexual overtones of U.S. punishments administered to Blacks have been recognized and are only now beginning to be studied.)[80]

During this era slave punishments spilled over into the medical sphere. These practices could be so brutal or bizarre that they could result in a slave's death or permanent injury. Whipping was a prominent feature of slave life in the South. Savitt describes the process in detail in *Science and Medicine in the Old South*:

> *From a medical point of view, whipping inflicted cruel and often permanent injuries upon its victims. Laying stripes across the bare back or buttocks caused indescribable pain, especially when each stroke dug deeper into previously opened wounds. . . . In addition to multiple lacerations of the skin, whipping caused loss of blood, injury to muscles (and internal organs, if the lash reached that deep), and shock.*[81]

The lash was not the only mode of whipping that slaves underwent. Savitt explains further:

> *The paddle jarred every part of the body by the violence of the blow, and raised blisters from repeated strokes. In addition to the possibility of death . . . there was the danger that muscle damage inflicted by these instruments might permanently incapacitate a slave or deform him for life.*[82]

Slaves were sometimes crucified, and castration was legal and common. Burning slaves alive at the stake was another legal method of punishment. Cutting off body parts such as ears or feet was sometimes utilized to impress other slaves. Masters wishing to avoid colorful or dramatic punishments resorted simply to starving slaves. Virtually any of these punishments carried to the extreme became a medical concern. In fact, after the Haitian slave rebellion in 1791 cruel public punishments became so common in slave-holding territories in the Western Hemisphere that the additional trauma altered the profile of slavery's illnesses. In areas of the South previously thought to be relatively safe and secure for Whites, slave patrols were also initiated.[83]

Although slave living and working conditions during the late eighteenth and early nineteenth centuries shaped the health profile and outcomes of African Americans, the effect of the health system's provision of institutions and health care resources to slaves also had a major impact. Thus, all of the external factors that affected slave health—from home and work to doctors, hospitals, health care and service provision, and clinics—were controlled and dictated by Whites and their infrastructure. How these institutional, professional, and logistical resources were distributed is the realm of health policy—the next area we will examine.[84]

An Emerging Dual Health System in Black and White

Poor slave health outcomes were virtually guaranteed by the health policies of the time. Miserly slave masters' stingy use of regular physicians indirectly encouraged the growth of the slave health subsystem. Black slave healers (sometimes in the frontier tradition of "kitchen physics"), conjure men, slave nurses and midwives, and "root doctors" provided the bulk of medical care and treatment provided to slaves. Often this was the choice of the slaves themselves, a cultural continuation of an ancient African healing tradition. The slaves often preferred these practitioners, who were friends or neighbors who usually looked like and related well to them. Although many masters frowned on the practice, such consultations were often sought by sick slaves. Planters sometimes considered such actions medically dangerous and as another means of delaying proper care to a slave. Other planters openly relied upon slave healers and midwives, sometimes allowing them to practice on other plantations in the region. Some planters even collected fees generated by their popular and talented "healer" chattel.

Some Southern physicians were contracted to care for a plantation's slaves, but this was not required nor uniformly adhered to. Often such "contract practice" was the way young and inexperienced White physicians got started and sustained themselves financially until their practices grew. Generally, slaves did not like these regular (allopathic*) physicians and resisted treatments, neglected their illnesses, or feigned being well in order to sever the doctor–patient relationship. Moreover, all these regular practitioners had to offer was the standard bleeding, cupping, purging, blistering, and vomiting that were consistent with the depletive therapies of the time. Slaves, along with the general public, observed that these treatments were usually unpleasant and didn't work. The most positive interventions physicians had in their armamentariums were connected with setting fractures, correcting obstetrical complications, or performing surgeries on surface structures (e.g., draining abscesses, extracting painful teeth, excising benign tumors). Formally trained or apprentice-trained physicians were most often called in when a slave was obviously in extremis or as a last resort. Doctors resented being called in under these circumstances, but there was little they could do to control the practice. This lack of formal care was often evidenced by the low immunization rates among the slaves. Unless an epidemic was raging, money was not often spent on slave immunizations.

The financial and social status of African Americans dictated that they were virtually never at the center of medical attention. Poor or compromised outcomes were tolerated and even expected. Moreover, wide and deep communication and class barriers generated more distance between a relatively elite and privileged medical profession and the nation's Black population. This was compounded by the fact that most of America's trained medical professional leaders were preoccupied with upward class mobility and the consolidation of professional prestige and status. The ideal patients these men desired in their practices were White, well-to-do, and middle to upper class. Another facet of the slave health subsystem was the treatment of slaves by their masters. Sometimes, these duties were assumed by the overseer, sometimes by the masters or slave owners' wives. Whether slaves saw trained physicians at all was totally dependent on the availability of resources. Medicine chests and self-help medical treatment books were common items in the plantation big house. Occasionally, to economize or avoid the heroic treatments regular physicians utilized, irregular medical practitioners from the outside were called in on complicated cases. It is clear that as far as the White medical profession was concerned, the Black population in the United States was a side line or peripheral issue—definitely outside the mainstream of medical practice.[85]

Another major demonstration of the separateness of the slave health subsystem was the establishment of a pattern of developing separate or segregated medical institutions based on race and class. As has been pointed out earlier, the colony's earliest institutions that were occupied with illness recovery and the delivery of health care—the public almshouses, poorhouses, maternity hospitals, and pesthouses in the larger cities—were already institutions on the margins of

---

*Allopathic (from the Greek word *alloin*, or *different*) refers to physicians who applied remedies whose effects differed from those of the disease. It also referred to "mainstream" physicians who tended to use *heroic* (e.g., bleeding, purging, depleting, vomiting) therapies.

society and the health system. Depending on local practices, Blacks were some-times able to use these facilities. There were also some eighteenth-century government-sponsored hospitals provided for sailors and the merchant marines, who were considered transients and burdens on local medical communities. These institutions were designed to house rootless, sick strangers without families to care for them. All such institutions relegated to the margins of the mainstream health system were considered inferior.

When being a member of the Black race was added to such a patient's plight, admission was often refused, or the person was assigned to an outbuilding, base-ment, or attic. Blacks were placed well away from White patients. Organization-ally, this health system policy prevailed nationwide. It is well documented that large and well-known early institutions such as the Philadelphia Almshouse (1731), Bellevue in New York City (1734), and Charity Hospital in New Orleans (1737) were racially segregated during the periods that they admitted Black patients at all. For the institutions opening later in the Republican Era, lines between private and paying patients were more rigidly drawn. For example, Leonard P. Curry noted in *The Free Black in Urban America 1800–1850*, "A physi-cian who admitted a black to the Massachusetts General Hospital in Boston . . . contrary to policy, was reproved by the hospital authorities, and . . . blacks seeking admission were turned away."[86] Clearly, policies allowing Black and White patients to share facilities within voluntary hospitals such as the Pennsylvania Hos-pital (1751) or the New York Hospital (1791) were out of the question. These same trends prevailed at the nation's earliest dispensaries and clinics.[87]

In the South, this racial separation was often carried out to greater extremes. However, in some communities where public hospitals, dispensaries, and clinics were established, Blacks were not denied access. As Curry observed, "In some cities free persons of color (and, in the southern urban centers, slaves as well) were received into public hospitals. This was not, to be sure, universally true."[88] In communities where Blacks were allowed admission, strict racial segregation was the rule. As Curry further explains:

> In New Orleans . . . not only had the original donation of Don Andres Almonaster y Roxas, which formed the basis for the development of the renowned Charity Hospital, specified the admission (on a segregated basis) of free persons of color, but by mid-century there was also a sepa-rate charity hospital for free persons of color.[89]

Therefore, as was the case in the North, Southern Blacks were placed in out-buildings, attics, basements, or, at best, segregated wards. As Wade recorded when a foreign visitor toured the city institution, which was the most important facility in Louisville, Kentucky, he found "roomy and well aired apartments for the white patients, and in the basement, those for the negroes and colored per-sons."[90] These policies did not deviate much from those in force north of the

Mason-Dixon line. None of these facilities were staffed by African American caregivers. Ironically, Black slaves, whose masters often assumed financial responsibility for this substandard care, were usually better off than the few free Blacks. Unenslaved Blacks were the truly disconnected in the system and their health status, the poorest of all Americans, reflected this reality.[91]

Similar to the West Indian experience, some Southern plantation owners built their own slave hospitals. (See Figure 4.2.) This was a prominent trend on large plantations with 100 or more slaves. All levels of providers staffing the slave health subsystem were mobilized to serve these facilities. Physicians from the area were sometimes contracted to make rounds and supervise the organization and operations of the plantation hospital. Such affluent circumstances were relatively rare.[92]

Dispensaries and clinics were scarce in the eighteenth century. As Lyons and Petrucelli stated in *Medicine: An Illustrated History*, "[O]nly the very wealthy could be assured of the services of a qualified doctor of medicine, and this of course forced the general public into the hands of mountebanks, quacks, and others poorly prepared to offer rational treatment."[93] Even people who were not actually poverty-stricken had no place to turn for medical attention. With the opening of the Philadelphia Dispensary in 1786 at the behest of Dr. Benjamin Rush, this trend was officially addressed for the first time in America. This was followed by the opening of the Boston Dispensary in 1796. Other hospitals began establishing outpatient clinics by the late eighteenth century. Dispensaries became vital components of the health care infrastructure by the nineteenth century and grew in influence as sources of both training and care until the twentieth century. During the late eighteenth and early nineteenth centuries, from a medical professional viewpoint, dispensary service was considered vital for clinical advancement and as a source for attending interesting cases. In the South, segregated facilities that cared for Blacks and indigent Whites were opened to facilitate medical training. Ironically, free Blacks, most of whom were medically indigent, were more of a financial burden than were most slaves. These facilities were staffed at virtually no cost by physicians who served in exchange for professional advancement and training and participation in the care of surgical and rare cases. Moreover, many common conditions were more efficiently and economically managed with outpatient rather than inpatient care. Highly specialized fields such as otology, ophthalmology, and dermatology were especially well suited to dispensary and other outpatient methods of delivery. As Rosenberg remarked, dispensaries had "by the mid-nineteenth century become the principal form of institutional care for the working poor and the indigent."[94] For a variety of reasons associated with changes in health care financing, medical training and education, and medical sociology and politics, the dispensary movement was curtailed after the Civil War. A devastating effect resulted, further limiting access to care for working class, indigent, and Black patients. Not until the twentieth-century settlement house and community health center movements would corrective measures to address this problem be seriously undertaken.[95]

Figure 4.2   Magnolia Hill Plantation "Slave Hospital": Natchez,
Mississippi [Modern Photograph]

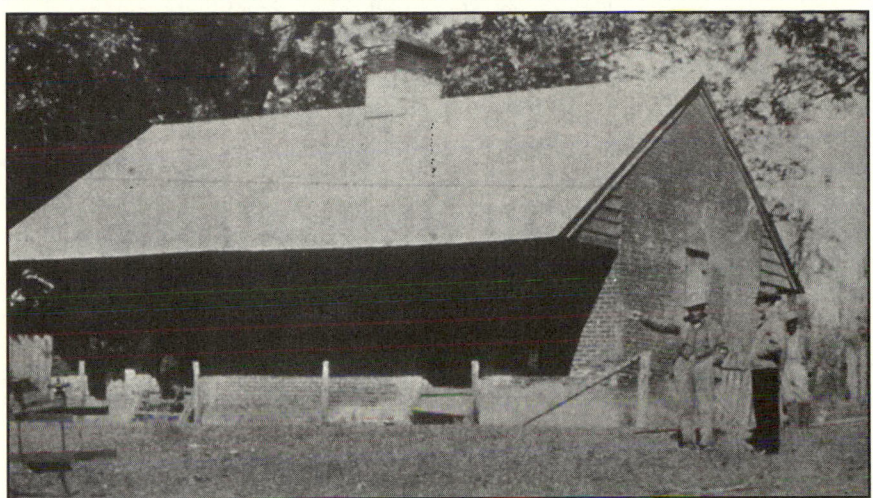

Though the debate on whether working slaves to death or maintaining and "breeding" them was never resolved during slavery, some plantation owners, thinking that maintaining slaves was cost-effective, built slave hospitals like the one here. Usually, these hospitals were staffed by the planter, his overseer, or the planter's wife who, with their medicine chest and domestic medical manuals such as Ewell's *The Planter's* and *Mariner's Medical Companion*, backed up slave caregivers. Regular physicians were usually called in for acute emergencies or as the last resort. The slave practitioners were often granny midwives, nurses, slave healers, root doctors, or occasionally conjure men or women. Such healers were sometimes granted official authority by the master. The slaves invariably chose these untrained healers if given a choice.

Between 1731 and 1812 other recognizable components of the health system developed. Private hospitals appeared. A medical-educational system developed simultaneously. By 1800 there were four medical schools. As their numbers increased in the nineteenth century, these schools immediately took advantage of Blacks and the poor in the health system by establishing mechanisms and institutions to overutilize them for training and demonstration purposes. Black participation at the policy or professional levels in these activities was absent.[96]

Race Medicine: Real or Imagined Differences?

It is well known that human groups living in relative isolation in particular environments not only demonstrate differences in appearance but also manifest differing disease susceptibilities and relative immunities. Human groups under certain circumstances demonstrate genetic adaptations to special environments, thereby producing specific disease states such as sickle cell anemia, thalassemia, and others. These facts in no way challenge the unity of the human species from biological, physiological, pathological, or medical-therapeutic standpoints. That is why there are no separate disciplines of medicine or medical treatments for various racial or ethnic groups.

In America, a great deal has been made of Black "differences" relative to Whites and other groups for nearly 400 years. There has been no more important arena for this ongoing polemic regarding these differences than that of health care. Not only have these "differences" been used from a biomedical perspective to account for existing hierarchies and stratification of society (including the medical profession), but they have also been used as rationales and yardsticks determining priorities and levels of resource allocation for health care. Moreover, issues such as unethical experimentation, surgical exploitation, and sterilization; the culture of racism and discrimination in the health system; and overt discrimination in the health professions are all influenced by this "difference" factor. Myrdal even suggested that America's traditional policy of health care nilhism regarding African Americans may represent an underlying public policy of eliminating the Black race in the United States.[97] Many of these concepts, beliefs, and practices became institutionalized in our health system during the nation's Republican Era.[98]

There has always been a great deal of variety in the human family. However, the human species shares the same basic genes, biology, and physiology and suffers from the same diseases. On the other hand, different racial and ethnic groups, including Blacks, exhibit different incidences and risks of certain health problems. For example, as medical historian Todd Savitt has repeatedly noted in his research and writings, "Jews are less prone to contract tuberculosis, but more subject to Niemann-Pick Disease and Gaucher's Disease."[99] He has documented that Swedes exhibit vulnerabilities to sarcoidosis, porphyria, and pernicious anemia, while South Africans of Dutch descent are prone to porphyria cutanea tarda. Eighteenth- and early nineteenth-century physicians took note of these trends—especially as they related to Blacks. After all, it was in their financial as well as political interest.

Physicians who cared for large numbers of African Americans began noticing that Blacks seemed to possess immunity to various fevers. The resistance seemed more prevalent in newly arrived Africans after the "breaking-in" period. Although differentiating the various fevers according to cause was beyond the capabilities of eighteenth- and nineteenth-century medicine, historians retrospectively make educated etiological guesses today. The major fevers that Africans seemed to have resistance to were yellow fever, sleeping sickness, and malaria. Presenting clinically as intermittent fevers, they were often confused with each other.

Yellow fever is a viral disease of men and monkeys transmitted by the bite of the Aedes mosquito. The disease has over 100 names but is commonly referred to as "yellow jack"; the "Bay of Benin Fever," because of its points of origin; the "black vomit," referring to a prominent clinical sign produced by vomiting digested blood; and "bilios remittent," referring to its pathophysiological course. Medical men called it yellow fever because of the jaundice (a yellow tint to the skin produced by high circulating levels of bile pigments) it produced. After much historical and epidemiological debate, the general consensus now is that the disease originated in Africa and was carried across the Atlantic following Columbus's landing in America. Both the disease and the mosquito, which is a highly domestic species living and breeding in artificial containers of water, were disseminated to the Americas over the long years of the Atlantic slave trade. Symptoms of yellow fever are the acute and sudden onset of fever followed by a severe headache. Agonizing pains are followed by vomiting large quantities of greasy, black blood produced by the action of gastric juice. Half the susceptible victims vomit themselves to death over several days. Survivors are immune for life. Providentially, infected children have a mild form of the disease through which they acquire permanent immunity. Black slaves from the endemic areas in West Africa were relatively resistant to the ravages of yellow fever. Eighteenth- and nineteenth-century physicians in this instance were correct in their intuitive conclusions.

Sleeping sickness—now known to be caused by microscopic, spindle-shaped parasites with undulating membranes named *Trypanosoma gambiense* and *T. rhodesiense*—was called the "narcotic dropsy" and "the sleeping distemper" by slavers on the West African coasts. The victim is bitten by the tsetse fly *(Glossina)*, which injects the organisms with its proboscis (a sharp, tubular mouthpiece). The dread disease begins as an intermittent fever, headache, and pain in the limbs. Injected organisms spread to lymph glands in the back of the neck (which the slavers used to identify as a marker to screen out infected victims), after which the victim becomes lethargic. After spreading to the brain the patient sleeps, cannot care for himself, becomes covered with sores, and dies of pneumonia, dysentery, or starvation. Infected natives were thought to be mentally slow and lethargic or extremely homesick when the disease was observed during the Atlantic slave trade. It is possible that the behaviors and mental acuity associated with this illness may have encouraged misconceptions of White superiority and African inferiority by Europeans. Africans residing in the disease's endemic areas in West Africa and the Congo developed some immunity to the disease. Once more, astute eighteenth-century medical observers were not far off the mark.

Between 1730 and 1812, malaria was known as intermittent or remittent fever. Its other names were fever and chills, marsh fever, and autumnal fever. Science has subsequently proved that malaria is a parasitic disease caused by a one-celled animal, the plasmodium, that colonizes red blood cells. After being injected into the human bloodstream from an infected anopheles mosquito, the immature parasite enters liver cells, multiplies, and reenters the bloodstream by rupturing host cells. They multiply and then reinvade red blood cells, rupturing and destroying them. This event corresponds with chills and fever. As the body defends itself with phagocytic white blood cells, which ingest the plasmodia, blood vessels in the lymph glands, spleen, and vital organs can become clogged with red cell debris, phagocytes, and large numbers of parasites leading to organ damage and death. The three major forms of the disease are due to *Plasmodium falciparum* (infection lasts 6–8 months), *P. vivax* (infection multiplies for 5 years), and *P. malariae* (infection can last up to 30 years).

The clinical onset of the disease is characterized by a period of severe chills unrelieved by even large numbers of blankets, followed by paroxysms of extremely high fever, frequent nausea, vomiting, and severe headaches. Profuse sweating for up to 5 hours accompanies the break in the fever, which is followed by severe weakness and prostration. The break in the fever can last from one (*P. falciparum*) to four (*P. vivax*) days while the parasites multiply again in the host's bloodstream. This cycle can recur for several weeks, and then recur months or years later depending on the victim's condition and the type of parasite causing it. After each paroxysm of disease the host is weakened and prone to other infectious diseases.

Physicians were usually the only ones worried about the esoteric mechanisms of slave resistances to various diseases. As far as the fevers were concerned, planters only knew that initial episodes could kill his slaves, incapacitate his laborers during harvest season, and could relapse, causing time away from work and even death to his chattel. Science has later confirmed that some acquired immunity to malaria was possible if slaves were exposed to repeated infections of the disease over several years. However, the major reason for Black immunity to vivax or falciparum malaria related to selective genetic factors. Recent medical research has revealed that red blood cells lacking a factor called the Duffy antigen are resistant to *P. vivax*. Up to 90 percent of West Africans lack Duffy antigens on their red blood cells, as do approximately 70 percent of African Americans. This hematologic condition is asymptomatic and is very rare in other racial groups.

Two other abnormal hemoglobin conditions, sickle cell disease (a serious form of anemia) and sickle cell trait (the asymptomatic carrier form of the anemia that can be transmitted to future generations), confer decreased severity of illness and lesser mortality from the falciparum form of malarial disease. Deficiency of the enzyme glucose-6-phosphate dehydrogenase (G-6-PD deficiency) also affords some malarial resistance. Since up to 22 percent of Africans transported to the Americas brought sickle cell genes and up to 20 percent brought G-6-PD deficiency genes, probably 30–40 percent of the slaves were protected from some forms of malaria by these mechanisms alone.

Southern physicians also observed that Blacks were more prone to cold injuries (e.g., frostbite) and seemed more resistant to heat injury (e.g., heat prostration and heat stroke) than were Whites. Both observations have supporters for these impressions as medical fact.

Even today there is confusion among medical authorities regarding Black susceptibility to severe pulmonary infections. There is also evidence that Blacks may be more prone to severe tuberculosis infections. These phenomena are explainable by the fact that Black exposure to these illnesses began only 500 years ago through contact with Caucasians. Caucasian and Asian immune systems have adapted to handling these types of infections for millennia and may have milder clinical responses to the disease.

Another condition that seemed to affect slaves almost exclusively was the sudden and unexpected death of Black infants by "smothering," "overlaying," or "suffocation." Retrospective evaluation of these incidents indicates that most of them were probably attributable to what we know today as SIDS. The cause of SIDS is unknown; to this day it has a much higher incidence in the African American population. The reasons for the increased risk remain unknown.

Other clinically obvious conditions that were more prevalent in African American slaves were polydactyly (extra fingers), umbilical hernias, and lactose intolerance (wherein the ingestion of cows' milk causes gastrointestinal upset, cramping, and diarrhea). Since milk was very seldom included in slave diets, the latter condition probably rarely manifested itself clinically. Hypertension, another disease more commonly afflicting Blacks, is usually clinically asymptomatic until end organ complications such as renal failure, heart failure, or stroke occur. Black slave life spans were very short. Thus, they seldom lived long enough to manifest these clinical syndromes.[100]

Other biological, anatomical, and medical "differences" presented by eighteenth- and nineteenth-century physicians and natural scientists have not withstood the rigors of scientific scrutiny, deteriorating into the category of scientific racism in the process. Maturation of scientific racism in English North America was built upon the compilation and "documentation" of racial differences in the European biological, anthropological, and ethnological sciences of the late eighteenth and early nineteenth centuries. Both Northern and Southern physicians made and wrote statements and treatises contributing to the deluge of scientific racist mythology of the era, "documenting" the Negro's "differences." (See Table 4.1.) In fact, several influential physicians and academicians in the United States devoted significant portions of their professional careers examining this question. This body of work, and the effects it had socially and politically on the Black population, was extremely important, for it had a great deal to do with influencing and determining the health policy for and thus the health care provided to slaves

Table 4.1   Republican Era "Negro Diseases"

- Chronic leprosy . . . sometimes results in blackening of the skin and a "smell"
- Locked jaw . . . caused by heat and smoke of slave cabins
- Hipochondriasis . . . attributed to grief over enslavement
- Difficult parturition . . . caused by heavy burdens and kicks of the masters

Source: Jordan WD. *White over Black: American Attitudes Toward the Negro, 1550–1812.* New York: W.W. Norton and Company, Inc., 1968, 517–521.

and free Blacks. Additionally, scientific racism served as the scientific justification for enslaving 95 percent of more than 2 million people of African descent
during this period and for cruelly dominating and subjugating the rest.[101]

The Black Medical Profession: 1731–1812

African American exclusion from formal health professions and training during
this period was the rule. However, African American healers and medical practitioners were practicing all over America during these years, especially in the
South. Most of these practitioners constituted the slave health subsystem of self-
trained or informally trained healers, conjurers, root doctors, and slave midwives.
Social conditions and financial status during the late Colonial and Republican
eras kept free Blacks from formal medical training in the new Republic's few
medical schools. Slaves were not educated to read or write, thus precluding their
being considered for professional training—in many states, educating a slave was
against the law. Recording African American history in any field of endeavor for a
people under such restrictions was out of the question. Therefore, the record of
these practitioners is understandably sparse.[102]

The first Black acknowledged as a healer in North America may have been
an elderly Southern slave who was granted his freedom by Lieutenant Governor
Gooch of Virginia in 1729. Gooch recorded that he:

> met with a negro [sic], a very old man, who has performed many wonder-
> ful cures of diseases. For the sake of his freedom, he has revealed the med-
> icine, a concoction of roots and bark. . . . There is no room to doubt of its
> being a certain remedy here, and of singular use [in the treatment of
> syphilis] among the negroes, it is well worth the price (£60) of the negro's
> freedom, since it is now known how to cure slaves without mercury.[103]

The first Black healer to reach public notice was recorded in the Philadelphia *Pennsylvania Gazette* in 1740 for escaping from slavery. His name was
Simon, and he was credited with being able "to bleed and draw teeth, pretending
to be a great doctor among his people."[104] This last statement was emblematic of
the relationship between Black healers and the medical establishment, setting a
demeaning tone for delineating the status of African American healers in English
North America. As Kenneth Ludmerer observed about Black access to health
professions training in *Learning to Heal*:

> Blacks . . . faced much greater obstacles that mirrored the problems they
> encountered elsewhere in . . . American life. Before the Civil War, physi-
> cians in the North openly denied blacks entrance to the profession. In
> the South, blacks were sometimes permitted to practice folk and herbal

remedies on fellow slaves but were not allowed to receive formal medical instruction.[105]

In such a professionally negative environment, Bousfield remarked that he was amazed that any African Americans overcame the social, educational, and professional obstacles to practice medicine before the Civil War.[106] A Negro slave, Caesar, wrote the first medical publication by an African American about a remedy for snakebite, which was published in the *Massachusetts Magazine* in 1792. There must have been thousands of traditional healers, conjure men, root doctors, spiritual healers, granny nurses, and slave midwives who served and delivered the hands-on care necessary for African American survival in a hostile land. Medical historians such as John A. Kenney, Leslie Falk, Herbert Morais, W. Montague Cobb, Todd Savitt, Kenneth Kiple, Richard Sheridan, and others have resurrected some of them from obscurity. They served as the medical work force for the slave health subsystem, which was the cornerstone of health delivery for Black slaves, and also served as a continuation of the established health policy that Blacks had to be treated "differently" than others. Thus, this vital subsystem that served 20 percent of the U.S. population was relegated to the periphery of the "mainstream" health system. That in no way diminishes the fact that these unsung Black health pioneers had a great deal to do with providing health care services and, ultimately, contributing to the survival of the Negro people.[107]

After the appearance of Lucas Santomee (a Dutch-trained Black physician) in the 1660s in New Netherlands, there was no other university-trained Black physician practicing in the United States until James McCune Smith (1813–1865) returned to New York City from the University of Glasgow with his B.S., M.S., and M.D. degrees in 1837. There is no historical evidence that other Blacks were fully trained in university settings during this time. The 177-year gap in these two African American physicians' professional accomplishments tell a story. As far as a voice from university-trained African American healers in English North America in the intervening years is concerned, the silence is deafening. The facts are emblematic of the relationship between the mainstream health providers and the Black population and Black healers. A national pattern of health care involving Black dependency on trained White health providers, rather than self-sufficiency, was established and remains today. Although the exact social mechanisms, medical educational deficiencies, and political economic landscapes have changed, the end results have been the same. The representation of Black physicians has remained at the 2–3-percent levels for the past century, and proportional and equitable representation for African Americans in the prevailing health policy environment has been a structural impossibility.

Meanwhile, in the North, self-trained and informally trained Black practitioners were rare. One instance of an apprentice-trained African American physician from Philadelphia, James Derham, is well documented. It should be made clear that less than 10 percent of the new republic's physicians held the M.D. or university degrees. Of the remainder, the next most desirable level of training was apprentice training, constituting between 25 and 50 percent of the remainder. Understandably, these percentages increased over time. Thus, Derham, though not university trained, was in the mainstream as far as eighteenth-century medical training in America was concerned. Bought as a child by well-known Philadelphia physician John Kearsley, Jr., the bright, lively boy endeared himself to the physician, who decided to teach him medicine. After Kearsley's death in 1777 (related to treasonable activities), Derham was owned by several physicians. Seemingly they taught him how to mix drugs and treat patients. He became an excellent physician along the way. Dr. Robert Dove of New Orleans, his final owner, was so impressed by his medical competence that he permitted the young man to purchase his freedom. He was so well trained and erudite that he greatly impressed Dr. Benjamin Rush, the colony's most famous physician, who wrote and spoke copiously about him.[108]

The vertical and condescending relationship between Rush and Derham serves as another example of the relationship between the Black and White medical professions. Upon interacting with Derham, Rush was shocked and effusive with praise. Rush said of Derham's professionalism:

> I have conversed with him upon most of the acute and epidemic diseases of the country where he lives, and was pleased to find him perfectly acquainted with the modern simple mode of practice in those diseases. I expected to have suggested some new medicines to him, but he suggested many more to me.[109]

Rush was one of the best trained and most highly respected physicians of his generation, with degrees from both the University of Pennsylvania and Edinburgh buttressed by extensive formal European training and prestigious U.S. academic faculty appointments. Derham was, by comparison, an apprentice-trained slave during the greater part of his medical career. Although only approximately 10 percent of American physicians possessed medical school degrees and less than one-third were apprentice trained at that time, physicians of Rush's ilk were the medical leaders charting the course of the profession. All of these men were White. The early Rush–Derham relationship was emblematic of the most positive aspects of Black and White medicine professionally. Rush praised Derham, but was condescending and even paternalistic toward him. Moreover, Rush's previously discussed conflicting and schizophrenic ideation relative to Blacks as totally equal human beings precluded his acceptance of Derham as a true equal. Moreover, Derham's absence of a formal liberal arts background and medical school training placed him in an inferior professional caste even before the veil of race was superimposed. Nevertheless, no other Black physicians before the second quarter of the nineteenth century arose to challenge this Black versus White professional caste relationship, remnants of which remain today.[110]

The White Medical Profession: 1731–1812

The years from 1730 to 1812 were pivotal for the White medical profession. However, the period offered few practical therapeutic breakthroughs. The ancient techniques of bleeding, cupping, and purging remained the mainstays of medical practice. Syphilis and venereal diseases continued to be treated with huge, often fatal, doses of mercury. Theriac, the ineffective cure-all of antiquity, was still in use. One effective therapy was John Huxham's (1692–1768) cinchona bark concoction against fevers of all kinds. Its usefulness was widespread.

The most important drug to be introduced in the eighteenth century was digitalis for the treatment of dropsy (swelling of the limbs). After many years of study based on a folk remedy, William Withering (1741–1799) introduced the active ingredient from the herb *Digitalis purpura* as foxglove in 1785. Treatment of the insane was advanced through the practices and writings of Frenchman Phillipe Pinel (1745–1826), Englishman William Tuke (1732–1822), and Benjamin Rush (1745?–1813). Of public health significance was the 1798 scientific discovery of vaccination for smallpox (a procedure dating back to the 1721 presentation to the Royal College by Cotton Mather) by Edward Jenner (1749–1823). However, credit for transferring Jenner's contribution into clinical practice by 1800, which led to the control of smallpox, goes to his English countryman, Dr. Benjamin Waterhouse (1754–1846). British Royal Naval Surgeon James Lind (1716–1794) proved the efficacy of citrus fruits and vegetables in preventing scurvy in 1747. This nutritional deficiency disease had killed a million sailors between 1600 and 1800. Despite the growing body of biomedical science and technology alongside the growing corpus of racist anthropological, biological, and ethnological information emanating primarily from Europe, no separate medical treatments proved applicable to Blacks or any other racial or ethnic groups. Meanwhile, on the health policy front, Johann Peter Frank (1745–1821) devised a prescient approach to cradle-to-grave health care delivery similar to the British model of today.[111]

The lack of proven utility of medicine kept patients in the new republic skeptical of physicians and formal health care. Americans continued to suffer high death rates from tuberculosis, respiratory diseases, nervous system diseases, diarrhea, scarlet fever, dropsy, and old age. Dreaded epidemic diseases such as influenza, cholera, yellow fever, and typhoid fever took heavy tolls. Physicians could do little to help. Therefore, in America home medical manuals became, and remain, extremely popular. John Wesley's *Primitive Physick* (1747) was enormously successful. Of more lasting and pervasive influence until well into the nineteenth century was Scottish physician William Buchan's (1729–1805) *Domestic Medicine*, which went through innumerable editions and joined the Bible on bookshelves all over America. Not surprisingly, self-reliance also proved to be the foundation upon which the slave health subsystem was built. Planters and their wives treated slaves based on these self-help references just as other Americans did. However, their treatments were supplemented to some extent by medical articles in periodicals and publications targeting the plantation South.[112]

Although most medical-scientific advances had little practical application to patient care, the theoretical foundation of modern medicine made significant progress during the eighteenth and early nineteenth centuries. George Ernst Stahl (1660–1734) debated with Friedrich Hoffmann (1660–1742) at the University of Halle over whether medical systems should be based on vitalism or mechanistic theories. Hermann Boerhaave (1668–1738) advanced the clinical teaching of bedside medicine, placing the University of Leiden at the forefront of scientific, pathology-based medicine. His proteges Gerhard van Sweiten (1700–1772) and Anton de Haen (1704–1776) spread the method over Europe, establishing a renowned medical center in Vienna. Alexander Monro (1697–1767) reinvigorated the ancient University of Edinburgh through his teachings. Albrecht von Haller (1708–1777), one of Boerhaave's Swiss pupils, conducted groundbreaking medical research on the nervous system while helping to establish the University of Gottingen in Germany. Perhaps the greatest eighteenth-century advance in the basic medical sciences of pathologic anatomy, comparative anatomy, and embryology was the contribution of Giovanni Battista Morgagni (1682–1771), whose five decades as professor of medicine and pathology at Padua were crowned by the 1761 publication of *On the Sites and Causes of Diseases*, which established the relationship between specific, localized pathology and clinical diseases. Major clinical advances in surgery and anatomy were made by the British brothers John (1728–1793) and William Hunter (1718–1783) and Frenchman Pierre-Joseph Desault (1744–1795). These legitimate medical and scientific advances would later benefit mankind and all patients regardless of color.[113]

During the 1713–1812 period in America, the White, university-trained medical elite based in urban centers were able to open medical schools, lay the groundwork for medical licensing laws, and gain control of the embryonic health delivery system. Most of the efforts of men such as John Morgan (1735–1789) and William Shippen (1736–1808) were based on their emulation of European medical training at Edinburgh and London. These two Edinburgh graduates opened the first American medical school in the colonies in 1765 at the University of Pennsylvania. Largely due the efforts of physicians such as Samuel Bard (1716–1799), the second American school opened as the Medical School of King's College, New York (Columbia) in 1768. Significantly, Bard was also instrumental in organizing New York's first voluntary hospital in 1771. Harvard Medical School was founded in 1783 through the efforts of Dr. John Collins Warren (1753–1815), who also helped found Boston's first voluntary hospital. In contrast to the British medical school models, which were affiliated with hospitals, Colonial American schools were full-fledged university departments reminiscent of the University of Edinburgh or numerous schools on the European continent. Creation of these academic health centers represented some of the most important contributions made by the White medical profession during the Republican Era.

For a struggling medical profession and a cadre of wealthy community leaders, control of both private and public health institutions assumed increasing importance. As Rosenberg states in *The Care of Strangers*, "[T]o that handful of elite urban physicians who staffed them and those philanthropists who supported and administered them, these pioneer hospitals were significant indeed."[114] Moreover, European-trained specialists gained control and stewardship over the growing public health care sector required to provide minimal services to expanding urban, poor populations by the late eighteenth century. These findings give pause to the impression projected by Paul Starr and others that the early medical profession was virtually powerless. More proof of that power is evidenced by the fact that European medicine, through its American trainees, was shaping bedside and hospital training for U.S. physicians throughout this period. Through the establishment of new institutions and utilization of old ones for new purposes, America's elite physicians and their lay allies were able to provide adequate, if not state-of-the-art, medical training domestically. Thus, the amalgamation and affiliation of the early medical schools with institutions such as the Philadelphia Almshouse, Bellevue in New York City, and Charity Hospital in New Orleans was an almost inevitable result of the political clout these local medical leaders wielded. Although they weren't able to carry out all of their wishes in the give-and-take political processes so characteristic of the United States, their individual and personal influence must have been substantial. These developments and events reinforced the European relationship between medical training and charity care, with all of the class implications for the poor that entailed. Addition of the American race factor to this mix had grave implications for African Americans, rendering them a particularly and peculiarly vulnerable and disadvantaged caste in the new health system.[115]

Beginning in the early Colonial Period, the poor were placed in categories in English North America. The White medical profession facilitated the process. As extensions, if not exaggerations, of Protestant, Puritan, and Calvinist traditions regarding the poor that dominated the Colonies, they were divided into the "worthy" poor and the "unworthy" poor. Facilities and provisions for these two classes were assigned different levels of responsibility by society and received graded levels of resources. The "unworthy" received the worst. Being Black in most communities automatically meant belonging to the "unworthy" category. Thus, in an American health system already dividing along class lines, with a stringent if not draconian moral perspective plagued by pervasive race and slavery problems, negotiating such a system was incredibly difficult for Blacks, whether slave or free. African Americans were not only burdened with the stigma of low socioeconomic status and "unworthiness," but they also underwent health system abuse, exploitation, segregation, and discrimination on the basis of their race. These policies were implemented and enforced by members of the medical profession charged with the stewardship of a growing network of socially, morally, educationally, and racially defined institutions.[116]

Despite their efforts, the medical profession's leaders were frustrated in their attempts to organize and officially regulate the medical profession. The formation of weak, often transient, medical societies took place. The nation's first hesitant efforts to regulate the practice of medicine in a European manner started during this era. Colonial physicians proposed to do this on several levels. The legal and regulatory level would require anyone practicing medicine to be licensed. New York City passed the first medical licensing law in 1760. Physicians in Norwich, Connecticut, submitted a request to their Colonial legislature to authorize medical societies to license practitioners in 1763. It did not pass. Medical educators wanted to require professional university training to practice medicine. John Morgan, upon his 1765 founding of the University of Pennsylvania's Medical School, also proposed the profession's obtaining licensing authority through the new school. Other than New York's ineffective and unenforced law, these proposals were rejected. The first provincial medical societies were organized in Boston as early as 1721 and in New Jersey in 1766. Internal regulation of the profession through medical societies was first attempted with the 1781 incorporation of the Massachusetts Medical Society. A ceremonial licensing law was passed at the same time. Having no discernible meaning or effect on the practice of medicine, the Massachusetts licensing law would be rescinded by the mid-nineteenth century along with New Jersey's. Therefore, few of the recognizable legal and regulatory components of the U.S. health care system that would mature into today's system emerged in the Republican Era. It was not until the late nineteenth century in America, after medicine had proven itself to the American public, that vigorous medical licensing and regulation laws were permanently enacted.[117]

Major reasons for medicine's lack of official authority and power strongly reflected America's culture. The republic spouted egalitarian rhetoric that resonated positively with the masses. Thus, an upper class–oriented and privileged profession such as medicine received little political or public support. Rosenberg observed the relationship between the realities of social class and a successful nineteenth-century medical career in the United States, noting, "A mixture of academic accomplishment, social advantage, and the tenacity needed to piece together an ad hoc assortment of part-time and short-term clinical appointments were elements that brought professional success."[118] Another reason physicians were denied the privilege they sought was the clinical ineffectiveness of medicine at that time. Doctors could describe and prognosticate about a number of disease processes. There were elaborate systems of disease classification. But there was very little effective treatment for most serious disorders. The U.S. public was simply not convinced of medicine's effectiveness. Only after the triumphs in basic science, surgical anesthesia and antisepsis-asepsis, and laboratory medicine would the medical profession convince the public of its necessity. During this period, Blacks were either excluded from the organized White medical profession or submerged as practitioners in the primitive slave health subsystem, thus prohibiting their participation in the domestic medical-social conflict.[119]

American physicians have always been interested in Black biological and medical "differences." However, this polemic has continually been framed in terms of White superiority and Black inferiority and has had a very deleterious effect on American culture and society. During the Republican Era, the White medical profession became heavily involved in the promotion and promulgation of scientific racism. In the American republic little was documented or written about racist involvement in books or scholarly venues, largely because there were scant academic or research institutions with publishing outlets. Instead, racism permeated the day-to-day delivery of health care and practice of medicine. White superiority and non-White inferiority became incorporated into the American life science ethos and academic and delivery structures. Thus, scientific racism wrought deleterious and long-standing effects on the U.S. health system and the American medical education infrastructure during their formative stages.[120]

Documentation that derogatory biological material alleging White superiority and Black inferiority had entered the American medical school curriculum by the early nineteenth century is provided by the lectures delivered in 1808 by Dr. John Augustine Smith (1782–?), a lecturer in anatomy and surgery in the College of Physicians and Surgeons of the University of New York. Citing European authorities, from whom he had received postgraduate medical training, he espoused Black racial inferiority based on the latest anthropometric, anthropological, and Biblical data. His influence was far reaching in that he later become president of the College of Physicians and Surgeons of the University of New York and the College of William and Mary.[121]

Racial inferiority dogma was also widely disseminated in academic medical circles and curricula by Dr. Charles Caldwell (1772–1853), student of Benjamin Rush, graduate of the University of Pennsylvania, and professor of natural history at the university. A nationally renowned lecturer and medical academician and leader, later in his career Caldwell became one of the most eminent phrenologists in America. Caldwell, an effective debater, wrote and lectured long and hard against Reverend Samuel Stanhope Smith, the early nineteenth-century champion of a single creation (monogenesis) and environmental causes of racial differences. He considered himself "the first introducer of true medical science into the Mississippi Valley,"[122] based on his founding of two Southern medical schools in Kentucky, one at Transylvania University in Lexington and the other at the University of Louisville.[123]

The new mechanism of designating Blacks and other groups (i.e., Native Americans and other non-Whites) as inferior and subhuman emerged through the foundations of modern science. Although Western culture was already racist on the basis of its cultural mythology and religious traditions, the potential for this new tool, the natural sciences, was frightening. Rather than relying upon faith and belief systems, science had the guise of rationality, being of the physical concrete world, and objectivity. Older theological models that had previously explained the differences between Blacks and other Christians were in the process of becoming secularized in terms of the biology of race. Even the unitary origin of man through Adam and Eve purported by the Bible and the egalitarian ideology promoted by the European Enlightenment and the American Revolution were not powerful enough sociopolitically, ethically, or intellectually to counteract the onslaught of scientific racism. By the end of this period even abolitionists and anti-slavery advocates had come to believe in the racial inferiority of the Negro. As Stephen Jay Gould noted in *The Mismeasure of Man*, "[W]e must first recognize the cultural milieu of a society whose leaders and intellectuals did not doubt the propriety of racial ranking—with Indians below whites, and blacks below everybody else."[124] Gould goes further in his dissection of the relationship between science and society, stating, "[T]he pervasive assent given by scientists to conventional rankings arose from shared social belief, not from objective data gathered to test an open question. Yet, in a curious case of reversed causality, these pronouncements were read as independent support for the political context."[125]

For the 185 years since the Republican Era ended in the United States, African Americans, Native Americans, and the poor have been major foci of scientific racism in English North America. It must be understood that this work in America was no fringe movement or the product of some group of ignorant, poorly educated extremists. It is deeply embedded in the mainstream of Western and American scientific culture.[126] Thus, the concept of biological determinism, "the notion that people at the bottom are constructed of intrinsically inferior material (poor brains, bad genes, or whatever),"[127] became central to the American worldview. The White medical and health professions promoted and promulgated these concepts. These ideologies had, and continue to have, profound effects on the health and social systems. Uneasiness and even remorse about the conflict between republican notions and the social milieu generated by these commonly held beliefs in English North America were expressed in the writings of Thomas Jefferson, Benjamin Rush, and Benjamin Franklin. Alexis de Tocqueville would later confirm how prevalent these social views of White superiority and manifest destiny, juxtaposed with Black and Native American inferiority, had become. Seemingly to the founding fathers of the republic, racial hierarchies were a small price to pay for an enlightened American republic of free White men. The consequences and impact this movement wrought on medicine and the healing professions and on African Americans vulnerable to their effects is only now being uncovered. Modern social scientists, anthropologists, and behaviorialists have also sounded an alarm that should be reverberating throughout the entire medical-social milieu.[128] That this emerging late eighteenth-century movement laid the foundations for the burgeoning scientific racism of the nineteenth century, including the American school of anthropology, has been clearly documented.[129]

The "differences" that late eighteenth- and early nineteenth-century American physicians and natural scientists saw in the Negro slaves, and other allegedly inferior groups, was shaped by the previous biological and scientific work emanating from Europe. As we have discussed, the work of men such as Linnaeus, Blumenbach, and Buffon was at the forefront of modern eighteenth-century natural sciences and dominated the life sciences. Most of the anthropological and ethnological work of American physicians such as Benjamin Rush and John Augustine Smith was often imitative, an extension of work previously done in Europe. In fact, the authors quoted in the overwhelming majority of academic lectures and writings presented by Americans were Europeans. The landmark work of Samuel George Morton, Samuel Cartwright, Louis Agassiz, and Josiah Clark Nott, which followed during the 1830s and 1840s, constituted the first efforts emanating from U.S. soil.

These American developments in the biomedical sciences between 1730 and the early nineteenth century complemented and reinforced slavery and would lay the groundwork for the American school of anthropology. The dense corpus of theories, illustrations, computations, and tabular data, later identified as the American school of anthropology, which blossomed during the Jacksonian and antebellum periods after 1830, constituted a new, distinctively American anthropological and sociobiological movement that was recognized internationally. Physician-scientists led the way. The school explained racial differences and hierarchies in pseudoscientifically derived quantitative terms within a paradigm of polygenic, separate development based upon innate and genetically determined levels of competence, and presumed a consensus regarding White European racial superiority and eventual hegemony over the "lesser" races. This was the first American academic work that was taken seriously by the international scientific community. Between the second quarter of the nineteenth century and the intellectual and social earthquakes created by the 1859 publication of Darwin's *Origin of the Species* and the American Civil War, this stream of polygenic scientific scholarship purportedly quantifying Black, Native American, and non-White inferiority held sway over the entire biological and anthropological world. Endorsement and promotion by the U.S. medical profession shaped the scientific movement's domestic character, its effects on American society, and its health system dimensions.

Another by-product of the scientific activity promoting racial difference and inferiority in America was the creation of a lexicon of "Negro diseases" and physiological peculiarities by physicians and natural scientists. (See Table 4.2.) This creation of separate, racially determined diseases and physiology was largely an American phenomenon. In many ways it reflected the unique and distorted relationship that existed between Black patients and the White health professional community. On a more basic clinical level it represented a unique, if not unwholesome, doctor–patient relationship. Beginning with Benjamin Rush's special 1792 session of the American Philosophical Society in Philadelphia, wherein he presented his "scientific" theories and medical findings on race,

Table 4.2   Republican Era "Black Physiological Peculiarities"

- Blacks have larger penises and breasts than Whites . . . signs of their indecent and unbridled sexuality
- Blacks tolerate pain better than Whites . . . a sign of their close relationship to lower animals
- Black women have less copious menstruation . . . confirming their close association with apes who bleed even less or not at all
- Blacks have stronger body odor than Whites . . . in lieu of their sweating less
- Blacks engage in social relationships with apes (i.e., it was alleged that apes captured and enslaved Blacks and abused them sexually)

By the end of the Republican Era, U.S. physicians were already assigning people of African descent a set of physiological peculiarities. These "findings" were not only specious but derogatory, and justified Black stereotypes and mistreatment.

Source: Gould SJ. *The Flamingo's Smile.* New York: W.W. Norton & Company, 1985, 281–290.

"Black medicine and physiology" were pernicious American forces.[130] His attribution of diseases such as "chronic leprosy" and a "smell" that "continues with a small modification in the native African to this day"[131] to an entire race was irrational and regrettable. His "research," dating from 1788, on "Negro diseases" such as "locked jaw," purportedly caused by the heat and smoke of slave cabins, "hipocondriasis," attributed to the grief over enslavement, and "difficult parturition," caused by heavy burdens and kicks of the masters, set precedents.[132] Explaining differences in appearance such as skin color, hair texture, and facial features; investigating brain size, cranial contours, and mental capabilities and characteristics; and hypothesizing and describing previously unrecognized "new" diseases, disease susceptibilities, and unique responses to illnesses and treatments when applied to African Americans became "legitimate" scientific research. Significantly, some of the first major efforts in this new area of American scientific interest emanated from Philadelphia, which at that time was the leading medical city in the new republic.[133]

During the next era, the Jacksonian Period (1813–1861), republican strengths and faults reached maturity. Industrial and market revolutions fueled unprecedented prosperity, but inattention to social policies embodied in a nation divided by slavery led to a catastrophic Civil War. All of these major developments profoundly affected the health care system. The differential effects they had on Black health is the next subject of our inquiry.

🝆 PART III

Race, Medicine, and Health in the United States from 1812 to 1900

✕ CHAPTER FIVE

Black Health and the Jacksonian and Antebellum Periods, 1812–1861

Growth, Change, and Manifest Destiny

The period from 1812 to 1861 was dominated by the Age of Jackson. It was an era of explosive expansion for the United States. The policies of President Andrew Jackson (1767–1845), a Tennessee-born soldier, politician, and planter, were especially important from an African American perspective. Jackson was largely responsible for resolving the national political and Constitutional debate about conflicts between the notions that "all men are created equal" and permanent Black chattel slavery and the rights of Native Americans. Jackson determined that both groups were to be subjugated to permanent slavery and dispossession under the aegis of official national government policy. For these non-White minorities, he shaped the political economy and social fabric of the United States for almost 200 years.[1]

Between 1803 and 1860 the new nation more than quadrupled in size while the economy grew even faster. The market and technological revolutions swept the new nation with tidal waves of triumphant expansion, progress, and change. However, these revolutions also generated sectional conflict and animosity between the North and the South that led to the Civil War. All of these events would have profound and complex effects on the health system. Despite generalized health progress for most Americans, African Americans would suffer health status stagnation followed by deterioration. Despite national expansion and prosperity, between 1812 and 1861 African American longevity, mortality, and fertility showed only slight signs of improvement for the first 18 years and then deteriorated after 1830. The mythology of the contented well-cared-for slave is refuted by the *slave health deficit* that continued, and deepened, during the Jacksonian and Antebellum periods. The Antebellum Period demonstrated that the widely accepted principle of public health—that improved health status goes hand in hand with generalized prosperity—did not apply to Americans of African descent. We will investigate some of the complex interactions and explanatory hypotheses that clarify and lend perspective to these health findings while elucidating and examining some of the social, political, and historical forces leading to them.

To fully comprehend the dramatic health and health system changes that characterized the period, a brief background in the history of the period is required. The successful outcome of the War of 1812* buttressed the new nation's confidence and transformed Andrew Jackson (known as "Old Hickory") into a nearly mythical national hero identified with jingoism and Indian fighting. The period began with an advantageous peace with America's traditional enemy, Great Britain. These events, combined with Jackson's spectacular victory over the British in 1815 at New Orleans, positioned the United States for expansion across North America. Occupation of lands acquired in the Louisiana Purchase (1803) combined with expansion in the 1840s led to the occupation of all of the United States' present territories (except Alaska and Hawaii) by 1850. This runaway expansion set the tone for social and health system development—a perpetuation of frontier conditions.

Politically, the 1828 election of Andrew Jackson symbolized an almost total rejection of Alexander Hamilton's concepts of Federalism, which emphasized a strong centralized national government in favor of almost total reliance on the individual and the repudiation of so-called elite rule. It also embodied the ruthless national policies of Native American displacement and elimination for the sake of national expansion, and entrenchment of the slave system for commercial and ideological reasons. The rhetorical facade of moral certitude and implied egalitarianism belied the nation's growing aggressiveness, exploitation, socioeconomic inequalities, and militaristic domestic and foreign policies. American character development based on individualism and survival of the fittest was also reflected in and permeated the health system. More fundamental than the adverse health effects on the two subjugated and allegedly inferior subpopulations, however,

---

*The War of 1812 between the United States and Great Britain lasted from June 18, 1812, to December 24, 1814 (the last battle was actually fought at New Orleans on January 8, 1815). War began because of British naval policies of seizing and inspecting ships at sea and impressing U.S. seamen into service. For the British it was an extension of a far greater continental war with Napoleon; for the United States, the Anglo-American War, as it was sometimes called, was one of survival, national assertion, and potential expansion.

Indian extermination and Black chattel slavery helped fuel the United States' westward expansion and the conversion from an agricultural-commercial to an industrial corporate economy.

The formation of a new Democratic Party in 1826 represented, in fact, not only a symbolic rebirth of rule by the "common man," if he was White, but also a new round of relentless national expansion. Presidents Jackson, Tyler, and Polk promoted the activities of free-booting quasi-official privateers such as Army Captain John C. Fremont, General Stephen Kearny, and ambitious Navy Commodore Robert F. Stockton, ensuring a national growth outcome. Annexation of Texas (1845), the Mexican War (1846), confiscation of the short-lived Bear Flag Republic (as California was called in 1848), and fabrication of a diplomatic impasse over Oregon territory leading to territorial incorporation were some of the results. The deeper meanings and mechanizations undergirding these policies would cause North–South sectional conflicts to intensify, bring the nation's founding principles into question, and lead to the bloodiest civil war in history.[2]

These events had both direct and indirect effects on the health system. Westward expansion perpetuated frontier conditions in health care in most places in the United States and institutionalized the general practitioner as the archetype of American medical practice for another three generations. Besides perpetuating traditions of health care delivered in the home and by traditional healers, geographic expansion also generated harsh health care conditions for all patient populations on the frontier. Moreover, whether by direct or indirect mechanisms, U.S. medical specialization and scientific progress was slowed. Additional health system caste arrangements were erected for Mexican Americans and Native Americans, augmenting those traditionally provided for Black and poor populations. Meanwhile, the Northeast grew into the educational and technical headquarters of national medical advancement.[3]

The increasingly divergent Northern and Southern economic systems generated unprecedented profits. Simultaneously, they also produced political and cultural clashes that would prove to be self-destructive. From both regions' perspectives expansion of the nation was not the question, but rather expansion for whom and for what. Slavery was at the crux of the issue. Progress stemming from developments in technology, transportation, communication, and manufacturing spurred Northern industrialization. This was described succinctly by Takaki in *Iron Cages: Race and Culture in Nineteenth-Century America*:

> *The shipping boom of the early 1800s allowed merchants such as Francis Lowell to accumulate the capital needed to invest in manufacturing enterprises. The proliferation of banks and the expansion of the credit system enabled farmers to borrow paper money and acquire land for commercial agriculture. Government intervention in the form of protective tariffs and internal improvements also contributed to the advance of the market. Technological progress transformed manufacturing from*

> household to factory; machinery became the main means for the produc-
> tion of manufactured goods and an urban population was increasingly
> organized around the machine. The transportation revolution laid vast
> networks of turnpikes, canals, and railroads throughout the country;
> between 1815 and 1860, freight charges for shipments of goods over
> land had been reduced by approximately ninety-five percent.[4]

Removal of the Indians and the expansion of Black slavery were largely responsible for the market revolution. Runaway change and differentiation between an increasingly urban North and rural South literally tore the new nation apart. Economic pressures wrought by the new industrialization and the creation of a market economy forged political and economic agendas for the competing regions and interest groups that proved irreconcilable. One major factor driving these conflicts was the pattern of economic "inter-regional specialization," to use Takaki's term, that had developed.

Nevertheless, profits from cotton grew dramatically and still proved to be the decisive factor in the national economy. As Takaki noted, "[C]otton constituted thirty-nine percent of the total value of exports from 1816 to 1820, sixty-three percent from 1836 to 1840, and over fifty percent from 1840 to 1860."[5] Du Bois placed this expansion of the cotton economy in more concrete terms in *Black Reconstruction in America*:

> Cotton grew so swiftly that the 9,000 bales of cotton which the new
> nation scarcely noticed in 1791 became 19,000 in 1800. . . . The cotton
> crop reached one half-million bales in 1822, a million bales in 1831,
> two million in 1840, three million in 1852, and in the year of secession,
> stood at the then enormous total of five million bales.[6]

Creation of the cotton kingdom had been based on the expansion of both White settlement and Black slavery into Indian lands of the Southwest. Louisiana in 1812, Mississippi in 1817, and Alabama in 1819, the major cotton states, had been carved out of Indian territory. Nevertheless, Southern planters wanted the growing nation to continue providing them with an ever-expanding empire for slavery. The annexation of Texas in 1845 followed by the taking of California and other Mexican territories after the Mexican War gave them heart in this regard. Northerners, most of whom still did not like Blacks, wanted free labor, dignity of work, and laissez-faire capitalism. Melding frontier territories into a single nation with such stresses and dichotomies proved impossible. Paradoxically, the two regions, along with a growing western economic unit, were economically interdependent. Some estimates indicated that as much as two-thirds of Northern economic growth was directly related to the growing Southern agricultural system. As laissez-faire market-based capitalism flourished in the North, feudal capitalist-agrarianism in the South expanded, built upon the ancient institution of chattel slavery. As economic growth continued, scientific breakthroughs also increased the efficacy of medicine and facilitated the founding of dentistry as a separate discipline in the United States. Some areas of the United States also began to see the hospital practice of medicine in a positive light.[7]

By the nineteenth century Europeans had strong feelings of superiority, as J. Marc Roberts points out in *The Triumph of the West*:

> *Even if they were not always clear why, those of European stock often behaved as if they were not merely right, but were actually superior beings. The West knew it was superior. This is what lay behind the nineteenth-century's idealization of the way white men were expected to behave. They were expected to show confidence, courage, dignity because they represented a higher civilization.*[8]

White Americans felt no differently, considering themselves transplanted Europeans in a new land. However, one peculiarly American phenomenon set the United States apart from other slave-holding societies. During this period a cadre of Southern scholars and opinion leaders promoted Black slavery and subjugation as a positive social good. This was a new turn in Western culture-driven European superiority. Roberts observed, as had other scholars and historians, in his television documentary *The Triumph of the West*, that during this period in the South an elaborate justification for slavery emerged. A great deal of this "new" justification emanated from the field of medicine and the biologically related sciences. Moreover, in virtually every other nineteenth-century society, including Cuba and South America, slavery was on the decline. In contrast, the U.S. slave system was growing geometrically in both financial and numerical terms. In English North America the Black population had grown from the original 20 Negroes in 1619 to 757,181 by 1790, 1,002,037 by 1800, 1,771,656 by 1820, and 4,441,830 by the time of the Civil War.[9]

During the post–Revolutionary War period chattel slavery was hotly debated by the Founding Fathers, who perceived a natural conflict between the national creed of the United States and human bondage. Southern representatives in the Congress saved the slave system. By the early nineteenth century, the invention of the cotton gin in 1793 by Eli Whitney, potentially increasing cotton output a hundredfold, made slavery profitable once more. As Roberts observed, "[S]lavery . . . came to be regarded as the essential core of a particular civilization."[10] Anything preserving and strengthening the institution of Black chattel slavery had the effect of perpetuating the inferior slave health subsystem and, thus, exerted profound effects on Black health. As far as Blacks were concerned, writes Kenneth O'Reilly in *Nixon's Piano*, "[T]he Jacksonian movement invented a party and a style of presidential leadership that knew no higher purpose than protecting slavery forever."[11] The profitability and success of these policies for the dominant White majority were clear—and they continued. This latest configuration of U.S.

democracy seemingly had no patience or place for the Indian and could only predict further exploitation of, and dependency upon, Black labor and Mexican and Indian land.[12]

An indicator of the mixed national feelings toward slavery and the deterioration of the status of Blacks after American independence was the formation of the American Colonization Society in 1816 and the American Anti-Slavery Society in 1833. Both organizations had strong religious ties and overtones. The American Colonization Society proposed to solve the "Negro problem" by removing all Blacks and "returning" them to foreign locations in Africa or the Caribbean. The American Anti-Slavery Society also posited various foreign destinations for slaves after they had been freed. Neither body considered Blacks as equal citizens or as future permanent and full-fledged Americans. Emblematically, efforts at significant Black participation in these organizations at other than the lowest levels met stout resistance. The same could be said of the Abolitionist Movement (starting in the 1830s) to free the slaves. Abolitionists, also in the midst of a golden age of influence and importance, seemed at first to rage and rant at each other, as evidenced by the original body splitting into two groups over women's rights and several other policy differences by 1840. However, the cacophony the abolitionists generated piqued the public conscience, subtly raising opposition against slavery on religious and moral levels. This movement dovetailed with the growing anti-slavery "free labor" political movement evinced by the Northern White working classes. As Takaki observed, "During the 1840s and 1850s, northern working class antagonism toward blacks . . . helped generate strong opposition against the extension of slavery into the territories."[13] Ironically, this movement was fundamentally anti-Black.

In response to Northern anti-slavery campaigns—which grew highly organized after the 1830s—the South found it necessary over the next 30 years to orchestrate a positive justification for slavery. Led by politicians such as John C. Calhoun, sociologists such as Henry Hughes and George Fitzhugh wrote books and papers attacking the basic assumptions of capitalism and democracy. They synthesized political-economic systems based on a reactionary seigneurialism and the patriarchal plantation, which were suggested as alternatives and improvements for the working classes in both the Northern United States and Great Britain. Some went to the extreme, positing that if 90 percent of Whites were unable to care for themselves in capitalist systems, Black slaves certainly needed masters to care for them.[14] Health care delivery within the framework of the slave health subsystem would take care of itself. Both Northern and Southern physicians such as John Van Everie, Samuel Cartwright, Josiah Clark Nott, and Samuel George Morton fell prey to the scientific fallacies of *reification* and *ranking*,* which, aggravated by their racism, allowed them to twist, distort, and manipulate the biomedical sciences into disciplines supporting and promulgat-

---

*Reification (from the Latin res, or thing) is the tendency to convert abstract concepts into entities. Ranking is the tendency of scientists to order complex variation as a gradual ascending scale.

ing racial inferiority. Other Southern intellectuals such as Edmund Ruffin, William J. Grayson, and George Frederick Holmes expressed aristocratic justifications for slavery that were repugnant to the society they were attempting to persuade, for, as George Fredrickson pointed out in *The Black Image in the White Mind*, "Some of these theorists severely limited their own influence by openly manifesting aristocratic revulsion to the values and practices that resulted from the extension of democratic procedures and attitudes during the Jacksonian period."[15] Southern regional justification for slavery based on Black racial inferiority and White social superiority became so intense and hysterical that this specious worldview and ideology formed the primary foundation upon which the Southern Confederacy was built. Such an extreme social paradigm built upon racial hierarchies was unprecedented in world history. Some historians chose to label this antebellum phenomenon of the 1830s and 1840s the Great Reaction:

> [T]he South, threatened it seemed by internal and external enemies, became a closed, martial society determined to preserve its slave-based civilization at whatever cost. If Southerners had once apologized for slavery as a necessary evil, they now trumpeted that institution as a positive good.[16]

In his famous "Cornerstone Speech" of 1861, Alexander H. Stephens, newly elected vice president of the Confederacy, articulated the ultimate political effect this ideological and pseudoscience-based justification movement had on Southern culture as it spilled over into the Confederate Constitution:

> Many governments have been founded on the principles of subordination and serfdom of certain classes of the same race; such were, and are in violation of the laws of nature. Our system commits no such violation of nature's laws. . . . Its foundations are laid, its cornerstone rests upon the great truth that the Negro is not equal to the white man, that slavery—subordination to the superior race—is his natural or normal condition. [emphasis in original][17]

The South not only adopted the ancient institution of slavery but also projected it as the foundation of their entire society. Unsound social and economic theories and scientific racism were brought forward to prop up the delusion and myth of race. A civil war would be necessary to clear the atmosphere and restore a semblance of Western civilization–based rationality and reality.[18]

The only mechanisms offering possibilities for reconciliation between the North and South, ensuring preservation of the Union, came to be political ones. National turmoil grounded in the national character, sectional, and political conflict played itself out as a series of political events emphasizing compromise and reconciliation between 1812 and 1860. For a while nationalism and "manifest destiny,"* embodied in the facilitation of national expansion, triumphed over sectionalism. The Missouri Compromise (1820) was the first such measure. Northern and Southern factions in Congress, possessing equal numbers of slave and free states (11 each), agreed that Missouri, already heavily involved in slavery, would enter the Union as a slave state and Maine as a free one. In the future, although balance could be maintained in the Congress, slavery would be limited to areas south of the lower (southern) border of Missouri (the 36°30′ parallel). The 1850 Compromise followed. This consisted of admitting California as a free state; admitting other lands acquired from Mexico without restrictions on slavery; abolishing the slave trade, but not slavery, in the District of Columbia; settling border disputes and debts with Texas and the New Mexico territories; and a strong national fugitive slave law.** It was considered a Southern victory. The uneasy truce created by this compromise, based on self-interests instead of genuine agreements, disintegrated in four years, punctuated by the Kansas-Nebraska Act of 1854, which opened up new territories in the Midwest by violating Indian treaties and expropriating millions more acres of land from Native Americans. It also created the potential states of Kansas and Nebraska, maintaining the slave state/free state balance while implementing the principle of squatter sovereignty.†

However, traits in the American character such as individualism, independence, and egalitarianism, noted during the period by Tocqueville in *Democracy in America* (1835), served to tear the new nation asunder despite these compromises. Tocqueville noted, "The Americans believe that in each state supreme power should emanate directly from the people, but once this power has been constituted, they can hardly conceive any limits to it."[19] The Monroe Doctrine (1823) warning Europeans not to interfere in American continental or hemispheric affairs was an international extension of that point of view. Extremes of local commitment to such ideals, evidenced in Americans as early as the Revolutionary Era and the Continental Congresses, generated irreconcilable regional differences and conflicts built around the issues of chattel slavery and free labor. Northerners were increasingly committed to "free land" and "free labor," feeling that slave labor limited a competitive labor market, and was immoral besides. Tocqueville's observation of fierce individualism and regional independence in the American character also had the effect of vitiating the possibilities of centralized support of progressive social institutions and policies regarding poor and disadvantaged Americans. He observed about the American character: "Such folk owe no man anything and hardly expect anything from anybody. They form the habit of thinking of themselves in isolation

---

Manifest destiny was the belief that America was destined by both God and history to expand its boundaries over a vast area. The area included, but was not restricted, to the North American continent.

**The *fugitive law* was a national law upholding and enforcing Southern slaveholders' right to have their slave "property" returned to them after they had escaped to Northern states.

†*Squatter sovereignty* embodied the principle that settler states had the right to choose to become slave or free. This, in effect, vitiated the Missouri Compromise limiting the expansion of slavery.

and imagine that their whole destiny is in their own hands."[20] Insular and conservative social attitudes and policies yielded truncated and half-hearted development of separate systems for the "haves" and "have nots," including a mainstream health system alongside flagrantly insufficient health provisions for Blacks and the poor. Local poor relief and an expanded slave health subsystem proved inadequate vehicles toward improved health for all Americans.[21]

Expansion, sectional greed, competing interests, and differing national visions according to Northerners and Southerners (free soil and free labor versus slavery and states' rights) led to a series of confrontations and conflicts threatening either Southern secession or civil war. By the time of Polk's presidency (1845–1849) with the acquisition of the Oregon territory (1846), Texas (1845), California (1848), and the spoils of the Mexican War (1848), sectional conflict to maintain the balance of slave and free states (15 states each in 1849) and a national fugitive slave law further battered the integrity of the Missouri Compromise. Conflicts over the fugitive slave law and the Dred Scott decision (1857)* endangered and undermined the truces between North and South. As North-South conflagrations escalated, Brinkley noted, "an increasing number of Northerners, gradually becoming a majority, came to believe that the existence of slavery was dangerous not because of what it did to blacks but because of what it threatened to do to whites."[22] Secession or civil war seemed inevitable.[23]

The multiple and confounding layers generated by the numerous tumultuous events that marked this dynamic period pose a challenge to any meaningful efforts to resurrect the African American health experience. Innumerable changes occurred in the health system between the early nineteenth century and the Civil War. In many ways they reflected what was happening in the country as a whole. Technically, American medicine came of age in the first half of the nineteenth century, as if the rosy enthusiasm and general good fortune smiling on the new country blessed its biomedical sciences as well. For African Americans this medical flowering would bear little fruit. This tumultuous period would presage the most revolutionary period in U.S. health history up to that time—the Civil War.[24]

Beginnings of a Health System: Black Subjugation, Dependency, and Separate Development

From a population in the early eighteenth century of approximately 400,000 Whites and 40,000 Blacks, the 13 colonies of English North America and later the United States grew to 9.6 million in 1820, 23 million in 1850, and 31.5

---

*Dred Scott was a slave who had lived in free territories for more than four years. Upon returning to Missouri, a slave state, he sued for his freedom. The Supreme Court ruled that Blacks were a lower form of being and, thus, Scott could never become a citizen of the United States. The Court ruled that Blacks "had no rights a White man was bound to respect."

million in 1860 across 33 states. Blacks grew to constitute 20 percent of the population by 1800. The overwhelming majority of Americans lived in rural and frontier areas, small towns, or settlements. As J. M. Roberts observed about the United States in lieu of its spectacular growth, as late as 1850 "the only cities with more than 100,000 inhabitants were the three great Atlantic ports of Boston, New York and Philadelphia."[25] While all this transpired, the new nation's expansion helped create the Deep South and Southwest. As one historian stated, "After 1815 the American economy began to expand rapidly. The cotton boom in the South spread settlements swiftly across the Gulf Plains: the Deep South was born."[26]

As the U.S. expanded westward the health system responded to these changes. What might have been viewed as a pragmatic approach to health care in the burgeoning frontier areas could be viewed as backward approaches to health care in cities. After all, self-reliance in areas without physicians or hospitals could be, and was, projected as a virtue. In the Northeast and in urban areas, distrust of the medical elite led to continued American reliance on home remedies and self-help medical books. Lack of faith in both regular and irregular practitioners and medical "quacks" grew even though patients continued to visit them. Self-reliance and self-help remained the cornerstones shaping health system development among an individualistic and frontier-oriented people. Deterioration of professional standards during the first half of the nineteenth century, which we will explore in more detail later, exacerbated these low trust levels. The slow growth of the voluntary hospital system itself reflected these health policies and public attitudes. After the Civil War, as industrialization and urbanization proceeded westward, the health system as a whole largely duplicated the same stages of development experienced in the East.

Slavery's expansion into frontier areas automatically increased the boundaries and complexity of the slave health subsystem and was a major factor in modifying the profile of slavery's illnesses. It would take a civil war to convince the American public that hospitals and formal medical care were necessary for all classes of people. Through the decades leading up to 1860, racial and social stratification of the health care institutions and system as a whole continued. The slave health subsystem became more elaborate and institutionalized, as did the entire health system.[27] (See Figure 5.1.)

With increased industrialization and the urbanization that accompanied booming economic development, large poverty-stricken and displaced populations became generalized phenomena. As cities grew, this occurred earliest in traditional Northern centers such as Boston, New York, and Philadelphia. However, it also became a problem in Southern urban centers such as Charleston and New Orleans. Concomitantly, the need for charity and welfare services increased. In most nineteenth-century cities, the almshouse was the only place that could be likened to a hospital. Thus, building upon a scant foundation of almshouses, pesthouses, poorhouses, and isolation facilities, hospitals evolved in many cities. As Rosenberg observed in *Care of Strangers*, "Although envisioned as a 'receptacle' for the dependent and indigent, the almshouse had by the late

Figure 5.1   Antebellum Broadside Announcing Slave Sale: Evidence
of Slave Health Subsystem Influence and Sophistication

Sale of Slaves and Stock.

The Negroes and Stock listed below, are a Prime Lot, and belong to the ESTATE OF THE LATE LUTHER McGOWAN, and will be sold on Monday, Sept. 22nd, 1852, at the Fair Grounds, in Savannah, Georgia, at 1:00 P. M. The Negroes will be taken to the grounds two days previous to the Sale, so that they may be inspected by prospective buyers.

On account of the low prices listed below, they will be sold for cash only, and must be taken into custody within two hours after sale.

No.	Name.	Age.	Remarks.	Price.
1	Lunesta	27	Prime Rice Planter,	$1,275.00
2	Violet	16	Housework and Nursemaid,	900.00
3	Lizzie	30	Rice, Unsound,	300.00
4	Minda	27	Cotton, Prime Woman,	1,200.00
5	Adam	28	Cotton, Prime Young Man,	1,100.00
6	Abel	41	Rice Hand, Eyesight Poor,	675.00
7	Tanney	22	Prime Cotton Hand,	950.00
8	Flementina	39	Good Cook. Stiff Knee,	400.00
9	Lanney	34	Prime Cottom Man,	1,000.00
10	Sally	10	Handy in Kitchen,	675.00
11	Maccabey	35	Prime Man, Fair Carpenter,	980.00
12	Dorcas Judy	25	Seamstress, Handy in House,	800.00
13	Happy	60	Blacksmith,	575.00
14	Mowden	15	Prime Cotton Boy,	700.00
15	Bills	21	Handy with Mules,	900.00
16	Theopolis	39	Rice Hand, Gets Fits,	575.00
17	Coolidge	29	Rice Hand and Blacksmith,	1,275.00
18	Bessie	69	Infirm, Sews,	250.00
19	Infant	1	Strong Likely Boy,	400.00
20	Samson	41	Prime Man, Good with Stock,	975.00
21	Callie May	27	Prime Woman, Rice,	1,000.00
22	Honey	14	Prime Girl, Hearing Poor,	850.00
23	Angelina	16	Prime Girl, House or Field,	1,000.00
24	Virgil	21	Prime Field Hand,	1,100.00
25	Tom	40	Rice Hand, Lame Leg,	750.00
26	Noble	11	Handy Boy,	900.00
27	Judge Lesh	55	Prime Blacksmith,	800.00
28	Booster	43	Fair Mason, Unsound,	600.00
29	Big Kate	37	Housekeeper and Nurse,	950.00
30	Melie Ann	19	Housework, Smart Yellow Girl,	1,250.00
31	Deacon	26	Prime Rice Hand,	1,000.00
32	Coming	19	Prime Cotton Hand,	1,000.00
33	Mabel	47	Prime Cotton Hand,	800.00
34	Uncle Tim	60	Fair Hand with Mules,	600.00
35	Abe	27	Prime Cotton Hand,	1,000.00
36	Tennes	29	Prime Rice Hand and Coachman,	1,250.00

There will also be offered at this sale, twenty head of Horses and Mules with harness, along with thirty head of Prime Cattle. Slaves will be sold separate, or in lots, as best suits the purchaser. Sale will be held rain or shine.

By the Antebellum Period the economics of slavery were shaped by health issues and concerns. Concrete evidence of the increased sophistication of the slave health subsystem is suggested on examination of this 1852 broadside announcing a slave sale. Slaves with provider skills are outlined (lines 2 and 29); African Americans with health conditions compromising them in the slave system are named in lines 3, 6, 8, 16, 18, 22, 25, and 28.

eighteenth century become in part a municipal hospital in function if not in name."[28] In most communities, these institutions served multiple functions, including those of orphanages, pesthouses, workhouses, and poorhouses. Governed by local politicians and elite community leaders as acts of charity, expenditures for these facilities were cut to the bone.[29]

These public facilities had poor physical plants, and sanitation was very primitive. The stench from such institutions and the tattered sheets hanging on their lines were prominent features characteristic of the public health care infrastructure. Inmates' diets were so poor that accounts of nutritional diseases such as scurvy were commonplace. In virtually all of these institutions the ambulatory patients were forced to work. Inmate coercion for performance or janitorial and nursing care tasks in most of these facilities was routine. Moreover, some of the facilities became diversified enough to provide punishment services for insane patients and Black slaves.[30]

Isolation of patients with contagious diseases such as plague or leprosy was one of the important functions performed by public health care facilities. Quarantine had become standard Western medical practice since the Venetians reinstituted the ancient practice in the fourteenth century. Thus, despite the lack of specific disease therapies such as antibiotics, most Western societies had made the connection between improvements in sanitation and improved community health. This approach was scientifically supported by the miasmatic and contagion theories of the time. Therefore, virtually all urban communities had begun to provide both public hospital facilities and isolation and quarantine facilities and policies. By the early nineteenth century community leaders and regulatory bodies felt compelled to provide these public health services and institutions.[31]

Between 1813 and 1860 public health care facilities grew in both number and complexity. In response to growing medically needy but indigent populations, the old poorhouses established in the seventeenth and eighteenth centuries began to treat an increasing number of sick patients. An 1810 description by Rosenberg of the New York City almshouse follows:

> [Though] it was in fact the largest hospital in a thriving port city (its private competitor, the New York Hospital, was far smaller) the internal logic of the almshouse allied it more closely to the hospice of the Middle Ages than to the twentieth-century hospital. . . . It housed the insane, the blind and crippled, the aged, the alcoholic and syphilitic, as well as the ordinary working man suffering with an extended siege of rheumatism, bronchitis, or pleurisy.[32]

Therefore, functionally, by the end of the period, many of these institutions had transformed into general hospitals for the poor and underserved, including Blacks. The transformation would not be complete for many of these facilities until the late nineteenth and early twentieth centuries. Prominent examples are

Bellevue Hospital in New York City and the Philadelphia General Hospital in Philadelphia. They would not shed their other functions as poorhouses, workhouses, pesthouses, and orphanages until late in their histories.[33]

As these facilities grew in size and complexity, they changed both in character and how they were governed. As their hospital and health care functions increased, their social welfare functions received less emphasis. Their governance became slightly more democratic, although elite community boards still attempted to micromanage their operations. Nevertheless, letters of recommendation on behalf of patients from hospital board members, subscribers, or community leaders increasingly were dropped as requirements for admission. Medical decision-making came to determine who was admitted to the hospitals instead of the traditional social and class considerations. However, there was still a struggle for control between hospital boards and commissions and the hospital's administrator, whose orientation, if not his training, was medically oriented.

Trainees in the form of medical students, house pupils (equivalent to resident house staff physicians of today), and nursing students served as cheap professional labor. Some of them either worked without pay or paid the institution for being allowed to train there. Their hours were long and grueling. Class, racial, and ethnic differences often led to poor communication between the staff and patients. Such differences were the predecessors to the sociocultural insensitivity often demonstrated by health care providers and institutions toward African American, other disadvantaged minority, and poor populations today. Conflicts and abusive incidents were not uncommon at the time.

The senior medical staff who worked in these facilities for the prestige or the practice usually assumed the responsibility for instructing the trainees. Many of the senior physicians were highly respected specialists who were faculty members at local medical schools. They perfected their clinical skills and techniques in these facilities in order to better serve their private paying patients. Although these practitioners had private practice patients whom they regarded and treated in a deferential and respectful manner, the quality of work in the public facilities varied from neglect and abuse to eleemosynary and paternalistic dedication. For these elite, often European-trained academic faculty physicians, working in the public health care infrastructure was expected. Their private patients were either treated in the early private voluntary hospitals, which were separate facilities; in special wings of the public hospital, usually with more luxurious accommodations where trainees were not allowed; or at home. The latter was still the most common situation.[34]

As the Civil War approached, a significant percentage of the facilities that provided care for Blacks, both slave and free, were affiliated with medical school teaching in some manner. This transformed the Black disadvantage due to U.S. health policies of racial hierarchy into fertile soil for medical exploitation. There is relatively abundant evidence that unethical experimentation and medical exploitation for training and research purposes took place on Black, mostly slave, patients in many of these facilities. There are also accounts of how Blacks dreaded entering them. One of the earliest of the city institutions to open that admitted Whites and Blacks was the College Infirmary of the Hampden-Sydney Medical Department in Richmond, Virginia, which opened in 1838. Other groups of Thomosonian and botanical physicians operated teaching hospitals at various times in the 1830s and 1840s in Richmond, Petersburg, and Norfolk, Virginia. Some private hospitals such as Bellevue in Richmond and Montaeri in Petersburg provided some free care for lower-class members of society, including Blacks. Slaves not lucky enough to live near urban areas where most of these public and teaching hospitals existed had to make do with the poorer quality care rendered at their lodgings or in the kitchens of private citizens. Some communities, especially smaller ones, used jails as hospitals for Blacks and the insane.[35]

Some Southern areas had dispensary care available to Black patients—on a segregated basis. One of the earliest dispensaries that provided care to Black freedmen opened in Charlottesville in 1826 as part of the University of Virginia Medical School. Alexandria, Virginia, operated a busy dispensary from the 1830s until the Civil War that provided care to Blacks. More of these facilities opened throughout the Antebellum Period as Southern cities acquired city services and Southern medical schools became more numerous.

As time passed and the Civil War approached, the tendency in the health system seemed to be toward more, not less, segregation of the races. This pattern was especially evident in the South. In some areas as the need arose, slave hospitals served as alternatives for the provision of health care to Blacks. New Orleans had two such facilities, Dr. Warren Stone's Maison de Sante and the Circus Street Hospital. But the tendency over time, as Richard C. Wade observed in *Slavery in the Cities*, "was always toward exclusive and separate treatment."[36] Savannah eventually opened a Negro Infirmary. Natchez opened and supported a two-story Negro hospital across the street from the town's slave market. Slave hospitals would open in numerous cities in the South as the Antebellum Period approached.[37]

Private hospitals before the late nineteenth century were rare. In addition to the Pennsylvania Hospital (founded 1752) and the New York Hospital (founded 1771, received patients 1790s), the Massachusetts General Hospital opened in 1821. (See Figures 5.2 and 5.3.) As Rosenberg points out, "In 1873, the first American hospital survey located only 178."[38] Unlike the public facilities, these private institutions were usually small. By 1850, outside of large cities such as Boston, New York, Philadelphia, or New Orleans, few Americans were even familiar with large hospitals such as those common in London, Paris, or Vienna. The small private facilities available were headquartered in private homes and usually owned by physicians, individually or in groups. Very few of these facilities were integrated into the medical education system unless the participant physicians had apprentices. However, the medical culture of the era, especially the educational component, was the formative element involved in shaping all of these hospitals, both public and private. As was common practice in Europe and America, incur-

Figure 5.2   New York Hospital

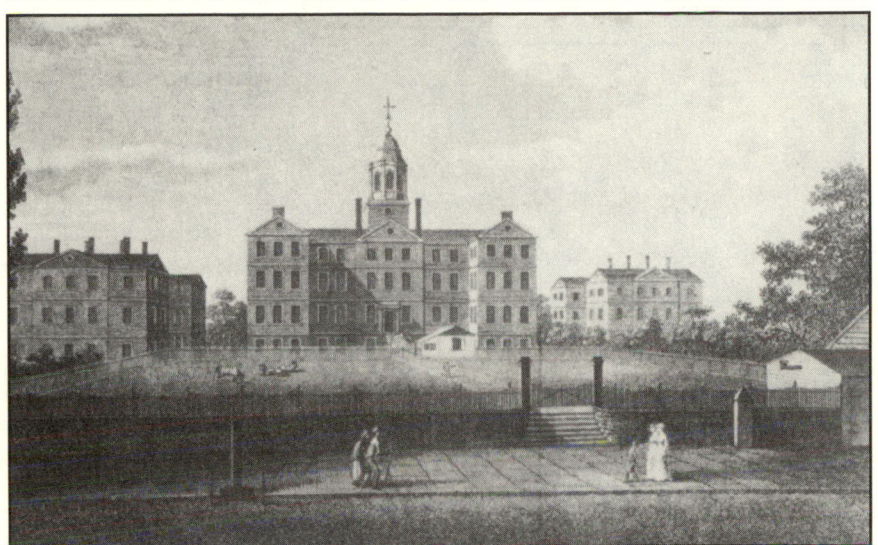

Public-spirited New Yorkers were as proud of their new hospital as they were of their new nation. This view, embodying a sense of order and social responsibility, dates from approximately 1820. Its segregation along race and class lines was not remarkable for the period—it was considered standard practice.

ables, venereal disease patients, or people of dubious character were refused admission to any hospitals—unless they were paying patients. The new voluntary hospital routinely transferred these undesirable or incurable patients to the almshouse facilities or jails. Sailors had a special status in the early system. After 1798, based on an act of Congress, sailors were either admitted to their own facilities or were provided guaranteed care in private hospitals. In 1811 the U.S. Navy initiated its own medical service. If Black patients were admitted into the private facilities at all, they were provided segregated, inferior accommodations.[39]

By 1810 five medical schools were functioning in the United States. This tiny number of schools was inadequate to supply trained practitioners for the entire U.S. population, which by then numbered 7,239,000. Significantly, the first proprietary school was opened in Baltimore in 1807. It was affiliated with the University of Maryland and was a jointly sponsored private venture organized by a few local physicians. It represented the first of dozens of proprietary schools to open under state charters during the nineteenth century. Before the twentieth century began, there was a great interest in expanding the capacity for medical education in the United States. The number of schools grew from five in 1810 to the opening and existence of more than 400 by 1900 (no more than 175 to 200 existed at any one time). With the exception of the University of Pennsylvania and a few others, most of these schools provided perfunctory 8- to 14-week school

Figure 5.3 Washington, D.C., Slave Pen and Hospital, Judiciary Square, Southwest Corner of G and 4th Streets, NW

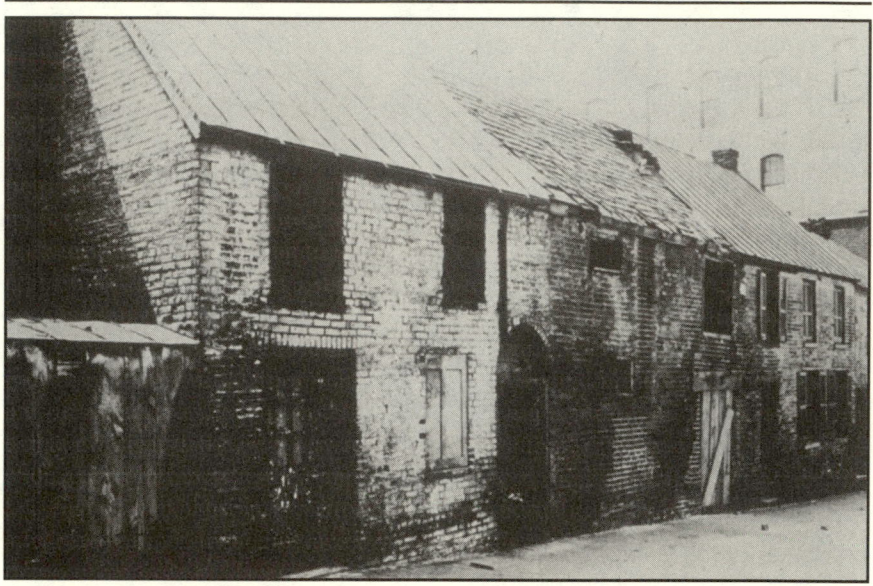

Used as a jail and slave pen since 1801, it was much feared by Blacks before the Civil War. Beginning in 1844 the "Washington Infirmary," a type of slave hospital, was located here. Such facilities grew alongside the private hospitals serving as hospitals and health facilities for the dispossessed of American society—including Black slaves.

terms. A few of the proprietary schools issued diplomas after one year, while most required attendance for two years. Most of these institutions were diploma mills.

Medical educational reform thus became a top priority of medical professionalization, though legislation and implementation of medical licensing laws and effective medical educational reform would not take place until the late nineteenth century. All of these successes would be spearheaded and shepherded by the formation and flourishing of an effective, lily-White national professional organization that emerged during the Jacksonian and Antebellum periods. Culmination of the medical professional society movement that had taken hold in the eighteenth century resulted in the establishment of the American Medical Association (AMA) in 1847. For the first 23 years of its existence, the AMA would informally exclude African Americans based on medical-social custom. In 1870 that discrimination became a formal AMA policy that stood for most of the following century. Medicine remains one of the nation's most rigidly segregated professions today.[40]

To many medical historians the nineteenth century marked the rise of modern U.S. medicine. This is especially true from a European perspective in that many U.S. medical schools affiliated with universities for the first time, and several hospitals and research laboratories appeared. European medical schools had initiated and capitalized upon such institutional ties since their late medieval beginnings. Some European-led medical advances occurring in the first half of the nineteenth century included:

- Advances in basic sciences such as chemistry, pathology, bacteriology, histology, physiology, and pharmacology
- The introduction of statistics and the numerical methods that forever changed the nature and scope of clinical medicine and public health
- The clinical acceptance of vaccination for smallpox
- Introduction of the stethoscope
- Simmelweis's contribution to controlling puerperal fever
- Rapid advances in clinical schools such as Paris, London, Dublin, and Vienna, where medical specialization evolved and new technologies were adapted to aid the clinician at the bedside
- Laboratory medical advances that became essential allies to clinicians previously totally reliant upon, and limited by, medical teleological systems and bedside medicine
- The publication of Percival's *Code of Medical Ethics*

Although the U.S. public had to experience the Civil War to learn the value of Western medicine's technological and scientific advancements, the modern hospital, now offering more than a location for rest and recovery and ineffective therapies, emerged. By the end of this era hospitals began offering a few laboratory diagnostic modalities, some surgical interventions, and access to knowledgeable specialists without the concomitant dangers of exposure to contagions. Unfortunately, most of the medical progress emanating from Europe would be cumulative and would produce benefits only in the future. American clinicians and their public sought something different. To impress Americans, medical progress had to be practical and palpable, yielding immediate and measurable benefits. From another perspective, the United States was an isolated pioneer environment encouraging bold and colorful individual medical actions and scientific pursuits.

The United States' lack of emphasis on esoteric research was emblematic of the rise of its unique medical-social culture. The United States did not have large cadres of scientists, research laboratories, and universities. In light of this, the rather unique character and nature of American medical contributions that began surfacing by the Civil War becomes somewhat more comprehensible. As Bender observed in *Great Moments in Medicine:*

> *New World doctors of the early 1800s followed the practice of European physicians, to whom they looked for leadership in medicine. They were importers of ideas; seldom exporters. However, there were a few, but*

> *important, exceptions. Rugged physicians, faced with the myriad med-*
> *ical problems of the new American frontiers, and without consultants or*
> *publications to fall back upon, were forced to improvise, to invent, to*
> *experiment, to take chances. Out of their experiences, when they could*
> *find time to write them down, came some remarkable contributions to*
> *medical knowledge; and medical communication across the Atlantic*
> *began to acquire a two-way flow.*[41]

For African Americans locked in the slave health subsystem and the few free Blacks having access to even less health care, this progress had a hollow ring with ominous overtones. Black isolation from the evolving mainstream health system increased exponentially during the Jacksonian and Antebellum periods. Partially as a result of this development, Black/White differences in health status and outcome increased. Moreover, by then African American legal and social status had deteriorated to such a degree that Blacks were fertile targets for medical and scientific exploitation, even abuse. Sadly, other than those involved with the marginal White abolitionist movement, very few Americans empathized with their plight.[42]

A *Unique Health System Culture's* Modus Operandi: *Sensationalism, Pragmatism, and Race and Class Exploitation for Scientific Advance*

From a European perspective, American physicians were engaging in bold, occasionally brilliant, clinical medical feats that were not being performed anywhere else on earth. The American character and the circumstance of an evolving multitiered and unequal health system hierarchically based on race and class facilitated these developments, as did prevalent and pervasive professional and scientific isolation. The Black social condition and the racial nature of U.S. slavery along with the unfortunate medical-social position of so-called "unworthy poor" patients offered White physicians unprecedented possibilities for experimentation and research along with the potential for exploitation and unethical behavior relative to these powerless patient populations. Moreover, the United States had broken loose from the aristocratic and clerical moorings that grounded European health professions and systems in paternalistic and protective stewardship regarding the poor and unfortunate. The alleged presumption that every man in America was "free" to fend for himself relegated misfortunes to the category of "individual concerns." For Blacks this abnegation of social culpability was compounded by their legal designation in most states as chattel—therefore, due no more legal consideration than hogs, sheep, or cattle. Weak and powerless "dependents" in the United States (Black chattel slaves were the epitome of helplessness) were rendered vulnerable to privation or abuse while simultaneously being

excluded from the concern of powerful protectors. These factors set the stage atti-
tudinally, institutionally, and circumstantially for a certain unrestrained variety of
medical heroics and exploitation. Physicians in America performed on a medical
stage where there was little scrutiny or concern when Blacks or the poor were
involved. This created a world of "sliding-scale" medical ethics and health system
performance evaluation. All this was compounded by the fact that "these people,"
the unfortunates, were felt to be personally responsible or predestined by birth or
race to embody their dependent and vulnerable positions. America from its beginnings had an aggressive strain of condescension and disdain for welfare or its recip-
ients—and receipt of this care was often considered a form of welfare.[43]

Word spread around the world of heroic American surgical exploits. In 1809,
Ephraim McDowell (1771–1830), a Danville, Kentucky, general practitioner,
successfully removed a 20-pound ovarian tumor from a 45-year-old woman who
went on to live to the age of 78. Danville was an isolated frontier outpost from a
medical standpoint, and such surgery was considered a virtual death sentence for
patients during this period. Though McDowell was a well-trained Edinburgh
Medical School graduate, such an operation would have been considered dangerous and radical in Europe where he trained. It is documented that a significant number of McDowell's surgical patients were Blacks. John Richmond
(1785–1855), a frontier physician in Newtown, Ohio, successfully performed the
first Caesarian section west of the Allegheny Mountains in 1827. Forced to take
action due to a clinical emergency, he operated under primitive conditions with
common instruments. Although it was not the first time C-sections had been performed by any means, it did stretch the limits of acceptable circumstances under
which a major procedure like this could be performed in Western medical circles. Such positive results and the quasi-heroic accounts of them stirred the
American imagination, simultaneously convincing many citizens that modern
medicine was beginning to attain some practical value.

Between 1845 and 1852 in Montgomery, Alabama, J. Marion Sims
(1813–1883), manipulating and exploiting the exigencies of slavery, perfected
the techniques for repair of vesicovaginal fistulas and vaginal gynecologic
surgery. His experiments and techniques were developed almost entirely on
Black slave women. Without them, Sims would not have achieved his medical
and surgical breakthroughs. White women would not have been available for
these brutal (no anesthesia) and repeatedly futile (there were huge numbers of
failures requiring repeat surgeries) procedures (see Vignette). Evidence that
Sims, however dimly, perceived some moral culpability for this unethical experimentation is demonstrated by his behavior. During the 1850s when Sims was
harvesting fame for his breakthroughs in New York and Europe, he covered up
the fact that his pioneer work had been done on Black slaves in numerous writings and presentations. Even his illustrations and surgical diagrams were of fic-
tional White women. Such deceptions serve as evidence for Sims's awareness of
the medical-ethical aspects of what he was doing.

A New Perspective on a Medical Icon

J. Marion Sims, M.D. (1813–1883), a nineteenth-century gynecologist, is portrayed as a medical hero in virtually every medical school in the United States. In the field of obstetrics and gynecology, he bears the sobriquets of the "Father of Gynecology" and the "Father of Vaginal Surgery." Born in South Carolina, Sims practiced in Mt. Meigs and Montgomery, Alabama (1830s–1850s), New York City (1850s–1880s), and throughout Europe (1860s–1880s). Little known is the fact that many of his accomplishments developing innovative gynecologic techniques and surgical procedures and instrumentation were obtained at the expense and surgical exploitation of Black women.

The essence of Sims's contributions lies in the field of gynecologic surgery. His discovery of successful methods for the repair of vesicovaginal fistulae and his invention of various instruments and techniques for the performance of vaginal surgery laid the technical foundations for the present field of gynecology. His serial discoveries, concentrated over four years of intense human experimentation, consisted of standardizing the Sims position for exposure of female pelvic anatomy for diagnostic, surgical, and therapeutic purposes; the invention and perfection of the vaginal speculum and several female catheters; and pioneering the utilization of silver wire sutures and other special vaginal surgery techniques. Sims's promotion of the treatment of "women's diseases" varying from infertility to painful female conditions or disabling ones such as fistulae, along with the creation of a worldwide coterie of physicians expert in these areas, made gynecology as practiced in the United States a medical specialty with a particular place and utility. These were important accomplishments.

However, the medical-social aspects of Sims's career are seldom mentioned. As Richard Shryock pointed out relative to American medical contributions in general, and Sims's accomplishments in particular, in *The Development of Modern Medicine:*

> American surgery was notable not only for the introduction of anesthetics, but also for the development of difficult operations rarely attempted in European practice. This was particularly true in gynecology. Local conditions, in the form of the "peculiar institution" of slavery, were a factor in making possible Marion Sims's epoch-making operation on vesico-vaginal fistula (1849). Sims first experimented upon slaves, and it is interesting to find him remarking that in one case he had to purchase his patient in order to operate upon her.[44]

It is acknowledged that male-dominated medical stewardship and patient exploitation on the basis of race, gender, and class have changed a great deal since the mid- and late nineteenth century when Sims practiced. However, closer examination of his career reveals that his faults in medical-social and ethical areas were extreme.

Realistically, Sims's surgical breakthroughs correcting vesicovaginal fistulae (an abnormal opening between the urinary bladder and the vagina, then most often caused by traumatic childbirth) would likely not have occurred as rapidly without aggressive and cruel surgical exploitation of three Black slave women named Betsy, Lucy, and Anarcha. As has been mentioned, he even purchased one of the women to continue operating upon her. The moving Robert Thom painting in Bender's *Great Moments in Medicine* (see Figure 5.4) captures his subjugation of these Black women as he performed repeated major surgical procedures (Sims admitted operating on Anarcha on at least 30 agonizingly painful occasions), exposing their genitals to the public, without anesthesia—believing Blacks did not have morals or perceive pain as Whites did. Moreover, to manipulate their postoperative healing

Figure 5.4   Sims About to Operate on a Slave Woman

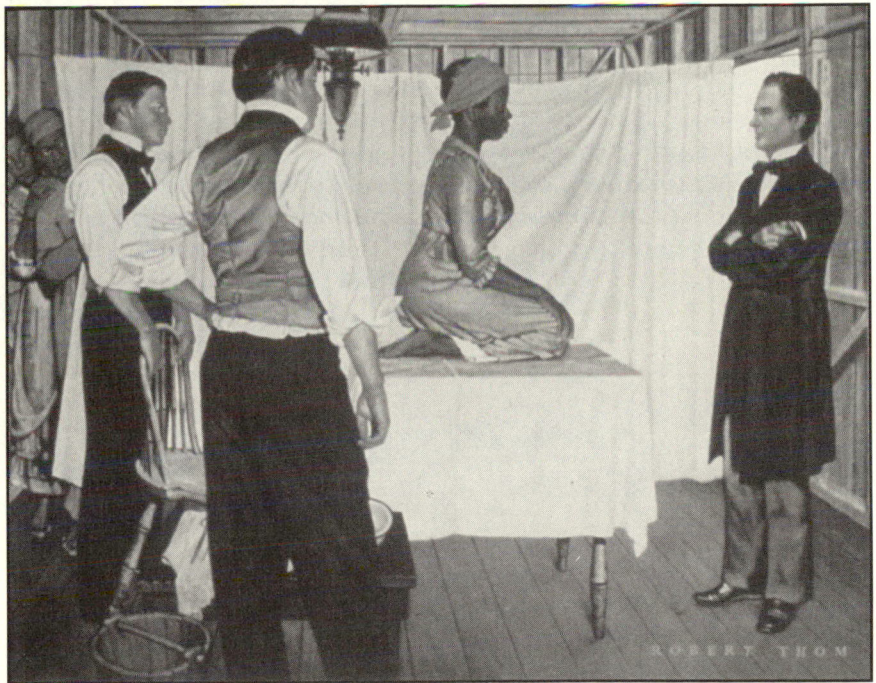

A Thom painting of J. Marion Sims, the "Father of Gynecology," about to operate on a slave woman named Lucy. Betsy and Anarcha peep from behind the curtain at Dr. Sims and his assistants. Sims exploited both Black slaves and poor White women to further his surgical career. He purchased slave women in order to operate experimentally on them. Giving them no anesthesia due to their racial "differences" (Blacks purportedly did not feel pain), he addicted them to opiates to regulate their bowel and bladder function. He operated on several of these women 20 or 30 times before obtaining the results he wanted. When he attempted to transfer his hierarchical, individualistic, medical ethical practices to New York, Dr. Sims ran into professional trouble.

process he addicted them to opiates (equivalent to morphine or heroin) to modulate their bowel and bladder function. Medical exploitation of the Black slaves was accepted without comment. This would not have been acceptable medical ethical practice on upper-class white women. Significantly, his continuation of this pattern of gender-based hierarchical thinking, individualistic and self-serving medical ethics, and experimental surgical exploitation of Black, poor, and Irish women after his relocation to New York led to controversy and professional problems for Dr. Sims.

Sims's attitudes did not change after moving to New York in 1853. Deborah Kuhn McGregor identifies Sims as an example of America's class bias in the exercise of medical school teaching at Women's Hospital in New York City: "Without a doubt, class was a powerful agent of discrimination. Women whose diagnoses and presences were part of clinical lectures were poor patients receiving charity. Education for medical students was the fee exacted from them."[45] McGregor revealed Sims's attitudes and behavior toward Black and poor patients later in his career relative to an African American woman who died after a dangerous, highly experimental surgery he performed at Women's Hospital of New York: "Clearly, from Sims' point of view, the life of the patient in this case was expendable. Her body in many ways had become his even before she died. . . . [W]hile he placed his findings on the 'altar of science,'. . . her class and race placed her at Sims' disposal."[46] As these incidents multiplied in his New York practice they caused Sims trouble from his peers and eventually led to professional sanctions.

Although the existence of the South's "peculiar institution" was no fault of his, Sims's behavior was emblematic of the European contention identified by Shryock, Walker, Savitt, and McGregor that American physicians were known for performing reckless and dangerous experiments and surgeries on Black slaves. Many Europeans attributed U.S. leadership in surgery and anesthesia on practices that would not have been fully condoned outside the confines of slavery and American medical-social practices. According to McGregor, Sims seemingly tried to hide the racial status of his female experimental subjects based upon the text and illustrations in his numerous scientific articles on experimental female surgery. McGregor concluded that hiding the fact they were in bondage or, later, charity patients implies culpability on Sims's part at the very least. Sims's chauvinistic approach and his somewhat cold, egotistical, calculating, obsessive-compulsive personality, combined with U.S. social and scientific conditions in the areas of race, gender, and class, may have encouraged the potential for his "soulless scientist" persona. These facts cannot be ignored.

Although the social milieu relative to race, gender, and class has changed dramatically since Sims practiced, continuing to portray him as an icon to American physicians without exposing all the facts surrounding his achievements does not provide a complete and accurate picture of him as a physician-scientist or human being. Classical and conventional medical history literature has portrayed Sims as an unqualified scientific hero without human dimensions or frailties. This is especially relevant to a U.S. medical profession with an unfortunate medical-social history and an arrogant and detached approach to the race and class problems in the United States. The contemporary aspects of this circumstance are exemplified by the

Tuskegee experiment and the Helen Lacks controversy (the Black cancer patient whose cervical tissue [HeLa cells] has been utilized experimentally for decades without her, or her family's, permission). This calls for a reassessment of the relationship between race, gender, class, medicine, and health care in the United States. McGregor's book serves as an excellent beginning.

Notes

Bender GA. *Great Moments in Medicine.* Detroit: Northwood Institute Press, 1966, 236–244, 237.

Byrd WM, Clayton LA. *A Black Health Trilogy* [videotape and 188 page documentary report]. Washington, D.C.: The National Medical Association and the African American Heritage and Education Foundation; 1991.

Fausto-Sterling A. Anatomy. *Encyclopedia of African American Culture and History.* Eds. Salzman J, Smith DL, West C. 5 vols. New York: Macmillan Library Reference USA, 1996.

Jones JH. *Bad Blood: The Tuskegee Syphilis Experiment.* New York: The Free Press, 1981.

Lewis JH. Contribution of an unknown Negro to anesthesia. *J Natl Med Assoc* 1931; 23:23–24.

Lyons AS, Petrucelli RJ. *Medicine: An Illustrated History.* New York: Harry N. Abrams, Inc., Publishers. 1978, 523, 531.

McGregor DK. *Sexual Surgery and the Origins of Gynecology: J. Marion Sims, His Hospital, and His Patients.* New York: Garland Publishing, Inc., 1989.

Morais HM. *The History of the Negro in Medicine.* Under auspices of The Association for the Study of Negro Life and History. New York: Publishers Company, Inc., 1967.

Savitt TL. The use of blacks for medical experimentation and demonstration in the old south. *J Southern History* 1982; 48:331–348.

Shryock RH. *The Development of Modern Medicine: An Interpretation of the Social and Scientific Factors Involved.* Madison, Wisconsin: The University of Wisconsin Press, 1974, 177.

Walker HE. *The Negro in the Medical Profession.* Publications of the University of Virginia Phelps-Stokes Fellowship Papers. N.P. University of Virginia, 1949, 7.

Washington HA. Of men and mice: Human guinea pigs: Unethical testing targets Blacks and the poor. *Emerge* 1994 (October, No. 1): 6:24.

Simultaneously, as early as 1842 Crawford Long (1815–1848), a University of Pennsylvania–trained Southern physician practicing in Jefferson, Georgia, was experimenting with ether after discovering its anesthetic properties at social "frolics." He was probably the first physician to utilize the agent as a general anesthetic specifically to perform surgeries. Despite Long's successes, patients were leery and persuasion was necessary to convince them to use the new technique. As Bender pointed out in *Great Moments in Medicine*, "Dr. Long used ether whenever he could persuade surgical or obstetrical patients to permit it."[47] Significantly, a large percentage of Long's early experimental patients were Black slaves. It is unlikely that he obtained their consent. A few years later, formal demonstration of ether as a general anesthetic was publicly demonstrated at the Massachusetts General Hospital in Boston by dentist William T. G. Morton (1819–1868) on October 16, 1846, at what is now known as the ether dome. A major case under ether anesthesia, an amputation, was performed at the same institution on November 7, 1846. Touted as "surgery without pain" and named "anesthesia" by Oliver Wendell

Holmes, the technique had spread to Europe by December 21, 1846, when Dr. Robert Liston performed an amputation at University College Hospital of London. Meanwhile, the only major pre–Civil War U.S. medical contributions lacking the American flair for daring, impetuosity, and public appeal were the solid contribution to the burgeoning science of physiology by William Beaumont and Oliver Wendell Holmes's contribution to obstetrics.[48]

An obscure apprentice-trained U.S. Army surgeon, William Beaumont (1785–1853), took advantage of frontier circumstances and serendipity at Fort Michilimackinac in northern Michigan to conduct landmark physiological experiments documenting mechanisms of digestion beginning in 1822. Alexis St. Martin, a French Canadian, suffered a gunshot wound to his upper body, opening large areas of his chest and upper abdomen. After miraculously healing, the wound left a permanent communication between his stomach and the exterior. Beaumont, being his attending physician on a frontier post in relative professional isolation, conducted careful experiments on the man's stomach and published his results in *Experiments and Observation on the Gastric Juice and the Physiology of Digestion* in 1833. It caused a sensation in Europe, where it was hailed as a major medical breakthrough. The quiet nature of discoveries such as Beaumont's, no matter how important, however, didn't pique the American public's curiosity nor promote the value of medical science. Another example of a quiet American contribution without any evidence of race or class exploitation that would only receive notice and credit decades after its occurrence was that of Oliver Wendell Holmes (1809–1894). This famous medical practitioner, medical educator, poet, and essayist was the first to recognize the contagious nature of puerperal or childbed fever, hypothesizing that it was transmitted by the examinations and manipulations of women's attendants during labor and delivery. His correlation antedated the germ theory by some 40 years, and Holmes was soundly criticized by other physicians for his explanatory hypothesis. His presentation in 1843 preceded by at least four years the work of Ignaz Semmelweis (1818–1865) at the Allgemeines Krankenhaus in Vienna that statistically proved the relationship. He would belatedly receive minor credit for these discoveries, largely from within professional circles. Only after pioneers such as Pasteur and Koch had established bacterial pathogenesis would the significance of Simmelweis's and Holmes's discoveries be appreciated. However, the net result of all these discoveries began a gradual change in America's estimation of the value of medical science.[49]

These medical landmarks were the fruit of the peculiar medical and health system environment of early America. They are not indicators of the frequency of exploitive or unethical medical practices exercised on Black or poor patients in this country, which undoubtedly occurred thousands of times. This serves as a serendipitous and random catalog of some of the most important and famous incidents. Whether all or some of these discoveries, all of which could be viewed as contributing to the general good through the beneficence of medical progress, could have taken place in Britain or on the continent is questionable.

There are several reasons for raising this issue. Certain patterns are discernible here that serve as explanatory hypotheses and reveal basic currents that help define today's unique American medical-social culture and health dilemma. Such an inquiry also reveals some of the underlying dynamics and root causes of the U.S. health system's race and class problems. These factors loom in the background and help block equitable health reform today. Many medical breakthroughs themselves, or their conceptual or experimental antecedents, occurred on the frontier. The urban centers were the headquarters of professional American medicine and science at the time. In some ways analogous to the Royal Society in London, some scientific professional interchange occurred at professional and scientific society meetings in Philadelphia, Boston, and New York as early as the late 1700s. Though not at the same level of sophistication as scientific communities in London, Paris, or Rome, frontier isolation nevertheless insulated and isolated these discoveries from outside scrutiny. These biomedical scientific breakthroughs also took place in a medical-social environment peculiar to America. This environment was influenced and in some instances shaped by the interaction produced by frontier conditions and American attitudes regarding the disadvantaged and the South's "peculiar institution"—Black chattel slavery. The potential for manipulation and exploitation of this environment, a moral price extracted for this "dark side" of medical progress, was enhanced by a longstanding European tradition of overutilization of criminal and poor populations for medical demonstration, dissection, and experimentation purposes. Virtually all authorities agree that European medicine has a long history of overutilization of poor and criminal classes for medical dissection, educational demonstration, and experimentation purposes. These origins stretched back to ancient and medieval times. Only recently have ethicists begun examining and questioning that tradition.[50] Hierarchical ranking and the assignment of disadvantage based on poverty, social disadvantage, and often dependency is nothing new to Western medicine. As has been observed, some of these tendencies toward hierarchical ranking of the "worthy" and "unworthy" poor may have been less codified in America but were just as extreme as in Europe. Unlike Europe, where these rankings were often the result of birth or ancestry, in North America they were often pragmatically based on the present access to visible and palpable wealth; moral evaluation, standing, and judgment by the community; and social circumstance and standing. Superimposed on these conditions for Blacks was the uniformly unfavorable effects of being of African descent and most likely a slave in a Western, predominantly White Protestant, culture.[51]

Two other major factors contributing to the unique American medical environment was the medical isolation and the pressure on practitioners to succeed in healing their patients. The first factor differentiated this country from Europe on organizational and institutional grounds, while the latter was probably more extreme due to the worship of pragmatism in the American character. For example, physicians such as Beaumont, Sims, and Richmond were faced with extreme clinical circumstances that stretched beyond, or to the extremes of, the limited capabilities of the medical science of that time. Some of the disease conditions were either emergent or incurable. Faced by an ever-doubting American public reticent to trust in medical practice, they were pressured by the impulse to "do something." Shryock noted this timeless factor, quoting Roger Bacon: "The operative and practical sciences which do their work on insensate bodies can multiply their experiments till they get rid of deficiency and errors, but a physician cannot do this because of the nobility of the material in which he works."[52]

Relative isolation meant there were no professional societies or colleagues with which to discuss these complicated cases. Improvisation and innovation were also encouraged by the fact that the bounds of American medical practice were not defined legally or professionally at the time. Each practitioner, thus, worked as a separate entity—virtually on his own. Legal or professionally defined divisions of labor such as those that existed between European physicians, surgeons, apothecaries, or midwives were nonexistent. Everyone considered a "doctor" in America had the leeway to do anything he had the nerve to try. His work or what he did to patients, especially poor or Black ones, was, thus, not subject to professional, practical, or moral scrutiny. The final unique ingredient in many of these American contributions to world medicine was the total medical dominance over and subjugation of 20 percent of their patient population, the overwhelming majority of whom were Black slaves. As has been explained earlier, the relatively small number of free Blacks were worse off and more vulnerable in many ways than the slaves from a medical-social perspective. The Black sociocultural condition and the nature of U.S. slavery offered White physicians untold possibilities for experimentation and research along with the potential for exploitation and unethical behavior relative to powerless Blacks. As Black patients came to be increasingly defined as a group apart and "different," from medical-social, biological, and ethical perspectives, American physicians engaged in the entire gamut of dubious professional possibilities.[53]

These exploitative medical-social tendencies were reinforced in the U.S. health system during the Jacksonian and Antebellum periods. Whether Beaumont would have been allowed to observe and experiment upon Alexis St. Martin if the patient had been wealthy enough to seek and maintain a private physician is unlikely. There is evidence he objected to and resisted the way Beaumont managed him while he was conducting his experiments.[54] There are several allusions in the literature to Crawford Long's performing a major percentage of his early anesthetic experiments on Black slaves—patients who were easily coerced or without choice in the matter.[55] These and other examples raise the question of whether these breakthroughs may have been paradoxically related to, or at least facilitated by, race- and class-based medical-social flaws in the Antebellum health system. In short, the Jacksonian and Antebellum health system's scientific and medical progress was obtained at an exorbitant medical-social price.[56]

Entrenchment of a Black Health Deficit

Despite the social and scientific progress for the White population in the United States, Black health remained terrible during the Jacksonian and Antebellum periods. This was a paradox in a country undergoing an economic and political boom when improvements in health status and outcome for all populations should have been expected. Moreover, the South, strongly based in a plantation economy and home for more than 90 percent of the nation's Blacks, was responsible for more than two-thirds of the nation's profitable exports by 1860. Because of "difference" disadvantages suffered by African Americans in the health system due to their slave status and racial subordination, expected health status and outcome improvements did not accrue. Slavery had grown from 700,000 slaves when George Washington assumed the presidency in 1789 to 1.5 million in 1820 to more than 4 million by 1860. Conventional wisdom and much of the mythology passed down to us claims that owners (planters) would treat their property (slaves) well to protect their economic investment. However, many students of slavery such as Kenneth Stampp, Kenneth Kiple, and Todd Savitt have documented that such was not necessarily the case. Investigation reveals that the poor health status and outcomes of most African Americans was dependent upon a complex mixture of factors related to deprived and stressful health environments, inadequacies in the health system, and changes affecting the institution of slavery itself. The few free Blacks, denied institutional support, suffered the worst health status of all.[57]

Many external factors in the changing political economy of slavery between 1813 and 1860 helped determine the profile and outcomes of slavery's illnesses. A majority of these forces were outside the purview of the health care system of the time. One major determinant of the health status of the Black population was that plantation slavery in the Antebellum Period expanded into the Western territories. This had many ramifications on health in general and African American health in particular.

Implementation of the Southern plantation system in the Western and Southwestern territories involved a profound change in the nature of the work required of slaves and the environment in which they were forced to work. This was some of the most brutal and heavy work imaginable and had many ramifications on Black health. Not only was it physically taxing, but it was also dangerous from an accident and disease perspective. Land clearance, tree removal and burning, swamp drainage, and planting virgin land with staple crops such as cotton, sugar cane, and rice was grueling, back-breaking work. This brutal overwork in rustic conditions, often overexposed to the elements, took a heavy toll on slaves.[58]

Primitive living quarters and marginal logistical support in these areas meant more overexposure risks. Poor sanitation imposed by frontier conditions translated into more disease risks from the various forms of dysentery, typhoid fever, and worm infestations. Work in low and undrained swampy areas such as the recently settled cotton and rice lands around New Orleans increased the risks from the various fevers. Transfer to these areas from the East was dreaded by slaves. It was known that slave owners in old plantation states such as Virginia and North Carolina could threaten recalcitrant chattel with the threat of selling them "West" or "to Texas." Rustic agricultural and environmental factors combined with brutal work conditions, especially in the "boom areas" of the Deep South and Southwest, translated into poor slave health status during the late Antebellum Period. Based on the upturns in the economy and living conditions and health status for the general population, one would have expected slave health status to improve, but it is understandable why it declined instead.

The seeming paradox becomes more comprehensible when one factors in the overall effects that British abolition of the Atlantic slave trade in 1807 had on Black health. This major factor affected Black health but was outside the purview of the health system itself. Effects of the abolition of the Atlantic slave trade were compounded by the impact of various states' abolition of manumissions as well as state abolitions of slave trading in the North following the American Revolution. These events forced America to become increasingly dependent on the domestic slave trade if adequate manpower to capitalize on the new commercial possibilities the cotton gin opened up were to be realized. Despite the illegal importation of African slaves up to the end of the Civil War, westward expansion of the system and concomitant increases in the slave population depended on domestic slave fertility and fecundability.* Therefore, slave breeding became both profitable and necessary for the first time. This traffic in human beings had profound adverse maternal and child health consequences, the details of which will be discussed later.[59]

Another effect of the rapid geographic expansion on Black health is that the care provided African Americans, both slave and free, would be much more disorganized and chaotic on the frontier than that rendered in stable and settled areas. The establishment of health delivery institutions and the provision of adequate numbers of trained health professionals were pressing problems in newly settled and frontier areas. What had been a generalized problem for seventeenth- and eighteenth-century North American English colonies was just beginning to be addressed in the newly settled areas of the United States. In the lower South and Southwest even the slave health subsystem was handicapped by the absence of adequate back-up medical providers and slave hospitals and dispensaries that were present in more developed areas such as Virginia, Charleston, or New Orleans. Moreover, the absence in these new areas (e.g., Alabama, Mississippi, Texas) of a significant public health care infrastructure anchored by almshouse hospitals and dispensaries was a significant handicap. These institutions became prominent health delivery resources for working poor and Black people (slave and free) by

---

Fertility is the ability to become pregnant. *Fecundability* is the probability of conceiving during a monthly cycle. It provides the basis for estimating fertility over time.

this period. Their absence differentially affected largely dependent slave, poor, and free Black populations. Thus, not only were these groups' risks increased by the primitive environmental conditions of the frontier, but they were also positioned to receive virtually no health care or services in these developing areas.[60]

Beginning in the early Colonial Era in both the North and the South, corporal punishments for Black slaves, such as public branding for punishment and burning alive, were relatively common. The frequency of such punishments increased geometrically with the prevalence of slave rebellions and revolts. Although the Haitian slave rebellion in 1791 sent shock waves across the entire Western Hemisphere and redefined and transformed subsequent slave uprisings as legitimate revolts by the most stringent criteria, Genovese reminds us there was a vivid English North American experience:

> The most important slave revolts in the English-speaking North American states occurred in New York City in 1712; at Stono, South Carolina in 1739; in southern Louisiana in 1811; and in Southhampton County, Virginia under Nat Turner in 1831. To them might be added the conspiracy at Point Coupee, Louisiana, in 1795 . . . and the conspiracies of Gabriel Prosser in Richmond, Virginia, in 1800 and of Denmark Vesey in Charleston, South Carolina, in 1822.[61]

The specter of organized bands of Black slaves marching over the countryside from plantation to plantation was impressed upon the minds of the White South with the slave rebellion that occurred in the Pointe Coupee section of Louisiana in January of 1811. This triggered a White civilian mass migration into New Orleans. Several hundred Black slaves participated and were defeated by well-armed planters, numerous militiamen, and almost 300 U.S. Army troops.[62] As Stephen Oates observed before the Nat Turner revolt in 1831, "Virginia was . . . almost a military garrison, with a militia force of some hundred thousand men to guard against insurrection."[63] After the Nat Turner rebellion, perhaps America's most terrifying slave uprising, this situation became worse throughout the South. Local militias were strengthened and the severity of slave codes increased. Medically, this translated into more physical repression and torture, cruel public punishments, and bodily injuries.[64]

The political economy of slavery was already built upon the lash. Terror was the main incentive for labor and control of slaves, who were whipped and punished for those reasons. Extreme punishments were common enough, but when associated with rumors or acts associated with slave rebellions, insurrections, or suspected plots, they became gruesome. These brutal incidents and punishment practices had a tremendous impact on the prevalence and incidence of trauma for slave populations. Punishments for transgressions by Black slaves were brutal and often public. Floggings, castrations, amputations, nose splittings, and a variety of other mutilations added to the slaves' already high injury burdens related to

Figure 5.5   Detail of Inventory of Female Slaves: Slave Breeding
            Practices

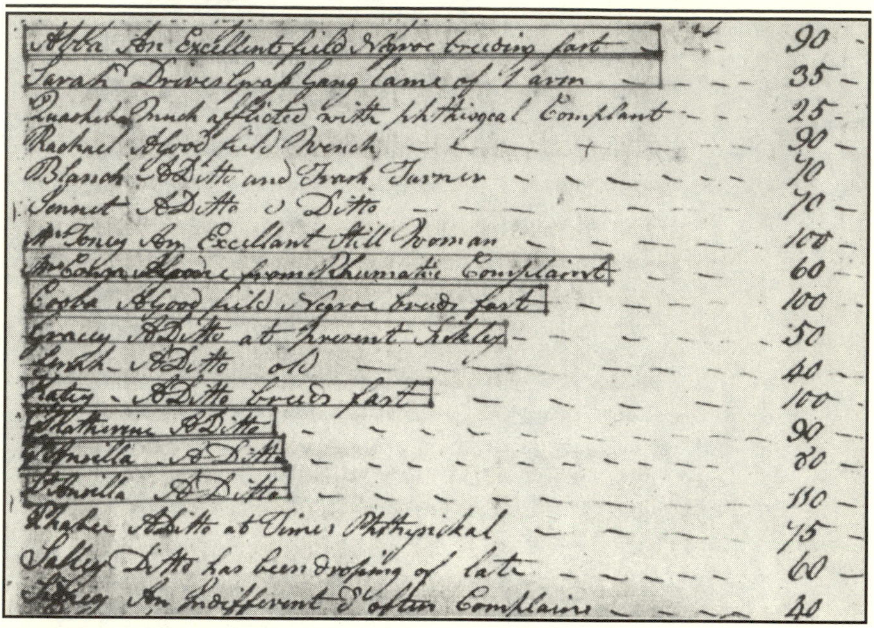

A detail of an inventory of female slaves. There are six slave women with notations "breeding fast" or "breeds fast" on this inventory list (∗). Three others are noted to have either medical or chronic illness complaints (≠).

agricultural and industrial work and punishments associated with the workplace. The myth of the idyllic and classic Southern slave paradise dissipates within the realities of the lash, hangman's noose, and the axe.[65]

Because of the elimination of the Atlantic slave trade, U.S. dependency on its domestic slave trade to increase the slave population became absolute. Slave breeding became necessary to raise the number of slaves to expand the system westward. (See Figure 5.5.) All facets of women's health suffered. Overworked slave women were encouraged, if not coerced, to have excessive numbers of children. Some planters did not even alter the work schedules of pregnant slaves. Apologist scholars since the time of Ulrich Phillips have tried to deny that slave breeding took place, but the weight of the evidence and professional opinion has affirmed its existence. Slave women were encouraged, cajoled, and coerced by their owners to become pregnant. For not complying, some were whipped or sold. Some female slaves were purchased specifically for breeding. Women were often forced to engage in intercourse with strange men or males to whom they were not attracted. Some studies document that 4–8 percent of slave children were the products of intercourse (or legal rape) between masters and slaves—which also increased slave populations. The practice became more prominent during slavery's last days.

It is well documented that maternal mortality was much higher for Blacks than for Whites. This may be related to the heavy work burden imposed on African American slave women. Katz reminds us that women slaves were routinely expected to work as much as men:

> Women worked as hard as men, one recalling, "I had to do everything dey was to do on de outside. Work in de field, chop wood, hoe corn. . . . I have done everything on a farm what a man done 'cept cut wheat. I splits rails like a man, I drive the gin, what was run by two mules."[66]

Childbearing was always a risky undertaking for slave women. Numerous accounts document that women were forced to engage in heavy work until they delivered and were returned to the fields soon thereafter. Moreover, this risk was accentuated by the fact that slave women did not receive formal medical attention unless they were in extremis, in most cases, and/or were owned by exceptionally humane masters. Prenatally they were at risk, and parturition itself was dangerous. Postpartum they were often overworked and given inadequate time to recover or provide care for their newborns.

Another dimension of this reproductive health problem was the risks to which the unborn or recently born children were exposed. Slave women during the Antebellum Era, more than ever considered breeding machines, were often poorly fed. Very seldom were they given the supplementary dietary support pregnant and lactating women require. Most White women of the era could "self-select" their diets, rendering them adequate. For slave women this was impossible. Thus, slave women received the already inadequate slave diet relatively high in calories (4,000 to 6,000 calories) but low in niacin, riboflavin, vitamin A, thiamine, and sometimes iron and vitamin C. Calorie supplementation along with these and other essential nutrients are critical to pregnancy and lactation. Overwork and the lack of prenatal care translated into a high risk of both spontaneous abortions (pregnancy loss before viability) and low birth weight (caused by being born too early or not growing properly in the womb). These factors had tremendous impact on the fetal death rates, stillbirth rates, perinatal death rates, infant mortality rates, and childhood mortality rates. Improper handling of the umbilical cord by untrained slave midwives dramatically increased the incidence of neonatal tetanus in the slave quarters.

Slave infants were neglected routinely when their mothers were forced back to work immediately after their birth. There are many records documenting that this adversely affected the slave women's ability to adequately breastfeed. Many authorities document that childhood was a dangerous period for slave children. Not only was their nutrition compromised, but they were also exposed to many diseases in their immediate environments. Even in developed areas, most slave quarters had no basic sanitation. The surrounding environment near the cabins was utilized as a privy even when formal accommodations were available. Periodically, the wastes were raked up and added to the compost heap and eventually utilized as night soil or fertilizer. This usually occurred once or twice a year. Meanwhile, the slave children played in these areas, displaying regular childhood behavior, including hand-to-mouth contact. These children were at extremely high risk for contracting enteric diseases such as dysentery, typhoid fever, and hepatitis. They were also at risk for contracting worm diseases and infections from any stool-transmitted larvae. Slaves' astronomical child and infant mortality rates during the Antebellum Period reflect these facts.[67]

Although it is difficult to obtain quantitative data on Black health outcome before the Civil War, a few general conclusions can be reached based on some of the rare sources that are available. It does seem clear that the slave health deficit identified in previous periods of our nation's history continued, and worsened, during the Jacksonian and Antebellum periods. Some comparative racial mortality data were collected during the period from 1813 to 1860. Mortality, measured as the numbers of deaths in a population during a specified period, also reflects the standard of living and is in part determined by the availability of high-quality medical care, income, nutritional status, environmental quality, and cultural habits. These are the major variables that affected slave mortality in the Antebellum period and still affect Black mortality today. Therefore, studies of racial differences in mortality provide useful and important information on the determinants of mortality rates in historic populations. Utilizing the work of Ewbank and others we attempt to place the history of Black mortality into the context of the broader history of the decline in mortality in the United States.[68]

The first survey and tabulation of deaths by disease and race was taken by the U.S. Census Bureau in 1850. Ironically, it is extremely difficult to determine White antebellum mortality rates from available government data. Seemingly, some data is obtainable on the Black population from plantation records maintained on slaves. Experts such as Reynolds Farley and Walter Allen in *The Color Line and the Quality of Life in America* interpreted and compared national and regional mortality data on domestic Whites, Western European Whites, and all available data on Blacks and concluded, "Mortality conditions among blacks prior to the Civil War were worse than those of some western European nations and probably worse than those of American whites."[69] This corroborates findings by Ewbanks, who compared mortality trends between Blacks and Whites between 1800 and 1840 and found that for all the periods studied Black mortality rates were "substantially higher" than those for Whites. When Curry compared mortality rates between Blacks and Whites in four antebellum cities in *The Free Black in Urban America, 1800–1850*, he stated, "It appears almost certain that the death rate among urban blacks . . . was, with rare exceptions higher than for whites."[70] Savitt, who surveyed 1850 Virginia government census data comparing White, Black slave, and free Black mortality rates in *Medicine and Slavery*, found "a higher death rate for free blacks (140/10,000) than for Whites (111/10,000), though the rate for slaves remains the highest (178/10,000)"[71] (see Table 5.1). However, when Savitt evaluated the locally gathered county health data collected in Virginia between 1853 and

Table 5.1   Mortality Rates from Two Sources Compared, for White,
             Slave, and Free Black Virginians (per 10,000 of Each
             Group in Population)

Year	Whites	Slaves	Free Blacks
		Rural and Urban	
1850 [a]	111	178	140
1853 [b]	111	172	80
1855 [b]	105	151	71
1857 [b]	97	152	65
1858 [b]	95	146	65
		Urban	
1850 [a,c]	205	133	222
1853 [b,d]	120	80	87
1855 [b,e]	97	54	41
1857 [b,f]	121	109	112
1858 [b,g]	76	74	49
		Rural	
1850 [a,h]	106	180	127
1853 [b]	111	184	79
1855 [b]	106	156	76
1857 [b]	93	154	58
1858 [b]	93	150	70

[a] Calculated from mortality returns of Seventh Federal Census, 1850.

[b] Calculated from published tabulations of the State Auditor; not all cities or counties submitted returns.

[c] Alexandria, Norfolk, Richmond, Portsmouth, Petersburg.

[d] Fredericksburg, Lynchburg, Norfolk, Petersburg, Richmond, Staunton, Williamsburg.

[e] Danville, Fredericksburg, Lynchburg, Petersburg, Richmond, Staunton, Williamsburg, Winchester. Norfolk was excluded because excessive mortality during the yellow fever epidemic would have distorted the figures.

[f] Danville, Lynchburg, Norfolk, Petersburg, Richmond, Staunton, Williamsburg, Winchester.

[g] Danville, Fredericksburg, Lynchburg, Norfolk, Richmond, Staunton, Williamsburg, Winchester.

[h] Includes several urban areas which could not be isolated from the figures—e.g., Lynchburg, Fredericksburg, Danville, Winchester, Staunton, and Wheeling. Only Wheeling was attacked by cholera.

Source: Savitt, *Medicine and Slavery*, 140–141, Table 8, p. 141.

1858 comparing the three populations, he found the raw data and the results to be so poor as to be useless for reaching solid conclusions regarding comparative mortality. He did find it useful for delineating the prevalence and patterns of disease. Ewbanks found more reliable child mortality data covering the years 1786–1863. During that period he found that the range for child mortality in Black slave

Table 5.2   Estimates of Child Mortality, Life Expectancy at Age 10,
and Life Expectancy at Birth, U.S. Blacks, 1850–1940

| | | | Life Expectancy at Age 10 | | | | Life Expectancy at Birth |
| | | | Census Survival | | DRA Estimate | | |
	q(5)	From e(10)	Male	Female	Male	Female	
1850	280–320	37					
1880	264	39					35.5
			36	36			
1890	264	39					35.5
			40	42			
1900	264	39					36.5
			39	39			
1910	235–255	40					
			39	39			
1920	186	45					
1930	126				44.3	45.3	48.5
1940	90				48.3	50.8	53.8

Notes: The proportion of all live births that survive to their fifth birthday is generally termed q(5), expressed as numbers per 1,000. The index of Adult Mortality used as e(10) is the expectation of life at age 10 expressed in years.

Source: Eubank DC. Black mortality and health before 1940. *Health Policies and Black Americans*, Table 1, p. 105, Estimates of Child Mortality.

children was 280–320 per 1,000 live births. This was 42–56 percent higher than the White child mortality rates from other representative samples (see Table 5.2).

Another parameter most authorities have surveyed is longevity. Based on several studies, Black male longevity at birth during the Antebellum Period was approximately 30 years; females lived 32 years. Even for this historical period this was an extremely short lifespan. Clearly, using conservative estimates from available mortality data, antebellum Blacks lived at least five to eight years less than Whites based on the best estimates available. Moreover, Fogel and others noted a halt in a century-long decline in Black mortality during the 1810s and 1820s, after which it began to rise. Utilizing mortality data as a "gold standard" of health status, it is clear that antebellum Blacks suffered not only a slave health deficit during the period under study, but also a *decline* in health status and outcome.[72]

It is a basic principle of public health that social and economic progress are usually benchmarks associated with improvements in the health status for a given population. The plunge in Black health status during the Antebellum Period is, therefore, an enigma. It is likely that too little data exist to document exactly why

Black health status deteriorated during the late Antebellum Period. Nevertheless, as we examine the changing disease prevalences, altered medical-social practices, and changed environmental circumstances that altered the profile of the illnesses of slaves and possibly affected Black slave mortality during the Antebellum Period, examination of some contributing environmental health factors* seems indicated.

It was a standard practice that a different health system was provided for the slaves. The poorer health of free Blacks is often attributed to the fact that even the inferior resources and services provided by the slave health subsystem were denied them. Therefore, left on their own to deal with the mainstream system administratively and financially, they most often received no care at all. Other factors contributing to the higher incidence and prevalence of illnesses among African Americans were the stressful health and work environments to which they were exposed. Expansion of slavery into Western frontiers exaggerated the effects exerted by all of these factors. As has been pointed out, slaves had access to very few trained health providers. Because of the paucity of physicians in these areas generally, this automatically cut the access to medical care for slaves. Therefore, during the Antebellum Period slaves became more dependent on the informal, sometimes acknowledged, network of Black health workers. As Bousfield noted, "A knowledge of African herbs was probably an advance upon . . . medicine for quite some time."[73] Thus, in terms of efficacy, these untrained village healers, slave midwives, granny nurses, root doctors, and, occasionally, conjure men may not have been much more dangerous than the mainstream medical profession. Regular physicians were still closely tied to "heroic" therapies such as bleeding, purging, cupping, and depleting** until late in the nineteenth century. What may have been more important, and would certainly become a major medical outcome factor as regular medicine became more effective, was establishing the pattern, along with the expectation of and acceptance of, a different level of medical professional care and services for Blacks. The physical, psychological, and medical-social effects of this health policy on Black and disadvantaged minority health have not been totally overcome today. Resignation and acceptance of "difference" in health delivery between Blacks and Whites in the United States was established in the minds of the public and the medical establishment.[74]

Black health in the Antebellum Period was affected by a number of environmental health factors. Economic demands generated by huge increases of cotton

---

*According to Moeller, one way to view the health environment is from the *chemical, biological, physical,* and *socioeconomic* standpoints. The latter three, including food and water contamination, vector transmission of diseases, excessive heat and cold, nutritional adequacy, stressful social conditions, and access to medical services and care, are the principle foci here.

**Purging* is the use of cathartics to cause a free evacuation of the bowels. *Cupping* is the application of a small glass cup to the skin with a vacuum to cause slow bleeding. It was a popular early heroic medical therapy. *Depleting* is the removal of accumulated bodily fluids of solids through bleeding, purging, or vomiting. This was an old-fashioned heroic medical therapy.

production and the creation of the Cotton Kingdom were daunting. As a result of this changing socioeconomic environment, slave work schedules, especially in frontier areas, became even more pitiless and demanding. Slaves typically worked from first light until darkness fell. If there was a full moon, this could amount to 16–18 hours. As Loren Katz notes, one planter stated his slaves "work[ed] all night by the light of the full moon during some heavy periods."[75] Working slaves to exhaustion was not uncommon, and many contemporary biological anthropologists allege that slaves were literally worked to death. Slave punishments increased to coerce and enforce these brutal work schedules. Obviously, overexposure to the elements such as extremes of heat or cold under such circumstances increased the risk of heat exhaustion, heat stroke, or cold injury such as frostbite, trench foot, or immersion foot. Heat injuries could terminate in central nervous system damage, coma, or death, while cold injuries could result in gangrene, amputations, sepsis, or death. The quality of slave housing was variable. This was extremely important in those areas that did not experience tropical or semitropical climates. Most slaves lived in inadequately ventilated, poorly heated cabins. Most of these buildings had leaky roofs, holes around doors and windows, and dirt or clay floors, accounting for the high incidence of viral and bacterial respiratory conditions afflicting the slaves. If nutrition was compromised, the risks were increased. To combat the cold, especially in the upper South where snowy winters were common, slaves habitually built huge fires in the primitive fireplaces. The incidence of fires and their accompanying injuries and deaths was high. Compounding the health risks of this situation was cabin overcrowding, based on the standards printed in pro-slavery magazines such as *De Bow's Review*. According to several sources, the average slave cabin was some 15 square feet, housing an average of five to seven people. Therefore, contagious conditions such as Streptococcal respiratory infections or tuberculosis, transmitted by air droplets, spread throughout the slave quarters.

Closely related to the housing situation in a temperate climate was the quality and adequacy of clothing issued the slaves. Again this was variable, but based on the accounts available, the slaves were properly dressed only some of the time. This was due to the fact that the issue of two to three outfits per year presumed warm Southern winters by the planters and allowed little leeway for clothes washing. Many owners issued only one outfit annually. In many instances, as William Loren Katz writes in *Breaking the Chains*, "Clothing was a crude cloth outfit issued in the spring and another in the fall. Shoes were handed out once a year, a blanket every three years. Boys and girls younger than thirteen were not given clothing."[76] The discomfort and inadequacy of slave clothing extended to slave shoes, which were stiff, uncomfortable, and poorly made. In many instances a slave bed was a shelf or a few rags. Sometimes sleeping on the floor was required and mattresses were rare. As a result, most slaves suffered many uncomfortable days and nights, especially when harsh turns in winter or rainy weather occurred. Frontier conditions and migratory status made all components of a westward expanding slave system vulnerable to economic or climatic fluctuations, rendering even these conditions worse.

Another important environmental factor directly affecting Black health during the Antebellum Period was the lack of reliable logistical support. Food supplies, for example, were at risk in the unpredictable frontier environment. In many areas markets and transportation were not stable. Thus, harsh turns in the weather or economic downturns could have catastrophic effects on newly established plantations or farms. Once more, the dislocation and disorganization of the westward expansion of the slave system would have negated the progress of organization and civilization manifested by the established Southern slave system. This could be one explanation contributing to the downturn in Black health status, outcome, fertility, and longevity in the late Antebellum Period.[77]

Commercial factors combined with the exigencies of expanding the Black slave population independent of a legal Atlantic slave trade changed the profile of antebellum slavery's health agenda. Expansion of the Cotton Kingdom came at a heavy health cost. Some of the health consequences of these developments were related to the implementation of slave breeding, which became profitable and necessary. The fecundity of the Black population became a pivotal, if often unspoken, health policy issue and economic concern profoundly affecting female and child health. Growing insecurities of slaveholding areas along with increasing emphasis on commercial agriculture forged a militaristic, autocratic, social environment. This less humanistic, more dictatorial environment resulted in more injuries and permanently maimed casualties of the "war of terror" employed to protect slavery.[78]

Stewardship Denied: White Medicine in Jacksonian and Antebellum America

Paradoxically, the American medical profession, while gaining professional legitimacy based on advances in the biomedical sciences, was not granted the expanded social authority it expected and felt it deserved during this period. Early nineteenth-century medical advances were truly significant on a scientific level in lieu of their providing very little therapeutically. Many of these advances came from France, home of the new hospital movement and the focus of early nineteenth-century Western medical progress. Accompanying the restructuring of the French health system after the French Revolution, physicians questioned everything in the medical firmament, including classical medical theories. French physicians moved medical practice into hospitals and correlated disease syndromes with pathophysiology. Physicians such as Laennec created instruments with examining capabilities such as the stethoscope, and Louis statistically evaluated treatment regimens for their effectiveness. He documented that heroic therapy, upon which most Western medical therapeutics were grounded, was not only worthless but also could harm patients. American physicians who increasingly went to Paris for medical training in the first half of the nineteenth century brought back the new French scientific and quantitative approaches to medicine along with its scientifically based therapeutic nihilism. The fruits of these scientific medical advances would not become obvious until later in the century.[79]

Elite American physicians backed repeated efforts to regulate the practice of medicine through strict licensing laws and examinations by qualified peers. These efforts were thwarted by both politicians and public sentiment. However, at local and community levels physicians were growing in influence. In many ways these changes were subtle, with decision-making and policy determination made informally by community leaders and the elite public. Physicians, whether by "rights" of the profession or by qualifications, were automatically included in these deliberations. They were increasingly relied upon to determine public policy regarding public health and to structure the health system along scientifically sound lines. Covertly or overtly, decisions about health care or the community's health needs came to be determined by the physician class in virtually all communities. They also continued to be held responsible for the structural provision of health care services for the poor and underserved.[80]

Medical education was changing dramatically. Unfortunately, the infrastructure was out of control and proliferating in directions the profession often considered detrimental. Therefore, medical education reform became a top priority and a major component of medical professionalization. From the core of five university-based medical schools in 1810, proprietary medical schools began to proliferate at an alarming rate after the War of 1812. Some of these private proprietary institutions formed alliances with states and universities similar to the first such institution founded in Baltimore in 1807, which was affiliated with the University of Maryland; most would not. By 1850 there were 42 medical schools in the United States compared to three in all of France. By 1860 there were 47. These new schools only had two-year degree requirements, the terms lasting three to four months each year. Moreover, the second year was a repetition of the first—which increased their profitability considerably—until 1850. The expansion of the curriculum that occurred that year was considered a great reform. By mid-century, most U.S. medical schools, with virtually no entrance requirements, which encouraged large enrollments, and a financial interest in low standards and universal passage, had transformed into diploma mills. The deterioration of medical education standards in the United States had reached an alarming state. It expressed the medical profession's weakness and inability to overcome individual or small groups of physicians' advantages (plentiful medical student school fees, abundant licensure fees) for the greater overall good of the profession. Thus, in lieu of scientific medical advances pouring over from Europe, American medical school training continued to be viewed as supplementary to the apprenticeship system.

Despite these fundamental flaws and quality considerations in American medical schools, race and class considerations continued to remain exclusionary forces in American medical education. Blacks were systematically excluded from admission to even admittedly marginal medical educational institutions. James McCune Smith, an honor graduate of the African Free School in New York City who had so impressed Lafayette and other visiting European dignitaries in 1824 with his welcoming address and intelligence, was unable to gain entry to medical school in the United States. A similar state of exclusion also existed for women. However, by 1849, energized by the abolition and women's rights movements, Elizabeth Blackwell graduated from the Geneva Medical College in New York. However, Harriet Hunt, arguably the most successful early woman physician, was unjustly dismissed from the Harvard Medical School after initially being accepted in 1850. The era set a tone indicating that mainstream medicine in America was to be a White, upper-class, male-dominated profession with almost insurmountable barriers blocking the participation of African Americans and women.[81]

The proprietary expansion of the medical education system tended to lower medical educational standards and prolong the utility of the apprentice training system. As a result of the early rejection of the European approach to medicine, with its universities and scientific societies facilitating and promoting debates and discussions of intricate theoretical medical systems such as "vitalism," "iatro-chemistry," and "iatrophysics," American medicine acquired a unique character. The non-European flavor of U.S. medicine began manifesting itself, as Rosemary Stevens observed:

> *American attitudes to treatment, closely linked with botanical explo-ration in the New World, developed a strong emphasis on natural his-tory, and on conservative common sense. . . . [P]ride in the relative practicality of American medicine long outlasted the period of depen-dence on European theory.*[82]

The downside of this approach, as Stevens further observed, led to "the often unproductive insularity of American medical science in the eighteenth and nine-teenth centuries."[83] The most lasting effect would be the rise and persistent influ-ence of medical sects, natural remedies, and unconventional therapies in the United States. It would take the deficiencies in the medical system revealed by the stresses of the Civil War to shock both the public and the profession out of their torpor. Moreover, by the Civil War, regular physicians had abandoned most of the heroic therapies that U.S. patients feared and derided. Both the public and the profession began to sense, if not realize, that massive reform of the medical education system and the nation's health delivery system was needed to ensure the country's seemingly predestined place as a world power.[84]

Appropriately, the leaders of the profession persisted in their efforts to regularize and standardize American medicine. Energy for professionalization was generated largely as the result of a privileged U.S. medical elite's attendance at European medical schools. Consciously or unconsciously these men wanted to emulate and imitate the British and continental systems. Beginning with eighteenth-century efforts to pass medical licensing laws, organize medical societies, and open medical schools based on European models, American physicians adopted practices that would encourage the advance of medical science and the public health while implementing a code of ethics and acceptable behavior that would elevate the profession in the public's eyes. The net effect of these policies tended to gentrify the medical profession. Most of their successes resulted in their organization into state and national medical societies. Very little was accomplished in the legislative or regulatory arenas. As Rosemary Stevens observed, "After 1825, attacks on elitism at all levels of American society—and in all professional fields—led to demands for repeal of licensing laws and to the withdrawal of state recognition from medical societies. . . . [O]pen competition was the essence of Jacksonian politics."[85] All of these trends—socially elite measures from the profession itself and racially restrictive laws and regulations from Jacksonian and antebellum politicians—imposed drastic race, gender, and class restrictions on medical education and medical practice. Adverse effects imposed on women and minorities were ignored by the profession. However, their efforts did not go unnoticed by the public or their political representatives. Jackson's Age of the Common Man seemingly applied only in a White man's country, and organized medicine's professionalization efforts were openly criticized and rejected by most politicians and the public alike.[86]

The major breakthrough in the professionalization of the American medical profession during the Antebellum Period was the establishment of a national and influential medical association, the American Medical Association (AMA). As Haller noted in *American Medicine in Transition, 1840–1910* regarding the initial calls for the formation of a professional organization, "The initial calls for such an organization came not just from individuals but from colleges and medical societies concerned with the erosion of the physician's economic and social status."[87] The eighteenth century's pleas for action from a tiny core of elite, largely European-trained physicians concentrated in a few Eastern seaboard cities was joined in the nineteenth century by a chorus of concerned parties. However, the evolution of the organization of the American profession would differ significantly from the European profession's organizing principles, which were founded on stratification of the profession between formally trained and folk medical traditions; royal, religious, and aristocratic support of professional medicine; and traditional university-based training and regulation of medical practice. The AMA evolution embodied, as Haller observed, the typical clash, conflict, and contradiction of American institutions in that it "evolved through a process that was democratic in design, national in authority, and elitist in practice—much in keeping with many other developmental aspects of American society."[88] The strategy for controlling and then correcting the erosion in authority of organized American medicine was embodied in medical education reform, professional standardization, and medical licensing laws. The AMA would not accomplish all these ambitious goals until well into the twentieth century.[89]

The first substantial steps leading to the formation of a national medical association began early in the second quarter of the nineteenth century when the Vermont and New Hampshire medical societies convened a meeting of delegates from New England and New York to discuss medical educational problems in 1827. Concerns were also expressed by several colleges and physician groups in the 1830s. Because of abuses by teaching institutions, formal resolutions calling for the separation of the teaching and licensing of physicians from the Medical Society of the State of New York surfaced by 1845. Organizations of New Hampshire and Ohio physicians had also been formed. These variegated activities culminated in a meeting in May 1846 at the University of the State of New York. One hundred nineteen delegates from as far away as Louisiana attended. A consensus was growing that a national organization was needed to effectively address these serious educational, licensing, and standard setting issues. A meeting of some 250 delegates, many of whom had participated in the 1845 New York meeting, established the AMA in the hall of the Academy of Natural Sciences on May 5, 1847. The association would embark on the following mission:

> for cultivating and advancing medical knowledge; for elevating the standard of medical education; for promoting the usefulness, honor, and interests of the medical profession; or enlightening and directing public opinion in regard to the duties, responsibilities, and requirements of medical men; for exciting and encouraging emulation and concert of action in the profession; and for facilitating and fostering friendly intercourse between those engaged in it.[90]

This mission had little to do with improvement of the general status or outcomes of the public's health or with progressive medical-social policies to improve the profession's or the health system's race, class, and gender problems. (See Figure 5.6.) Instead, the AMA was concerned with social elevation and with increasing the power, exclusivity, and prestige of members of the medical profession. In many ways this mission resembled that of a guild or a union rather than a profession. A policy of encouraging the formation of local and state medical associations and consensus agreements on licensure policy was incorporated. Committees were established regarding problems surrounding the medical sciences, practical medicine, surgery, obstetrics, medical education, medical literature, and publications. Resolutions were aimed at abolishing quackery and nostrums; at the prevention of sectional dominance, including outlawing holding two consecutive meetings in one city; and at developing the groundwork for the

Figure 5.6   General Lecture Room, Women's Medical College of the New York Infirmary, c. 1870

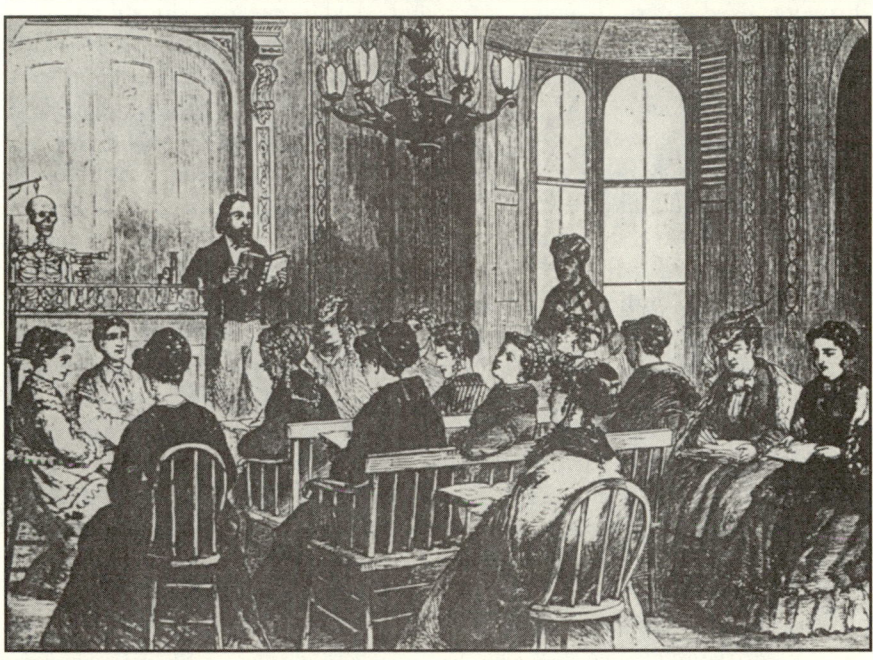

The founding of women's medical colleges was an offshoot of restrictive laws and regulations regarding race and gender in the medical profession passed down from the Jacksonian and Antebellum eras. Rebecca Cole, staff physician and second African American female medical school graduate (1867 graduate of Women's Medical College of Pennsylvania), stands near the window.

development of the *Association's Principles of Medical Ethics*. The strains of elitism, racism, and sexism that characterized the professionalization movement from its beginnings were not checked or corrected. By not addressing them their effects may have been enhanced. These problems would persist well into the late twentieth century.[91]

Medical professionalization, with the exception of medical licensing—probably because it had a minimal social component and was largely based on open examination—would remain racially segregated or profoundly discriminatory toward African Americans until the late twentieth century. During this era, Black and women physicians meeting the objective criteria of earning medical licenses remained professionally ostracized and isolated and continued to be the victims of covert and overt professional discrimination. Furthermore, none of these professional activities would prevent the decline of the quality of the medical profession in the middle of the nineteenth century until substantive regulation and reform took place after the Civil War. The decline of the apprenticeship system and the rise of abbreviated proprietary medical school courses as a substitute for legitimate training ensured medicine's poor performance and image. As competition between medical schools intensified in the Antebellum Period, courses tended to shorten, admission requirements declined, and tuition fees decreased. Schools that raised their admission or graduation standards suffered because of perverse competition. Medical school graduates would continue to fail Army and Navy Boards of Examiner for Surgeons standardized examinations for medical competence at rates of 50–75 percent. The progressive rot of the American medical professional and educational infrastructure continued until after the Civil War, which revealed the lack of preparedness, incompetence, and inconsistencies within the American medical profession. Obtaining competent surgeons to staff the Union Army's Medical Corps proved difficult with the astronomical competency examination failure rates. This development helped the AMA and the medical profession make their case and finally convince the American public that the time had come for educational reform.[92]

As Paul Starr observed about U.S. social conditions relative to professions at that time, if America was to have an aristocratic medical profession in the nineteenth century, it "would have required aristocratic patronage and legal protection; the social and political basis of the British and other European professional system did not exist in America."[93] American attitudes toward democracy and opportunity were antithetical to European concepts of medical professionalization in many ways. For White Americans many of these rules, regulations, and requirements would block "poor boys" from entering the medical profession. Moreover, they could potentially handicap the practices of the irregular practitioners such as midwives, bone doctors, Indian doctors, slave doctors, root doctors, and other healers who provided the bulk of the care in a frontier-oriented America. This was an extension of the colonial practice of labeling virtually any White person as "doctor" who engaged in any phase of the healing process. Even a few slave practitioners were given the title, more as a nickname, acknowledging their medical skills. Any rigid approach to medical practice with different levels of training, different titles, and assigned roles reminiscent of European systems would serve to limit the numbers of practitioners. Such actions threatened to adversely impact access to medical care, it was felt, and would also decrease the commerce in medical school tuition fees and fees generated by licensing. The medical profession had not acquired the necessary authority through society's dependency and earned legitimization to dominate American health as it wished. It would require a cultural transformation based upon the deification of science, which occurred by the second quarter of the twentieth century, before medicine would be placed upon its desired pedestal—sacrosanct and unquestioned.[94]

Aside from the inconsistencies bred by the U.S. "blind spot" relative to the accepted practice of class and race discrimination and egalitarian rhetoric and ideology, the heroic approaches to therapy practiced by regular physicians rankled American patients. Some of the sectarian approaches to medical theory and practice were contrary to classical medical theoretical systems and were also more naturalistic. Such approaches, along with self-help and naturalistic cures like hydrotherapy, appealed to the individualistic and naturalistic streaks so prominent in the American character. Popular nineteenth-century medical sects such as the Thomosonians and the eclectics emphasized botanical and herbal rather than mineral and chemical cures. They also decried the regular profession's reliance on heroic therapies based on bleeding and purging often to the point of the patient's clinical collapse. Therefore, some of the conflicts between the medical sects and the regular profession actually produced some positive effects by decreasing what would prove to be clinically dangerous and scientifically ineffective therapies.[95]

The medical profession was very cognizant of, and paranoid about, their situation. Aware of nineteenth-century scientific medical progress, the American profession was self-conscious of the public's lack of respect and their limited authority. Seemingly, in exchange for popularity and acceptance, physicians intensified their efforts to supply biological justifications for social and racial hierarchies. This was especially true regarding Blacks and Indians. In a democratic republic grounded in an egalitarian ideology, Black chattel slavery and Native American genocide had to rankle psychologically; therefore, some type of popular justification fulfilled society's psychic and moral needs. The abolitionist movement, women's rights movement, and defenses and protests against Indian atrocities are evidence that exposure of such ideological conflicts had the power to disturb and, even occasionally, transform. With the growth of the "American school of anthropology," which emanated from institutions such as the University of Pennsylvania and Harvard, the biomedical sciences increasingly "explained" Black, Native American, and female inferiority. In effect, the Great Chain of Being theory was justified again—this time on what appeared to be a quantitative basis.[96]

Leading U.S. academic physicians such as Samuel George Morton of the University of Pennsylvania; Louis Agassiz of Harvard University; Samuel Cartwright, graduate of the University of Pennsylvania School of Medicine; and Paris-trained Josiah Clark Nott, graduate of the University of Pennsylvania School of Medicine and faculty member of Louisiana Medical School in New Orleans, attempted to document non-White racial inferiority biologically. They dominated the fields of anthropology, ethnology, racial typology, and physiognomy internationally from the 1830s until Darwin published *The Origin of Species* in 1859. The American school of anthropology alleged, based on numerical documentary evidence of cranial measurements and skull configurations* along with other bodily dimensions, that Native Americans, South American

---

*The most influential set of craniometric data produced by Samuel George Morton could not be reproduced by Stephen J. Gould utilizing the same materials and methods. See Gould, *The Mismeasure of Man* (New York: W. W. Norton, 1981).

Indians, Blacks, and other non-European races were intellectually and culturally inferior. The basis of this inferiority was stated to be biologically predetermined and, according to the investigators, thus demonstrated separate origins of the various races of mankind (polygeny). This work undergirded and served as part of the theoretical basis for craniometry, the most influential numerical science of biological determinism during the nineteenth century. Craniometry was as important in this regard for the nineteenth century as IQ testing is for the twentieth. It also reinvigorated phrenology, which by 1850 was being discredited as a legitimate science.[97]

Louis Agassiz (1807–1873) a Swiss-born, German-trained physician, naturalist, and glaciologist, was considered the theoretician of the American school of anthropology. After beginning a fruitful academic career in Europe as Cuvier's protege, he became a major nineteenth-century Harvard biologist after moving to the United States in 1847. His presence elevated the status of American natural history and biology. Agassiz had never seen a Black person before his 1846 visit to America. He was shocked by the appearance of African Americans while visiting Philadelphia. This triggered what Gould calls "a pronounced visceral revulsion" in Agassiz.[98] This abhorrence, combined with his sexual fantasies surrounding miscegenation, caused him to immediately classify Blacks as a separate, subhuman, species. He spent a significant part of his career conducting pseudoscientific research to justify these subjective opinions. He wrote treatises and tracts speculating scientifically about origins of separate human species:

> These races must have originated . . . in the same numerical proportions, and over the same area, in which they now occur. . . . [T]hey cannot have originated in single individuals, but must have been created in that numeric harmony which is characteristic of each species; men must have originated in nations, as the bees have originated in swarms.[99]

After casting his racial arguments in scientific terms, Agassiz typically reverted to standard Caucasian cultural stereotypes to "prove" innate racial differences:

> The indomitable, courageous, proud Indian—in how very different a light he stands by the side of the submissive, obsequious, imitative negro, or by the side of the tricky, cunning, and cowardly Mongolian! Are not these facts indications that the different races do not rank upon one level in nature.[100]

However, taking pains to ensure that Blacks occupied the bottom rung of his "objective" ladder, he stated:

> It seems to us to be mock-philanthropy and mock-philosophy to assume that all races have the same abilities, enjoy the same powers, and show

the same natural dispositions, and that in consequences of this equality they are entitled to the same position in human society. History speaks here for itself. . . . [T]his compact continent of Africa exhibits a population which has been in constant intercourse with the white race, which has enjoyed the benefit of the example of the Egyptian civilization, of the Phoenician civilization, of the Roman civilization, of the Arab civilization . . . and nevertheless there has never been a regulated society of black men developed on the continent. Does not this indicate in this race a peculiar apathy, a peculiar indifference to the advantages afforded by civilized society?[101]

He clung to his beliefs about Black and non-White inferiority and biological "difference" and separateness even when polygeny had fallen prey to the scientific progress embodied in Darwinian evolution. Time and science passed him by. Gould writes, "Agassiz's world collapsed during the last decade of his life. His students rebelled; his supporters defected. He remained a hero to the public, but scientists began to regard him as a rigid and aging dogmatist, standing firm in his antiquated beliefs before the Darwinian tide."[102] It is unknown whether his advice to Lincoln's Inquiry Commission (1863) led by H. G. Howe* on the role of Blacks in a reconstituted nation (wherein Agassiz recommended racial segregation and separate development) was followed. He served as the theorist of polygeny within the American school of anthropology until his death in 1873.[103]

Agassiz collaborated with Samuel George Morton (1799–1851), internationally famous University of Pennsylvania Medical School graduate (1820) and faculty member and president of the Academy of Science. Utilizing his European training in statistics and phrenology along with his exalted medical school appointment, Morton served as the empiricist of the American school of anthropology. By 1830 he had collected, classified, and measured hundreds of human skulls, creating a racial classification in the process. Based on his elaborate skull volume and physical measurements, he graded the races' inherent intelligence and cultural potential—with Whites being superior, Indians intermediate, and Blacks on the bottom. He became the world's leading nineteenth-century empiricist of polygenesis and White racial superiority, the father of American physical anthropology, and author of *Crania Americana*. When this work was published in 1839 it was considered the world's primary ethnological-scientific reference "documenting" Indian, Black, and non-White inferiority. His later work, *Crania Aegyptica*, published in 1844, reinforced and buttressed the "scientific" basis for Black inferiority, alleging the Egyptian experience proved Blacks had not progressed in over three millennia and were predestined for slavery. It is documented that these false theories and princi-

---

*H. G. Howe is best known for his work on prison reform and education for the blind. His wife, Julia Ward Howe, wrote the "Battle Hymn of the Republic."

ples on racial inferiority, along with their numerical "justifications," were taught in U.S. universities and medical schools as part of the curriculum by men such as Morton, Agassiz, Josiah Clark Nott, Samuel Gliddon, George Combe, and Samuel Cartwright. This was a continuation of the American medical professional tradition established by Benjamin Rush, James Augustine Smith, and Charles Caldwell. All of these physicians and scientists helped codify, publicize, and translate these pseudo-scientific findings into components of the Black slavery and Native American public policy debates. The influence of these so-called scientific writings and didactic lectures in the nation's medical schools, academic institutions, and legislative councils cannot be underestimated. Public opinion, politics, and popular U.S. philosophy and ideology were also affected. It promoted and promulgated racism within the medical profession and American society that continues even today, at the dawn of the twenty-first century.[104]

Another active and nationally prominent physician participant in the American school of anthropology was Josiah Clark Nott (1804–1873), one of the most highly respected American physicians of the nineteenth century. After receiving an M.D. from the University of Pennsylvania's School of Medicine, America's top medical school of the period, Nott went to France for further study, as many well-to-do Americans serious about their medical training did at that time. Nott then returned South to Mobile, Alabama, to become one of the South's best-trained, most influential physicians. He became heavily involved in the slave system, opening a private slave hospital, owning slaves, and becoming one of the system's most able scientific defenders of the system. Nott unashamedly mixed his science with politics, designating his scientific defenses of slavery based on Black racial inferiority as "niggerology." Before the Civil War, Nott was granted a full professorship at the University of Louisiana Medical School at New Orleans.[105]

Perhaps the best known of the early nineteenth-century physician-scientists to influence the social issues surrounding the problem of race in pre–Civil War America was Samuel Adolphus Cartwright (1793–1863). His effectiveness was enhanced significantly by the fact that he was not only a knowledgeable physician, but also a pro-slavery propagandist. Cartwright spoke and wrote prolifically to a national cross-section of audiences. A nationally famous American physician-scientist born in Fairfax County, Virginia, he was a University of Pennsylvania Medical School graduate who practiced in Natchez, Mississippi, and in Louisiana. Cartwright was nationally recognized as a medical authority, ethnologist, and racial theorist. He theorized not only that Blacks were inferior, but also that they should be managed differently from a medical standpoint because of their nonhuman biological peculiarities. Heavily published in the scientific, medical, and popular press, writing on topics related to his racial theories and research, Cartwright and other pro-slavery and Southern physicians and scientists created elaborate theoretical systems to justify Black and Southern "difference," resulting in the creation of a lexicon of Negro diseases and physiological

Table 5.3   Antebellum Era Lexicon of "Negro Diseases"

Part 1

- Drapetomania . . . "the disease causing Negroes to run away"
- Typhoid pneumonia . . . "a severe form of pneumonia peculiar to Negroes"
- Cachexia Africana . . . "dirt eating" . . . Rx—wire masks or iron gags
- Struma Africana . . . "the Negro consumption"

Part 2

- Dyasthesia Aethiopis . . . "known to overseers as rascality"
- Chronic Leprosy . . . "accounts for dark color, big lips, flat nose, and wooly hair"
- Negro Consumption . . . "a severe pulmonary disease afflicting Blacks"
- Furor Sexualis . . . "Black men's resembled sexual attacks like bulls and elephants in intensity . . . the price . . . syphilis"

Source: Byrd WM, Clayton LA, *Documentary Report: Negro Diseases and Physiological Peculiarities.* Cancer Control Research Unit: Meharry Medical College, Nashville, Tennessee, 1990, unpublished data.

Table 5.4   Antebellum Era Lexicon of "Negro Physiological Peculiarities"

- " . . . deficiency of red blood in the pulmonary and arterial systems"
- Referring to Black's skin and body: " . . . 'shade of pervading darkness' throughout the skin and bone"; "black to the bone"
- " . . . defective atmospherization or arterialization of the blood in the lungs . . . seat . . . of Negro consumption"

Source: Byrd WM, Clayton LA, Documentary Report: Negro Diseases and Physiological Peculiarities, Cancer Control Research Unit: Meharry Medical College, Nashville, Tennessee, 1990, unpublished data.

peculiarities. (See Tables 5.3–5.4.) They also campaigned tirelessly for the establishment of separate and different Southern medical schools to provide a unique, Southern-oriented medical education. None of this withstood scientific scrutiny, and it appears ludicrous now. However, Cartwright's lexicon is an important reflection of the scientific community's rationales for the practices and policies conducted and implemented against Black people during the Jacksonian and Antebellum periods. There is no better example in history proving that science is an imperfect human endeavor strongly influenced by the society and culture in which it is submerged. The Jacksonian and Antebellum periods aptly demonstrate that science is laden with the values of its practitioners. It also serves as an important background for tracing and understanding the roots of the race and class problems plaguing the U.S. health system today.[106]

These antebellum developments simply reinforced the earlier corpus of Black racial inferiority pseudoscience that had been transmitted from Europe and incorporated into medical school curriculums by prominent academic physicians such as John Augustine Smith (1782–?) and Charles Caldwell (1772–1853), who appeared in the previous period. Significantly, Smith and Caldwell emerged to become nationally renowned medical and liberal arts college presidents, medical educators, and founders of several of the nation's medical schools during the Jacksonian Period. Smith subsequently became president of both William and Mary College and the College of Physicians and Surgeons of the University of New York. Caldwell was a professor of natural history at the University of Pennsylvania, where he received his medical training, and subsequently founded medical schools in Kentucky at Transylvania (1817) and the University of Louisville (1837).

The fact that racist material had entered highly respected and popular standard American medical school textbooks before 1850 is also extremely significant. (See Table 5.5.) Dr. Robley Dunglison's *Human Physiology with Three Hundred and Sixty-Eight Illustrations*, a popular and authoritative physiology textbook already in its sixth edition by 1846, cites physician-scientists Samuel George Morton, Johann Frederick Blumenbach, and Benjamin Rush as references in the section titled "Of the Varieties of Mankind." Some of Dunglison's textbook conclusions are highly derogatory toward Blacks, stating that compared to Whites, "This race is evidently of a less perfect organization than the last, and has some characteristics, which approximate it more to the monkey kind."[107] It was well known that Oliver Wendell Holmes, dean of Harvard's Medical School from 1847 to 1853, promoted and believed in the scientific value of the work of biomedical scientists such as Morton, Dunglison, and

Table 5.5   Table on Race Mixing from Dunglison's 1841 Physiology Textbook

Parents	Offspring	Degree of Mixture
Negro and white,	mulatto,	1/2 white 1/2 black.
White and mulatto,	terceron,	3/4 — 1/4 —
Negro and mulatto,	griffo or zambo, or black terceron,	1/4 — 3/4 —
White and terceron,	quarteron,	7/8 — 1/8 —
Negro and terceron,	black quarteron,	1/8 — 7/8 —
White and quarteron,	quinteron,	15/16 — 1/16 —
Negro and quarteron,	black quinteron,	1/16 — 15/16 —

A discussion on race mixing and racial "hybridization" included this table on the intricate systems of race mixing then being practiced. "As a general rule, the offspring of different races has an intermediate tint between that of the parents." Dunglison emphasized these systems were most common in countries "where negroes are common." There were numerous theories on the biological and physiological consequences of race mixing. Most of them were considered bad.

Agassiz, whose work pseudoscientifically documented non-White inferiority. As Takaki writes in *Iron Cages*, "Dr. Morton's *Crania Americana* which contained the Philadelphia physician's findings on the differential cranial capacities of whites and blacks, was in the private libraries of Harvard medical professors."[108] Takaki continues:

> *Dean Holmes had such a high regard for the writings of Dr. Morton that he considered Morton's research "permanent data for all future students of Ethnology. . . ." Thus, for Harvard students, black men might have had strong bodies, but mind or intelligence was a monopoly of the white race, especially males of that race.*[109]

The unjustified expulsion of Black and female students from Harvard Medical School in 1850 reaffirmed the race- and gender-exclusive attitudes of the medical school faculty, led by nationally renowned physicians such as Holmes, John Ware, and John Jacob Bigelow. More significant is the fact that Harvard represented American medicine's apogee. Any physician of this period graduating from an American medical school with an open mind and healthy attitude toward Blacks, or Native Americans for that matter, after exposure to such curricula and faculty attitudes would have to be exceptional indeed.[110]

American medicine became and remains one of the most rigidly segregated professions. The period between 1813 and the Civil War is very important in that organized medicine began defining itself as a profession during this time. It also began crystallizing its relationships with Blacks and women in the profession. The era associated with the founding of the AMA in 1847 can be viewed as a sociocultural watershed for the United States and for an emerging medical profession.

The Health Professions' Color and Gender Lines

Some of American medicine's major steps toward professionalization took place in the decades before the Civil War. Systematically excluded from the medical-professional mainstream based on access to training, social status, and professional authority, the institutionalized pattern of African American and gender marginalization, discrimination, and exclusion in medicine became entrenched. Factors that affected the status of Blacks and women in the profession were some of the same social and cultural factors defining multiracial relations in Jacksonian America. As Tocqueville noted in *Democracy in America* and as Takaki expounded:

> *During the age of Jackson, blacks were not regarded as "sons of nature" or the subjects of "melancholy reflections"; nor were they "obstacles"*

which had to be removed beyond the Mississippi River or destroyed. Rather, blacks lived in the settled areas of the United States, within white civilization, in physical proximity to whites. As workers, blacks possessed the labor slaveholders appropriated in order to cultivate the "vacant lands" they had taken from Indians and to produce surplus for the market. Thus, blacks had a unique future in America: Unlike Indians, they were not to be expelled but to be even more securely chained to white society and its political economy....."Free" in the North and enslaved in the South, blacks had different regional relationships to the process of production.[111]

In response to increasing social pressures and change-producing anxieties bred by ongoing market and technological revolutions, Blacks were branded as "children" and "savages." These actions purportedly justified White policies and practices and defined a racial hierarchy comforting to a dominant White culture. However, as Takaki writes, economic factors reinforced and speeded up these developments: "As the economy of the Market Revolution became dependent on black labor, as the southern planter class escalated its defense of slavery, and as industrial cities and a white proletariat developed in America, the racial ideology of the black 'child/savage' served both caste and class functions in an increasingly complex way in the North as well as the South."[112] One must be reminded that this was an era of nationwide racial lynchings, race riots throughout the North and Midwest, and increasing *de facto* segregation in all non-slaveholding areas. A primary reason White working-class people increasingly opposed the extension of slavery in the 1840s and 1850s was fear of its competitive effects on free White labor and economic opportunity. Their self-interested and self-centered approach to restricting expansion of slavery dovetailed with the Abolitionist Movement, which gained full steam by the 1830s. Meanwhile, as Blacks were enslaved and segregated, White women were restricted in a narrow role of domesticity and dependency on male providers. Professionalization was defined in terms of White male exclusivity. The nation was caught in a web of cultural mythology involving race and gender that defined the American transformation from an egalitarian-driven republic of the late eighteenth century to a market and technological revolution–driven nineteenth-century culture based on Indian extermination, the exploitation of Black labor, and the new race and gender roles this process produced.[113]

During the second quarter of the nineteenth century, a tiny, trained Black physician class emerged for the first time. The time had come for redefining relationships between Blacks and Whites practicing medicine in the United States. For the first time formally trained Black physicians with medical degrees and first-rate training were reviewed from a professional standpoint. A similarly endowed group of women physicians also emerged. These developments were diametrically opposed to, and were sure to generate conflicts with, the racial and gender relationships carved out in American society during this period.

Many of the professional disparities reflect the poor educational back-grounds of Black and female applicants. However, the disparities related to more than training and credentialing. When these were not factors, the color line was drawn, as exemplified by James McCune Smith, a Black man who, as mentioned earlier, was an early nineteenth-century honor student at the renowned African Free School of New York City. Smith, who was denied admission in his own country, went overseas to the University of Glasgow for his medical training. The American medical education system, which was consistent with American politi-cal and social systems generally, had traditionally excluded groups based on race (Blacks, Native Americans, Hispanics), gender (women), and religious affiliation (Jews). Therefore, the only leveling factors allowing disadvantaged or so-called undesirable groups into the medical and other health professions were the pro-prietary schools, the rising medical sects,* and the inability of White organized medicine to prevent informally trained physicians and healers from practicing. Black practitioners created by the slave health subsystem represented one aspect of a paradoxical opportunity borne of failed regulation, combined with strong economic incentives for slave owners who saved money while caring for their chattel.[114]

The emergence of this "new Negro" on the medical scene between 1813 and the Civil War raised an entirely new set of issues. This handful of Blacks, mostly from privileged free African American backgrounds, possessed the requi-site education and training to enter the legitimate medical profession based on merit. It is documented that some of them, such as Smith and John Van Surly de Grasse, possessed skills far superior to many of their White peers. Whether they would be admitted into medical societies, permitted to practice in the few hospi-tals then in existence, or accepted as colleagues and peers professionally and aca-demically were now legitimate questions. The standards of professional and social relations outlined in the AMA's constitution and Percival's code of medical ethics did not mention race. Moreover, Percival's code was foreign to the Ameri-can social fabric. Would a race of people, the overwhelmingly majority of whom were designated legally as slaves, who were increasingly cast as socially and bio-logically inferior, be allowed full participation in the formally defined social intercourse necessary to function within the medical profession? Professional clashes and confrontations following the Civil War would provide the answers. Unfortunately, they would take an almost universally negative turn.[115]

This tiny handful of professionally trained individuals in no way substituted for, nor represented, the huge numbers of Black healers providing hands-on care for the Black communities in the urban North and in the slave health subsystem from 1813 until the beginning of the Civil War. However, their conflicts and

---

*Medical sects such as the Thomsonians, Eclectics, and Homeopaths, who opened medical schools during this period, had more liberal admission policies, allowing occasional Blacks and women access to health professions training.

occasional clashes with the medical professional system acknowledge and highlight the tiny number of privileged slaves and minuscule numbers of free Blacks, concentrated in the Northeastern and border states, who channeled their talents into the medical profession. Considering their social circumstance and educational handicaps, as Midian O. Bousfield stated in his article about Black physicians in the *Bulletin of the History of Medicine*, "It is astonishing that Negro doctors should have practiced medicine before the Civil War."[116]

As previously noted, the first African American to have a formal medical education in the United States was James McCune Smith (1811–1865). (See Figure 5.7.) Born of a free mother in 1811 in New York City, Smith's father, an ex-slave, was a successful merchant. Young James received his primary education at the New African Free School on Mulberry Street, which had been established by the New York Manumission Society in 1787. As early as age 11, Smith obtained notoriety by delivering the welcoming address when General Lafayette visited the school in 1824. Lafayette's visit was a manifestation of his advocacy of educating Negro youth for productive citizenship. Nevertheless, after being denied admission to institutions of higher learning in his own country, Smith entered the University of Glasgow in 1832. While there he earned the B.A. degree in 1835, the M.A. degree in 1836, and the M.D. degree in 1837. He immediately returned to New York, engaged in an extremely successful medical practice, and opened two highly regarded apothecary shops. Smith was extremely successful financially and professionally and established a traditional pattern for Black physicians that Bousfield describes: "He set a pattern generally followed by colored doctors ever since: he became a leader of his people, and was an ardent abolitionist."[117] Historians and social scientists such as Carter G. Woodson, Leslie Falk, Edward H. Beardsley, Dennis Dickerson, W. Montague Cobb, and the authors have traced these traits and tendencies in Black physicians into the late twentieth century.

As a result of his extra-medical activities, Smith's social significance far outweighed his formidable clinical contributions. This is not to say that his large and busy practice was unimportant to him or his patients. Smith became a nationally respected abolitionist, scientist, speaker, writer, and political organizer. His contributions do not end there. The impact he had on the social and political world of his time will be forever etched in the history of the world at large. One example of Smith's medical professional contributions is the first formal "Letter to the Editor" submitted to a U.S. medical journal by an African American (*The Annalist* in 1874). More significant was the fact the submission was based on his assessment of a previous statistical analysis he disagreed with. Smith had proven his mastery of the new field of statistics with his 1844 "Memorial to the U.S. Senate," refuting the racist use of the fraudulent U.S. census by the Secretary of State, John C. Calhoun. More significantly, within less than a decade of his return from Europe, Dr. Smith was acknowledged as the most able defender of the Negro people against racial inferiority myths. He proved this by soundly defeating John C. Calhoun—a confirmed racist and defender of Black slavery who had received

Figure 5.7   Black physician: James McCune Smith, M.D. (1811–1865)

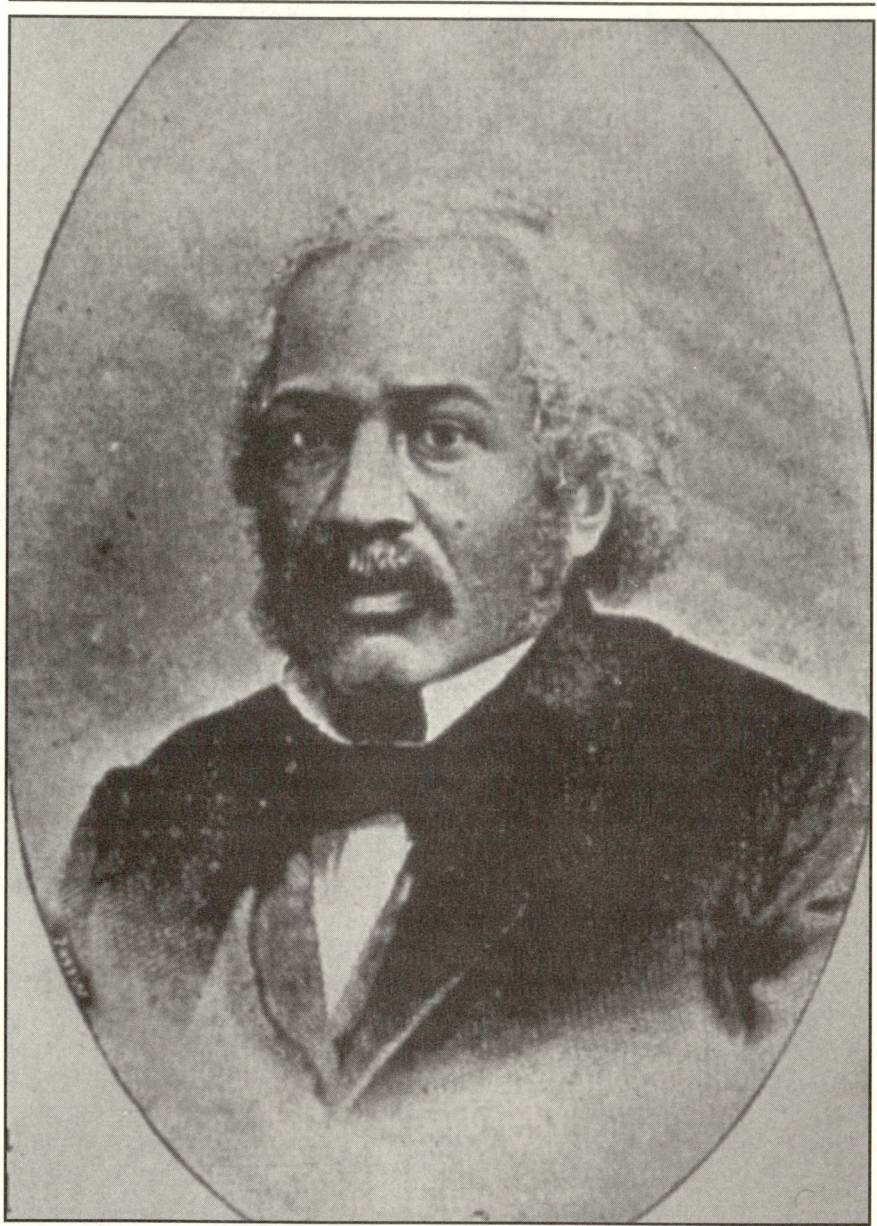

Smith was the first African American to earn a formal medical degree from the University of Glasgow, Scotland, in 1837. This is an engraving of abolitionist Smith. He was born in New York, NY, and was an honor graduate of the African Free School.

prior medical training himself—in public debates in Brooklyn in 1843. He also published several scientific works in the medical and scientific literature. His professional and statistical expertise was so well established and acknowledged by 1852 that he was invited as a founding member of the New York Statistics Institute. By then Smith's career was dominated by his work for the Negro people in abolitionist and anti-slavery political activities. Before his death in 1865, he had given up the practice of medicine.[118]

While Smith emerged as one of the singular national representatives and leaders of the African American population, David John Peck became the first African American to earn an M.D. degree from a U.S. medical school. A native of Pittsburgh, Pennsylvania, he was a protege of Martin Robison Delany who practiced medicine and was a dominant Black community leader and abolitionist in that city. Peck was a member of several youth groups inspired by Delany, such as the Juvenile Anti-Slavery Society, organized in Pittsburgh on July 7, 1838. Peck later entered Rush Medical College in Chicago, Illinois, and graduated in 1847. Based on what we can gather from peripheral sources including Delany's biographers, Peck had a difficult time establishing a medical practice in Philadelphia or New York. For example, it was reported, "In February 1848 when another of Delany's young men, David Peck, left for Philadelphia to practice medicine and was kicked out of Thomas' Auction Store at a sale of medical books, Foster had the comment: 'We presume this gross insult was perpetrated on a young man of education, simply to curry favor with the southern students who were in attendance.'"[119] Another sign of Peck's difficulties was his experience in New York during the winter of 1851–1852, where, "Like many another young black, then and now, he was asking, 'Education—for what?' His difficulties in establishing a medical practice were much like those of young George B. Vashon practicing law, with all public facilities denied him."[120] Eventually he immigrated to Nicaragua, where, upon Delany's invitation, he joined one of Delany's projects to establish a Negro republic in Latin America. He was immediately named Port Physician in Nicaragua, had a booming medical practice, and was named to a high post in the government. Peck remained for some time and successfully practiced medicine there. His absence from the United States for long periods may be responsible for his present status as a shadowy historical figure rarely referred to in references.[121]

Peck's story is emblematic of the difficulties confronting everyone but White males who entered medical practice in the U.S. during the Antebellum Period. Mary Roth Walsh describes in exquisite detail the difficulties facing early women practitioners such as Harriet Hunt, Elizabeth Blackwell, and Marie Zakrezewska. The parallel relationships between these groups is significant. The fact that a Black was graduated from an American medical school two years (1847 versus 1849) before the first woman, with both events taking place more than 82 years after the first American medical school was established (1765), is symptomatic of the U.S. medical education system's race and gender problems. Much of the activity to address and correct these problems sprang out of the Abolitionist

Movement and the Women's Rights Movement. Through the leadership of men such as William Lloyd Garrison, James Birney, and Wendell Phillips, "By 1840 the American Anti-Slavery Society listed 250,000 members, published more than two dozen journals and had about fifteen state organizations supervising 2,000 local chapters."[122] For Blacks interested in medical training in the 1840s and 1850s the usual arrangement required by the anti-slavery societies and the medical schools was a signed agreement that African Americans would practice overseas after graduating. Seemingly, for women it was worse because their rights movement did not gain significant momentum until after the 1850s. Blackwell and Zakrezewska, who were medical school–trained, degree-holding physicians, also encountered severe practice difficulties such that their careers were shaped and distorted by the professional gender discrimination they encountered. They experienced professional isolation; were restricted from hospital medical staffs, postgraduate and specialized training programs, and from participation in local and regional medical societies; were not invited or allowed to attend medical meetings; received less pay for equivalent work compared to their White male peers; and were downgraded in the professional community by their colleagues. These restrictions were similar to the experiences of trained Black medical men of the period and indicate the level of shared caste disadvantages within the profession.[123]

Harriet Hunt, one of these pioneer women physicians, was admitted to Harvard Medical School in the abortive "affirmative action" class of 1850 along with three Black men. The men, Martin Robison Delany, Daniel Laing, and Isaac Snowden, had been admitted under the mistaken impression that all three would subsequently immigrate to Liberia to practice. However, the redoubtable Delany had managed to avoid signing any such agreement. As Takaki writes, "Hunt's admission was also conditional: Allowed to attend lectures, she would not be permitted to take the examination for a degree."[124] When Dean Holmes caved in to pressure generated by the protests of some of the White male medical students — who alleged that graduating with the Blacks and a woman would "cheapen" their degrees — the Blacks and the woman were expelled. Walsh's research contends that Delany may still have received an M.D. degree from Harvard. Other historians also raise the possibility that all three Blacks eventually received their degrees. This possibility deserves more detailed research.[125]

On February 1, 1865, Dr. John Sweat Rock (1825–1866) was admitted to practice law before the bar of the United States Supreme Court. He was the first Black attorney admitted to do so — living repudiation of the infamous Dred Scott decision, which questioned Black claims to humanity, handed down by the Court in 1857. A little more than a year later, on December 3, 1866, he would be dead of tuberculosis. Although the crowning achievement of Rock's life takes place in the next period of our study, its true significance can only be examined in the context of what occurred during the Jacksonian and Antebellum periods. This single accomplishment would have been remarkable for most men, but John Rock was truly a Renaissance man.

Figure 5.8   Black physician: Engraving of Dentist, Author, Attorney John Sweat Rock (1825–1866)

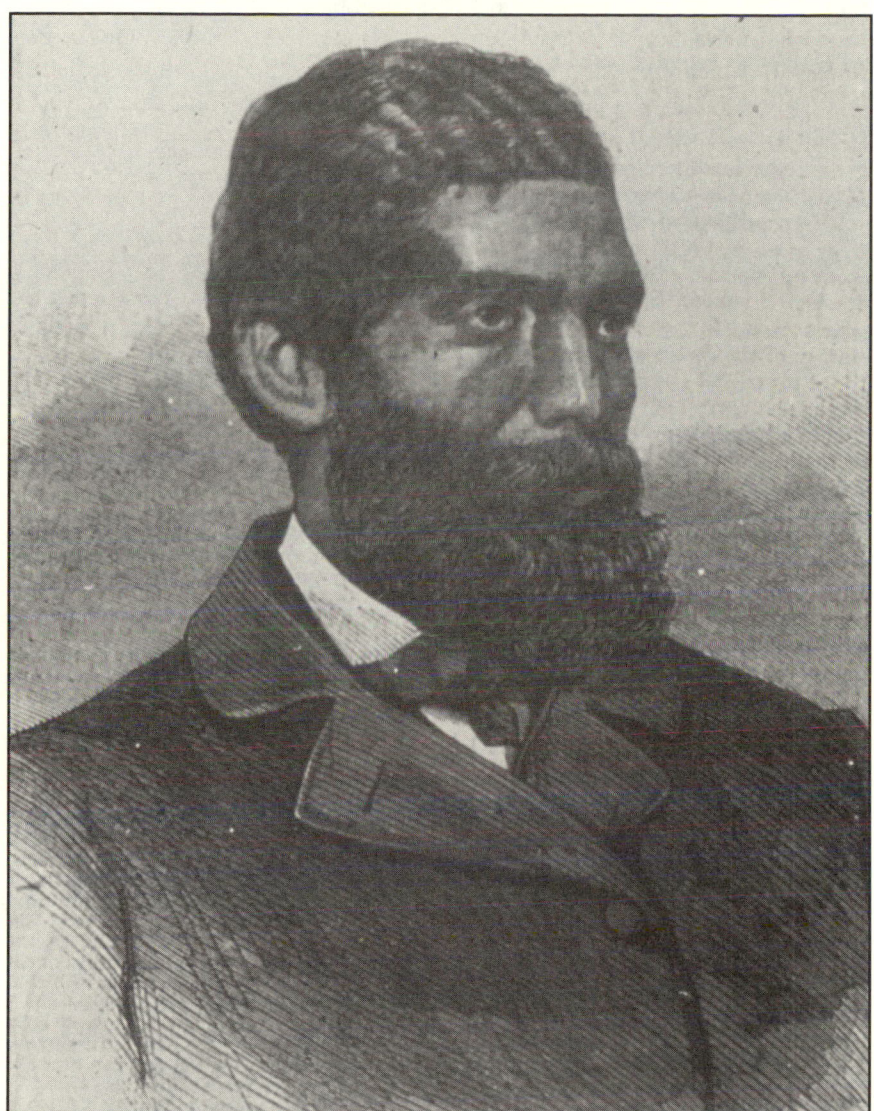

Rock was also an abolitionist and the journalist who coined the phrase "black is beautiful." Rock was both apprenticed and formally trained in dentistry and medicine, receiving a formal M.D. degree in 1852 from American Medical College in Philadelphia. Because of fragile health he was forced to discontinue the practice of medicine and dentistry. He would become the first African American attorney authorized to practice before the U.S. Supreme Court in 1864 or 1865.

Upon closer scrutiny we discover that Rock's legal career was only one of his three major callings. His first and abiding love was medicine. (See Figure 5.8.) During a medical apprenticeship with doctors Sharp and Gibbon in the area of his birth near Salem, New Jersey, between 1844 and 1848 while teaching school, Rock was denied admission to medical school, though he more than met the requirements of that era. By 1850, completing another apprenticeship with a Dr. Harbert, he mastered dentistry instead and set up practice in Philadelphia. Finally, he was allowed to attend the required two years of medical lectures at American Medical College in Philadelphia, earning an M.D. degree in 1852. By age 27 Rock was a fully trained teacher, dentist, and physician.

In pursuit of liberty, Rock moved to Boston in 1853, where he practiced medicine and dentistry for seven years. He was the second Black admitted to the Massachusetts Medical Society (mid-1850s) and became increasingly involved with the Abolitionist Movement and treated slaves in the Underground Railroad. Rock became a nationally famous orator, speaking on the "Unity of Human Races" before the Massachusetts legislature in 1856, on "The Light and Shadows of Ancient and Modern Tribes of Africa" in Philadelphia in 1857, and at Faneuil Hall in Boston for Crispus Attucks Day on March 5, 1858. In that oft-quoted speech, he coined the phrase and developed the theme that "Black is beautiful." Increasingly ill by the mid-1850s, Rock immigrated to France in 1858 for surgery by Auguste Nelaton and Valpeau before returning to Boston in 1859.

Rock, too incapacitated by tuberculosis and unwilling to compromise his high standards, discontinued his medical and dental practices by 1860 and began to study law. T. K. Lothrop, a White lawyer, motioned to have Rock examined by the bar in Superior Court on September 14, 1861. Rock passed with ease and was admitted to practice throughout the state the same day. He remained extremely active in the Negro Convention Movement that had begun in Philadelphia in 1830 and ended at the National Convention of Colored Men held at the Wesleyan Methodist Church in Boston, October 4–7, 1864. Rock and George L. Ruffin were the two publishers of the proceedings. Impatient and critical of Lincoln's conservative policies toward pursuit of the Civil War and slavery until the Emancipation Proclamation passed on January 1, 1863, Rock pushed Black participation in the war by recruiting a major portion of the 54th and 55th Massachusetts Infantry Regiments. His admission to practice before the U.S. Supreme Court led to his becoming the first Black lawyer to be received on the floor of the U.S. House of Representatives. This heady, but incomplete, chronicle of events epitomized the life of this medical warrior for civil rights.[126]

In 1849, the year that Blackwell, the first woman physician to graduate from a U.S. medical school, received her degree from the Geneva Medical College in New York, several Black men graduated from Bowdoin Medical College in Maine. John V. De Grasse (1825–1868) and Thomas J. White both pursued productive careers, with De Grasse distinguishing himself with formal training in Paris under Valpeau. He settled in Boston, where he excelled to such an extent in practice that he became the first African American admitted to a White professional society. De Grasse's admission in 1854 to the Massachusetts Medical Society was an American medical professional landmark. Charles B. Dunbar graduated from Bowdoin Medical School in 1850 and practiced in New York City. Kenney documents in *The Negro in Medicine* that Dunbar "was in active practice in New York until 1859, when he went to Liberia, pursuing his profession until his death."[127] Peter W. Ray (1823–?) of New York also completed his medical studies at Bowdoin during the early 1850s. He had a long and fruitful medical career in New York City. During the early 1850s, James J. Gould Bias graduated from the Eclectic Medical College in Philadelphia, and Robert B. Leach graduated from the Homeopathic College in Cleveland. Although it is poorly documented in the literature, David K. McDonough apparently obtained a medical degree from the University of New York sometime before 1852. He was born a slave and was the subject of an experiment on whether Blacks could benefit from academic training and absorb a medical education. After an argument between his owner and another planter over whether a Black could benefit from an education, McDonough was sent to Lafayette College in Pennsylvania, where he compiled an enviable academic record, finishing third in his class. He then begged his master to become a physician. He was then sent to New York under the tutelage of John K. Rodgers, one of the nation's most eminent surgeons, who facilitated McDonough's admission to medical lectures at the College of Physicians and Surgeons. After completing his training, he was appointed to the staff of the New York Eye and Ear Infirmary, where he achieved an excellent reputation. The first Black private hospital in New York City was named after him.[128]

At least one formally trained African American physician emerged in Canada during this period. Alexander Thomas Augusta (1825–1890) earned an M.D. degree from Trinity Medical College, Toronto, Ontario, in 1856. Born of free parents, Augusta obtained his early education from Bishop Payne by stealth. He had an early desire to practice medicine, so he underwent private tutoring in Baltimore, Maryland, and an apprenticeship in Philadelphia before moving to Canada. The move north was triggered by his inability to matriculate in U.S. medical schools. After graduation he supervised Toronto's public hospital, practiced several years in Canada and the Caribbean, then presented in Washington, DC, in 1862 for examination for the Army Medical Corps. Augusta was a man of many firsts. After being accepted as an Army physician, he became the first Black medical officer to be commissioned as a major on April 14, 1863. After suffering many racial indignities, including receiving enlisted men's pay, Augusta served with distinction with several Black units and as commander of the hospital at Camp Barker in Washington, DC, which would later become Freedmen's Hospital. Thus, he also became the first African American to command a hospital in the United States. His service was considered of such value that he was breveted a Lieutenant Colonel, U.S.V. in 1865. No other Black achieved this rank for 70 years. Subsequently, he became the first African American medical school faculty member, serving on Howard University Medical School's original medical faculty from 1868 to 1877. He practiced in the District of Columbia until his death in 1890. A few other formally trained Black physicians who practiced before the Civil War are not mentioned here. The total numbers of formally trained African American physicians gaining medical degrees during this era were far too few to exert much medical impact on the health of the population, but as can be seen from the chronicles of their careers, their social impact was profound.[129]

Martin Robison Delany was Black medicine's Spartacus. Delany (1812–1885), editor, author, physician, abolitionist, Black Nationalist, explorer, colonizationist, and Union Army officer, was born free in Charles Town, West Virginia. (See Figure 5.9.) He was an impeccably qualified physician by the standards of his day, having apprenticed with the leading White physicians and attended more than a term of classes at some of the nation's leading medical schools. But whether he ever received a medical degree is a matter of debate. His standard apprentice training under doctors such as Andrew N. McDowell, F. Julius LeMoyne, and Joseph P. Gazzam—some of Pittsburgh, Pennsylvania's, finest physicians—was first rate. They recommended Delany for admission to several medical schools. Harvard, after a struggle, finally accepted him in 1850, but subsequently expelled him and two other Black male students and a White female student. Delany openly debated White politicians and scientists and debunked the myth of Black biological and racial inferiority. He also wrote books on the question of race and ethnicity and crusaded for Black rights throughout his life. His indomitable spirit and brilliant intellect combined to mark Delany as one of America's first Black Nationalists and a father of militant politics. As the 1850s progressed, Morais observed, "His interest in medicine was overshadowed by his intense desire to crush slavery and elevate his people. . . . [H]e joined white abolitionists in castigating the Fugitive Slave Act of 1850."[130] However, his publishing and political activities never supported him or his large family—medicine always did.[131]

As we have seen, Black social and educational disadvantages had profound effects on the race's medical educational potential and circumstances. This relationship was described by physician-historian Leslie Falk in the *Bulletin of the History of Medicine:*

> *Since all U.S. blacks—slave and free—had serious problems of access to education, there was a continuum of training—the folk healer, the self-made practitioner, the nurse-midwife, the bleeder-cupper, the dentist, the barber, the apprenticeship-trained, and finally the medical school graduate.*[132]

Because of the oppressive social conditions confronting African Americans, very few Black medical school graduates emerged between 1813 and the Civil War.

Figure 5.9   Martin Robison Delany: Physician, Editor, Explorer, Ethnologist, Abolitionist (1812–1885)

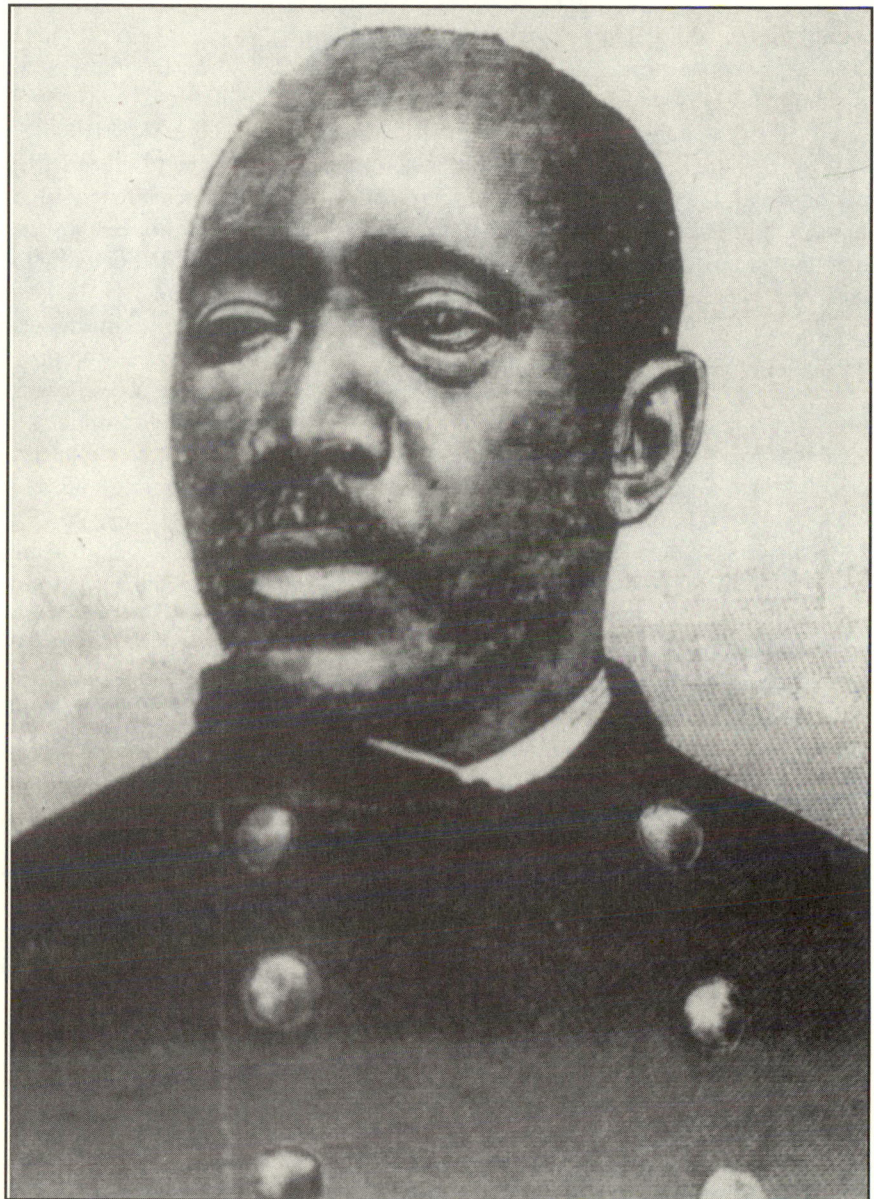

Delany was an author, ethnologist, abolitionist, and Union Army officer who was free born in Charles Town, West Virginia. A multifaceted scholar and activist, he is best known as a father of Black nationalism and a Harvard-trained physician.

Moreover, the lower the level of training, the less documentation of the nature and length of the practitioner's activities. Thus, professional participation at the level of medical school acceptance or graduation, passage of state boards or licensing requirements, or membership or participation in formal medical or professional societies serve as means of identifying and characterizing health professionals. Black exclusion based on segregation and discrimination at all these levels handicap the documentation of the African American health professions' experience.

Even though apprentice training was much less prominent during this period—with the proliferation of American medical schools—there are records of some African American, apprentice-trained physicians. Two prominent apprentice-trained physicians from the Washington, DC, area were Drs. William Taylor and John H. Fleet. Another apprentice-trained physician, Dr. James H. Wilson, mentioned in John A. Kenney's *The Negro in Medicine,* studied privately and was admitted to practice in Pennsylvania sometime before 1847. Many of the other physicians previously mentioned, such as Delany, served as apprentices prior to their formal medical training. Charles Dunbar, for example, studied under Dr. Childs during the 1840s before attending Bowdoin. Before their admission to Harvard Medical School in 1850, Daniel Laing, Jr., and Isaac Humphrey Snowden worked under Dr. Clarke in Boston. It has been previously mentioned that Dr. John S. Rock studied medicine under Dr. Shaw and Dr. Gibbon before being admitted to medical school and receiving a degree. Bousfield recalls that prominent practitioner Dr. John P. Reynolds gained fame for a number of years as a doctor in Vincennes, Indiana, and was evidently apprentice trained. Also mentioned is Dr. Lewis G. Wells of Baltimore, who was a phrenologist, orator, and minister. He combined all these assets to become a most successful physician. By all accounts he was apprentice trained. These are just a few of the apprentice-trained African American physicians practicing during the Antebellum Era. Although records of their existence are scant, they outnumbered the trained African American physicians possessing medical degrees. Based on the extant accounts of the difficulties encountered by the formally trained African American physicians, who eventually positioned themselves through dogged determination and sacrifice to earn medical degrees, these practitioners encountered staggering levels of professional discrimination, obstruction, and frustration.[133]

William Wells Brown (1816–1884) could technically be categorized as an apprentice-trained physician. However, his fame as an escaped slave who became internationally known as an abolitionist, reformer, author, and historian overshadowed his medical career. His contributions as the first African American to publish a book on travel, the first Black novelist, and the first Black foreign newspaper correspondent will be remembered forever. Nevertheless, after 1865 during the end of his active life, Brown listed himself as a physician and practiced intermittently. His interest in medicine stemmed from his teenage years in slavery under his master Dr. John Young of St. Charles County and later St. Louis, Missouri. This early interest was buttressed by his relationship with Dr. John

Bishop Estlin in Europe between 1849 and 1854. Estlin gave him medical books and advice on resuming practice. After his 1860 return to Boston he studied medicine and attended some private medical courses. During the Antebellum Period he was another African American physician who utilized his scientific knowledge to combat the myth of Black racial inferiority. Attacking the pro-slavery thesis that Blacks were racially inferior to Whites, he wrote in *The Black Man: His Antecedents, His Genius, and his Achievements* (1863):

> *There is nothing in race or blood, in color or features, that imparts susceptibility of improvement of one race over another. . . . Knowledge is not innate. Development makes the man. . . . The majority of the colored people of the Northern States [are] descended from slaves; many of them were slaves themselves. In education, in morals, and in the development of mechanical genius, the free blacks in the Northern States will compare favorably with any laboring class in the world. And considering the fact that we have been shut out, by a cruel prejudice, from nearly all the mechanical branches, and all the professions, it is marvellous that we have attained the position we now occupy.*[134]

After 1865 he opened a medical office in Boston and divided his time between medicine, temperance work, lecturing, writing, and publishing.[135]

Of the other categories of self-trained African American healers, the overwhelming majority resided in the South and functioned in the slave health subsystem. As has been previously noted, the slave folk healers, root doctors, nurse-midwives, and bleeder-cuppers were the first line of defense for sick or injured slaves. For almost two centuries Africans had brought a healing tradition with them from Africa to English North America. Due to a combination of cost-effectiveness, convenience, and cultural competence, reliance on slave healers had become a slave system tradition. Other economic and demographic factors were also responsible for expansion of this subsystem. As slaves became more expensive and more essential for Southern economic development, attention to slave health grew in importance to the South's political economy. Moreover, as the slave system matured throughout the Antebellum Period with larger slave communities owned by fewer masters, the slave health subsystem became more prominent and better organized. Historian John B. Boles identified this changing demography in *Black Southerners 1619–1869* by using a cohort of 10 slaveholders based on 1850 and 1860 census data. If one sampled this cohort the result would be "eight owning two slaves apiece, one owning twenty-four, and the tenth owning sixty."[136] His detailed analysis went further:

> *Obviously most slaveholders (80 percent) would own fewer than five slaves, but most slaves (84 out of a 100) would reside in units of more than twenty. . . . In 1850, when 73.4 percent of the slaveholders held*

> fewer than ten slaves, exactly 73.4 percent of the slaves lived in units numbering more than ten. Over half, 51.6 percent resided on plantations of more than twenty bondsmen. These figures were more pronounced in the Deep South, and still more so in 1860, when fully 62 percent of the slaves in the Deep South lived in plantation units, and one-third on really substantial plantations of more than fifty slaves.[137]

This growing concentration of slaves during the Jacksonian and Antebellum periods is more pronounced, as Bole's research reveals: "Remembering that 2.4 million of the South's 3.9 million slaves lived in the Deep South, it is clear that most slaves lived on plantations in close proximity to numerous other slaves. . . . [T]his proved to be a cultural fact of great significance."[138] Several health care phenomena can be explained if these data are properly interpreted.

With larger agricultural units generating more monoculture crops, more income, and more elaborate plantations, this growing concentration of slaves was significant to the slave health subsystem. More plantation hospitals were built to serve the expanding and more concentrated slave system, more slave hospitals were built in the cities, and the slave health subsystem grew more elaborate and more organized. According to medical and health historians Postell, Savitt, Horsman, McGregor, Vlach, and Sheridan, this is precisely what occurred. These developments required an expansion of personnel. Not only were more regular (both medical school and apprentice-trained) physicians contracted, more slave health personnel engaged in health care delivery in the form of granny midwives, granny nurses, and slave healers. On the informal level, larger slave colonies able to preserve more African healing traditions encouraged more spiritual healers, conjure men, root doctors, and voodoo doctors.[139]

Officially, the planter or his wife was responsible for attending sick slaves. On some plantations, the overseer took on this function. A medicine chest and health books such as *Gunn's Domestic Medicine, or Poor Man's Friend; The Planter's and Mariner's Medical Companion;* and physician John Steinbach Wilson's projected *The Plantation and Family Physician; a Work for Families Generally and for Southern Slaveowners Especially; Embracing the Peculiarities and Diseases, the Medical and Hygienic Management of Negroes, Together with the Causes, Symptoms, and Treatment of the Principal Diseases to Whites and Blacks* were prominent and pervasive components of the subsystem. However, on most plantations, reliance was placed on certain slave doctors, root doctors, or granny nurses to provide the initial illness encounters or the time-consuming, labor-intensive hands-on care required by the sick and afflicted. Obviously, none of the healers at this level of the system were trained in a formal sense. Community physicians were sometimes summoned for difficult cases, obstetrical emergencies, or when slave-patients were in extremis, as a back-up to the system. All too often, slaves died unattended by any trained personnel. Some planters formally contracted with local physicians to care for their slaves on a regular basis. Moreover, though some of the facilities were

A Slave Hospital on a "Good" Plantation

The following is one of the few personal descriptions of a slave hospital and infirmary. The location was a large property named the Butler's Island Plantation on the Georgia coast near Savannah. It was the property of Pierce Butler, a Southern planter. The description is excerpted from a letter from Fanny Kemble, a well-known stage personage of the Antebellum Period who was recently married to Butler. She writes to Elizabeth Sedgwick, sometime during 1834.

The infirmary is a large two-story wooden building containing four large rooms. The first I entered was half dark; some of the windows are glazed but encrusted with dirt and the shuttered openings were closed to keep out the cold. In the enormous chimney a few feeble embers glimmered and here many of the sick women were cowering on wooden settles, the poor wretches too ill to rise lay strewed about on the earthen floor without bed, pillow or mattress. Here, in their hour of sickness and suffering, lay those whose health and strength are spent in unrequited labor for us, those whose husbands, fathers, brothers and sons were, at that hour, sweating over the earth whose produce was to buy for us all the luxuries which health care revel in, all the comforts which can alleviate sickness. . . . Here lay women expecting the agonies of childbirth, others who had just brought their offspring into the world, others groaning over the pain and disappointment of miscarriages—here lay some burning with fever, or chilled with cold and aching with rheumatism upon the cold hard ground, in droughts and dampness, dirt, noise and stench—here they lay like brute beasts, all absorbed in physical suffering. . . . I told old Rose, the midwife, to open some of the shutters and myself went to the fireplace to build up the fire, but as I lifted a log, there was a universal cry of horror, and old Rose tried to snatch it from me, exclaiming: "Let alone, Missis—let be! what for you lift wood? you have nigger enough, Missis, to do it!" I made Rose tidy up the miserable apartment. It was all I could do. The other rooms, one of them for sick men, were in the same deplorable condition of filth, disorder and misery; the floor was the only bed and scanty begrimed rags of blankets the only covering. And this is the hospital of an estate where the owners are supposed to be humane, the overseer efficient and kind, and the negroes well cared for! I left this refuge for Mr. Butler's sick dependents with my clothes covered with dust and full of vermin. . . . I went again today to the infirmary and was happy to perceive there had been some faint attempt at cleaning, in compliance with my desires. I remonstrated with one of the mothers, a woman named Harriet, who was ill herself, upon the horribly dirty condition of her baby and she assured me it was impossible for the mothers to keep their children clean, that they went out to work at daybreak and did not get their tasks done till evening and then they were too worn out to do anything but throw themselves down and sleep. . . . In another room a woman was lying on the floor in a fit of epilepsy, barking most violently; she excited no particular attention, the women said was subject to these fits; she lay barking like an enraged animal. I stood in profound ignorance, sickened by the sight of suffering which I knew not how to alleviate. How I wished that . . . I had been taught something of sickness and health, that I might have known how to assist these poor creatures and direct their ignorant nurses. The swarms of fleas are incredible; I never come away from the infirmary without longing to throw myself into the water and my clothes into the fire.

Notes

Armstrong, M. *Fanny Kemble: A Passionate Victorian*. New York: The Macmillan Company, 1938, 220–222.

Byrd WM, Clayton LA. *A Black Health Trilogy* [videotape and 188 page documentary report]. Washington, D.C.: The National Medical Association and the African American Heritage and Education Foundation; 1991.

Byrd WM, Clayton LA. The "slave health deficit": Racism and health outcomes. *Health/PAC Bulletin* 1991; 21:25–28.

Joyner C. "The World of the Plantation Slaves." 50–99. In: Campbell EDC Jr, Rice K., eds. *Before Freedom Came: African-American Life in the Antebellum South*. Charlottesville, Virginia: The Museum of the Confederacy, Richmond and the University Press of Virginia, 1991, 58.

Morais HM. *The History of the Negro in Medicine*. Under auspices of The Association for the Study of Negro Life and History. New York: Publishers Company, Inc., 1967.

Savitt TL. *Medicine and Slavery: The Diseases and Health Care of Blacks in Antebellum Virginia*. Urbana: University of Illinois Press, 1987.

Sheridan RB. *Doctors and Slaves: A Medical and Demographic History of Slavery in the British West Indies, 1680–1834*. Cambridge: Cambridge University Press, 1985.

Ransford O. *Bid the Sickness Cease: Disease in the History of Black Africa*. London: John Murray (Publishers) Ltd., 1983.

adequate, many slave hospitals were truly "hell holes," as described by Fanny Kemble, a prominent British-born Victorian actress, who married into a slave-holding family and described her sojourn on a large Southern plantation (see Vignette).

Most slaves preferred being seen by their own healers and distrusted Western medicine and the White doctors representing that medical tradition. They sometimes expressed these sentiments, but often were too intimidated by the system to speak out or express their wishes. Nevertheless, the slave health subsystem not only functioned but expanded until the Civil War. Despite the medical profession's increases in specialization, complexity, and resource allocation, slave health status and outcomes deteriorated during the Jacksonian and Antebellum periods. What would substitute for this obviously inferior health subsystem, which had been firmly institutionalized to serve the Black third of the South's population after its Civil War breakdown, is the subject of the following chapters.[140]

One woman nurse and folk-healer, famous for her role as an "engineer" on the Underground Railroad, was Harriet Ross Tubman. She was in an intermediate position between the slave health subsystem and the health care provided by the abolitionists for the escaping slaves. It is well known that the abolition and anti-slavery societies often hired physicians to provide care to escapees at various major stops on the trip North. Tubman evidently provided some care before these safe havens were reached. Tubman (1821–1913) is well known as an abolitionist and engineer in the Underground Railroad. She escaped from slavery in 1849 and subsequently returned to the South at least 19 times over the next 10 years to lead more than 300 blacks to freedom in the North. Tubman became a hero to all who respected freedom, dignity, and human worth and was often referred to as "a woman called Moses." Often unacknowledged is the fact that Tubman also functioned as a nurse during the journeys with escaped slaves and at contraband hospitals to such an extent that the supervising physicians of these facilities came to rely upon her. Some even wrote memoranda requesting that she be issued medications from other physicians at the other end of her journeys. She also compounded herbal and root medications that she administered, and obtained cures for patients ill with some forms of "malignant disease" or dysentery. Interestingly, she ended her career running a "hospital," which would be categorized today as a long-term care facility, in her adopted home community of Auburn, New York. Another giant in the abolitionist and feminist movements during this era, Sojourner Truth, also functioned quite often as a nurse and health care provider.[141]

Meanwhile in the North there were a few informally trained African American practitioners. Since the recent wave of scholarship describing the slave health subsystem, this small group's activities are the most difficult to document. Because of their absence of imprinting on any institutional infrastructure, compounded by their small economic significance, their contributions were left totally to generic history taking by an impoverished and unlettered racial minority group. There was a tiny cadre that history has recorded, beginning with James Still (1812–1872?), whose contribution survived because he self-published his memoirs in 1877, *Early Recollections and Life of Dr. James Still*. His parents were ex-Maryland slaves who purchased their freedom and migrated to New Jersey. After being vaccinated as a child, young James had a lifelong desire to become a physician. Still became a well-known, self-trained physician who practiced in and around Lumberton, New Jersey. He represented the small but growing number of self-trained, free African

American healers that had arisen by the nineteenth century in response to Black medical needs, health profession discrimination, and Black socioeconomic conditions. Overt racial neglect, discrimination, and segregation plagued the health system and combined with still surviving African healing traditions to energize the growth of this healer population. Although Still was known in his region as a physician, his brothers William and Peter became nationally known because of their writing, speaking, and participation in the Abolitionist Movement. William authored *The Underground Railroad*, and Peter wrote *The Kidnapped and Ransomed*. Around 1843 Dr. Still began making his own medicine, selling it, and affecting cures. He practiced for more than 34 years and had a prosperous practice. No doubt he expanded the dimensions of the health care system to African American and other underserved populations in the "Down Jersey" area where he practiced. There were many other unacknowledged African American healers who did much the same good for African American and medically underserved communities where they practiced.[142]

David Ruggles (1810–1849) was a self-trained hydropathic physician and abolitionist. Suffering from severe chronic illnesses, he opened a water cure establishment in Northampton, Massachusetts, in 1846 and successfully practiced hydropathy for three years. Ruggles is better known as a militant abolitionist, editor, and publisher.[143]

Another self-taught African American practitioner was John P. Reynolds. He practiced in both Zanesville, Ohio, and later in Vincennes, Indiana. He was trained in the late 1820s by an "Indian physician" and later became a member of the "eclectic school" of medicine.* Dr. Reynolds was highly respected and became an influential citizen in the communities where he practiced.[144]

Although trained antebellum African American physicians were few in number, their contribution was enormous. America was on the verge of becoming a world power, and Western medicine was on the threshold of carving out its niche as a basic human need. Biomedical science was also to emerge as a major cultural influence in the late nineteenth and twentieth centuries. African American participation in these developments and events, even if relegated to a subsidiary position, meant pioneer efforts had been made. Moreover, the appearance of such dynamic and brilliant personalities as James McCune Smith and Martin Robison Delany made an imprint on the American medical and medical-social scene that would prove irreplaceable. A new tradition of health practitioner whose focus was on the community at large and who actually lived by lofty medical ethical principles was begun. A group emerged whose emphasis was on health rather than wealth, on actively doing good rather than just doing no harm, and on health care for all rather than health care for a privileged few. They would

---

*The *eclectic school* of medicine was made up of a group of pre–Civil War physicians tracing their origins to the Indians and the Colonial Period. They believed in native remedies including herbs and plants. The Eclectic Medical Association formed in 1840 survived for 30 years.

pioneer a tradition unique to Black healers in America—a tradition of caring for the underserved. This new breed of physician was not staid and conservative, but courageous and committed. These physician-scientists used their training to confront the pundits who preached the false doctrine of Black biological inferiority. Those to follow would have strong role models and an ethical foundation upon which to build.

As for the slave health subsystem, it collapsed along with the rest of the South after the Civil War. Moreover, its major medical-social function, the provision of health care for enslaved African Americans of the South, was dead. The termination of the slaves' legitimate claim to health care as chattel, albeit inferior in character and quality, would raise a major challenge to the U.S. health system. Jacksonian "democracy's" attempt to constitutionally shape American society into legitimate and permanent strata of slave and free failed. Although the Jacksonian legacies of racism and radical individualism remained, the Civil War ended the U.S. slavocracy. Large numbers of Black slave healers, one of the foundations of that system, would be thrown out of work and largely cast aside—or at least into obscurity. If the African healing tradition was to survive it would have to assume a new role in the U.S. health system. It would have to continue under new circumstances and new conditions. However, chaos and conflict loomed ahead as the Black health odyssey continued. The grumblings of discontent surrounding the Lincoln election in November 1860 transformed into the April 1861 rumblings of the guns off Fort Sumter.

CHAPTER SIX

The Civil War, Reconstruction, Post-Reconstruction, and Black Health, 1861–1900

Southern artillery batteries fired on Fort Sumter in Charleston Harbor at 4:30 AM on April 12, 1861. The Civil War, called by some "The War Between the States," had begun. Nearly four years later on April 9, 1865, the guns were silent. Confederate General Robert E. Lee surrendered to Union General Ulysses S. Grant in Wilmer McLean's parlor at Appomattox Court House in Virginia. It was the bloodiest war in the nation's history.[1]

As we will explore, the Civil War and its aftermath had revolutionary effects on the U.S. health system. During this period health care in Western industrialized countries was increasingly universal and egalitarian. But in the United States the health system's race and class relationships set a course to resist the influences of medical-social changes that positively reshaped the industrialized world's health systems over the next 150 years. The Civil War forged major changes in the perception of health care and health care delivery in America. Universal access and egalitarian treatment for all patient groups remained foreign. Despite Lincoln's "new birth of freedom," virtual race and class apartheid would remain in place in the U.S. health system more than 125 years after the Civil War.[2]

The Reconstruction Era covered the period from 1865 to 1872 according to many historians, 1865 to 1877 according to others. During this period following the Civil War the seceded states were reorganized for readmission to the Union according to a congressional program. Military occupation and strict rules regarding political organization and participation during the Reconstruction Era made the federal government a dominant force in the nation.

Immediately after the Civil War ended, President Lincoln was assassinated. Under the supervision of the Congress and President Andrew Johnson, reassertion of private sector dominance and White Southern resistance followed. It was an expansive and dynamic period for institutions and citizens located in the North. For Southerners it was a mixed bag. As is characteristic of most post-revolutionary periods, the Reconstruction bred conflict and adversity. Following late President Lincoln's suggestions, the Congress struggled and passed the Thirteenth (enacted 1865, ratified 1865) and Fourteenth (enacted 1866, ratified 1868) amendments to the Constitution, which abolished slavery and began the process of ensuring citizenship and civil rights for all citizens. The Fifteenth Amendment to the Constitution followed (1870), guaranteeing ex-slaves' right to vote. Rights granted African Americans by these amendments were soon vitiated by nonenforcement by the federal government and rulings by the courts.

The South, in alliance with President Andrew Johnson, resisted the substantive social and political changes proposed by the Northern-dominated Congress. Historians Lincoln, Hughes, and Meltzer described the congressional response:

> Aroused by the refusal of most Southern states to ratify the Fourteenth Amendment protecting Negro citizenship, by the revival of the Black Codes of slavery days and by growing violence against the Negro, the Stevens Committee won Congressional approval for its Reconstruction Act of 1867.[3]

This committee represented the so-called Radical Republicans. They imposed martial law, divided the South into five military districts, and proclaimed universal manhood suffrage. They also required the drafting of new state constitutions and required ratification of the Fourteenth Amendment by all states for readmission to the Union. The committee proposed weak efforts, which never came to fruition, to sell or lease abandoned federal lands acquired as spoils of war to the freedmen.

A firestorm of White protest erupted in the South, along with turmoil, racial violence, and mythology, which surrounds today's discussions of the Reconstruction Era. In response to massive social and institutional collapse and dislocation in the South disproportionally affecting Blacks and poor Whites, Congress passed the Freedmen's Bureau legislation on March 3, 1865. The first large-scale government aid program, it emphasized education, the provision of rations for the destitute, and enforcement of the freedmen's newly won legal and citizenship rights. Medical programs grew out of the necessities of the battlefield and, later, urban crises.[4]

Ex-slaves were the flashpoint of many controversies during the enactment of Reconstruction and Freedmen's Bureau legislation. Nevertheless, they were forced to sit on the sidelines as the issues played themselves out in Washington. This goes a long way toward explaining why, as far as African American health was concerned, the Reconstruction and post-Reconstruction eras were a disaster. As new waves of epidemics, poor health, sickness, and death swept through the postwar South, along with a recrudescence of tuberculosis, African Americans were differentially affected. J. O. Breeden summed up the Black health situation: "[A] higher incidence of tuberculosis was only one indication of the deteriorating health of the former slaves. Left to fend for themselves after the collapse of Reconstruction, freedmen experienced excessively high rates of sickness and death."[5] President Lincoln viewed abandoned Negroes as "[a] laborless, landless and homeless class" caught "in a hazy realm between bondage and freedom."[6] Having no worldly possessions, the few ex-slaves with craft skills were almost universally blocked from using them by working-class Whites. Less than 10 percent of the freedmen could read and write. Lacking access to education or training, virtually no Blacks engaged in professions.

A large percentage of African Americans were heartened as they listened to, and believed, their Republican Party allies, abolitionists, the Freedmen's Bureau, and Freedmen's Aid Society friends. These powerful groups and institutions reassured them repeatedly. They told Blacks they would be rendered financially solvent at the end of the war through the provision of farmland deeded by the government to each ex-slave family. These groups also told Blacks they would be granted full citizenship and suffrage rights. President Andrew Johnson, politicians, and Northern and Southern capitalists blocked most of these efforts and returned confiscated lands to rebel planters.

When sent to South Carolina by President Johnson to inform the freedmen of the failed fulfillment of Republican promises of "forty acres and a mule," General Oliver O. Howard, the appointed head of the Freedmen's Bureau,

> who had no stomach for the mission, called a huge assembly on Edisto Island, but the words wouldn't come. How does one tell a people who have known nothing but betrayals, that they have been betrayed again? Howard couldn't say it; and he asked the freedmen to sing one of the good old Negro spirituals. The freedmen knew. They sang "Nobody Knows the Trouble I've Seen," and Oliver Otis Howard broke down and wept.[7]

By November 5, 1865, at the New Orleans Theater, a resigned General Howard had no such difficulty delivering that same disappointing message to a Black audience gathered there.[8]

Government Reconstruction programs were massive and multifaceted efforts from a health care perspective. Although the government had begun providing health care for small groups (e.g., merchant seamen) in the previous century, the Freedmen's Bureau efforts were unique in the young nation's history. These health programs represented the first large government venture into the provision of health services for huge numbers of largely civilian populations.

Aimed primarily at the newly freed slaves, these programs also served the needs of war-shocked Southerners and refugees of all kinds.[9]

Overlapping and often conflicting with these developments and events both chronologically and sociopolitically was the nation's entry into the Gilded Age (1870s–1890). The year 1870 marked the waning of Northern zeal or concern for African Americans and their problems, a shutting down of most of the Freedmen's Bureau programs, and a resumption of the dominance by American business of governmental, political, and economic institutions that had been attained during the Antebellum Period. In many ways, it was as if the Civil War had served as a brief interruption of "business as usual."

After the Civil War the scientific and social influence on Western culture by Charles Darwin's theory of evolution, detailed in *The Origin of Species* (1859) and *The Descent of Man* (1871), took hold in the United States—which increasingly worshiped the new science. An almost irrational social optimism gripped America despite increasing suffering of industrial workers, African Americans, displaced Native Americans, southern sharecroppers, and immigrant and Catholic groups. Herbert Spencer had arbitrarily stretched Darwin's scientifically sound biological theories to encompass society as a whole in *The Study of Sociology* (1873). He coined and popularized the term and concept of "survival of the fittest." His American disciples, sociologists William Graham Sumner of Yale, Charles Ellwood of Missouri, and John Fiske in New York, facilitated and promoted a mood of intolerance and unquestioning social hierarchy as they linked biological predestination with the social performance of the indigent and downtrodden. Widespread popular and scientific acceptance of Spencer's flawed hierarchical ranking and predestination theories and concepts was especially detrimental to African Americans, who were arbitrarily and automatically assigned to the bottom ranks.[10]

After the Hayes-Tilden Compromise of 1877,* everything moved in different directions. Weary of the war and its aftermath, the nation moved toward conservative retrenchment and the withdrawal of Union troops from the South. The "Black problem" was handed back to Southerners and was transformed into "states' rights," or a series of problems to be dealt with locally. This included providing health care to an impoverished and unlettered population whose medical services had previously been the responsibility of their private owners. Most Southern charitable and publicly supported institutions for the indigent such as hospitals, dispensaries, and mental institutions refused to serve Blacks. Poor Black health outcome was, thus, in many ways predetermined. Freedom's sun wouldn't

---

*The Hayes-Tilden Compromise of 1877 was a political deal cut between conservative Southern Democrats and Republicans to resolve a disputed 1876 presidential election in the electoral college and Congress. Elected president despite the popular vote, Hayes agreed to formally end Reconstruction and to withdraw Union troops from the South. This threw the African American population on the mercies of their former slavemasters, pragmatically ended Black suffrage, facilitated enactment of Jim Crow laws, and enabled the imposition of a reign of terror on the Black community. Politically, the "solid South" was born.

break through the darkening clouds of oppression, segregation, and discrimination for Blacks in the health care system until after the mid-twentieth century.

Falsely projected by most Whites as massive government experiments that failed, Blacks and poor Whites would continue to benefit from the fruits of the Freedmen's Bureau movement and the Reconstruction into the twenty-first century. Provision of universal basic and advanced education that spawned professionals to staff and administer schools; a Civil Rights movement; and vital community-based institutions such as banks, hospitals, and businesses were major accomplishments and legacies of the Freedmen's Bureau. Concrete evidence of this beneficence has lingered into the twenty-first century in the form of a viable network of Black colleges still graduating almost half the nation's African American college graduates.

A Black medical profession, separated from the White profession through no fault of its own, burgeoned to upgrade African American health status several notches and to begin leading its communities politically and spiritually. Nevertheless, tiny and usually underfunded organizations, institutions, and efforts could not reverse the tide nor correct the entire burden of poor Black health status, an outcome that was borne of a hostile national health system environment compounded by segregation and neglect. Effects of the mainstream health system's policies and practices of racial exclusion, disregard, and discrimination would prove impossible to overcome. Nevertheless, creation of the new "Negro medical ghetto" for African Americans locked out of the mainstream health system represented a valiant compensatory endeavor.

The need for both African American physicians and health facilities became clear, and more than 10 Black medical schools and a network of Black hospitals opened by 1900. (See Table 6.1.) After the withdrawal of the Union Army troops that had been placed throughout the South to protect ex-slaves in 1877, the Redemption, the term used for the political and social reinstitution of White superiority and dominance over the South, proceeded. Racial antagonisms and violence through Ku Klux Klan activity and lynchings reached all-time highs. African American civil, suffrage, and public accommodations rights were stripped away by Southern legislatures and the courts. As Beardsley observed in *A History of Neglect*, "By the 1890s, with the codification of segregation in the South, white racism was once again as virulent as it had been during slavery."[11] He noted that White physicians of the era, who were responsible for the health of the late nineteenth-century South—where over ninety percent of all Blacks lived—had not adopted more enlightened racial attitudes. In fact:

> *Until the early twentieth century most white doctors believed, as had their antebellum counterparts, that blacks were biologically inferior and subject to a different pathology from that governing whites. Further, they regarded blacks as psychologically unfit for freedom and for the most part uneducable in the ways of better hygiene. Among many white doctors, the thinking was that it was futile even to try to rescue black health.*[12]

Table 6.1 Black Medical Colleges, 1865–1923

	City	Year Organized	Year Discontinued	Affiliation
Howard University	Washington, D.C.	1869		
Lincoln University	Oxford, Pennsylvania	1870	1874	Presbyterian (local)
Straight University	New Orleans	1873	1874	Congregationalist
Meharry Medical College	Nashville	1876		Methodist, Episcopal
Leonard Medical School of Shaw University	Raleigh	1882	1918	Baptist
Louisville National Medical College	Louisville	1888	1912	Proprietary
Hannibal Medical College	Memphis	1889	1896	Proprietary
Flint Medical College of New Orleans University	New Orleans	1889	1911	Methodist, Episcopal
Knoxville College Medical Department	Knoxville	1895	1900	Presbyterian
Chattanooga National Medical College	Chattanooga	1899	1908	Proprietary
State University Medical Department	Louisville	1899	1903 (Merged with LNMC)	Baptist (Ky.)
Knoxville Medical College	Knoxville	1900	1910	Proprietary
University of West Tennessee College of Medicine and Surgery	Jackson (1st location)	1900	1907	Proprietary
	Memphis (2d location)	1907	1923	
Medico-Chirurgical and Theological College of Christ's Institution	Baltimore	1900	?	?

At least fourteen Black medical schools existed between 1865 and 1910. Between 1910 and 1970 Meharry Medical College and Howard Medical School were virtually the sole sources of Black physicians and dentists.

Clearly a worsening racial climate, nihilistic and negative health policies, and the reinstitution of Black codes* and economic oppression had begun by the 1880s and 1890s. These factors had profound and adverse effects on the delivery of health care and services to African Americans and thus on Black health status.[13]

Black Health 1861–1900: A Roller-Coaster Ride to Nowhere

Tracking the Black health experience from 1861 to the turn of the century is a daunting task. Thirty-nine years is a short time from a historical perspective. Although African Americans have never shared the same health status or outcomes as European Americans, during this period Black health status plunged precipitously at least three times in conjunction with massive political, social, and economic upheavals and events that typically affect the status of public health and health systems.

Race-based health disparities assumed the status of a basic health system assumption during this period. Nineteenth-century adult and child mortality data are crude measures of comparative Black/White mortality. Douglas Ewbank, Reynolds Farley, and Jitsuichi Masouoka have identified shortcomings in the available data between 1800 and 1940 because of inaccuracies in collection, improper sampling, and failure to perform modern statistical analyses on the raw data. Nevertheless, reexamination of the Census and other data between 1850 and 1900 by modern methods reveals markedly higher mortality rates among Blacks than had been previously identified. It also reveals higher Black infant mortality rates, higher child mortality rates, and markedly shorter life expectancies experienced by African Americans throughout the nineteenth century.

The 246-year health "roller-coaster" of health disadvantage suffered by African Americans during slavery continued. During this period there were no appreciable improvements in Black health or health care in either relative or absolute terms. Virtually all authorities agree that Black health status plummeted during the Civil War, Reconstruction, and the 1890s. Several experts noted that during certain parts of this 39-year period Black/White health disparities actually increased. Toward the end of the period, while the health status and outcome for European Americans improved rather dramatically, significant and measurable improvements in Black health status did not occur until just before World War I.[14]

Black codes were laws implemented by Southern legislatures after the Civil War, attempting to regulate the lives of the former slaves. African Americans could not testify against Whites, vote, serve on juries, or in state militias. They were forced to sign yearly labor contracts or be declared vagrants, arrested, fined, and hired out to White landowners. This helped trigger the Radical Reconstruction.

Social and political events generated by the Civil War devastated, then forever changed and reshaped, the health delivery system generally and Black health specifically. The South was particularly affected:

> The Civil War and its aftermath had a disastrous effect on health in the South. On the one hand, the hostilities left untold thousands of southerners in precarious or weakened health. On the other, the conflict's legacy of poverty exacerbated the region's tradition of poor health. As a result, old diseases increased in incidence and virulence, and new health problems arose.[15]

For Blacks, there is compelling evidence that the Civil War worsened the *slave health deficit,* defined as the dramatic and deleterious Black/White differentials in health status and outcome presumed to be the consequence of slavery and subordinate racial status. In addition, Black health status deteriorated further during the Reconstruction Period. Presumably the trauma and dislocation of war exacerbated these adverse effects.

The Southern economy was in such shambles by 1863 that it couldn't support the war effort, much less provide peacetime levels of health care for a dependent slave population. The deleterious effects this situation had on Black health care have been well documented by several institutions established to help the freedmen. The short supply of White physicians and hospitals and an inadequate public health care infrastructure in the South were accentuated by the war. By war's end poverty, refugee status, and poor sanitation and housing placed the entire Black population at risk. The Freedmen's Bureau, which included health provisions, was the government's official response to deal with an emergency situation.

The end of the Civil War plunged the health of the Black population into what may have been its worst state since the forced African migration to North America. By the late 1860s Black health status had deteriorated to levels worse than it had been during the war. Abandoned by the modicum of care offered by the inferior slave health subsystem, emancipation threw African Americans into a social cauldron of illiteracy, poverty, racial segregation, exploitation, and national hostility. The health system was no oasis from this unfavorable environment. It was an extension of the period's racially hostile social milieu. Moreover, when chattel slavery ended, the social and political justification for Black existence, which had been based on slaves' material role in the U.S. political economy, was over.

In contrast to other slave emancipations,* no educational or logistical preparations had been made to cushion the blow of newly acquired freedom in

---

*In Egyptian, Sub-Saharan African, Greek, Roman, and Moslem slave systems, many bondsmen were highly skilled teachers, physicians, administrators, or craftsmen. At emancipation, many slaves held exalted positions or were entrepreneurs and property owners.

America's competitive market system. Moreover, Blacks were not popular among either Northern or Southern Whites. With mass exportation to Africa, South America, or the Caribbean being too expensive and the role and rights of Blacks thrown in question, the deleterious results and outcomes of ex-slaves' clash with an absent or hostile health system were no surprise. The well-intended Freedmen's Bureau efforts were underfunded, inadequate, and ended far too soon to have a long-lasting positive impact on Black health.[16]

The end of the Freedmen's Bureau and the beginning of Southern Redemption, in effect, pushed Black health to the side — off the mainstream health policy agenda. Blacks were segregated ideologically and structurally from the rest of the American health system. Moreover, this development was consistent with and reinforced trends that were already dominant. The new political economy and ideology generated by the Gilded Age, based on White corporate domination and social Darwinism, activated and accentuated already unwholesome, apartheid-like trends and developments. Health discrimination based on race and class apartheid, and medical-social, health policy, and institutional infrastructural boundaries, was institutionalized in the period from 1870 to 1900. Complementing these trends were the medical and anthropological professions' leadership in the link to biological determinism, Nativism, and scientific racism. (See Figures 6.1 and 6.2.) This development was extremely detrimental to Black, immigrant, female, and other non-White Americans as it supplied pseudoscientific justification and rationalization to the era's racist and caste-ridden social hierarchies.

These developments, occurring in clear view of humane and egalitarian European Americans such as General Oliver Howard and former Union Army medical corpsman and abolitionist school teacher George Whipple Hubbard, demanded some type of corrective strategy. (See Figures 6.3 and 6.4.) Their approach, reinforced by ancient medical traditions lying dormant in a beleaguered African American community, pointed to the establishment of health care and academic institutions that would produce Black physicians, nurses, dentists, allied health professionals, and hospitals.

This "self-help" approach was also in sync with Gilded Age ideologies and practices and might, therefore, be positively received by certain elements of the policy and institutional establishment. Their hunch was correct. By 1900, out of 10 Black medical schools that had opened, seven were functioning. At least 40 Black hospitals were operational throughout the country. Although this movement was vital to the Black community, and in some instances ensured and increased African American survival and outcomes from disease, it also paradoxically served to further institutionalize health system apartheid in the United States.

Many of today's health system's lingering race, gender, and class problems emerged during this turbulent period. The persistence of the slave health deficit

Figure 6.1   Racist Illustrations of Evolution

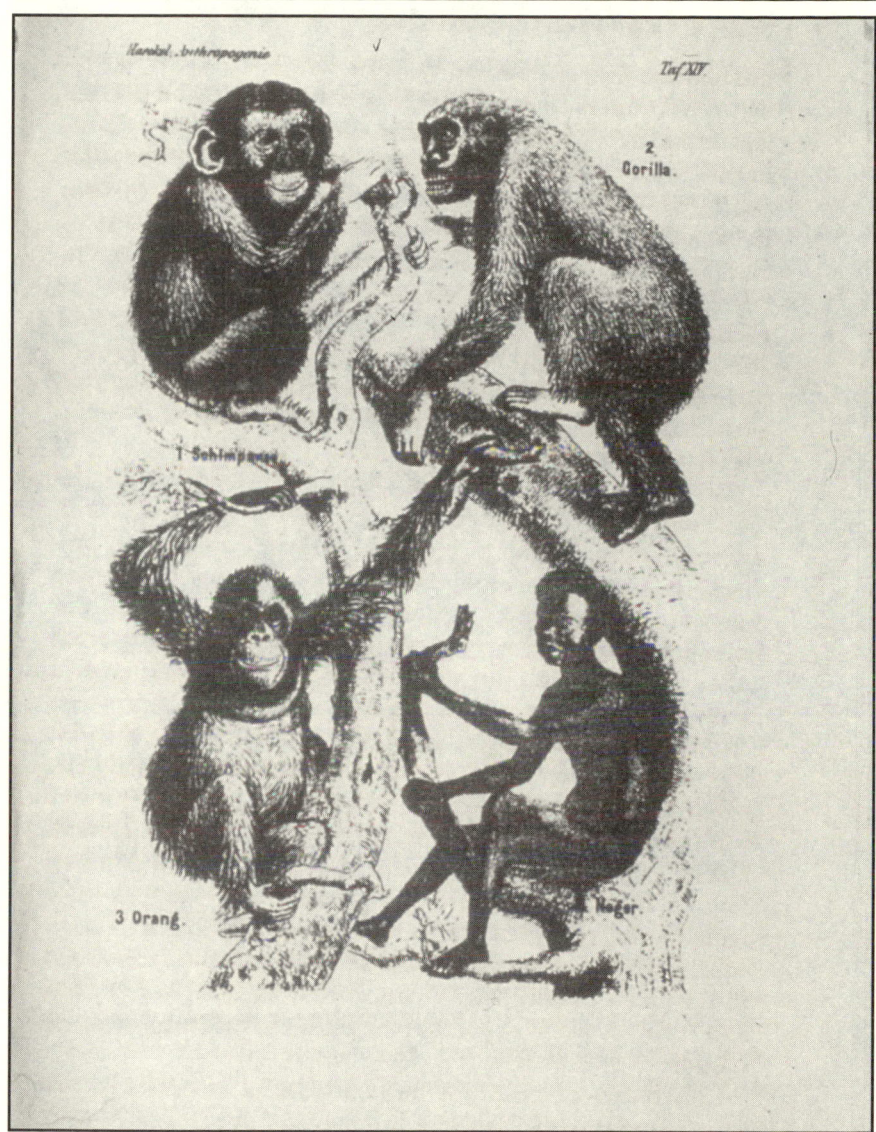

This illustration from Ernst Haeckel's 1874 textbook *Anthropogenie* suggesting the biologic classification of Blacks as subhuman "things" depicted them in trees with apes. This racist illustration is from the files of the American Museum of Natural History. Haeckel was one of the leading late-nineteenth-century biological scientists and social Darwinists, and his work was later recognized by the Nazis in their efforts to justify Jewish extermination on the basis of Aryan superiority and "racial inferiority."

Figure 6.2   The Zulus: A Typical Anthropological Display

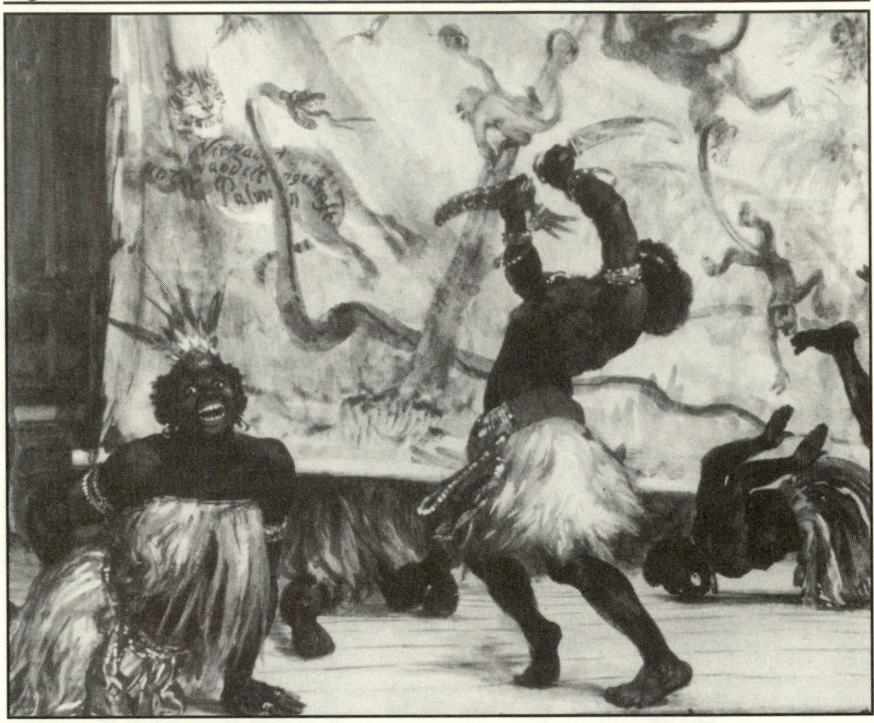

Late-nineteenth-century anthropologists and ethnologists, through elaborate museum displays, sponsorship of exposition and world fair programs and activities, and academic conferences and writings, promoted and popularized derogatory racial images, White superiority, non-White inferiority, and racial and cultural hierarchies (Caucasian Europe was the standard). Exhibitions of up-to-date "science" such as this one were typical of expositions and fairs conducted throughout the United States between the 1870s and the 1920s.

into the twentieth century was one of the legacies of the Reconstruction, Gilded Age, and early Progressive periods.[17]

The Civil War and Black Health

To obtain a feel for the Black health experience during the Civil War, in the cataclysmic years from April 12, 1861, to April 9, 1865, one must assess both African American military and civilian health. The relationship between the African American population and the Union and Confederate armies was more intimate than is usually projected. Dudley Taylor Cornish in *The Sable Arm*

Figure 6.3   General Oliver O. Howard (1830–1909)

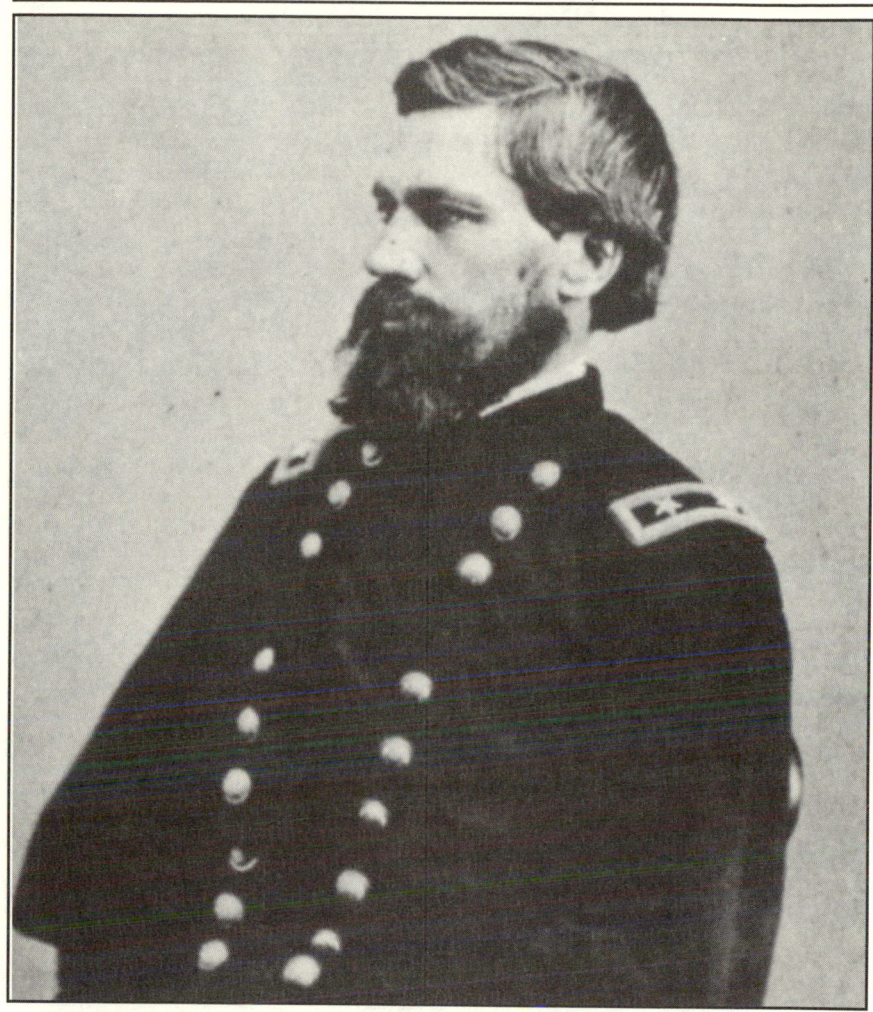

A photograph of Howard at the time he was helping lay the foundations for Black education. He profoundly influenced Black health care, helping found the two major African American medical schools (Howard and Meharry), over 100 Black hospitals, and health clinics over the entire South. Most of this occurred during his tenure as director of the Freedmen's Bureau between 1865 and 1872.

states that as many as 200,000 Black troops may have served in the Union Army. However, virtually everyone accepts "the figure of 180,000 as probable," meaning that "Negro troops made up between 9 and 10 percent of the total number of Union soldiers"[18] at the very least.

Figure 6.4   Dr. George Whipple Hubbard, Young Medical School
              Founder and Dean

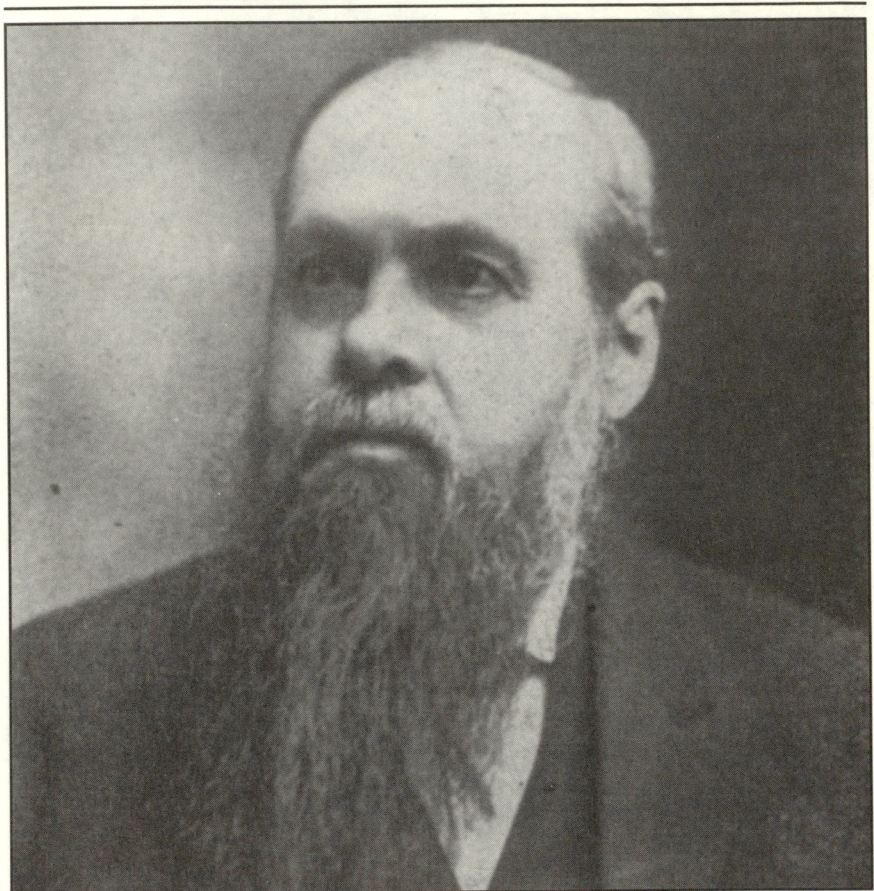

George Whipple Hubbard (1841–1924), a native of Charleston, New Hampshire, was the primary of
the three founders of Meharry Medical College, of Nashville, Tennessee, in October 1876. Meharry
was the first American medical school opened specifically to train African American physicians and
subsequently trained more Black physicians and dentists than any other institution on earth. The
dream behind this school was to correct the horrible health status and outcomes of the recently freed
ex-slaves who were locked out of any health delivery system after the collapse of the slave health
subsystem.

A second major component of the Black population was a large population
of slaves who escaped to the Union Army lines and encampments, thus ending
their bondage. Throughout the war this may have amounted to 1 million slaves
entering the refugee and contraband populations. This huge group created significant logistical problems for Union Army generals, who consistently com-
plained about the "contraband" inundating their camps. These "unofficial"

people required not only rations but also health care. The third and largest group was the 3 million African Americans who remained in the Confederacy as either rural or industrial slaves for the duration of the war. Finally, the last group was the 480,000 free Blacks concentrated in the Northern and border states, but living throughout the United States.[19]

Although African Americans had participated in virtually all of America's wars—the colonial wars, the Revolution, and the War of 1812—according to Cornish, "until the American Civil War, the American Negro was never an official part of the military establishment of the United States."[20] Delineation of official status of African American soldiers in the Civil War was extremely important. Defining such a covenant between Black soldiers and their government highlights the later neglect of the Black troops as a glaring example of the peculiarly racist nature of military health policies and the health system relative to African Americans. One of the most fundamental and precious relationships is the health care covenant that exists between a government and its soldiers during war. Care for sick or wounded soldiers is a first priority that instills confidence and high morale in the troops.

It is well documented that the health of Black soldiers was worse than that of Whites in the Union Army. In his comprehensive study of Blacks in the Civil War, Cornish pointed out that, "Losses among Negro troops were high: 68,178 from all causes reported or over one-third of the total enrolled. Of these, 2,751 were killed in action; the balance died of wounds or disease or were missing."[21] Barbeau and Henri record a slightly higher death toll (2,894).[22] A Confederate officer in the field recorded his observations about the high Black Union Army casualty rate:

> As usual with the enemy, they posted their negro regiments on their left and in front, where they were slain by hundreds, and upon retiring left their dead and wounded negroes uncared for, carrying off only their whites, which accounts for the fact that upon the first part of the battlefield nearly all the dead found were negroes.[23]

Thus, both military and health policy accounts for poor African American outcomes during the war. The paucity of Black doctors may have been another factor. Henri and Barbeau observed that, although no accurate record of Black officers was maintained, "at least eight surgeons* . . . held commissions from the United States Army."[24] This is a tiny number compared to the number of Black troops enlisted in the Army. If higher numbers of Black physicians had been recruited to the Medical Department and assigned to Black units, the health outcome of the Black Union Army soldiers most likely would have improved.[25]

Health care may have been a glaring example, but it was not the solitary manifestation of racism and discrimination African Americans endured in the

---

*The U.S. Army Medical Corps designated all physicians as "surgeons."

Union Army. Black troops were victims of outright exclusion and discrimination in other areas of Army life until late in the war. African Americans received $7 per month instead of the standard $13 pay until protests and lobbying changed the policy. They were given menial and undesirable assignments and were routinely discriminated against and slighted at Army posts and activities. Blacks were often denied standard equipment issues of clothing and supplies. Clearly, the medical-social relationship between the U.S. Army and its African American troops was as distorted as the racial discrimination in assignments, logistics, and pay—if not more so.[26]

For the tens of thousands of African Americans who joined the Union Army, many of them ex-slaves, the induction physical examination was their first encounter with the formal Western medical system. Having a fully trained White physician perform and record a comprehensive history and physical examination was an unheard of experience for many Blacks of the period—slave or free. Pioneer gastroenterologist Leonidus Berry supplies a detailed description of such an initial medical encounter experienced by one of his ancestors in his book *I Wouldn't Take Nothin' for My Journey*.

For several thousand Black soldiers their interaction with formal Western medical systems took an unwholesome turn. It predicted many aspects of the sometimes deceptive relationship between the White research community and African Americans that played itself out later in the infamous Tuskegee syphilis experiment. For a large cohort of Black soldiers, this first mainstream medical encounter was misused by the U.S. Army and the government to provide racially derogatory and biased anthropometric data. This data would be used for generations to pseudoscientifically disparage and discredit people of African descent.

The mechanism for the research abuse was created by the amalgamation of two bodies, the Provost Marshal-General's Bureau and the United States Sanitary Commission. The latter, as Fredrickson and Haller note, was, before obtaining its political clout and legitimacy during the Civil War, "a semiofficial organization made up of predominantly upper-class . . . patrician elements which had been vainly seeking a function in American society."[27] The elevation of these and several other civilian welfare organizations such as the Christian Commission and the Western Sanitary Commission to official status by President Lincoln in 1861 led to many positive and a few negative results. The new Sanitary Commission infrastructure influenced and enlightened U.S. Army personnel and governmental and civilian health care policy makers on the importance of sanitation and public health measures. They improved military camp sanitation standards and practices, making Union Army efforts in these areas the envy of the world. Ambulance service for the Army was upgraded. The crude and inadequate Army hospital system was reorganized into a modern system of regimental and divisional hospitals. Innovations by these policy makers extended hospital care to the entire Army at the field level. Their promotion of innovative pavilion-type hospitals rendered these the dominant models for hospital construction for the next 50 years. They also encouraged the emergence, female dominance, and professionalization of the vitally important nursing profession.

The United States Sanitary Commission also became singularly and internationally famous for conducting large-scale, racially comparative, anthropometric studies of Civil War soldiers. Funding for the project was governmental and private. The insurance industry aggressively underwrote the study, feeling it would generate and supply much actuarially useful data on the general population and specific racial groups. Therefore, the Civil War, through the United States Sanitary Commission Studies, also turned into a watershed for nineteenth-century anthropometric and anthropological "sciences."[28]

The study was designed as an investigatory tool to discern the physical and moral status of the Union troops, measure them anthropometrically, and make suggestions to expand their capabilities. It was supposed to create an objective, scientific, biomedical yardstick to enhance military capability. Anthropometry was espoused by a cadre of scientists led by Belgian statistician, sociologist, and astronomer Lambert Adolphe Jacque Quetelet (1796–1874) in the 1830s. The discipline consisted of measuring and tabulating such items as physical body measurements, demographic items, mortality rates, and even moral qualities compiled as numerical data sets. The latter included indices for drunkenness, insanity, suicides, and crime.

This mass of quantitative information was utilized to statistically arrive at a theoretical model Quetelet referred to as the "average man" (*l'homme moyen*). He attempted to lay the groundwork for a social physics based on discrete versions of his average man altered to represent specific groups. The Caucasian male was the established standard. This formed the basis for "objectively" evaluating and comparing members of various groups. Physical, social, and moral items were compared. It was used by many as scientists and laypersons use IQ tests today. In fact, it was considered the comprehensive "test" of its age.

The Civil War, according to the social "progressives" of the time, provided an excellent opportunity to conduct large-scale, comparative racial studies with resources Quetelet and other European anthropologists had previously lacked. From contemporaneous biomedical and anthropological viewpoints, opportunities were even greater late in the war. Congress initially authorized the deployment of Black troops on July 17, 1862. Lincoln decided to officially admit Blacks into the Union Army in 1864. These events created unparalleled opportunities to compare the races quantitatively based on the latest scientific methodology. Such a study could also serve to satiate the appetites of the European anthropological societies and interested American scientists. These groups had heard about the United States Sanitary Commission Study and were excited by prospects of a so-called scientific comparison of the races.[29]

Because of the Union Army bar on Black soldiers early in the War, the first and smaller arm of the study involved 8,004 White Union and Confederate troops. Between July 1864 and the end of the war, 15,900 examinations, 15,781 of which were considered valid, were performed. Negro inclusion in the new sample was considered so important that both the equipment and the forms for the data collection and entry for the study were changed. Modifications were made such that Black/White differences would be easily discerned.

As Haller observed, by 1864, "No examination of the negro troops seem to have been made yet . . . and the importance of such inspections needs no comment."[30] The new and larger sample included 10,876 White soldiers, 1,146 White sailors, 68 White Marines, 2,020 "full-blooded" Negroes, 863 mulattoes, and 519 Indians. Instruments were selected to measure "the most important physical dimensions and personal characteristics."[31] The instruments used by the Commission were the andrometer, spirometer, dynamometer, facial angle instrument, platform balance, calipers, and measuring tape.

The study was based directly on Quetelet's methodology. He had performed several statistical analyses of human physiognomy in Europe. Although they served as a baseline, none had been as thorough or comprehensive. Quetelet's studies included examinations of 900 Belgian draftees, 9,500 Belgian militia, 69 convicts, and 80 Cambridge University students. Included in the U.S. Sanitary Commission Study methodology were the flawed scientific rituals outlined by Samuel George Morton for measuring skulls and Petrus Camper's specious facial angle measurements. Gross flaws were inherent in categorizing such a high percentage of Black study subjects as "full-blooded" Negroes. Experts such as Du Bois estimated that less than 25 percent of the African American population was of unmixed African descent by the twentieth century. How such a high percentage of "full-blooded" Negroes could have preceded them by only one generation is impossible to determine. The generalizability of the Native American data to all Indians is questionable when only one, largely Iroquois, prisoner-of-war group of Indians was measured. Realizing there were more than 200 distinct tribal groupings of American Indians inspires less confidence in the data. The accuracy of the raw data must be questioned when many of the field workers performing the measurements were untrained and unfamiliar with the instruments being used in the study. A few of the other basic flaws in the Sanitary Commission investigation were revealed much later by scientists of the twentieth century. Nevertheless, the influential study reached several damaging conclusions.[32]

Not surprisingly, the Gould Sanitary Commission Reports, based on the Sanitary Commission data published in 1869, found physical differences between the races. Whites were found to have longer heads and shorter forearms. The Indians possessed long forearms and wide lateral dimensions except at the shoulders. Blacks had greater arm lengths and shorter body lengths. Blacks also were found to have smaller chests, with Indians in between and Whites possessing the largest. These findings were not new, and any trained biologist or anthropologist of the era could have predicted and expected them. What was considered significant was the size of and scientific weight attributed to the Sanitary Commission Anthropometric Study. It was unprecedented in scale and had impressive resources devoted to it. Purportedly, the larger numbers, standardized equipment, and methodology based strongly on Quetelet's advanced statistical work enhanced the scientific validity of the results. It was a fertile garden for the scientific speculation that ensued.

As Haller recognized, "The evidence offered an immediate refuge for both hereditarians and environmentalists,"[33] monogenists and polygenists, racialists and egalitarians; anti-Black and anti-Indian scientific speculation abounded. Transparent and specious attempts to establish close relationships between people of African descent and apes were revisited. If results of the Sanitary Commission Anthropometric Study were taken at face value, the relationship between Black arm and body lengths, long considered to be closer to anthropoid (ape-like) development, now had stronger "scientific" foundations when they were linked to retarded levels of human development. Attempts to link Blacks and remote tribal peoples biologically to apes dated back to such biomedical luminaries as Linneaus, Cuvier, and White and to travelers' accounts before that. This latest effort, however, had the panache of the most current numerical and statistical methodology.

Later utilization of the Sanitary Commission anthropometric data, such as J. H. Baxter's *Statistics, Medical and Anthropological, of the Provost Marshal-General's Bureau* released in 1875, concurred with the original Gould Sanitary Commission Reports published six years earlier. The Gould Reports concluded that mulattoes probably were less vigorous than the "original" races. The reports also concluded that although Blacks were sound physical specimens, their mental abilities were virtually untested and probably limited compared to members of "higher civilizations." Both studies also served as barometers of contemporary medical professional opinion on race and biology. Baxter analyzed a survey answered by the Army physicians in the study. Their answers reflected contemporary lay and scientific opinion as well as the medical school curriculums of the time.

Baxter noted a common set of professional conclusions that, "The Negro in America, by reason of his contact with a higher civilization, lost most of his 'grosser peculiarities.'"[34] Some of the physicians alleged that in lieu of few objective physical limitations, Negro mental development was limited. They also alleged that some of the physical peculiarities of Blacks (e.g., smaller facial angle) were evidence of their possession of brute force rather than intellect. In general, the physicians also felt that mulattoes were physically inferior and less vigorous than racially "pure" individuals in a survival sense. Doctors documented in their writings that both Blacks and mulattoes were imitative, rhythmical, and obedient by nature. Such opinions polluted the minds of health professionals who cared for particular racial and ethnic groups clinically. It has been proven repeatedly that such culturally insensitive and incompetent attendants automatically skew the caregiving process against disadvantaged minority groups.[35]

Sanford B. Hunt, a surgeon in the United States Volunteers, performed many autopsies on soldiers during the Civil War at various sites. This constituted one arm of the U.S. Sanitary Commission Anthropometric study. Based on his analysis of 405 autopsies of Black (n = 381) and White (n = 24) soldiers, brain-weight analysis revealed that Blacks' brains weighed 5 ounces less than Whites' brains. Hunt concluded that small amounts of racial admixture decreased Black brain weight even further while the large infusions of White blood in mulattoes decreased the differential by 2 ounces. Hunt further concluded that these findings corroborated those of Samuel George Morton, conducted in the 1840s and 1850s. Hunt published these findings in the *Quarterly Journal of Psychological Medicine* in 1867 and the *London Anthropological Review* in 1869. This was added to a collection of brain weight data that has repeatedly been falsely correlated with race, intellect, and gender differences for more than a century. Information gleaned from pseudoscientific physiognomic investigations conducted on Black Civil War soldiers collected by the War Department was used as "proof" of Black inferiority, provided a rationale for the social hierarchy, and justified institutional racism in health care and all other areas of American life for more than half a century.[36]

After the struggle to admit African Americans into the Union Army, it is well known that Black troops faced blatant discrimination while serving in the military:

> Afro-American soldiers were only gradually accepted. As members of a segregated unit, the first Afro-American volunteers were given a great deal of fatigue duty, which tended to underscore the idea that they were only laborers in uniform. . . . [O]ther problems . . . remained. The Afro-American soldier received six dollars a month less in pay and uniforms than whites. He was armed with poor or obsolete weapons and received inferior medical care.[37]

For African American soldiers, maintenance of difference in medical treatment distorted even the doctor-patient relationship. It is well documented that Black Civil War soldiers died and suffered excessively compared to Whites. Negro battle casualties during the war numbered more than 37,000, which was, depending on the sources cited, equivalent to a casualty rate between 35 and 50 percent higher than that of the other troops—even though African Americans did not serve in the Army until 18 months after fighting and dying had begun. As Shryock noted in "A Medical Perspective on the Civil War," "Illness was always more common and more fatal among Negro than white troops: the lung infections which killed 6 white men per thousand annually, resulted in no less than 28 deaths among a corresponding number of Negroes."[38] W. Montague Cobb made further observations regarding the racially discriminatory medical corps policy: "The excessive casualty rate suffered by the colored troops was due in significant part to the poor medical care they received. It was difficult to find qualified white surgeons to serve with Negro troops and the War Department was reluctant to commission available Negro physicians."[39] Despite these facts and the statistically significant racial disparities in risks and outcomes, the racially discriminatory medical corps policy was allowed to continue to assuage White physicians' social and racial proprieties.

Few acknowledge that part of the responsibility for these results belongs to the Union Army Medical Department, which allowed its physicians to behave in prejudicial and discriminatory ways toward African American units and troops. Its encouragement of and engagement in institutional and individual racism is a strong argument for its culpability. Prejudiced attitudes and behaviors of individual White doctors were also prevalent. Another result of these policies was that untrained and unqualified personnel were allowed to care for, and even perform surgery upon, Black troops. In this regard W. Montague Cobb cited one Union general's observations and protests about the Black troops' deplorable health care situation resulting from criminal and unethical practices:

> In many cases Hospital Stewards of low order of qualifications were appointed to the office of Assistant Surgeon and Surgeon. Well grounded objections were made from every quarter against the inhumanity and surgical operations from such men. It was an objection that could not be disregarded without bringing discredit upon the Army and the Government.[40]

Therefore, the multipronged policy of allowing White physicians to reject assignments to Black units based on their social preferences, refusing to recruit and retain as many Black physicians as possible for assignment to those units, and allowing unqualified personnel carte blanche in the medical treatment of Blacks created an Army-condoned medical disaster for Black Union Army soldiers.[41]

The exclusion of qualified Black physicians from service in the Medical Corps was sometimes by commission and often by omission. One example of a qualified Black physician not even allowed to take the qualifying examination for medical service was Martin Robison Delany, who wrote the War Department to volunteer for physician's duty on at least two occasions. Delany had trained at Harvard Medical School. As Victor Ullman, a Delany biographer, pointed out, "Delany attempted to join the Army himself. He wrote to apply for a post as Army surgeon, and the War Department replied that his letter had been received and the application was 'under consideration'... but Delany never heard from the War Department."[42] He actually tried twice—hearing nothing from the War Department in both attempts. After spearheading recruitment campaigns of several Black Union Army units—Delany's vision being an army of 40,000 Black troops commanded by Black officers moving irresistibly through the South and bringing the war to a speedy conclusion—he was mustered into service on February 15, 1865, as a major in the infantry. Sent to Charleston too late to recruit an "armée d' Afrique," Delany served the Freedmen's Bureau in Hilton Head Island, South Carolina, where he made great contributions to Reconstruction efforts.

The terrible consequences this exclusionary policy wrought on Black units sorely in need of medical attendance makes the War Department policies all the more reprehensible. The few Black physicians who were accepted (some eight physicians documented) were the butt of discrimination during their service. African American physicians were physically attacked and abused in public when wearing their uniforms, received enlisted men's pay though they were officers, and were assigned exclusively to Black units unless an oversight had occurred. Despite such obstacles these men served with distinction. Nevertheless, this matrix of policies pursued by the Union Army's medical support system adversely affected Black troops at all levels—administrative, professional, and patient.[43]

Evidence of the racially discriminatory medical care rendered Black Civil War soldiers was not only discernible at the battlefield level. At the more subtle policy and administrative levels, the adverse effects of discriminatory actions of the Medical Bureau of the Army had profound effects on Black troops. The Bureau created roadblocks during the organizational phase of raising Black Civil War regiments. Before African American troops were officially assigned to the field, Daniel Ullman, a White general charged with raising and organizing four regiments of Black Louisiana volunteer infantry, encountered some of these difficulties. (See Figure 6.5.) According to Cornish in *The Sable Arm*, General Ullman stated, "[T]he work of organizing moved more slowly than was agreeable because of the delay in some of the Government Bureaus in filling requisitions."[44] Writing about the Union Army bureaucracy's response to the needs of Black troops, the General stated, "It required sharp letters from the Secretary of War . . . to stimulate action of several of them, especially the Paymaster and Medical Bureaus."[45] The detrimental effects of these discriminatory activities and policies resulted in unacceptably high Black mortality and morbidity rates in the Union Army.

Meanwhile, outside the military another story was emerging. The health care and health status for nonmilitary, refugee, or contraband Black populations during the Civil War reflected the health status of their living environments and the availability of health care. Blacks who worked as agricultural or industrial slaves in Confederate or border states were affected by one set of circumstances. In that instance they were vulnerable to the vagaries of the slave health subsystem, the economic collapse of the South, and the crumbling Confederate States Army health system. For the million or so slaves that escaped bondage, becoming either refugees or entering Union lines to become contraband, medical care depended on Union Army military surgeons or on the care provided by the Freedmen's Bureau contraband camps.

Since over 90 percent of Blacks lived in the South, our focus concentrates on that region. As Mohr discussed in *On the Threshold of Freedom: Masters and Slaves in Civil War Georgia*, health affairs in the South, along with other social conditions, were profoundly affected by the military situation experienced in particular geographic areas. Whether or not the Union Army invaders were close by or whether a particular area of the South was militarily secure dictated the

**Figure 6.5   Brigadier General Daniel Ullmann and the
            Dysfunctional Medical Bureau**

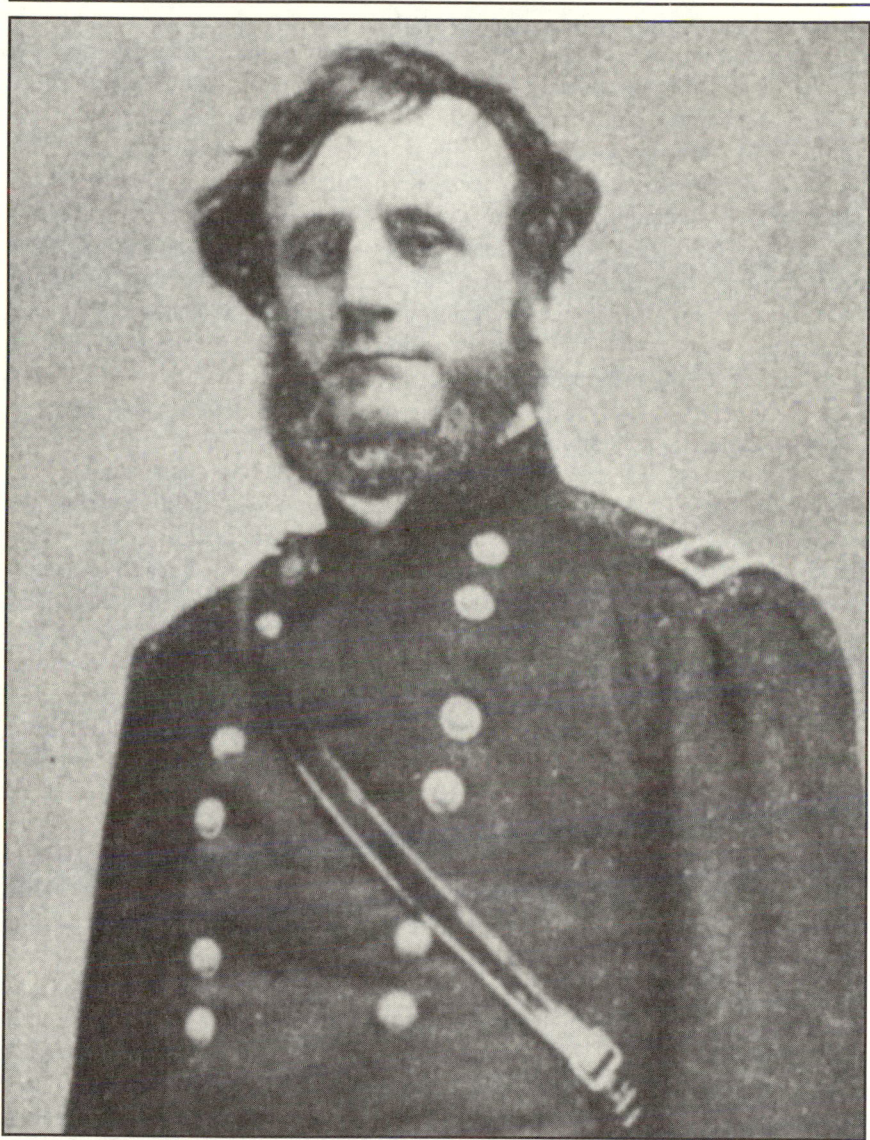

After urging President Lincoln to utilize Black troops in the Union Army, General Ullman was charged with organizing African American units. Some of the strongest resistance in marshalling routine support for Black units in the Union Army arose from the Medical Bureau. Secretary of War Stanton had to intervene, forcing this branch of the Army to render Ullmann reluctant medical support.

functioning of health and all other social systems. As Mohr pointed out, "In a purely physical sense, the already meager living standard of most slaves deteriorated even further during the war, particularly after 1861 when the Federal blockade tightened around Southern ports and local merchants exhausted stocks of Northern goods."[46] The breakdown of the Southern health system along with its economy and labor system energized a health crisis across the South. By 1863 starvation, poor housing, inadequate clothing, and inadequate sanitation became social problems with health care effects and implications throughout the South. The medically dependent slave population was adversely affected by these events.[47]

As slave nutritional status deteriorated, infectious diseases became more prevalent and epidemics of smallpox and measles appeared among the bondsmen. Increasingly, rural slaves were impressed for industrial labor, producing large numbers of previously rare occupationally related health problems. As Mohr noted, "The inexperience of many black workmen, together with less supervision and dangerous working conditions, resulted in a number of industrial accidents. Bondsmen fell from scaffolding, were struck by trains, and injured themselves while lifting heavy objects."[48] Thus, slave injury rates increased as the Southern health system collapsed around them. These trends were more severe in the rural areas and on the plantations than in the cities, where medical care was more readily available. The already sketchy infrastructure of the slave health subsystem became weaker and less functional and the health status of bondsmen deteriorated. The slave health subsystem, dependent on the planters' medicine chests and supplies, contracts with local back-up physicians, and attendance by the planters' wives or overseers, broke down as the war progressed. Moreover, most of the qualified physicians were serving in the Confederate Medical Corps, which by all descriptions rendered excellent service to the Confederate States Army. Their principal handicap was insufficient professional manpower and medical supplies.

The social disorganization and chaos generated by the war adversely affected everyone in the South. Economic collapse of the monoculture agricultural system based on chattel bondage, intensified by the depletion of an already sparse civilian physician population, created a hardship on the Southern health system. The difficulty in obtaining medicine because of the Union naval blockade exacerbated the ill effects. Even the industrial slaves employed at vital armaments factories, whose care was a direct responsibility of the Confederate government, were placed at greater medical risk as the war progressed. Slave hospitals became increasingly understaffed and hospital medications unavailable. Confederate officials recruited civilians to collect roots and herbs from which to make medicines. Conditions were so compromised that planters felt that sending slaves to the hospital was futile.[49]

The runaway slave population appeared at the doorsteps of the Union Army from the very beginning of the war. As Bremner noted in *The Public Good: Philanthropy and Welfare in the Civil War Era*, "Before the war was over nearly a quarter of a million former slaves came under direct control of military authorities and more than one million were within Union lines."[50] Running away from their plantations was a traumatic experience for the bondsmen, who often undertook dangerous and debilitating journeys to escape their masters. Not only did it mean leaving family and relations behind, but these trips were especially hard on slave children and the elderly. Upon arrival at Army facilities the ex-slaves were usually destitute and malnourished. They were not always well received, as Mohr observed about the Northern troops: "Many of the white enlisted men . . . surpassed Southern slaveowners in the depth of their anti-Negro sentiments. Reluctant liberators at best . . . troops greeted . . . bondsmen with profane epithets and physical abuse at least as often as they reached out to blacks in a spirit of brotherly concern."[51] The rations provided by the army and the private Northern voluntary agencies, such as the missionary associations, were enough to relieve the immediate deprivations of the slave refugees, but were never adequate to sustain the runaway slaves forced to linger around the camps.

Ex-slaves often received urgent health care services from Union military health personnel but were left on their own otherwise. Moreover, the commitment of the Union Army units to the welfare of the refugees varied with the attitudes of the commanding officers. Some, such as General Butler in New Orleans, were supportive of runaway ex-slaves from the very beginning. Others, such as General William Tecumsah Sherman, remained aloof and were occasionally hostile to what they sometimes considered slave interlopers and hindrances to their military operations. Sherman expounded on his legitimate concerns, stating, "We cannot now give tents to our soldiers and our wagon trains are a horrible impediment, and if we are to take along and feed the negroes who flee to us . . . it will be an impossible task."[52] Bremner commented on the sensitivity levels of Union commanders: "Providing shelter and rations for thousands of fugitive or abandoned slaves was an unwelcome and onerous burden for army commanders, who often lacked supplies for their troops and were more interested in getting on with the war than in devising relief and rehabilitation projects."[53] Lincoln anticipated the problems with refugee slaves as early as September 22, 1862, before issuing the preliminary Emancipation Proclamation. Afraid of the potential influx of ex-slave refugees, he queried, "What should we do with them? How can we feed and care for such a multitude?"[54] One major strategy was the establishment of contraband camps.[55]

The Union Army herded "former slaves into a series of 'contraband' camps scattered from the outskirts of Washington, D.C., down the Atlantic seaboard to South Carolina and along the Mississippi and its tributaries from Cairo, Illinois, to New Orleans,"[56] according to Bremner. Although a few of the camps were clean, organized, and well provided for, "Most of the camps . . . provided crowded, makeshift accommodations in which the refugees suffered and succumbed to exposure, unsanitary surroundings, lack of medical attention, and want of food and clothing."[57] One slave recalled his experience in one of these refugee camps, stating, "We was freed and went to a place that was full of people. We had to stay in a church with about twenty other people and two of the babies died on account of the exposure. Two of my aunts died, too, on account of exposure."[58] This was a typical experience.

Such circumstances meant that slaves may have often received services to meet their immediate crisis needs, but this did not bode well for the long-term health status or outcome of the ex-bondsmen. There is increasing evidence that morbidity and mortality rates were high in this segment of the Black population during the war. James Yeatman, an inspector for the Western Sanitary Commission, submitted a report concerning the horrible conditions at contraband camps at Helena, Arkansas, and other locations throughout the Mississippi Valley. "It would seem, now, that one-half are doomed to die in the process of freeing the rest,"[59] he wrote.

Free Blacks, already the least healthy American subpopulation, numbered approximately 480,000 by the onset of the Civil War. Virginia's 58,042 free Blacks were the largest concentration in any one state, with Maryland ranking second and North Carolina third. Locked in a world of segregation, discrimination, and economic exploitation buttressed by strictly enforced legal and social second-class citizenship, Blacks were overwhelmingly subject to poverty and illiteracy.

Free Blacks could theoretically vote in only five states by 1860. They could vote in Massachusetts, and in Maine, Vermont, New York, and New Hampshire suffrage applied if they met property requirements. Every free state admitted to the United States since 1819 had denied Blacks suffrage and severely limited or prohibited African American immigration. Blacks were denied employment and could only aspire to the most menial and unpleasant occupations. Whites refused to sit alongside them in schools, workplaces, or training programs. They were forced to live in the most undesirable and unhealthy neighborhoods.

Free Blacks were often denied access to health care even where it had been established for other poor populations. Some communities allowed Blacks access to public institutions such as almshouse hospitals or free clinics (e.g., New Orleans), but most did not (e.g., Nashville and Atlanta did not, while New York and Boston did only intermittently). Therefore, free Blacks suffered the highest morbidity and mortality rates. Theirs was a world of hostility and frustration. With education either segregated or unavailable and few menial occupations open to them, an 1819 valedictorian of a Negro school in New York City articulated the problem that still resonates today:

> Why should I strive hard and acquire all the constituents of a man, if the prevailing genius of the land admit me not as such, or but in an inferior degree! Pardon me if I feel insignificant and weak. . . . [W]hat are my prospects? To what shall I turn my hand? Shall I be a mechanic? No one will employ me; white boys won't work with me. Shall I be a merchant? No one will have me in his office; white clerks won't associate with me. Drudgery and servitude, then, are my prospective portion. Can you be surprised at my discouragement?[60]

Eighteenth-century discussions about colonizing free Blacks overseas had been begun earlier by Rhode Island Congregational minister Samuel Hopkins and by Thomas Jefferson. Previous efforts by the American Colonization Society (founded in 1816) to colonize the free Black population overseas had failed. Even President Lincoln's proposals to resettle Blacks in Africa or Central America met lukewarm receptions. Despite their gloomy circumstance and prospects, Black leaders encouraged African Americans to join the Union Army to participate in the fight for their freedom: "They responded to such appeals in astounding numbers. Constituting less than one percent of the North's population, blacks would make up nearly one-tenth of the northern army by the end of the war. Eighty-five percent of those eligible signed on."[61] A disproportionate number of free Blacks joined the Union Army and thus automatically enrolled themselves in another cohort of the African American health experience. Although wartime conditions precluded adequate health data collection, the period from April 12, 1861, through April 9, 1865, was a period of overall decline in Black health status.[62]

Black Health and the Reconstruction Era

The Reconstruction Era was a period of acute race conflict and the extension of postwar issues, turbulence, and concerns. The ascendancy of President Andrew Johnson transferred Southern attitudes and resentments from the war and the battlefield to the political arena. Rarely appreciated is the fact that the Reconstruction Era was the nadir of Black health in the United States. The country, especially the more urban North, was making a transition into the Gilded Age at the end of that period. Since health care activities involving most African Americans were lumped together with relief during this period, Reconstruction relief activities are a major focus in this section. Reconstruction, on the official governmental relief level, began in March 1865 with the passage of a compromise bill "which lumped supervision of refugees, freedmen, and abandoned lands in one agency located in the War Department."[63] Called the Freedmen's Bureau, Major General Oliver Howard, "whose reputation for piety had won him the sobriquet 'the Christian soldier'"[64] was appointed its head.

The next official milestone in Reconstruction history was the Congressional override of President Andrew Johnson's veto of a bill that extended the life of the Freedmen's Bureau for two years. The vote was held in July 1866, giving the bureau until January 1, 1869, "to complete all its activities except those connected with education and disbursement of moneys owed freedmen for military service."[65] The Army Appropriation Act of July 14, 1866, "recognizing the failure of land distribution as a source of income,"[66] granted the bureau approximately $8 million as a supplement.[67] Confronted with a total collapse of the postwar South, Congress adopted the basic Reconstruction Act on March 2, 1867. This resulted in the March 30 approval of a joint resolution expanding the Bureau's charge for the provision of relief without extra funding. After January 1, 1869, other than operating the educational and bounty divisions and the supervision of three hospitals and asylums, Freedmen's Bureau activities ceased. Congress terminated the Freedmen's Bureau in 1872, transferring responsibility for the Freedmen's Hospital in Washington, DC (which had already been transferred to Howard University's campus) to the Secretary of War.[68]

The Black health experience during Reconstruction is a far more human story. The precipitous and rapid deterioration in health status experienced by the Black population immediately after the war can be traced to a confluence of factors. The most important stem from slaveholders severing all ties with their former chattel. One ex-slave left this account in Ben Botkin's *Lay My Burden Down: A Folk History of Slavery*:

> When freedom came, my mama said Old Master called all of 'em to his house, and said, "You all free, we ain't got nothing to do with you no more. Go on away. We don't whup you no more, go on your way." My mama said they go on off, then they come back and stand around, just looking at him and Old Mistress. They give 'em something to eat and he say, "Go on away, you don't belong to us no more, You been freed." They go away and they kept coming back. They didn't have no place to go and nothing to eat. From what she said, they had a terrible time. She said it was bad times. Some took sick and had no 'tention and died. Seemed like it was four or five years before they got to places they could live. They all got scattered. . . . Old Master every time they go back say, "You all go on away. You been set free. You have to look out for yourselves now."[69]

Circumstances were exacerbated by the fact that Negro slaves in the United States were freed with no education, financial means, and very limited skills for a competitive market. Male heads of slave families were promised small land grants taken from confiscated and abandoned Confederate lands left with the Army. This promise was broken by the same government that gave away millions of both dollars and acres of land to giant corporations for railroad and commercial development. Millions more acres were given to White settlers in the West. Thus denied a promised toehold in agriculture, the slaves entered a highly competitive job market illiterate and with few marketable skills. These disadvantages were compounded by rampant racial discrimination. Du Bois objectively evaluated slave craftsmen as a paradigm of Black preparedness relative to the workers they faced in the free and competitive job market:

> The slave artisan was rather a jack-of-all-trades than a mechanic in the modern sense of the term — he could build a barn, make a barrel, mend an umbrella or shoe a horse. Exceptional slaves did the work exceptionally well, but the average workman was poor, careless and ill-trained,

> *and could not have earned living wages under modern competitive conditions.*[70]

One must also recall that such craftsmen were well prepared compared to the average ex-slave who had been a field hand. Exacerbating this situation was the fact that only 5 percent of ex-slaves could read and write. Bremner sketches out the paradoxical ways peace worsened the situation of the freedmen in *The Public Good:* "The immediate effect of peace was to increase rather than lessen the sufferings of freedmen."[71]

Black "contrabands" who held government jobs during the war were left stranded and unemployed when the Army demobilized. Civilian "contraband" camp jobs and military hospital jobs that had employed thousands of freedmen disappeared. The slave health subsystem abandoned the newly freed slaves. Bremner described this dissolution: "The old, infirm, and mentally defective no longer had any claim to support by former masters, who, even if charitably disposed, had no means to help."[72] This was exacerbated by a large population of orphan children, not "owned" by anyone, who were too young to work.

Between the Emancipation Proclamation and the Confederate surrender at Appomattox, more than 1 million slaves were freed in one way or another. With the adoption of the Thirteenth Amendment and the ending of the war, another 3 million were emancipated. As Morais portrayed the situation in *The History of the Negro in Medicine:*

> *With the countryside desolated—farms abandoned, bridges destroyed, river levees broken, railroads ruined—tens of thousands of emancipated slaves wandered about uprooted. . . . Free from the old quarter that once gave them shelter and a modicum of health care, they were turned loose, ill-clad, hungry and destitute, waiting and ever hoping.*[73]

These traumatic dislocations were accentuated by starvation, crowding in temporary refugee camps, and horrible sanitation conditions.

The exact numbers of deaths, illnesses, births, and epidemics documenting the health experience of the freedmen were not collected. However, accounts and sporadic data and surveys collected by local communities yield a vivid impression of the devastating health effects the Reconstruction wrought on African Americans. Morais summed up the accounting of that health experience: "From these and other figures, it is estimated that in some crowded and unhealthy Southern communities from one-quarter to one-third of the former slaves died during the first years of the Reconstruction."[74] Such mortality figures from a modern perspective are devastating. Black/White differences in mortality in cities such as Charleston, South Carolina, and Selma, Alabama, also indicate that the health gap between the races increased during this period. General conditions and health status were so bad in the refugee and contraband

Black populations that the situation alarmed the U.S. Congress, according to historians such as Herbert Morais and Howard Ashley White. As a result, "The gravity of the situation goaded a reluctant Congress to pass unprecedented legislation that was a significant forerunner of the disaster relief of the twentieth century."[75] Congress was virtually frightened by adverse Black health status and death rates into passing health care relief legislation. That evidence of this catastrophe was occurring on Congress's doorstep in Alexandria, Virginia, and Washington, DC, no doubt added urgency to the situation.

Epidemics of smallpox, yellow fever, and cholera swept through the South, including Washington, DC. They differentially devastated African American populations. Mortality rates for Black children were two to three times as high as those for White children. Tuberculosis was one of the worst predators in the Black community, with mortality rates reaching at least four times as high among African Americans as Whites. Black communities with horrible deficiencies of food, shelter, and clothing served as breeding grounds for the spread of this "white plague."[76]

A response from both the government and private sectors was mounted. In health care, the governmental response was the most important. As a result of Freedmen's Bureau programs, hospitals and clinics were established throughout entire areas affected by the war. Accounts tabulate that as many as 100 Freedman's hospitals were established from Washington, DC, to New Orleans, Louisiana. They were manned by civilian bureau physicians supplemented by local practitioners where they were available. The War Department was also charged with the responsibility of supplying physicians to the Freedmen's Bureau, but this seldom happened because of the demands of providing medical support to White military units in the field.

Financial constraints meant that Freedmen's Bureau health facilities were often dilapidated, makeshift, and marginal. However, they did offer, for the first time in the nation's history, a network of institutions serving African Americans with direct ties to the mainstream health system. The Bureau's focus was on serving the health needs of free, though impoverished, Black populations. This also symbolized the assumption of a new and unprecedented governmental responsibility in the future. These institutions, along with their affiliated outpatient facilities, provided more than 1 million medical treatments to freedmen and refugees over the five or so years of their existence.* In spite of this mighty effort, there were never adequate health services available. Although many of the Freedmen's Bureau hospital facilities were dirty, poorly maintained, and laced with corruption, they performed a yeomen service and probably blunted worst-case outcomes that would have occurred had they not been available.

---

*Although the Freedmen's Bureau health activities were officially stopped in 1872 with the transfer of Freemen's Hospital to the Secretary of War, the active network of hospitals and clinics were terminated in January 1, 1869, and phased out by 1870.

Significantly, these developments established a tradition among African Americans of the presence of hands-on health institutions founded and based on the needs and experiences of the Black community. This paradigm was emulated for the next 100 years, grounded in Black community self-help and the crushing health needs of the African American population. In the interim, many of the medical-social and public health lessons taught by the Civil War and Reconstruction were lost on the federal government, which dismantled its successful health programs. With the exception of Freedmen's Hospital in Washington, DC, congressional termination of all Freedmen's Bureau activities in 1872 ended a cost-effective, humane, epidemiologically sound health care experiment. It was too small, underfunded throughout its existence, and stopped far too soon, considering the realities of the U.S. medical-social environment, to have a permanent positive impact on Black health. Although the political and military aspects of the Reconstruction continued for another five years, the curtain came down on the most far-reaching and prescient health care program ever undertaken for African Americans.

Government withdrawal of concern and activity focused on Black health would defer to the private institutional sector to make the next strides toward a healthy African America. The overall result was perpetuation of a segregated and discriminatory "mainstream" health system and the formation of a racially separate and inferior "Negro medical ghetto" that lasted and served the Black population until the late twentieth century. The Civil War and Reconstruction did not emancipate Blacks in terms of health; the slave health deficit continued and in some ways deepened as the United States entered the Gilded Age.[77]

Black Health in the Gilded Age

The Gilded Age, covering the years 1870–1890, was a period of societal reaction and a general return to conservative, private sector politics and public policy. The vast reliance on government, represented by the Civil War and beneficial aid programs such as the Freedmen's Bureau health programs, ended. Covenants between Northern corporate forces in alliance with the Republican Party and Southern Democrat Redeemers representing post–Civil War planter-capitalists led to the Hayes-Tilden Compromise of 1876–1877. This handed Rutherford Hayes the presidency (1877–1881) even though he lost the popular vote. The essence of this massive political sell-out for power was that Union troops, who enforced civil rights, suffrage, and protective laws for Blacks, would be withdrawn from the South. Second, the federal government would turn a blind eye to events in the South and no longer concern itself with law enforcement or suffrage in that region. Third, a bevy of Southerners would be appointed to the Supreme Court and presidential cabinet. Fourth, Southern capitalists would be allowed to feed at the government trough for the first time since the Civil War.

What this intricate and multifaceted deal also meant was that it was open season on Blacks throughout the new White South. This was accompanied by blotting out the protections of the Fourteenth and Fifteenth Amendments by the Supreme Court rulings in *United States v. Cruikshank* (1875) and *United States v. Reese* (1876).[78] In *United States v. Cruikshank* the Supreme Court ruled that "the right of suffrage is not a necessary attribute of national citizenship," and in the conviction of the Louisiana rioters who had broken up a Black political rally, the plaintiffs had to prove they were harassed by the White mob because of their race. Moreover, the mob was a group of private individuals, not the state, and thus was not "state action." Only state action was covered by the Fourteenth and Fifteenth Amendments. In *United States v. Reese* the U.S. Supreme Court ruled that the Fifteenth Amendment was not a positive grant allowing Congress to regulate or control all state interference with a citizen's right to vote. Reese had to prove he was denied that right by the state of Kentucky solely because of his race. The reinstitution of the new "Black codes," the new sharecropping system, and new prison labor systems was also tantamount to the revocation of the Thirteenth Amendment, which abolished slavery. Black public accommodations rights would be lost and legal racial segregation established in *Plessy v. Ferguson* (1896)[79] before the Gilded Age and Progressive eras were over.

These events had drastic effects on the newly freed Black population. Around the turn of the century most African Americans would lose their right to vote. A rigid caste system based on race, unprecedented in the Western world until post–World War II South Africa, would be instituted. Black labor would be ruthlessly exploited and African Americans subjugated to social and economic peonage. The subjugation would be enacted by keeping the African American from voting "by force, by economic intimidation, by propaganda designed to lead him to believe that there was no salvation for him in political lines but that he must depend entirely upon thrift, and the good will of his white employers,"[80] according to Du Bois.

A reign of political and physical terror would be implemented and institutionalized throughout the South, increasingly buttressed by the legal and law enforcement establishments. Black leadership was intimidated into accommodation, and they redirected Black efforts away from participation and political representation toward industrial education and work. All the events represented by this multipronged assault on African Americans adversely affected the health system and Black health.[81]

The policy implementing a virtual health system apartheid, begun during the Reconstruction Era, became institutionalized during the Gilded Age. Reconstruction, including Freedmen's Bureau health programs, had offered the medical profession and the rest of the health system an opportunity to choose a progressive course. After the breakdown of the Southern health system and its slave health subsystem appendage, responsibility for Black health could have been assumed directly by either government or responsible private institutions. The network of

100 or more Freedmen's Bureau hospitals and clinics already established and functioning by the late 1860s was being operated and subsidized by a network of voluntary abolitionist and missionary associations. With appropriate leadership and policies a decent health infrastructure could have been built upon this foundation. The indirect strategy eventually chosen, which generated separate health professions and institutions, could have been integrated into such a system. However, such a direct health policy approach was rejected.

An indirect strategic approach to the Black health problem, which emphasized and cultivated racial isolation, separateness, and health system disparities was chosen. Such a strategy perpetuated the "difference" between the races from a health policy and institutional perspective and assuaged the U.S. health system's prejudiced medical-social attitudes regarding race and class. Moreover, it was predicated on almost complete withdrawal of mainstream White health system concern or support. With this approach, at least two levels of health care, health funding, and quality of care could be maintained, with Blacks and the poor continuing to receive the short end of the stick. The fact that these were the sicker populations did not matter. In fact, "coddling" these underprivileged classes with better medical care simply facilitated the survival and propagation of greater numbers of the "unfit," according to the increasingly popular Social Darwinism of the period. It took two White males who had been directly involved in Black health care delivery during the Civil War to appreciate the plight and crisis represented by Black health after the war—General Oliver Howard and George Whipple Hubbard. Their efforts forever changed the course of Black health and medical-social history in the United States.

General Oliver Howard was the commissioner of the Freedmen's Bureau from 1865 to 1874. He was as aware as anyone of the horrible state of Black health and the inadequacies of the system to deal with the problem. A New England Congregationalist born in Leeds, Maine, Howard had strong ties with the Christian missionary movement through the American Missionary Association. A graduate of Bowdoin College and the Military Academy at West Point (1845), he took command of the Maine volunteers in 1861 at the outbreak of the Civil War. By 1864, he commanded the Army of Tennessee. He led the right wing of Sherman's military march to the sea.

Howard witnessed the racist policies and practices of the Medical Bureau of the War Department regarding the provision of health care for Black Union soldiers. He experienced firsthand White physicians who refused assignment to Black units or to practice alongside Black physicians. He was aware of refusals by local city and county governments such as Nashville, Tennessee, and New Orleans, Louisiana, to assume responsibility for adopting vital public health programs and the care of destitute Black patients when Freedmen's Bureau programs were shutting down. Most important, he witnessed the suffering and excess deaths Blacks were experiencing because of these health policies and practices. Such human tragedies impressed Howard and guided his activities during and after the war. He was sensitized to the special medical and medical-social needs of the Black population.[82]

George Whipple Hubbard, the other White male protagonist in this sad but heroic drama, was born in Charleston, New Hampshire, with an abolitionist background. He was ideally suited to serve as one of the last of a generation of abolitionist missionary educators endowed with, as Hubbard would have said, the God-given mission of uplifting their Black brethren. Hubbard joined the Union Army, serving as what would be considered today a medical corpsman. He also had a background as a teacher. Typically, during wartime or military engagement, medical corpsmen (medics) were assigned to the "front line" of health care in Army units. Working in both field units and urban headquarters, young Hubbard witnessed all dimensions of the freedmen's health dilemma. After Congress effectively closed down the Freedmen's Bureau in 1869, Hubbard then witnessed the health care degradation of the large ex-slave population in Nashville, Tennessee. James Summerville relates Dr. Hubbard's experiences with Black patients: "Forced by poverty to live in the filthiest places in an unclean city, uneducated in health matters, and without doctors to treat them, blacks died in numbers far in excess of their proportion in the population. The mortality of black infants was also markedly greater than that of white infants."[83] Moreover, the city had closed the public hospital and disbanded the Board of Health by 1876. As Summerville relates and historian Don H. Doyle corroborates, "Nashville had the highest death rate of any city in the United States . . . and, of those reporting, the fifth highest in the world."[84] Hubbard was moved by the circumstances and suffering he witnessed; possessing a background of positive experiences with Black people through his teaching and medical service, he felt that training African American nurses and physicians was imperative for improving the health and medical care for Blacks. He earned a medical degree from Vanderbilt University Medical School in 1875 as a step toward fulfilling his dream. These events planted the seeds and supplied the roots for the Black educational activities that would dominate the rest of Dr. Hubbard's life.[85]

Both men had firsthand experience with the Black health crisis of that period, characterized by a rapid, war-related exacerbation of the slave health deficit. Both appreciated that the very survival of the Black population was at risk and that the health policies in effect at that time were insufficient to deal with the problem. The nation had rejected the idea of improving African American health by establishing conventional levels of White health professions personnel and institutions at the end of the war. Even Howard had been wary of encouraging African American dependency based on his Freedmen's Bureau leadership, as Bremner noted: "Like most of his countrymen in his own day and since, Howard had ambivalent feelings toward relief. Sympathetic and eager to respond to the need of 'our destitute wards,' he was suspicious of fraud and feared imposition."[86]

General Howard's hunch was right. Strains of Puritanism, Calvinist finger-pointing, and principles of Christian self-reliance regarding the poor and underprivileged are deep currents within the American character. As Churchill and others have subsequently pointed out, the provision of a publicly funded and operated charity health system for Blacks and the poor was probably unfeasible and unable to generate popular support at the time in spite of the successful example provided by the Freedmen's Bureau health programs. By contrast, Howard and Hubbard's vision, though ultimately suggesting popular self-reliant directions, was much more limited and individualistic in tone. Both men felt that training Black physicians and nurses to care for African Americans was an obtainable and viable approach to solving, or at least addressing, the Black health problem.

Both men founded Black medical colleges that eventually expanded into training in other health professions such as nursing, pharmacy, and dentistry. General Howard was a vital force in initiating and establishing the Medical Department of Howard University in 1868 in Washington, DC. Simultaneously, Dr. Hubbard initiated the process leading to the opening of Meharry Medical College of Central Tennessee College in 1876 in Nashville. Howard was the nation's first medical school open for admission to all minority groups, while Meharry was the nation's first medical school whose chief aim was the training of African American physicians.[87]

Most Black communities were denied any health facilities at all by the 1890s. Those that did allow a Black presence were rigidly segregated. Hospitals that admitted Black patients placed them in inferior outbuildings, attics, or basements. African American physicians were not allowed on hospital staffs, and professional standards were lowered when applied to Black patients even in the same facilities.

Most White doctors wouldn't treat Black patients. The few that did were often the marginal practitioners. For example, in 1883 in Charleston, South Carolina, Kenneth Manning described Dr. T. B. McDow in his book *Black Apollo of Science:* "He was one of the few white doctors who would treat poor blacks."[88] McDow's career was marked by a murder trial, expulsion from the county medical society, suspected sexual dalliances, practicing "under a cloud of suspicion,"[89] and eventual suicide. However, there was little choice for Black patients because, "In 1883 medical care was sadly lacking in the black community. . . . [T]here were few black doctors."[90] The new flowering of Black medical and health professions schools provided some partial solutions to these problems.[91]

Black Health Enters the Progressive Era

If the Gilded Age portended bad times for Blacks, the last decade of the nineteenth century lived up to its dour predictions. The Progressive Era, encompassing the years between 1890 and 1920, did not, contrary to its label, bring social, political, or programmatic progress to African Americans. Instead, the designation refers to a 30-year period of aggressive social and political intervention by White Americans, largely from the rich and powerful classes, who assumed that through the application of scientific and social knowledge they could solve the nation's social and financial problems. Their assumptions of White superiority and non-White inferiority remained intact. For African Americans the period represents one of the most racially oppressive episodes in the nation's history. A nation already inflicting punishment on a disadvantaged ex-slave population since 1870 almost unconsciously seemed to channel all its energies and newly acquired skills into its oppressive task.

Blacks, projected since the end of Reconstruction as an unimportant group relegated to the background of American life, now presented on center stage to suffer public abuse. As America entered the 1890s Benjamin Brawley, a scholar of this period, related in A Social History of the American Negro that "The Negro was already down; he was now to be trampled upon."[92] In 1886, in New York, Henry W. Grady, the prominent Atlanta Constitution newspaper editor and part owner, preached a doctrine of "The New South." He convinced the nation that the South was on the move politically and economically and that the Black problem was a local issue the North had concerned itself with for too long. The North was relieved and receptive to his message. For example, the Southern veneer of fairness enforced by the federal government was now stripped away as the state of Mississippi in 1892 protested the federal government's standard flood disaster relief for Black farmers. Southerners feared it would protect Blacks from economic intimidation and would encourage Blacks to reject miserly White planter buyouts for their farms. Booker T. Washington, in a series of speeches between 1894 and 1904, emerged as the new Black leader replacing Frederick Douglass, who died in February 1895. As Rayford Logan noted, "The Atlanta Compromise" speech delivered on November 18, 1895, marked Washington's ascendancy: "The national fame that Washington achieved overnight by his Atlanta speech constitutes an excellent yardstick for measuring the victory of 'The New South,' since he accepted a subordinate place for Negroes in American life."[93] Washington need not have delivered African Americans to the White South. The courts and the political system were already doing it. Disenfranchisement, beginning with Mississippi in 1890 and South Carolina in 1895 as examples, culminated in stripping away the Negro vote over the entire South. As a result, North Carolina's George H. White, whose term ended in 1901, would be the last of 22 Blacks since Reconstruction to serve in the U.S. Congress until the mid–twentieth century. Federal, state, and local court decisions stripped away Black public accommodations, voting, property, and civil rights. These events, along with the dissolution of the biracial Republican Party and institutionalization of the "solid South," placed African Americans back into virtual bondage.[94]

With regard to health care, the strategies suggested by General Howard, first president of Howard University between 1869 and 1874, and Dr. Hubbard, Meharry's founder, were successful. The production of Black health professionals yielded very positive results. Despite the desperate health conditions in which many African Americans found themselves as they entered the 1890s, there had been some health progress. In virtually all other areas they had been stripped of most of the material or human progress obtained by the Civil War or the Reconstruction.

Benjamin Brawley said that, by the beginning of the Progressive Era, "the pendulum had swung fully backward, and the years from 1890 to 1895 were in some ways the darkest that the race has experienced since emancipation."[95] Lynch law and the Democrats were in force, and by February 1893, Black lynching occurred almost daily. In this negative social environment it is truly amazing that African Americans obtained training and practiced medicine. Moreover, according to the historic accomplishments of the new cadre of African American physicians such as Daniel Hale Williams, Robert Fulton Boyd, and Nathan Frances Mossell, many were practicing it excellently.[96]

By 1900, there were more than 1,000 Black physicians practicing in the United States. Moreover, there were eight active Black medical schools, at least nine nursing schools, and at least two dental and pharmacy schools producing African American health professionals annually. As the work of physicians such as J. Edward Perry, R. F. Boyd, and George Cleveland Hall demonstrate, their active participation in placing Black health on the community agenda and upgrading health knowledge and awareness levels may have been as valuable to African Americans as their vital technical medical accomplishments. After being rebuffed several times during the Gilded Age by the American Medical Association (AMA), a Black medical profession organized nationally, forming the National Medical Association (NMA) in 1895. It also organized professionally at state and local levels. Although the Black physicians and the few Black hospitals they were opening could not completely reverse the horrible health outcomes African Americans were experiencing, they certainly upgraded the quality of medical life several notches in the Black community and began providing the medical leadership and organization required to address the black health crisis in the future.[97]

Health System Heal Thyself

The Civil War dramatically expanded the quality and capacity of the U.S. health system. As Novotny and Smith noted, "Although the Civil War records are not precise, the North reported 359,528 killed and 246,712 wounded, and the South 258,000 killed and 200,000 wounded."[98] A health system able to meet such a challenge had become formidable and was acknowledged as such by authoritative European academic physician Rudolf Virchow (1821–1902). Writing about U.S. Surgeon Generals Barnes and Crane's impressive *Medical and Surgical History of the War of the Rebellion* (1870–1888), Virchow noted:

> *Whoever takes up and reads the extensive publications of the American medical staff will be constantly astonished at the wealth of experience therein found. The greatest exactness in detail, careful statistics even in*

> *the smallest matters, and a scholarly statement embracing all sides of medical experience are here united in order to preserve and transmit . . . the knowledge purchased at so vast an expense.*[99]

Before the war the U.S. Army had virtually no hospitals or ambulances. With the aid of and coordination by the U.S. Sanitary Commission, hospitals and ambulances were systematically put into service. Similar efforts took place in the Confederacy under the direction of Dr. Samuel Preston Moore. By 1863, at the Battle of Gettysburg, the Union Army for the first time was able to retrieve and rescue, transport, and house thousands of battlefield casualties on the same day of the battle. Although handicapped by fiscal restraints, the Confederate Medical Corps performed just as well, if not better, until the end of the war. At the end of the war, both governments possessed impressive strings of field hospitals and health services delivery systems. Overall, not only had the health system performed impressively, it had reached another level of sophistication and changed forever the conception of the capabilities of the United States' health system.

As stated, the health system did not perform as well for Black Union soldiers, who suffered higher mortality rates, medical neglect, and medical abuse at the hands of unqualified medical personnel. In the South there was a sizable number of Blacks placed under the care of the Confederate Medical Corps as slaves working in war plants, on fortifications, and in hospitals. They too received lesser services compared to White personnel, and this neglect became very prominent near the war's end when Confederate medical supplies and resources ran thin. Black Union Army prisoners captured by Confederates were at the mercy of a government whose official policy until late in the war when Southern defeat appeared imminent was to re-enslave or murder them.[100]

While the U.S. health system did itself credit from technical and medical standpoints, it also took on the medical-social challenge of concerning itself for the first time with the overall health care needs and concerns of Black and underprivileged populations. Moreover, it approached these problems in new and different ways. Wartime necessities channeled the health system into modes of medical-social egalitarianism and high-priority health system involvement with indigent care. This was unprecedented in the nation's history in both the North and South. Regrettably, these positive lessons, which temporarily addressed some of the race and class problems in the health system, would be neither permanent nor long-lasting.

Another direct result of the war was that the Southern health system almost totally disintegrated. After simultaneously undergoing a rebirth and redirection back into the biomedical mainstream under wartime pressures, the Southern health system ended its 40-year detour into Southern distinctiveness.* Second,

---

*For example, one antebellum medical-professional movement alleged that Southern health environments, medical conditions, and patient populations (e.g., Black slaves) were so different that distinct training, diagnostic procedures, and medical therapeutics were called for.

the Southern health system allowed its own slave health subsystem to die a nat-ural death. However, one of the new consolidated health system's major failures was in not defining or creating an alternative. As this health system consolidation and expansion evolved under the duress of war, African American health emerged as a national problem requiring a response. Whites knew that totally neglected African American health would inevitably affect European Americans unfavorably through epidemics and disease transmission. This forced the system to fundamentally redefine itself and its institutions—if only on a temporary basis.

Was the health system to become an instrument of service to the entire com-munity serving a greater national good? Or was it to remain the exclusive tool of the privileged classes at both patient and professional levels? After a late start, would the progressive public health lessons drilled into the system by the sanita-tion commissions and the War Department be incorporated into the nation's health policy after the war? After the demise of the Freedmen's Bureau at the end of the Reconstruction, the U.S. health system deferred these questions for another century until they exploded into the twentieth-century consciousness during the Black Civil Rights and poor people's movements.[101]

In the nineteenth century, the U.S. health system had not matured into the multicomponent megastructure with the capacity for generating $1.5 trillion budgets and threatening to consume up to one-fifth of the nation's economic out-put. The Civil War had a great deal to do with creating many of the modern-day system characteristics recognizable today. During many decades following the war, the U.S. health system turned into a massive, multilayered, and interactive social mechanism designed to do many other things in addition to delivering health care. It evolved into a major corporate infrastructure, becoming a darling of Wall Street profiteers by the mid–twentieth century and a major U.S. growth industry with the potential to lead the nation's export economy into the twenty-first century, and it became a major scientific focus of biomedical research and technology, a defining element in a society medicalizing both its living space and workplaces. Charting its transformation into a major industry and cultural force in the United States is one critical focus of this study. Paul Starr, Eli Ginzberg, Vic-tor R. Fuchs, E. Richard Brown, Rosemary Stevens, Victor and Ruth Sidel, Charles Rosenberg, and Marc Roberts have explored many of the fundamental developments of this transformation. We do not intend to retrace covered ground. This work is simply a beginning effort to address some of the race and class dimen-sions of the U.S. health system that these scholars have not dealt with.[102]

The Civil War and its aftermath marked the beginning of the U.S. health sys-tem's exponential growth toward its immense size and complexity. For the first time familiar institutional networks, characteristics, and functions emerged that are recognizable today. Breaking this complex infrastructure into functional components is an invaluable and appropriate analytical tool. The U.S. health delivery system has structural components consisting of: (1) health care institu-tions such as hospitals; (2) health professions personnel such as physicians, dentists, and nurses; (3) a health professions education and research infrastructure; (4) state and local government functions related to health care; (5) outpatient facilities; (6) voluntary agencies; (7) the federal government and the health care system; (8) the pharmaceutical industry and medical supply and equipment industry; (9) the health care financing and insurance industry; and (10) the health care review and control infrastructure. This work extends the application of *component analysis* to the discipline of historiography.[103]

Some of these components, taken for granted today, were unrecognizable in the nineteenth century. For example, no structured and formal health care financing industry or review and control infrastructures, as we know them today, were identifiable near the turn of the century. Since the late nineteenth century, outpatient facilities have changed in character and have become so variegated that, with the exception of a few city hospital clinics, there are few discernible traces of the dispensaries and outpatient facilities of the past. In contrast, other components of the health system, such as the health institutional infrastructure, composed primarily of hospitals, became recognizable and began evolving into the dominant entity it is today.[104]

The Civil War represented the coming of age for hospitals in the United States. Modern hospital development had grown into a movement in Western Europe in the late eighteenth and early nineteenth centuries. The French Revolution is often arbitrarily used as the starting point. The Revolutionary and Napoleonic eras actually marked a renaissance in Western medicine. It was a unique period characterized by the discarding of medical dogma along with a simultaneous emphasis on hospital-based health care as a military, and later social, necessity. Nothing was taken for granted, and French empiricism guided scientific investigation. Statistical and hospital-based clinical methods, under physicians such as Louis, disproved the efficacy of medicine's traditional therapies. A generation of therapeutic nihilism resulted in Europe. Meanwhile, modern teaching hospitals such as the 30 great hospitals in Paris—including the Hotel Dieu, St. Louis, and the Salpetriere, with more than 20,000 beds; London, with Guy's and Saint Bartholomew's; and Vienna's Allgemeines Krankenhaus— became the foci of nineteenth-century medical progress.

A distinguishing characteristic of the modern hospital was the dominance of physicians and medical needs in the shaping of its institutional character. Many of the old domiciliary and stewardship functions were relegated to other institutions such as nursing homes, orphanages, isolation facilities, almshouses, and poorhouses. Even the traditional policies of screening out the terminally or chronically ill were more strictly enforced, emphasizing the new preoccupation with medical cures. Much of the granting of this new medical authority was related to real or perceived scientific medical advance by laypeople supporting hospital construction and operation. Deference to a scientific medical profession was rendered rational. Late nineteenth-century breakthroughs such as Pasteur and Koch's proof of the germ theory; successful treatment of rabies, syphilis, and diphtheria; and the efficacy of vaccinations impressed the public with the authority and progress of medical science. Safe and pain-free surgery augmented the public's regard for scientific, hospital-based medicine.

The U.S. response to this burgeoning international modern hospital movement and biomedical scientific explosion had unique characteristics. First and most important, America was very slow to respond to these new advances. Hospital expansion is one example. As Rosenberg notes in *The Care of Strangers*, "In 1873, the first American hospital survey located only 178, including mental institutions; they contained a total of less than fifty thousand beds."[105] By the early nineteenth century Paris alone contained nearly 30,000 hospital beds. The United States was also slow to adopt clinical hospital medicine and formal medical school curriculums as necessities for teaching medicine.

Only medical schools in Philadelphia and New Orleans around the time of the Civil War fully utilized clinical hospital medicine as a full-fledged teaching resource. These cities with their networks of hospitals served as magnets for young White physicians-in-training who could afford the time and expense of prolonged training cycles while generating no income. In fact, some institutions required trainees to pay them for the privilege of working there. However, by the 1890s even America began responding to the allure and promise of scientific medicine. A dramatic and discernible proliferation of a health care institutional infrastructure, increasingly dominated by hospitals, developed nationally. Meanwhile, the American medical profession's perpetuation of the society's segregated and discriminatory racial practices within the health system, including the emerging network of hospitals, was never questioned.[106]

Not all of the impetus for the growth of the hospital infrastructure came from science or education. By the late nineteenth century, White middle-class Americans began to think of hospital care as acceptable based on self-interest. As Vogel stated in *The Invention of the Modern Hospital*, "Social and medical realities were leading to the gradual but inevitable disappearance of prejudice regarding treatment in hospitals for all classes."[107] This change was energized by social and psychological as well as technological factors.

In burgeoning cities such as Boston, New York, and Philadelphia, exploding apartment house, boarding house, and lodging house populations made home care both remote and impractical for large numbers of Americans. For instance, 1885 Massachusetts census data found 15,938 boarders and 24,280 lodgers in Boston. By 1895 these figures were 9,496 and 44,926, respectively—a decline in boarders of 68 percent and an increase in lodgers of 85 percent. This represented a 35 percent increase in potential patients without homes in which to provide their illness care. It also represented a qualitative shift, from more household-connected boarders having a closer relationship to their landlords and receiving their meals, lodging, and often some illness care, to lodgers who only received a roof over their heads.

As Vogel pointed out, "The New York hospital survey recommended that the city's growing apartment population be considered as creating a disproportionate need for hospitals."[108] These dramatic demographic shifts and their sociological implications, as U.S. urbanization increased profoundly, altered the health care delivery environment. Mechanisms necessary to provide care for growing urban, industrialized populations dictated hospital development.[109]

As has been stated, community leaders and local governments had been providing health care for the poor since the seventeenth century in English North America. Almshouses, pesthouses, or poorhouses were the earliest identifiable institutions heavily committed to the delivery of health care. State and local governments, therefore, had been strongly involved in health care since the Colonial Era. As Paul Starr observed in *The Social Transformation of American Medicine:*

> *Some communities paid for medical treatment of the poor and maintained hospitals and pesthouses for contagious disease; some states gave small subsidies to medical schools, and by 1860 all the older states had constructed at least one mental asylum. The federal government maintained a limited system of compulsory hospital insurance for merchant seamen. But these functions were the extent of state intervention in the economics of medicine before the Civil War.[110]*

A new private hospital sector combined with the centuries-old public hospital network to push the United States along the road to modern hospital dominance that is seen today. Racial segregation of the new hospital system was almost universal.[111]

The medical profession and the medical education and research infrastructures began to come of age in the late nineteenth century. Physicians continued their efforts to regulate medical practice. Massachusetts had made some efforts to protect the public from quack doctors as early as 1649. In emulation of Europeans, this "paralleled the provisions of the 1649 Massachusetts law, the 1518 charter of the Royal College of Physicians in London, and the 1511 statute of Henry VIII that regulated provincial English practice."[112] These New England practitioners proposed a more comprehensive body of medical regulation in 1738.

Other states such as New York and New Jersey engaged in similar regulatory and medical licensing activities. Interestingly, initial attempts to regulate medicine and create medical standards failed. The American public of the eighteenth and early nineteenth centuries was unwilling to grant the medical profession the cultural authority to oversee the health care system at the legal and regulatory levels. Moreover, granting such authority to a trained cadre of elite physicians chafed at American ideals of egalitarianism and untrammeled opportunity. The public felt that the profession did not deserve such authority and that such actions would eventually limit entry into the profession based on class and restrict access to care for the general public.

The Jacksonian Period became the nadir of medical regulation in the United States, as Starr described: "[A]fter the collapse of licensure in the 1830s and

1840s, the state had almost nothing to do with the private transactions between medical practitioners and their patients."[113] As part of the Jacksonian attacks on elitism at personal and professional levels, many states repealed medical licensing laws and lifted restrictions on medical practice. Repeals occurred in the District of Columbia, Massachusetts, Maine, Connecticut, Illinois, Ohio, Mississippi, Maryland, Texas, Michigan, South Carolina, and New York between 1826 and 1845. In response to this potentially dangerous development, physicians increasingly organized at local and regional levels, eventually resulting in the founding of the AMA in 1847. Blacks were not in the position, nor were they allowed, to participate in these activities at any level.[114]

During the Civil War dramatic changes in the relationship of government to health care occurred. For the first time in U.S. history local government agencies took a back seat to federal governmental efforts to provide health care for both the Army and needy populations. Additionally, many benevolent society health programs developed significant roles in health care regulation and delivery. These programs were especially prominent in the North, where organizations benefitted from a windfall of increased funding during the war. The wartime emergency blurred class divisions and promulgated the provision of health care for all segments of society—including African Americans. Not only was national government care provided to Union Army troops, but the Freedmen's Bureau also expended up to 25 percent of its resources on health care. This massive effort has been described in great detail earlier in the chapter. Other developments that occurred after the war are more germane to this discussion.

In the North many of the public health efforts, especially voluntary activities, were redirected toward the war effort. After the war ended in 1865, most local health functions resumed where they had left off. Some of the Northern personnel and volunteers were now much more qualified and competent in public health matters and administration due to their wartime experience. Their greater expertise and influence led to their increased impact on public health. However, the South was a different matter. The South was relatively backward in implementing social service and public education programs compared to the North. Any type of government intervention in health care, which was already limited in the United States, was particularly scarce in the post–Civil War South.

On a national level, the federal government had been involved in provision of health services to the merchant marines since 1798 and had begun a few limited public health programs before the Civil War. At the state level, states would not even maintain medical licensing laws or educational standards. Traditions established by the English poor laws meant that some welfare services, including some health care, were provided for the poor at the local level though the range and quality of services differed for the "worthy" and "unworthy" poor. City and county governments along with community leaders and religious organizations considered the provision of these basic components of welfare as part of their stewardship. Though not as advanced as most Northern communities, many

Southern cities felt compelled to become involved in such activities during the Antebellum Period. However, the relationships regarding the social welfare institutions were peculiar in the South, as Rabinowitz observes in *Race Relations in the Urban South 1865–1890*:

> *Before the Civil War public officials had been spared the burden of supporting large numbers of ill and indigent blacks; slave welfare had been the responsibility of the master, while free Negroes had been left to fend for themselves. The growing number of antebellum local institutions such as orphanages, hospitals, and almshouses or state facilities such as insane asylums and institutions for the blind, deaf, and dumb were limited, with few exceptions, to whites.[115]*

Thus, as was the case in virtually all other areas of Southern life, there was a strong tradition of "difference" in policies and practices as far as Blacks were concerned. With regard to social welfare institutions before the war, this racial "difference" manifested primarily as exclusion.[116]

The Union Army occupied Southern "headquarter" cities such as Washington, DC, New Orleans, Louisiana, and Nashville, Tennessee, throughout the war. Intensive federal activity continued in these locations until the end of Reconstruction. As noted before, the Freedmen's Bureau implemented extensive health care programs for the newly freed slaves and refugee populations. While this effort delivered necessary and meaningful outpatient services and operated hospitals throughout the Southern and border states, it also provided health-related support services such as orphanages and care for the mentally ill. However, at war's end problems arose. According to Rabinowitz, "It proved difficult to transfer the responsibility for poor Negroes from federal to local officials."[117] He noted several reasons: "The beleaguered cities, short of funds sufficient to perform even their normal services and in any case determined to perpetuate antebellum welfare policy, initially sought to evade the responsibility of providing food and shelter to needy blacks."[118] Nashville closed its public hospital in 1876* due to lack of funds. Thus, by the 1870s "it was the Redeemers, many of them former slave owners and veterans of the Confederate Army, who determined the quality and quantity of welfare facilities for blacks."[119] The fact that Blacks were denied admission to either public or private hospital facilities in most Southern cities critically increased their health disadvantage. Squalid health conditions, contributing to catastrophic Black death rates, were part of the impetus leading Dr. Hubbard to pursue his idea of training Black physicians at Meharry Medical College in Nashville. Due to Federal cutbacks and racially biased Southern health policies and practices, the Freedmen's Bureau was unable to continue vital health programs in many Southern cities.

---

*This is the ancestor to Nashville General Hospital that reopened in 1892 and is now known as Metropolitan Nashville General Hospital.

There was unanimous agreement that Reconstruction and the programs initiated by the Freedmen's Bureau had spurred Southern activity in the public health arena. Before 1900, Southern cities such as Atlanta, Nashville, and Richmond* formally opened public hospitals. However, virtually all of these facilities were reserved for White patients. Even when Blacks were admitted to certain facilities such as the Ivy Street Hospital and Providence Infirmary in Atlanta, "which used charity patients 'for the promotion of medical teaching,'"[120] they were treated in segregated and inferior facilities under degraded and exploitive medical conditions.

The pressures of public health awareness and medical-social change forced the issue of acceptance of responsibility on the mainstream medical establishment and health system. "By 1890 white Southerners had been forced to accept responsibility for providing public and private welfare for blacks, although there were still many institutions which refused to admit Negroes. . . . [F]or in the years after the Civil War segregation became the norm in Southern welfare policy."[121] Although public policy and facilities regarding indigent health care were upgraded over the entire South after the Civil War, Blacks were never full-fledged beneficiaries.[122]

Outpatient facilities, a major and variegated component of our present health system, have undergone many metamorphoses in the United States over the years. The late nineteenth century was an important period in these developments. The growth and importance of outpatient health facilities for use by the entire population in the United States is a relatively recent phenomenon. Earlier in the nation's history utilization of outpatient facilities was very limited and had strong sociological and class implications. As Sardell reminds us in *The U.S. Experiment in Social Medicine: The Community Health Center Program, 1956–1986,* "For the middle and upper classes during the eighteenth and nineteenth centuries, physicians provided treatment in the patient's home."[123]

The first dispensaries, which could be considered the earliest formally organized delivery points for outpatient care, were established in 1786, 1790, and 1796 in Philadelphia, New York, and Boston, respectively. They functioned as free-standing outpatient clinics serving primarily the poor and urban working class. However, they were considered one step above outdoor relief. Many of these facilities were either racially exclusive or discriminatory. They provided services such as care of minor and acute illnesses, minor surgery, tooth extractions, and drug prescriptions for minor ailments. Most were privately run in conjunction with charitable organizations, except in New York where they received a state or city subsidy.

There was also a smaller network of public clinics, often associated with the almshouse or poorhouse hospitals, for the destitute and those considered the "unworthy poor." In communities free of racial exclusion or segregation, Blacks

---

*Richmond had a public hospital before the Civil War; thus, this was actually a reopening.

were often clients of these facilities. The growth of these outpatient institutions helped them become the major source of medical care for urban working classes and the indigent. Such expansion was related to increasing urbanization and expansion of poor and working classes. Rosenberg and Sardell indicated it was also directly related to their vital training function for physicians in both the apprentice and medical school education systems.[124]

During the late nineteenth century several forces encouraged the expansion of the outpatient infrastructure. The changing profile of the U.S. political economy, increasing industrialization and urbanization, and the great waves of European immigration were probably the most important factors. This created larger urban, working-class, and poor populations—the traditional clientele of outpatient facilities. A second force was changing demographics, which presaged a deemphasis on charity to the Black ex-slave population and a shifting of these efforts to European immigrant populations—populations White Americans tended to identify with more strongly. As has been noted, the hospital system expanded dramatically. For various reasons these institutions began providing outpatient services through affiliated outpatient departments or dispensaries. This increased and often diversified their patient loads. It enhanced their attractiveness to the elite specialty physicians seeking professional advancement and prestige. They were also provided with training "material" to fulfill their educational or teaching functions.

A third major force was medical specialization. Certain specialties such as dermatology or ophthalmology were ideally suited and configured for outpatient delivery in clinic settings. As Sardell points out, "By 1900 there were approximately one hundred dispensaries in the United States."[125] This does not take into account the scores of hospital-based outpatient departments. As Rosenberg observed, dispensaries were the major form of medical care for urban residents who could not afford to pay a physician during the nineteenth century. Some of these facilities were available to African Americans. When medical school teaching material was needed there was a direct relationship with declining racial exclusiveness. Ironically, as the medical profession became more organized and influential, it would attack and destroy much of this outpatient infrastructure by the 1920s, alleging unfair competition. When dominant outpatient infrastructures reappeared, instead of the nineteenth-century charity-oriented service for the indigent and working poor, by the middle and late twentieth century there were instead community health centers, surgicenters, and managed care outpatient facilities. The latter two were predominantly commercial in character with a middle- and upper-class clientele. These new reincarnations were co-change agents of choice used by corporate, profit-driven, managed care companies to take over a middle-class-dominated health system. Thus, one could reasonably state that the U.S. outpatient infrastructure would not fully recover and become vigorous again until the late twentieth century. Of course, in the process it completely transformed in role and character.[126]

The voluntary health agency infrastructure as we know it did not exist in the nineteenth century. As Wilson and Neuhauser point out in *Health Services in the United States*, *voluntary agencies* are composed of a "wide variety of nonprofit organizations that are supported in whole or in part by private contributions and whose activities are directed to specific or general health or social welfare problems."[127] The effects of scientific progress and social belief in sanitation measures were augmented by the pragmatic lessons learned during the Civil War. George Rosen suggests that up until the 1870s, America's public health leaders embraced an enlightened concept of "social medicine" that was a product of the U.S. population's physical and social environment. Thus, prevention and treatment strategies promulgated by voluntary health agencies targeted the cause of diseases during that period. Rosen concluded:

> It is clear that by the middle of the seventies [i.e., 1870s] considerable advance had been made in America toward a socially oriented view of health and disease. Physicians, lay sanitarians, and public administrators had come to recognize that health and disease were in considerable measure an expression of collective behavior, that social and economic conditions were inextricably intertwined with morbidity and mortality.[128]

This enlightened viewpoint was short lived and changed with emergence of the Social Darwinism and the racial Redemption that overtook the post-Reconstruction nation during the Gilded Age. The new public health orientation, which was rapidly changing and regressing,

> was empirical and pragmatic. It had no well-articulated system of ideas . . . into which such diverse problems as poverty and dependency, infant mortality, sweatshops, prostitution, tuberculosis prevention and tenement house reform could be fitted; . . . their uncoordinated attacks on specific diseases did little to advance a comprehensive formulation of the environmental and more particularly of the social relations of health and disease.[129]

Thus, by the 1890s individualistic and particularistic approaches to public health by settlement houses and other voluntary agencies fed into and promulgated the sociocultural and institutional isolation of the African American community. Because of the scientific irrationality and dangers inherent in this approach, the White community had to be constantly reminded that the health of contiguous African American populations profoundly affected their own health environments. Nevertheless, the voluntary agency trends during this era reflected the racial isolation and subordination of African Americans. Blacks, who had virtually no control of community resources, were increasingly on their own—if further health apartheid was possible.[130]

The emergence of the categorical disease, voluntary agency, which would dominate and revolutionize the private arm of the U.S. health and social welfare system through advertising agency–derived fund-raising techniques, did not arrive until the 1930s and 1940s. The origins of the American Lung Association, America's oldest categorical voluntary health agency, can be traced to the Pennsylvania Society for the Prevention of Tuberculosis founded in 1892. The rise of categorical voluntary agencies such as the March of Dimes and the American Cancer Society in the mid–twentieth century characterizes the watershed in this type of infrastructure's development. They would come to dominate the fields of public health education and information dissemination, and facilitate the public financing of the biomedical research infrastructure. These functions would be voluntarily handed over by the governmental, educational, and private health care sectors. Their goals and objectives were driven almost exclusively by middle- and upper-class agendas and concerns. This largely reflected the social and class orientation of their founders, leaders, and membership.

The voluntary agencies of the nineteenth century were small, discrete health system players unable to exert systemwide influence. Such groups were local charity agencies dominated by well-meaning groups of privileged women and religious groups. Health-related activities were considered one aspect of these groups' or institutions' community stewardship. In the instances where charity activities were desegregated, African Americans benefitted. Unfortunately, Black exclusion or discriminatory segregation was the general rule. In response, a corollary African American voluntary agency movement arose during the late nineteenth century alongside the Black hospital, nurse training, and health professions education movements. Their focus was on meeting the health care needs of the underprivileged in the African American community.

A lack of resources and the inability to mobilize the wealthy and dominant majority community in their efforts compromised the work and scope of African American charity and voluntary agencies. In the scattered places that they existed and were able to survive, these Black self-help groups did yeoman service within segregated Black communities. Black organizations such as the Phyllis Wheatley Club (1896) of New Orleans; the National Association of Colored Women's Clubs (1896); the Dorchester Home (1896) of Dorchester, Massachusetts; the Independent Order of St. Luke (1867) of Baltimore; and the Lucy Brown Club (1896) of Charleston, South Carolina, struggled to meet the social service and health care needs of their communities against great odds and under adverse circumstances. Many of their programs focused on supporting African American patients, hospitals, and nursing schools. These separate and very unequal voluntary agency infrastructures provided health care and health-related services and resources for indigent and dependent populations.[131]

In 1798, the U.S. federal government began providing health care when Congress passed the Act for the Relief of Sick and Disabled Seamen. The act imposed a 20-cent-per-month tax on seamen's wages for their medical care.

Later, the federal government began a policy of directly providing medical care, which continues today through clinics and hospitals for merchant marines in port cities. The government also played a limited role in quarantining ships to prevent epidemics. The Civil War represented massive involvement of the federal government in health care delivery at the military and civilian levels. In the late nineteenth century governmental withdrawal from certain aspects of public health and social medicine with handovers to private community agencies was a major movement in the United States.[132]

As the Civil War ended, federal involvement in the delivery of health care was quickly reined in, consistent with previous U.S. health policy and social ideology. State governments increasingly controlled health care delivery, implementing medical licensing laws, state health departments, and hospitals for mentally ill and retarded patients between the end of the war and the twentieth century. At the federal level even vital Freedmen's Bureau health care programs, which had irreplaceable and unanticipated positive effects, were terminated. After January 1, 1869, all Freedmen's Bureau programs, with few exceptions, were terminated. By June 1, 1869, only the Freedmen's Bureau hospitals at Richmond and Washington, DC, were operational. As Bremner noted in *The Public Good: Philanthropy and Welfare in the Civil War Era*, "[W]hen Congress terminated the Freedmen's Bureau in 1872, it provided the continuance of the Freedmen's Hospital and Asylum, under supervision first of the Secretary of War and later of the Secretary of the Interior. The hospital was still in operation more than a century after the bureau went out of existence."[133] Thus, by 1872, only remnants of the massive Freedmen's Bureau program could be found in the health care arena. And although the bureau's health programs were some of its most beneficial, its epitaph was written:

> *Notwithstanding these positive accomplishments, the shortage of doctors and personnel resulting from inadequate funds kept the medical department of the Bureau from rendering the service which conditions demanded. Neither in extent or activity nor in duration did the agency meet the health problems that followed emancipation of the slaves.*[134]

The Federal government would not make another major impact on the health care delivery system until the late twentieth century.[135]

Beyond the boundaries of public health and health policy, major changes were occurring in medical pharmacology and therapeutics. These developments had direct and indirect effects on the ongoing struggle between organized medicine and the drug and appliance industry. Pharmacology emerged as a distinct scientific discipline in the early nineteenth century. A plethora of plant and mineral drugs was available. Medical prescription of only a few of these were based on sound scientific or even empiric evidence. Quinine was available for malaria, digitalis was efficacious for treating heart failure, colchicine relieved gout, and opiates alleviated pain. Other traditional medications such as arsenic and antimony used for infections and other ailments fell out of favor.

Based on discoveries such as the chemical isolation of morphine in 1806 and the work of investigators such as Derosne and Seguin in France and Serturner in Germany, pharmacology developed into a science. French and German scientists furthered this process by chemically isolating strychnine, quinine, atropine, colchicine, and cocaine in the first half of the nineteenth century. Rudolph Buchheim (1820–1879) in Dorpat and Oswald Schmiedeberg (1830–1920) in Strassburg established pharmacology as an independent discipline in Europe and transmitted that knowledge to John J. Abel (1857–1938). Bringing his knowledge to America, Abel enlarged upon the foundation laid in pharmacology by H. C. Wood and Silas Weir Mitchell of Philadelphia. The Philadelphia College of Pharmacy, the first school of pharmacy in the United States, was founded in 1821. Next Abel headed the department of materia medica and therapeutics at the University of Michigan Medical School and later became the first professor of pharmacology at Johns Hopkins Medical School in 1893. Advances in pharmacology often led to the scientific evaluation of heroic therapies (bleeding, cupping, purging, blistering, and sweating) by the 1830s and 1840s. This process accelerated the devaluation of these therapies, so popular in preceding centuries. Medical directives issued by Union Army Surgeon General William Alexander Hammond further marginalized heroic therapies during the Civil War by outlawing their use in the military.[136]

Drug wholesalers and manufacturers successfully marketed remedies and patented medicines by the late eighteenth century in the United States. Nevertheless, during the early part of the period between 1861 and 1900 the pharmaceutical and medical supply infrastructures were virtually unrecognizable by current standards. Today, the more than 1,000 companies engaged in the manufacture of drugs yielding an annual shipment value approaching $40 billion would have seemed fantastical at the end of the Civil War. However, some of the events leading to the emergence of this infrastructure, or the mechanisms that facilitated its evolution, were either occurring or about to take place by the last third of the nineteenth century. The traditional European division of the healing professionals into physicians, surgeons, midwives, and apothecaries had long since succumbed to the tradition of the general practitioner who performed all these functions in the United States. American physicians, unlike their European counterparts, continued to prescribe, often compound, and sometimes market the medications their patients used. However, this practice began to wane in the nineteenth century.

Rosemary Stevens noted, "Urban practitioners had dropped their apothecary trade between 1790 and 1820 and were replaced by full-time druggists."[137] Drugstores proliferated and pharmacy grew as an independent profession with pharmacy schools and associations founded in Philadelphia, Boston, and New York City in the 1820s. In 1852 the American Pharmaceutical Association was established. With the geometric increase in nineteenth-century biomedical scientific knowledge and an exploding commercial market for drugs and nostrums after the Civil War, these relationships and practices changed. With the approach of the twentieth century, "ethical" drugs, preparations of known composition advertised only to the medical profession, and patent drugs* increased dramatically. Propri-etary, or patent, drugs and nostrums which are advertised and sold directly to the public would become more than a medical nuisance. They became the medical profession's nemesis.

African Americans, who in the United States were systematically excluded from most entrepreneurial activities, were excluded from mainstream participa-tion in the ethical or proprietary drug businesses. Only after the rise of a network of separate Black pharmacy schools in the late nineteenth century would Blacks participate in the distribution of medications, although at underrepresented lev-els. (See Figures 6.6 and 6.7.) Moreover, these trends toward mass production and formalization of the drug and pharmacy industry drove further underground the informal, community-based participation of Blacks as root doctors, voodoo priestesses and priests, and supernatural healers.[138]

Major Gilded Age changes in the pharmaceutical environment were the emergence of commercial advertisement, mass production of pills and other med-ications, and the possibility of widespread, even national, distribution. Thus, the more popular patent medicines were mass marketed and sold based on their highly successful advertising campaigns. In that most of these so-called medicines were composed of secret ingredients, they technically could not be legally pro-tected by U.S. patents. They often contained narcotics and other addictive agents. Some were Morrison's Universal Pills, Dr. James's Fever Powder, Lydia Pinkham's Vegetable Compound, and Radam's Microbe Killer. All were introduced by the late nineteenth century. The traditional sales of home remedies by neighborhood healers or root doctors, important up to the end of the eighteenth century, became minuscule in comparison. The regular medical profession, especially the elite academic factions, fought against these commercial companies from the begin-ning. Although able to be construed as based on self-interest, the battle could be framed as biomedical science, medical ethics, and public service commitments to the protection of patients. Increasingly, on this issue, the public sided with, and was supportive of, the White organized medical profession.[139]

Although the academic elite of the medical profession grumbled about the rise and public acceptance of patent medicines, the public was ready to accede to medical authority by the 1890s. However, there had been very few practical mea-sures taken to clean up the drug industry. By 1900, the political consequences of

---

Patent drugs is a loose term usually referring to proprietary medicines (drugs whose contents are pro-tected by copyright) or nostrums sold directly to the public through advertising and marketing. Their secret ingredients and unproven claims did not have to meet scientific muster of the "ethical" drugs promoted only to physicians and through the scientific literature.

Figure 6.6   Dr. Thomas W. Patrick: Pioneer African American
             Physician-Pharmacist

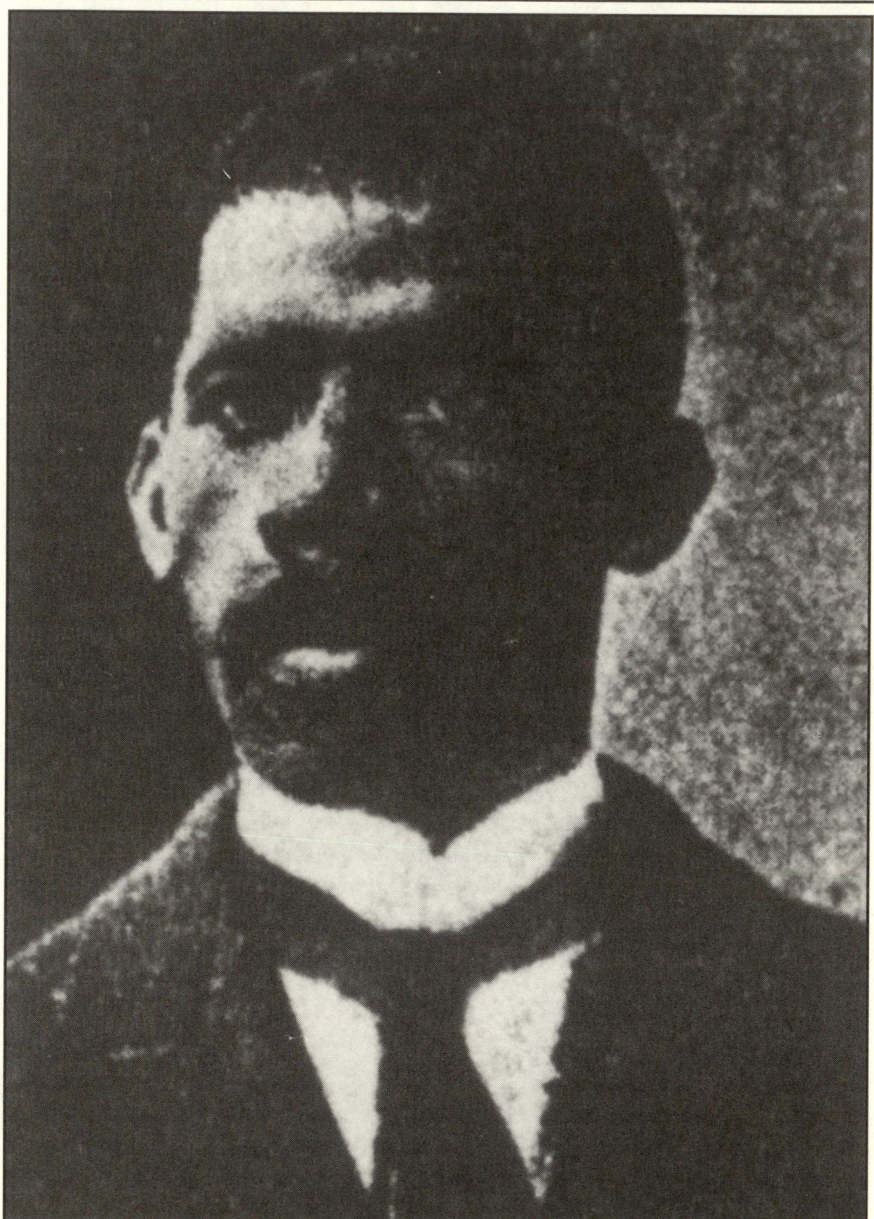

Patrick (1872–?) was a Trinidad-trained pharmacist who emigrated to Boston and graduated with an M.D. from the College of Physicians and Surgeons in 1894. He successfully opened and operated the Patrick School of Pharmacy in Boston from 1893 until at least 1910.

Figure 6.7   Black Drugstores

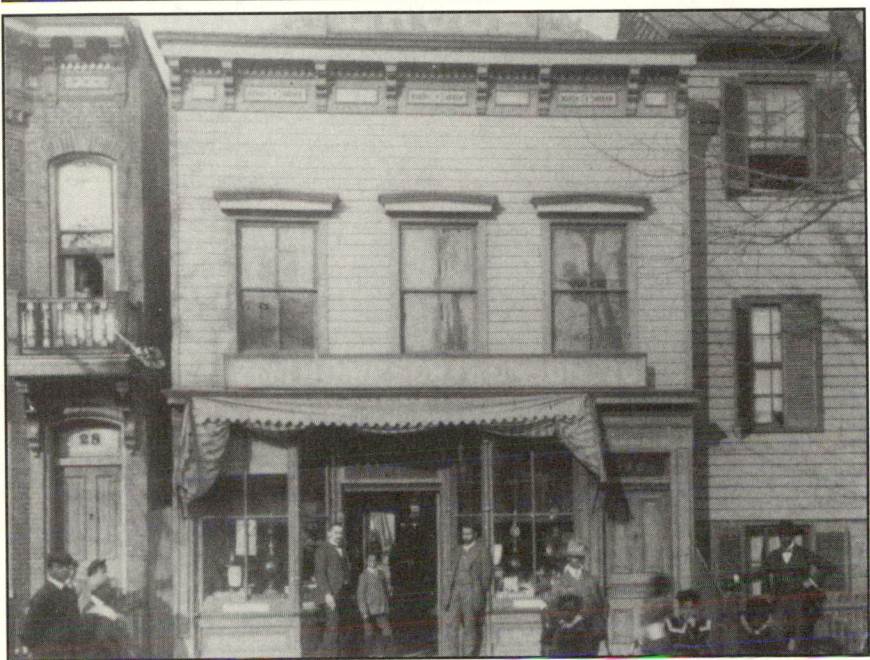

Nineteenth-century Black pharmacists often served as primary care providers in underserved communities and were also important centers of African American economic development.

the dramatic increase in AMA membership, enactment of medical licensing laws, and the physician-led clamor for regulation of the drug and infant food industries geared up the medical profession to win one of its first regulatory victories over a segment of the U.S. health system that it would grow to control—the drug and medical appliance industry. Black physicians, excluded from the AMA or its professional and official functionaries, had little direct participation in this struggle.[140]

The 50-year battle between the medical profession and the drug industry can be traced to a few well-defined steps during the late nineteenth century. Two years after its formation in 1847 the American Medical Association established an official board to evaluate drugs and nostrums. Due to lack of funding and the absence of legal or cultural authority, this effort yielded little results. With the growth of the drug manufacturing industry and the growing acrimonious relationship between physicians and pharmacists, the profession continued to condemn patent medicines, nostrums, and the progressive commercialization of the pharmaceutical industry over the next four decades. By the turn of the century, as Starr notes in *The Social Transformation of American Medicine:*

> In 1900 the AMA *launched a campaign to make the "legitimate" pro-*
> *prietary remedies "respond to the ethics of medicine" by forcing their*
> *manufacturers to disclose all formulae and cease public advertising. Its*
> Journal *announced that it would stop publishing all notices of offend-*
> *ing drugs when current advertising contracts expired. And it urged*
> *physicians not to prescribe, nor other medical journals to advertise,*
> *either secret preparations or drugs "advertised directly to the laity."*[141]

The gauntlet had been tossed down to the pharmaceutical industry. It would be another decade before the medical profession had the political clout or cultural authority it could convert into sufficient political and economic power to enforce its will on the drug industry.[142]

Between the end of the Civil War and the turn of the century there was no health care financing industry per se. The huge infrastructure of indirect payment mechanisms composed of more than 1,200 health insurance companies and hundreds of health maintenance organizations (HMOs) we are familiar with today did not exist. The only situation that even vaguely resembled such pre-paid arrangements for health care was the previously mentioned tiny, federally sponsored, prepaid merchant marine health benefits program.

The financial strains generated by the excessive number of physicians forced some to enter contract practice with lodge or fraternal organizations whereby care was paid for by the head for an agreed-on period of time. As Haller states in *American Medicine in Transition 1840–1910*, such arrangements had been more common in the South: "The contract system had thrived in the South from colonial days to the Civil War, providing cheap medical care for plantation families and their slaves."[143] Haller observed changes in these arrangements during the Gilded Age, noting, "In the latter half of the nineteenth century, benevolent societies throughout the nation negotiated for collective medical service and received it, largely because of the unwholesome competitive nature of medicine and the overabundance of doctors."[144] Although physicians despised and condemned these arrangements because of factors such as physician oversupply and cutthroat competition, they sometimes had to endure them. Otherwise, indirect mechanisms for the payment of medical fees did not exist. Black physicians were also drawn into prepaid fee arrangements with fraternal organizations or lodges on occasion. However, they had much less reluctance because of their less privileged circumstance and the daunting lack of access to health care experienced by the Black community.[145]

As has been previously noted, the review and quality control infrastructure as we now know it did not exist in the nineteenth century. States supervised the limited regulation of licensure of manpower, facilities, and quality control by governmental agencies. The private-corporate and governmental medical audit and quality assurance systems of today did not exist. Although the Civil War ended with the seeds of a universal and well-planned health system, by the close of the nineteenth century it was evident that this spawn had fallen on unyielding ground.[146]

The White Medical Profession Comes of Age

Paul Starr has made an excellent case for viewing the development of modern American medicine and the health system as two long movements. The first movement, the rise of a profession's sovereignty and control of the health system, took place between 1850 and 1930. The second movement, from 1930 to the present—the transformation of the health system into an industry as the profession lost power—is an incomplete and still unfolding story. However, Starr did not substantively include race and class dimensions, effects, and consequences implied in his analysis. While Starr's basic approach has veracity, everyone can agree that the Civil War certainly hastened, broadened, and redefined the rise of the medical profession in the United States. Thus the period from 1861 to 1900 was pivotal to the medical profession's unprecedented rise to power and authority in America. African Americans faced discrimination and systematic exclusion from the mainstream American medical profession legalistically and profession- ally throughout this period. Therefore, on a *de facto* basis until today, referring to the "White medical profession" is not a matter of polemics or ideology. It is a recognition and statement of fact. Revealing what Black physicians were con- tributing and experiencing in medicine in both technical and medical-social senses throughout this period is a journey into largely unknown territory. Exam- ining and evaluating this experience is a goal we take up in more detail later.[147]

After the mid–nineteenth century, and certainly after the Civil War, the White American medical profession became engaged in an upward spiral of cul- tural authority and power that would not wane until the mid–twentieth century. This was the result of several factors. Medical science was producing many break- throughs in the late nineteenth century, among them the provision of safe and humane surgery through antisepsis, asepsis, and anesthesia; proving and success- fully applying the germ theory; and preventing and curing diseases through immunizations and inoculations. Although most of these advances came from Europe, some of the more important ones, especially of a surgical nature, emanated from the United States. Moreover, the market and industrial revolu- tions had increased America's cultural dependency upon, and worship of, sci- ence. For many the medical profession was the day-to-day walking embodiment of their direct contact with the scientific world. This had much to do with medi- cine's growing hegemony over American society. Thus, the legal and political authority of the medical profession was increasing exponentially by the turn of the century.[148]

Despite the favorable environment created for the U.S. medical profession by scientific advance and the Civil War, there were several roadblocks to the assumption of professional authority. Most of the major problems could be grouped under the following categories:

1. There was an overabundance of White male physicians.
2. The medical education system was out of control with no regulations or standards.
3. The medical profession itself was disorganized and struggling with the process of specialization.
4. Regulation of the medical profession was inadequate with lax or absent licensing laws and no criteria for professional standards.
5. Sectarian wars were raging.

Significantly, during the period from the end of the Civil War to 1900, the White medical profession went a long way toward setting itself up to overcome all of these problems. The social and professional exclusion of the African American medical profession from participating in the conquest of all these system barriers would generate a peculiar professional contempt for Black doctors in the White profession. It would also generate a unique set of problems and disabilities that have been described by both African American professionals and students of the sociology of Black medicine.[149]

The most conspicuous result of the mainstream medical profession's inability to regulate the field of medicine either externally through legal regulation or internally by organized medical associations was the overabundance of White physicians. Moreover, many of these products of proprietary medical schools were marginally, if not poorly, trained. Patients suffered through perpetuation of these mechanisms. And the profession was unable both to fulfill its medical-social functions adequately by properly regulating and standardizing the growing U.S. health delivery system or to place American medicine on a sound scientific footing.

Between 1870 and 1900 the physician population increased by approximately 105 percent, from a population of 64,414 to 132,002, according to the U.S. Bureau of the Census. Of these there were more than 110,000 regular physicians,* 10,000 homeopaths, 5,000 eclectics, and more than 5,000 other practitioners. The medical student population more than doubled, rising 112 percent from 11,826 to 25,171 between 1880 and 1900. The White profession was outgrowing the population and concentrating unnecessarily in the cities. According to Starr, "Between 1870 and 1910, the number of physicians per 100,000 people grew from 177 to 241 in the large cities, while it fell from 160 to 152 in the rest of the country—this during a time when the overall ratio of doctors to population was still increasing."[150] Therefore, the medical profession was virtually cannibal-

---

Regular is a term usually applied to allopathic physicians. Allopathic physicians are considered members of the rational or regular school—which is erroneous from a purely comparative scientific standpoint—as distinguished from eclectic or homeopathic practitioners.

izing itself through oversupply and competition. These factors spurred the different medical factions, including specialists, academicians, homeopaths, eclectics, general practitioners, and the "regulars" to push for medical educational reform within a context of White male-dominated medicine. African Americans and women were considered separate and inferior professional factions of minimal significance. Paradoxically, the free and easy climate and lack of professional control by White organized medicine allowed the African American medical profession and a female contingent of doctors to survive through their most vulnerable period. The experience of the early part of the century did not hold out much hope that state licensing and standards could be depended upon as a mechanism to solve the myriad problems.[151]

America has had a marked predilection for opening medical schools. Rosemary Stevens reviewed the process historically in *American Medicine in the Public Interest*:

> *In 1800 there were only 4 functioning medical colleges; in 1825 there were 18. Between 1810 and 1840, 26 new medical schools were founded; between 1840 and 1876, 47; and in the great wave of immigration at the end of the century (1873–1890) 114 new schools were established. Altogether, it has been estimated, over 400 medical schools were founded between 1800 and 1900.*[152]

The Civil War seemed to delay the rampant process of medical school openings for 10 years. However, as Rosen notes in *The Structure of American Medical Practice 1875–1941*, "[T]he dislocations of the Civil War impeded the founding of new ones. By the 1870s, however, medical schools began to be established at an unprecedented rate."[153] Many of these proprietary schools were medical diploma mills with virtually no entrance requirements, two short and inadequate school terms, and assurance of graduation upon the payment of the fees.

In contrast to Europe, only the wealthy schools in the 1870s and 1880s established close ties with hospitals to ensure clinical training for their students. The lessons learned from the inadequacies of the medical professional education system during the Civil War sunk in. The profession continued its scientific advance modeled on the German medical universities. Therefore, educational reform became a pressing issue around which all the professional groups and sects rallied.[154]

Unlike the medical education system in Europe, which operated under the auspices of established universities, medical and health professions guilds, and the legal jurisdiction of a landed aristocracy, the majority of U.S. medical schools were private proprietary institutions operating under the jurisdiction of their small faculties—usually between 6 and 10 physicians. Moreover, these physician-owners profited based on high student enrollments; arbitrary entrance, academic, and graduation standards; and minimizing the amount of capital-intensive facilities such as laboratories, hospitals, and libraries required for the educational process. Many of these physician-owners, based on their own self-interest, fought against significant medical education reform efforts by organized medical bodies such as local or state medical societies or the AMA. Ludmerer described the typical mid-nineteenth-century medical course that held sway until the 1890s in *Learning to Heal: The Development of American Medical Education:*

> The standard course of instruction at the nation's medical schools in the mid–19th century consisted of two four-month terms of lectures during the winter season, with the second term identical with the first. The curriculum generally consisted of seven courses: anatomy; physiology and pathology; materia medica, therapeutics, and pharmacy; chemistry and medical jurisprudence; theory and practice of medicine; principles and practice of surgery; and obstetrics and the diseases of women and children. Scientific subjects received scant attention, the emphasis being placed on topics considered of "practical" value.[155]

Ludemerer goes on to say, "Whereas admission to medical school frequently involved no more than the ability to pay fees, these relaxed standards applied only to white males. Blacks and women faced much greater obstacles."[156] However, these lax policies and the chaos of nonregulation yielded unexpected side effects. The opportunities denied by White organized medicine allowed, even encouraged, the establishment and survival of Black and female medical schools. This enabled unanticipated African American and female entry into the medical profession by 1900.[157]

Until the twentieth century, most of the impetus toward medical school reform emanated from within the profession itself and not the AMA. Two mid-century White medical schools distinguished themselves by instituting significant innovative reforms into their curricula. The Civil War interrupted these efforts and the limited effects they had on the system. In 1857 the New Orleans School of Medicine introduced clinical teaching, based on the Parisian model, to include student externships with assignment of patients to students for their entire hospital course. It also introduced full history and physical examinations with presentations to their professors, discussions of case histories and case management, and daily morning rounds. Not until Johns Hopkins reestablished the clinical clerkship after 1893 would such modern reform grace American medical education.

In 1859, Lind University in Chicago (a forerunner of Northwestern University) established a graded curriculum with subjects being taught in order over two five-month terms. Harvard, the University of Pennsylvania, and the University of Michigan implemented similar changes in the 1870s. After the Civil War the AMA paid lip service to educational reform, projecting it as their only avenue for control of the professional market. Such pronouncements had little direct substantive impact.[158]

Between 1871 and 1893 a clash of divergent forces came together that would reform American medical education such that it would lead the world by the mid–twentieth century. The Civil War had revealed the obvious deficiencies in the U.S. educational system. Twenty-two top-ranked schools formed the American Medical College Association in 1876. It fell apart in six years after a dispute over establishing three medical school terms instead of two. During this period, universities such as Harvard, the University of Pennsylvania, the University of Michigan, and Johns Hopkins matured to become capable and willing stewards of the new scientific medical education process as they began to exercise their hegemony over the nation's medical schools.

Various states carved out educational requirements for medical licensing. A stream of scientifically trained academic physicians returned from Europe pushing for upgrading American educational standards to make them comparable to those in Germany, Austria, France, and Great Britain. Among a well-trained cadre of physicians strongly influenced by the empirical French clinical school, skepticism relative to the value and utility of scientific knowledge in clinical practice was still prominent. Despite the rhetoric, during the 1870s and 1880s the proprietary schools continued to provide superficial course lectures and exercise casual admission, academic, and graduation requirements. As Ludmerer observes, "[T]hese forces were to come into conflict at four pivotal schools: Harvard, Pennsylvania, Michigan, and Johns Hopkins. The result would be the first genuine, lasting improvements in medical education in the United States."[159] Harvard initiated significant reform in 1871 by making the medical school an integral part of the university. It lengthened the medical course to three terms, each nine months long, graded, over three years (the courses were not the customary two-year repetitive ones [e.g., anatomy preceded surgery]); added the basic laboratory sciences of chemistry, physiology, microscopic anatomy, and pathology to the curriculum; raised admission, academic, and graduation requirements; hired full-time medical school faculty physicians; and dramatically expanded student laboratory time.

Pennsylvania and Michigan embarked on similar reform programs in 1877. As Rothstein noted in *American Medical Schools and the Practice of Medicine,* "By 1880, 10 medical schools adopted a required three-year graded curriculum, and 26 adopted it by 1890."[160] In 1893, Johns Hopkins opened a medical school built upon a foundation of these reforms along with total integration of clinical hospital training with medical education. It pioneered laboratories and research facilities contiguous to and integral to the educational process at the medical school. To this were added layers of clinical postgraduate training programs whereby graduate physicians actively participated in medical school teaching, patient care, and research with an emphasis on a medical specialty—the first residency programs. With its full-fledged university affiliation and the medical school virtually located within the university hospital, Hopkins was a radical departure in medical education. It was the first modern medical school. Everything in medical education would be based on this model for the next century. From 1893 to 1963, its first 70 years and the era of its greatest influence on American medical education, Hopkins did not allow African Americans to attend, and all of its clinical services were racially segregated.[161]

While most of this medical educational reform activity took place, various states began to listen to the rhetoric of White organized medical opinion. Led by the AMA, physicians felt the time had come to reinstitute medical licensing laws and standards that had succumbed to the politics of the Jacksonian Era. As Starr observed in *The Social Transformation of American Medicine*, "The state, which had been indifferent to physicians' claims since the Jacksonian era, finally embraced the profession's definition of a legitimate practitioner."[162] The profession, largely through the efforts of the AMA, was also pushing forth with professional enrichment from scientific and technical perspectives and enhancing collegiality from within. Though the relationships were stormy, between 1870 and 1890 the AMA was able to mediate the wars between the specialists and the generalists to their mutual benefit. Thus, through the AMA's efforts, the specialty societies were able to advance medical progress in their fields autonomously while maintaining a united front with the rest of White organized medicine. Even the medical sects were embraced by the AMA. Only Black physicians were completely excluded.

Unlike European medicine, the U.S. profession did not have medically oriented universities, many dating from the Medieval Age, or medical guilds to serve as unifiers, standard setters, and organizers of the profession. Moreover, as Tocqueville had observed in *Democracy in America*, Americans virtually worshiped independence, and scattered frontiers did not lend themselves to cohesive political or professional movements. Rosemary Stevens and others have hypothesized that medical journals in the United States were thus forced to serve a unique role in unifying and uplifting the medical profession. They accomplished these things while serving irreplaceable educational purposes. This may be the reason that, regarding American medical journals, "By 1898 at least 275 periodicals were being published, most of them monthly."[163] Therefore, after its founding in 1883, the *Journal of the American Medical Association (JAMA)* may be indirectly responsible for the AMA's successful campaign of professional organization. First, JAMA helped control general practitioner versus specialist conflicts. Second, it resolved the unity-depleting, publicly demeaning, and professionally undermining sectarian wars. Third, it led to reforming the out-of-control, professionally limiting, and problem-generating medical education system. And fourth, it allowed the AMA to wage the political campaigns and forge connections necessary to force the introduction of, and shape the nature of, legislation regulating the health system while simultaneously protecting the public's interests.

Even the sectarian wars between the allopathic, homeopathic, and eclectic practitioners took a back seat to medical licensing and educational reform. As Starr noted, "Probably the most important sign of convergence between competing groups was their common support, beginning in the 1870s and 1880s, for the restoration of medical licensing."[164] Most states embarked on licensing in steps. First they enacted a statute requiring a medical school diploma. Later, after declaring that the diploma had to be inspected, the school issuing the diploma could be judged inadequate and the candidate rejected. Finally, all licensure candidates were required to present an acceptable diploma and pass a state examination. By 1901, the District of Columbia and 25 states required a diploma plus an examination, and there was no jurisdiction without a licensing law of some sort. The AMA's licensing and medical educational reform campaigns had helped resolve the old sectarian wars as all groups shared in the legal privileges of the profession and accepted the sanctity of scientific medicine. A new and stronger American Medical College Association had re-formed by 1895 to augment the AMA in the future to guide medical education.

The growing power of the late nineteenth-century medical profession also had some deleterious effects on the health care of the poor and underserved. White organized medicine gutted broad-based public health programs in cities such as New York and Chicago, which promoted free bacteriologic diagnosis, toxoid treatments, venereal disease therapy, and the diagnosis and treatment of children's diseases for the underprivileged. Newly empowered physicians blocked the building of rural health centers and eventually led the closure of the dispensaries so prominent near the turn of the century. Blacks and the poor were the prime victims of these nihilistic health care activities. Two new so-called outsider groups appeared during the 1890s, the osteopaths and the Christian scientists. The former were drawn in to share some of the legal and professional privileges of the medical profession early in the next century. The group the AMA and White-organized medicine cast aside during the Gilded Age—based on official rejection actions on June 9, 1869; February 1870; and May 6, 1870—was African Americans. Thus, Black and women physicians, whether qualified or not, were relegated to a virtually permanent, professional caste status in the American medical profession. Remnants of this professional caste status remain today.[165]

All of these developments had taken place or were well in progress by 1900. They set the U.S. medical profession in a direction of gentrification and gender- and race-based stratification. A focus of debate since the Colonial Era, the majority of Americans had previously chosen to level the medical profession, much to the chagrin of its leaders. "One way of looking at the changes that took place between the 1870s and the early 1900s is that the social distance between doctor and patient increased, while the distance among colleagues diminished as the profession became more cohesive and uniform,"[166] Paul Starr observed.

Raising admission standards to the medical schools, raising academic standards for schools and licensing, organizing the profession administratively, and creating a strong collegial environment pressured the profession toward European American upper-class or upwardly mobile homogeneity. Disadvantaged groups such as Blacks, women, and underprivileged immigrants bore the brunt of intensified pressure to exclude them. The educational system, evolving to support the country's industrial and economic expansion, was already producing a larger pool of well-educated students for medical and dental schools. Ludmerer points out in *Learning to Heal*, "In 1870, there were only 1,026 public high schools with 72,158 enrolled students; by 1900 the number of schools had increased to 6,005 and the number of students to 519,251. Fueled by the growth of the secondary schools, university enrollments also increased dramatically."[167] Again, a disproportionate share of these young people were privileged or upwardly mobile and White.

From a White patient perspective these trends were a mixed bag. For Blacks, they were devastating. Increasing exclusivity may have produced physicians with slightly more technical training, but it would make them less available numerically and more distant socially from the average patient. For African Americans, medical education reform and standardization would eventually close all but two of their medical schools and decrease their doctor–patient ratios for the next seven decades. Rosenberg, Savitt, Bullough, and others have documented that racial and class tensions between the privileged cadre of hospital-based physicians and the wards of the almshouse and public hospitals accelerated at times to the level of physical abuse or unethical medical experimentation. Fears that this new elevation of the profession would worsen these trends were well founded. For Blacks, however, who were already the victims of exclusion, discriminatory segregation, and differential victims of medical abuse at all levels of the health system during the Gilded Age and the early Progressive Era, things could hardly get much worse. These health policy changes and events virtually guaranteed that the slave health deficit would be carried into the twentieth century.[168]

For White physicians, the concentration of professional activities at specific institutions such as hospitals proved to be more efficient. Travel time and making rounds at a string of institutions were reduced and often eliminated. For example, factors such as physical proximity for the convenience of the medical staff and the availability of the parent institution's technological capabilities were pivotal in the configuration and founding of Massachusetts General Hospital's private hospital branch during the 1890s. Black physicians would not benefit significantly from these changes until the rise of the Black hospital in the next century. A changeover in financing mechanisms to a fee-for-service payment mechanism for hospital staff physicians also became necessary for the transformation of larger traditional hospitals into the newer private hospital configuration in U.S. cities. The old system in effect at many traditional hospitals such as Boston City Hospital, Pennsylvania Hospital, and Massachusetts General Hospital, which barred the paying of fees to attending physicians, proved to be increasingly inappropriate for a profession forced to live off income generated by their full-time practices. This grew more obvious, as increasing numbers of physician practices shifted to the provision of inpatient care in the hospital. As Vogel observed in *The Invention of the Modern Hospital*: "Increasing numbers of relatively affluent patients, making no attempt to disguise their finances, were paying the hospital its going rate for the private rooms they occupied and denying the attending practitioner the opportunity to collect for his professional service."[169] Thus, the manipulation of seventeenth- and eighteenth-century hospital rules of governance by patient influence on hospital infrastructure forced late-nineteenth-century changes in health care financing toward fee-for-service in hospital as well as office-bound care.

As the funds necessary to build, expand, and maintain these increasingly technical and labor-intensive institutions exploded exponentially, the traditional upper-class stewardship funding sources became inadequate. Therefore, the traditional health and hospital infrastructure embarked on structured fund raising throughout the community, including corporations, labor unions, citizens groups, and research foundations. Increasing affluence and upward mobility of White ethnic groups, coupled with the changing attitudes and the increasing demands for hospital care, triggered the founding of numerous ethnic hospitals in most urban communities. Saint Joseph's in Philadelphia (1849) and Saint Margaret's (1877), Carney Hospital (1880s), and Saint Elizabeth's (1880) in Boston are examples. Energy from this movement generated a few Black hospitals by 1900. Women, forced to start their own institutions to receive culturally sensitive care and training opportunities, founded institutions such as the New York Women's Hospital (1855), New England Hospital for Women and Children (1855), and the New York Infirmary for Women and Children (1860).[170]

During the 1880s and 1890s, when these dramatic changes were taking place in the health institutional infrastructure, African Americans were being increasingly isolated and segregated throughout the United States. Black codes were being enacted everywhere. African American suffrage was being taken away by various mechanisms, and social and residential segregation was rampant. Economic exploitation of Blacks in industrial and unionized urban settings and virtual rural serfdom in agricultural environments was universal. This translated into the absence of health facilities in many communities and inferior and segregated accommodations in nominally accessible institutions.

Black morbidity and mortality rates throughout this period remained staggering. In response to the health system effects of these sociocultural phenomena and the dynamics of increasing burdens of financing health care institutions, African Americans initiated self-help movements. Thus, they joined other disadvantaged ethnic minority groups such as the Jews and Irish Catholics in founding and financing their own hospitals, nursing schools, and health professions educational institutions. These would represent significant efforts to supply the health care and health professionals necessary to attempt to overcome the slave health deficit in the U.S. health system that was perpetuated and virtually imposed on African Americans through *de jure* and *de facto* segregation and discrimination as they entered the twentieth century.[171]

The Black Medical Profession: Practicing behind the "Veil"

Tracing the Black medical profession through the period of the Civil War, Reconstruction, Gilded Age, and the early Progressive Era, spanning the years from 1861 to 1900, is a surprising story of adventure and inspiration. Over this span of 39 years African American physicians transformed themselves from a tiny cadre of professional curiosities, whose careers were overshadowed by and kneaded into abolition and community activism, to full-fledged health professionals. Moreover, they became powerful enough from public health and medical-social standpoints to positively affect Black health status and health policy at the national level. Much of this experience was modulated by African American physicians being denied training, membership in professional societies, or practice privileges and collegiality because of their race. Only their patients and communities respected them as professionals, acknowledged their medical competence, appreciated their service to their communities, and admired them. Hence, we have the "veil," Du Bois's classic description, hovering over the health professional aspects of African American life.

During this period, African American physicians became a distinct and important arm of the U.S. medical profession. They made up more than 2 percent of U.S. physicians by 1910 and contributed deeply and profoundly to the health and medical-social fabric of their communities. Exercising their professional and social roles forever altered the profile of the U.S. health system. Black doctors benefitted indirectly, largely in their own communities, from many of the same scientific and social phenomena that were psychologically affecting White Americans. Although in some respects viewed differently than White physicians, Black doctors were considered the most prestigious men in their communities. However, the social and professional practices of the White medical profession set a pattern of separate and segregated medical professional development between 1870 and 1890 that remains today. But Black physicians, though forced into subordinate professional roles, often served as interface points and intermediaries between the mainstream health system, its scientific medical progress, and a separate and underprivileged Black community bludgeoned by racial discrimination.[172]

The existence of these physicians ensured that the cold medical facts of the health system's unwholesome response to the slave health deficit—characterized by compounding social deprivation with inhumane and unethical medical discrimination—would be scrutinized under the glaring light of professional and social awareness. Through the efforts of the Black medical profession, African American leaders and the lay population would be made aware of and kept informed about the Black health crisis and the slave health deficit that was its foundation. Unlike any other racial or ethnic group in the United States, health care would become, and remain, a civil rights issue as far as the Black community was concerned well into the twenty-first century. The unique seeds of a health care movement allied with the Black Civil Rights Movement were planted.[173]

Eight African American physicians recruited by the Union Army served during the Civil War. They were Alexander T. Augusta, Charles B. Purvis, Alpheus Tucker, John Rapier, William Ellis, Anderson R. Abbott, William Powell, and John Vancerlle DeGrasse. The mystery of how the U.S. Army acquired such a significant portion of the tiny cadre of East Coast, formally trained Black physicians can be solved if we recall W. Montague Cobb's revelation: "The recruitment of these officers appears to have resulted from a tour of the nation's medical schools, particularly those in New England, by Dr. J.V.C. Smith, a prominent physician of the time who sought to obtain competent young Negro medical graduates to serve as surgeons with the Negro units."[174] One must realize that these physicians were all Black but trained in and graduated from White medical schools before the Civil War. The available records, such as the detailed review by Dean Epps of the Howard University Medical School regarding the graduation of Black pioneer physicians from American medical schools, reveal that these men represented most of the formally trained African American medical manpower at that time. Similar to the African American civilians volunteering for Union Army duty, White medical school–trained Black physicians were overrepresented in the medical corps. These tiny numbers, totally incapable of improving the health outcome of 4.5 million African Americans, were emblematic of the minuscule representation set aside for Blacks in medicine in the Antebellum Period. This probably also represents the level of representation African Americans would have been ceded by White mainstream medicine in the future without the Black medical schools.

Despite their excellent training and credentials, these doctors were subject to the racial caste system that had been established within the profession for more than 200 years. Union Army African American physicians were all restricted to service with either Black units or to Freedmen's Bureau facilities serving Black populations. Significantly, while in the Army they were all subjected to frequent acts of overt and covert racial discrimination. Uniformly, they acquitted themselves well. Alexander T. Augusta, the Virginia-born Canadian medical school graduate mentioned earlier, was decorated and achieved the rank of Lieutenant Colonel, a rank not obtained by any other African American for 70 years.[175]

As the war proceeded and then ended, observers could interpret the developments regarding African American health in a positive light. Virtually all onlookers conceded that the Freedmen's Bureau health activities had a positive effect on Black health. As Howard Ashley White noted, "The medical services of the Freedmen's Bureau were among its most constructive activities. Frederick Douglass, a former slave who published a newspaper in Washington, gave the Bureau credit for lowering the national Negro death rate from 30 percent to 4 percent."[176] Although this estimate may have been overly optimistic, it attests to the astronomical African American death rates and the crucial and positive effects this first large-scale government health program had on them. The level of morbidity, pain and suffering, and disability this program prevented or relieved in the Black community is incalculable. Nevertheless, the Freedmen's Bureau health program represented a bold new government-based approach to a disadvantaged group's health care.[177]

The Freedmen's Bureau approach to African American health was a revolutionary phenomenon. Before the Civil War, the provision of health services to a dependent Black population had been an almost exclusively private affair. Substandard Black health status and outcome concerned only the slaveowner in most instances. He could decide to provide or deny decent health care for his chattel. When Union Army generals confronted the government with the provision of health and support services to the newly freed and contraband slaves, a new frontier was broached. Legislatively and logistically the U.S. Congress intervened for the first time. African Americans' health, and any other destitute racial or ethnic group's health, became an acknowledged national government concern. This preceded major European government interventions into health care in nineteenth-century Germany and England by several decades. If such programs had continued after the war, the slave health deficit conceivably could have been relegated to history.[178]

However, during and immediately after the war there were disturbing signs that this new commitment was not permanent. It was also distorted by overt and covert racism. White physicians spurned assignments to Black units and refused to work under the supervision of qualified African American physicians holding superior rank; the Union Army supported their breach of discipline. This was an insult to Black servicemen, and such policies represented a medical disadvantage for African American troops. The Army medical corps exacerbated this already perverse situation by assigning unqualified corpsmen to function as "surgeons" in the Black units. Although forced to provide medical support for African Americans in the Union Army, a substandard level of medical services was deemed officially adequate for Blacks according to Union Army Medical Department policy and practice. This barometer of the high levels of overt racial prejudice present in the White medical profession corroborated physician survey results later reported by the U.S. Sanitary Commission study.[179]

Despite the post–Civil War nadir in African American health status and outcome, the Freedmen's Bureau had discontinued virtually all their health programs by 1870. Howard Ashley White states, "Neither in extent of activity nor in duration did the agency meet the health problems that followed the emancipation of the slaves."[180] He made the following prescient observation:

> If the Republicans who appropriated large sums to be loaned to railroads had been equally interested in medical care for the indigent, the experiment could have been continued over a longer period of time, and the result might have been a system that would have served as a model

for succeeding generations. With all its limitations, however, the pro-
gram was a notable advance in governmental acceptance of responsibil-
ity in the field of public health.[181]

Although the Bureau and its functionaries knew there was nothing to replace the health programs, by 1872 government-sponsored health care for ex-slaves was over.[182]

Health Policy Born of Pragmatism

Abolitionist-educators Oliver O. Howard and George Whipple Hubbard were well positioned to witness the worsening Black health crisis. Both men saw Blacks decimated by deprivation and the lack of medical care, and both witnessed the refusal of the mainstream system to address the problem. Training Black physicians and nurses was a natural approach to solving a difficult problem that ultimately would extend beyond the good will of White people or the government.

Many of the negative attitudes regarding African American health emanated from the White medical profession. As James H. Jones observed about physician opinions on the effects of the Civil War and the emancipation of Blacks:

When the Civil War erupted, physicians in both the North and the South
warned that freedom would mean extinction for blacks. While other groups
discussed the future of the free blacks, physicians debated whether the race
as such had a future. They saw the emancipation of the slaves as a water-
shed in black health, the chief result of which was likely to be a decline in
health that was so drastic as to endanger the survival of the race.[183]

Such attitudes boded ill for African Americans and transformed the medical establishment's nihilistic health policies into self-fulfilling prophecies. In many instances White physicians actually became opponents of Black survival and good health. Therefore, opening Howard and Meharry medical schools turned out to be brilliant health policy strategies that tapped into the lingering abolitionist and relief agency infrastructure in Black education after the war. Moreover, it had the potential for expanding the most tangible and permanent infrastructure ever built to benefit African Americans in the United States—a network of schools.[184]

Although there were a few White medical schools that had allowed African Americans to enter and graduate by 1860, this was a rare and noteworthy event. As Morais pointed out,

By 1860 . . . nine Northern medical schools had admitted one Negro or
more to their lectures. The schools were: Bowdoin; the Medical School of

the University of New York; the Castleton Medical School in Vermont; the Berkshire Medical School in Pittsfield, Massachusetts; the Rush Medical School in Chicago; the Eclectic Medical School of Philadelphia; the Homeopathic College of Cleveland; the American Medical College and the Medical School of Harvard University.[185]

The devastating effects of professional segregation and discrimination can be found even in these few schools in that they did not necessarily graduate the Blacks they admitted. Harvard, though it admitted three African Americans in 1850, for example, did not actually graduate its first Black physician until 1869.* Moreover, as if to restrict Black admissions even more, some of these more liberal schools would not survive medical school reform. The situation was further compounded because one-third of all medical schools—which eventually were located in the South—would not admit Blacks until after 1948. Another consideration was that practically all African American practitioners before the war were trained in White medical schools on condition that they would emigrate to Africa to practice. As Cobb notes in *Medical Care and the Plight of the Negro*:

> *Before the Civil War, there was objection to professional education for Negroes if they intended to practice in the United States, but it was permissible if they proposed to go to Liberia, which was then being colonized. In this way, Dr. William Taylor and Dr. Fleet of Washington, D.C.; Dr. John V. de Grasse of New York and Dr. Thomas White of Brooklyn received their training.*[186]

Even the tiny output of trained Blacks was never intended to serve African Americans in the minds of antebellum White physicians and health policy makers. This tiny cadre of graduating Black physicians, who could not have possibly provided care for 5 million people, illustrates the gravity of the health system's problem. These policies were evidence of the insensitivity of the White medical establishment regarding the urgent medical needs of the African American population.[187]

The Medical Department of Howard University was incorporated on March 2, 1867, and opened its doors on November 9, 1868. Its stated purpose was to assist agencies already at work in the relief of ignorance and personal suffering in the District of Columbia and in the country at large. It was the first American medical school with an open admissions policy to all U.S. racial and ethnic groups. Emblematic of Howard, one of the entering class of eight was a young White man from Brooklyn named Bennit. From its very beginnings Howard was a worldly and cosmopolitan institution, and its early classes were heavily populated by a widely diverse student body from many states, foreign countries, and the West Indies. All

---

*Edwin Clarence Howard (1846–?) was the first African American to graduate from Harvard Medical School.

ethnic groups were represented, and most of the African American students hailed from the Northern states. Thus, most of Howard's students were the beneficiaries of decent secondary and advanced educations. This was unusual for Blacks at the time. From the feminist perspective, "Howard Medical School recognized very early the close relationship between the equal rights movement for Negroes and for women."[188] Therefore, early in its history, Howard began graduating women physicians; the first was Mary Dora Speckman in 1872.[189]

Howard University's first medical school faculty was predominantly White, headed by Dean Silas L. Loomis, professor of chemistry and toxicology; Joseph T. Johnson, secretary and professor of obstetrics; Robert Reyburn, professor of surgery; Lafayette C. Loomis, professor of physiology and microscopy; and the sole African American, Alexander T. Augusta, demonstrator of anatomy. A second African American physician, Charles Burleigh Purvis (1842–1929), a graduate of Wooster Medical College (now Western Reserve University), was recruited as professor of materia medica and therapeutics and assistant surgeon in 1869. Howard's White physicians were highly sought after and respected medical personnel in the District—many of whom were on other medical school faculties. Both Drs. Reyburn and Loomis were full professors at Georgetown Medical School. Because of his affiliation with Howard, Dr. Loomis had been terminated from Georgetown, and it was quickly rumored that Dr. Reyburn's dismissal was imminent. This was symptomatic of the pathological relationship that existed between Howard and the White medical profession in the District. As W. Montague Cobb observed:

> It is not to be assumed, however, that even in the beginning, the noble purpose and distinguished figures associated with Howard were able to secure for it the approval and respect of the medical profession. Ridicule and contempt, in part emanating from the jealousy of a sister school in Washington, were quickly pointed at the institution and the white physicians who dared associate themselves with it.[190]

Because of Howard's unique location in the nation's capital, having the support of able and representative citizens and governmental funding and connections, it could attract the nation's top Black physicians. These included physicians such as Daniel Hale Williams of Chicago, who served as surgeon-in-chief of Freedmen's Hospital from 1893 through 1898 (see Figure 6.8), and Austin Maurice Curtis, who served as surgeon-in-chief at Freedmen's from 1898 to 1902 and later as the first Black chairman of surgery at Howard between 1928 and 1936. Howard gained a reputation for excellence, however, even among those who begrudged its existence. Interestingly, Howard's faculty remained predominantly White until just before 1900. Howard remained the District's highest-rated medical school throughout the late nineteenth century, outscoring other local medical schools, according to the Flexner Report of 1910.[191]

Figure 6.8 Dr. Daniel Hale Williams at Howard: African American
Medical Leader

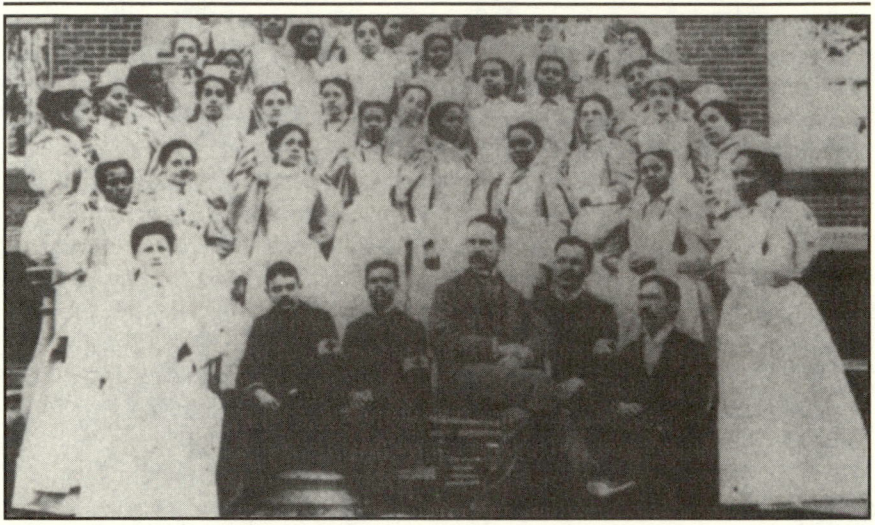

Fresh from his performance of the first successful open-heart operation in medical history (1893),
surgeon Daniel Hale Williams (1858–1931) was appointed Chief of Surgery at Freedmen's Hospital
in Washington (1893–1898). He strengthened Howard Medical School's clinical educational
programs and established a nurse training program at Freedmen's. This rare 1897 photograph shows
him amid interns and nurses at the hospital. He is the seated figure in the center of the first row.

During the shocking decade of the Radical Reconstruction and its effects on
the health status and outcomes of the African American community in Washington, DC, Howard began graduating professional health providers. The medical
school produced 238 Black male physicians and 14 women physicians by 1890.
Nevertheless, the new school had a disappointing effect on the health of the
Black community as a whole. The racial health disadvantage was systemic and
pervasive and virtually the entire health care establishment was ranged against
Howard's efforts.

Major socioeconomic factors also mitigated the medical school's impact on
the nation's capital, especially after the onset of the depression of 1873 and the
Southern Redemption during the Gilded Age. Initially, after the abolition of
slavery in the District in 1862 and the establishment of free schools for Blacks
in 1863, the District's Black population exploded to more than 30,000 by 1866.
Government-sponsored freedmen's health and aid programs in the District had
also been a magnet for Black in-migration. These circumstances bred huge
shantytowns prone to epidemics of typhoid, smallpox, yellow fever, and
cholera. Infant and childhood mortality rates in these areas were astronomical.
However, for the African American community during the Gilded Age in

Washington, "The early bid for first-class citizenship was made and was over-whelmingly crushed."[192] Segregated schools were implemented in 1875, suffrage was lost in 1878, and the Civil Rights Laws were nullified in the District until 1952.[193]

At least six Black doctors were practicing in the District at the end of the war: Drs. Anthony Bowen, George Brooks, William Johnson, Alexander T. Augusta, Charles B. Purvis, and A. W. Tucker. According to Cobb, "[S]ome of these men were very able and well trained according to the standards of the time."[194] Nevertheless, because the medical profession and health facilities in the District were rigidly segregated, they were excluded. There was an understandable early nineteenth-century tradition of fully trained Black practitioners who never practiced medicine, presumably because of the hostile atmosphere, restrictions, and logistical difficulties. Dr. John H. Fleet, for example, whose training was sponsored by the American Abolition Society under condition that he emigrate, never practiced medicine. The difficulties of practicing medicine experienced by Black physicians such as David John Peck, Martin Robison Delany, and Robert F. Boyd suggest that future research into the number of Black practitioners who actually succumbed to the racism and professional pressures is needed.

Cobb observed that Howard's appearance in the post–Civil War environment in Washington "accentuated a hostile attitude toward Negro physicians in an already prejudiced community."[195] If prejudice and discrimination did not force large numbers of African American physicians in the Washington, DC, area to leave medical practice, it certainly forced them to practice part-time. Facing many obstacles, they found it impossible to make a living practicing medicine. Many of these physicians, most of whom had regular jobs in the government bureaucracy, practiced medicine in the evenings after the government day ended between three and four o'clock. Thus, they became known as "sundown doctors."* This was a very common phenomenon for Black doctors until the 1900s, and it also explains why many of them earned extra degrees in dentistry and pharmacy as a hedge against failing financially as physicians. Dr. Hubbard of Meharry and Dr. Meserve of Leonard Medical School unintentionally revealed the extent of the problem by repeatedly bragging that more than 90 percent of their graduates practiced medicine or dentistry full-time as late as 1900.[196]

During the Gilded Age, Black physicians in the District of Columbia were denied hospital privileges. White physicians unethically refused to consult with African American doctors, virtually stealing their patients from them. Highly qualified Black physicians such as Alexander T. Augusta related "that members of the medical society have repeatedly refused to consult with him, alleging as a reason that the laws of the society prohibited them from so doing."[197] He added

---

*"Sundown doctors" was a disparaging term used to describe physicians unable to make a living practicing medicine. These practitioners kept days jobs teaching, preaching, or portering and saw patients in the evenings or after sundown.

that one White physician "has taken two of my patients while I was attending them, and without any notice to me, except that my next visit I was informed that Dr. Garnett was attending."[198] On patient stealing, Dr. Charles B. Purvis relates, "It is not an uncommon experience of mine to have physicians take my patients, they knowing I had not been dismissed, doing me a direct injury."[199] This was only one aspect of the crushing professional discrimination inflicted at the personal level by White doctors. Official and systematic exclusion and discrimination had more serious consequences for African American physicians.

After the Civil War Black and a few fair-minded White physicians presumed the medical profession would open its arms to all qualified physicians. When three of the most qualified and deserving Black physicians were placed as candidates before the Medical Society of the District of Columbia in 1869, two of whom were Howard University Medical College faculty members, they were rejected solely because of their race. Drs. Alexander T. Augusta, Charles B. Purvis, and A. W. Tucker did not realize they had become the flash-points of a professional policy issue that would chart White organized medicine on a course of discriminatory treatment of African American physicians into the twenty-first century. The Medical Society of the District of Columbia decided to exclude these three well-qualified African American physicians between June 9 and June 23, 1869.

Since membership in a medical society was a prerequisite to obtaining hospital privileges, being consulted by professional colleagues, and enjoying access to training and continuing medical education activities, systematic exclusion was devastating to anyone in practice. As Cobb pointed out, "[T]he actual exclusion of the colored physicians precipitated a bitter four-year controversy in this Society which was carried to the United States Senate and the American Medical Association."[200] After a second round of rejections, the Black physicians, spurred on by Howard's mostly White medical school faculty, formed the racially desegregated National Medical Society on January 15, 1870. From May 3 to May 6, 1870, at the twenty-first national AMA convention in Washington, DC, the AMA refused to seat the racially desegregated delegation of the National Medical Society. They also condoned the racist actions of the Medical Society of the District of Columbia on the basis of ethics! When a similar biracial delegation, which had been renamed the Academy of Medicine, challenged the AMA at their Annual Convention in Philadelphia in 1872, they were rejected again. (See Figure 6.9.) Professional racial discrimination remained virtually unchanged until 1968 when some token reform measures were introduced.[201]

After being apprised of these events, Senator Charles Sumner of Massachusetts was outraged. When he heard of the Medical Society of the District of Columbia's actions the Senator said, "Thus do members of the society constitute themselves a medical oligarchy. . . . [I]n my opinion these white oligarchs ought to have notice, and I give them notice now, that this outrage shall not be allowed to continue without remedy. . . . The time has passed for any such pretension."[202]

Figure 6.9   Dr. J. M. Kellar in His Confederate Uniform

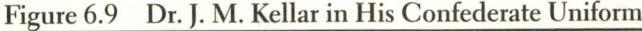

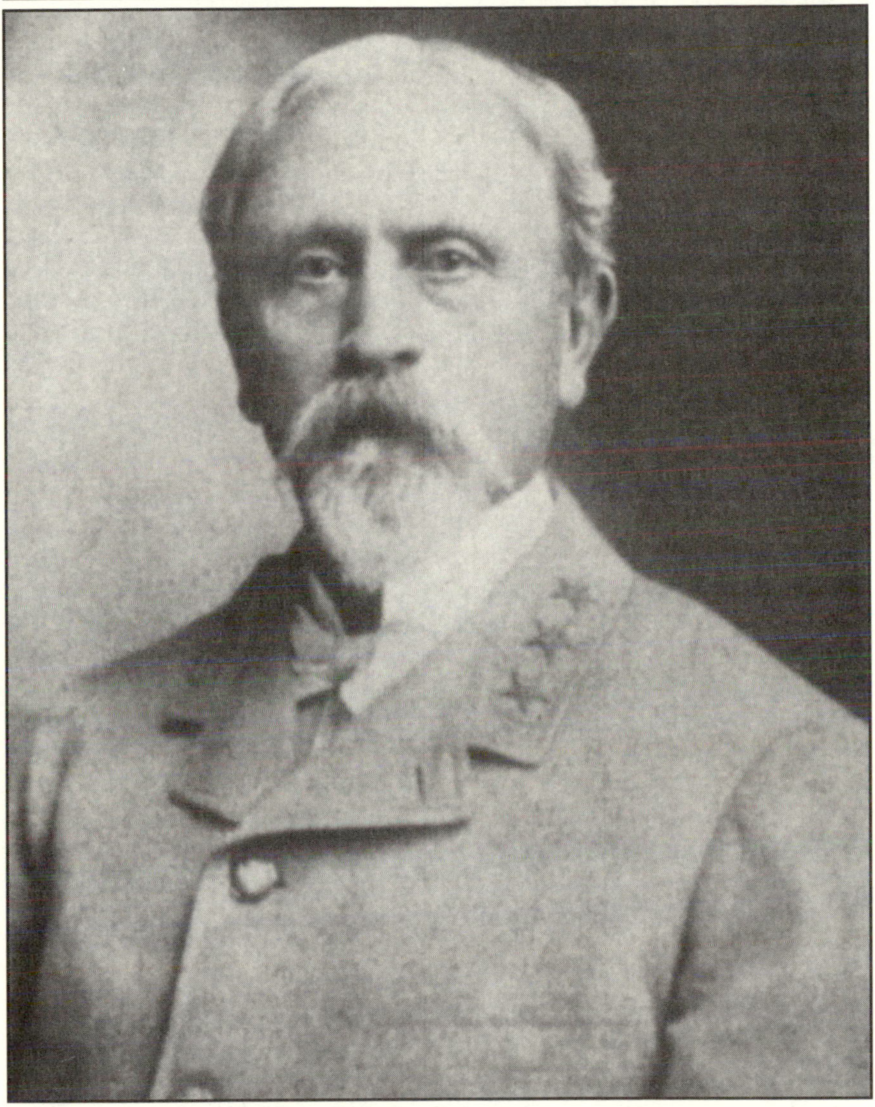

Kellar was a distinguished physician in the Confederate States Army. He later became an influential AMA Ethics committee member who voted down African American participation in that professional organization. This policy remained in effect for more than a century. This man being chosen to decide the fate of the physicians serving the African American population, the effects of which lasted for over a century, is symbolic of the degree of justice and fair play Black doctors faced within the post–Civil War, U.S. medical profession.

The efforts of Senator Sumner culminated at the Congressional level with the introduction of bill S.511 to repeal the charter of the Medical Society of the District of Columbia. Introduced on February 8, 1870, the bill assailed the organization's discriminatory policies toward African American physicians. Enacting the bill was blocked. Legislation to repeal the Medical Society's charter was brought four times to Capitol Hill, the final bill occurring on December 18, 1871—to no avail. Nor did the protests of fair-minded White physicians, congressmen, or Black physicians curb the unprofessional or racist actions of the Medical Society of the District of Columbia.

Another factor, besides their small numbers, that dampened the impact of Black physicians produced by the medical school was that most of Howard's students and graduates were concentrated in the North, where less than 10 percent of the Black population lived at the time. Global factors, such as the economic depression of 1873, caused Howard's medical department to almost close due to lack of funds. Had it not been for the leadership and emergency financial support of Black physicians such as Charles B. Purvis and Alexander T. Augusta and several sympathetic White physician-faculty members, the medical school at Howard would have been lost. These Howard physicians reorganized and shouldered the finances of the medical department for several years, risking their own resources in the process.[203]

Although culturally a Southern city, because it was the nation's capital and was situated contiguously to the urban northeast, Washington, DC, housed what was considered the Northern arm of Black higher and professional education. Howard became the apogee—the Harvard—of Black academia. The medical school—with its White faculty orientation, its multinational and multicultural student body, and growing tendency to identify itself with the urban American dream and mainstream medical and educational trends—set Howard apart from its Southern counterparts. Thus, Howard was very aware of and sensitive to medical education's new scientific trends and movement toward specialization.

Against great financial and logistical odds, Howard struggled to remain open and abreast of medical progress. Lincoln University of Chester County, Pennsylvania, the other Northern Black medical school, opened in 1870 but was virtually stillborn with no known graduates. Meharry, the first successful medical school (Straight had opened in New Orleans in 1873 but closed the next year) for African Americans to open in a Southern ex-Confederate state, represented the reorientation of American medical education, based on the needs and experiences of the Southern Black masses—still 90 percent of the African American population. Thus, from their very beginnings, Howard and Meharry, the two major Black medical schools, were different from each other, complementing rather than competing.[204]

From its origins, Meharry Medical College was organic to the Black community. Although two other unsuccessful efforts to open Black medical schools had preceded Meharry, the Nashville school spawned one of the two dominant branches of the African American medical profession both numerically and socioculturally. Meharry would eventually train and graduate more Black physicians than any other institution in the world. Meharry's forte was producing grassroots, primary care–oriented practitioners with folksy manners and the common touch, almost deceptively combining professional skills and new medical technology with the imagery of the Old South's Black healer roots. The college's White founders, Dr. George Whipple Hubbard, Reverend John Braden, and Dr. William Joseph Sneed, represented a strange sociocultural mix of New England abolitionism, the Northern missionary education movement for ex-slaves, and Southern paternalism, responsibility, and stewardship. They emphasized training physicians who would serve the community. Keeping up with technical advances, new educational requirements, and movements toward medical specialization were not prioritized for intellectual aspirations or attainments—they were means to an end of fulfilling Meharry's mission.

As previously noted, Dr. Hubbard, the ex–Union Army medical corpsman, Vanderbilt Medical School graduate, and abolitionist educator; Reverend Braden, the mainstream philanthropic cleric, Black education professional, and Freedmen's Aid Society missionary school principal of Central Tennessee College; and Dr. Sneed, the highly respected ex–Confederate Army surgeon who sacrificed a lucrative and professionally prestigious and influential White medical career to train Black doctors in a hostile post-Reconstruction South, produced the peculiar social and educational chemistry that enabled the financial gift of the Meharry brothers to breathe life into Dr. Hubbard's and Rev. Braden's dream of producing Black medical professionals. Hubbard predicted this army of Black men and women, after being equipped with health professions training, would embark on missions of medical service and sacrifice for a health-deprived Southern Black population. In many ways, their dream bore fruit.

Fate combined with circumstance to help George Whipple Hubbard found Meharry Medical College. After a deep and devoted friendship with young Dr. Sneed, which began during the Civil War and culminated in their lifelong sharing of careers, Hubbard, with Sneed's sponsorship, completed his medical training in 1876 at Vanderbilt University Medical School. Before his graduation, Hubbard and Sneed committed themselves in 1875 to open a medical department at Central Tennessee College to train Black physicians and nurses. This had also been Reverend John Braden's dream since around 1870. Thus, Hubbard was poised in 1876 to live out his shared vision of training African American health providers to serve the Black community. Meharry became the nation's first long-lived medical school specifically designed to train African American physicians.[205]

As a general rule, Meharry's entering students were not as well prepared academically as Howard's were during its formative years. Many were barely literate ex-slaves when they presented for medical school. Largely products of the substandard Southern educational system, remedial work and retention in grade were rules rather than exceptions. As Morais observed, "For the most part they came from the South and had only the rudiments of a preparatory education."[206] Moreover, Black students usually received less than their share of the already educationally inadequate resources allocated to ill-prepared Southern White public schools. Often, Dr. Hubbard and his faculty had to teach students to read, write, and count; they would refer students to Central Tennessee College, Fisk, Roger Williams, or other local institutions that provided these preparatory services. Morais described these students in *The History of the Negro in Medicine:*

> *Ex-slaves or the sons of ex-slaves, they were largely without means and, hence, had to work their way through medical school. They took jobs of every kind, including the most menial, all the while devoting themselves to study. That many of them after graduation remained in the South, developing lucrative practices and rising to eminence in their communities, was a testimonial to their perseverance and ability.*[207]

How, indeed, was Meharry able to address the educational handicaps of their students? It was standard practice during this era of proprietary medical schools to graduate virtually everyone who attended classes and paid tuition. Failing to graduate students threatened the financial viability of the school.

As Dr. C. V. Roman, an 1890 Meharry graduate, pioneer faculty member, and historian stated in his voluminous writings, "Meharry was different." What he meant was that in contrast to the rash of medical diploma mills that dotted the nation, Meharry was built and operated on the highest levels of integrity. For example, of the first class of 11 medical students, only one—James M. Jamison— graduated in 1877. Three of the 18 who started the next class received degrees in 1878. There were three graduates in the medical class of 1881. Clearly, this pattern, indicated by the statistics and close reading of the commencement addresses and accounts about the school by Reverend John Braden and others, reveals that a tremendous selection process was at work. Educational miracles were being performed. Although Meharry was private, it could not be considered just another proprietary medical school. There is evidence that not only Meharry but also other Black medical schools, in their efforts to compensate for the deprived African American educational backgrounds, went to such extremes to maintain standards. Some set such rigorous criteria and standards that they literally put themselves out of business.

The abortive Lincoln University Medical School, which functioned between 1870 and 1873 and did not officially close until 1876, is a prime example. Lincoln set strict entrance requirements of a bachelor's degree for admission—which was unprecedented for the time. They required a three-year, nine-month-long, graded curriculum. Lincoln recruited a highly trained White faculty that included nationally prestigious academic physicians. They also required written examinations in each course before passing to the next level and required not only certification in anatomical dissection, but also attendance on their rural campus for at least a year and completion of a thesis for graduation. Such requirements and standards were almost unheard of in 1870—even among White schools. Only Harvard and Chicago Medical College had similar stringent requirements and standards. Lincoln's isolated Chester County, Pennsylvania, location, the school's lack of finances, and the school's lack of prestige—compounded by the caste-like status conferred by educating African Americans—doomed the medical school from its inception.

The little-known Louisville National Medical College (1888–1912) had stringent admission and curricular standards that kept it financially vulnerable. By elevating standards and performance levels, Dr. Henry Fitzbutler (1842–1901) had not a single graduate who failed state licensing examinations while he lived. He even conducted a year-long primary course, which he included in the curriculums of some of his least-prepared students. His wife, struggling to keep the school open after his death in 1901, was evidently unable to duplicate her husband's excellent administrative performance. Louisville National graduates' performance on state boards declined to the levels of other proprietary schools.[208]

Black medical schools in the United States, according to Todd Savitt, the leading authority on these institutions, can be categorized as missionary or proprietary. Howard, although it received some intermittent church support, doesn't fit neatly into either category since it was subsidized by the federal government from its inception. Meharry was a project initially funded by the Methodist Episcopal Church, although it depended strongly on the tuition paid by its students, similar to other medical colleges of the era. A gift from the Meharry family was critical to starting the school, and repeated gifts proved necessary for the school's survival and modernizations to meet rising standards. Central Tennessee College, Meharry's parent institution, also received support and resources from the Freedmen's Bureau. These nonproprietary origins, buttressed by Dr. Hubbard's and Reverend Braden's input, might help explain Meharry's integrity and commitment to the ideals and standards of medicine often absent from purely commercial health professions schools. That students persisted and arrived prepared to make the sacrifice for medical, dental, and pharmacy training was truly a miracle. Morais recorded Georgetown University Medical School's petulant faculty statements regarding their fears of Howard and other Black medical schools surpassing them "because of the 'determination on the part of the "Niggers" [*sic*] to be educated, and on the part of their friends throughout the North that they would be educated.'"[209] There was no one better equipped to facilitate that process than George Whipple Hubbard.[210]

After Meharry's 1876 opening, there was a lapse of several years until 1882 when Shaw University in Raleigh, North Carolina, opened what amounted to a proprietary institution under the umbrella of a missionary school. Although the

American Baptist Home Missionary Society (ABHM) authorized Shaw to operate a medical school on their campus, they never assumed financial responsibility for it. This lack of financial support by the ABHM, the foundations, the state, or the other missionary associations, compounded by the demands for medical educational reform by AMA-driven educational committees and state medical licensing boards, would force the Shaw University's Leonard Medical School to close by 1918. At its closing, the Medical School was enjoying state board passage rates of 70–80 percent, which was as high as the national average. Despite overwhelming African American health needs, medical educational reform—driven by the AAMC, the AMA, and wealthy, White male–dominated, upper-class and corporate interests that were oblivious to the health needs of Black and poor patients—closed institutions that were vital sources of African American physicians and health professionals. Approximately 1,000 African American physicians were trained by Black medical schools other than Howard and Meharry before their closure due to medical educational reform. Leonard trained almost half of them. As McBride noted, it "produced many distinguished black doctors," including a pivotal figure in American medicine—John A. Kenney (1874–1950).[211]

Over the 45 years after Howard University's Medical Department opened in 1868, more than a dozen Black medical schools attempted to emulate Howard and, later, Meharry's mission of training Black health professionals. This next wave of openings of Black health professions schools, beginning in 1888, would be almost wholly proprietary. Although not energized purely by monetary gain, they represented the entrepreneurial efforts of the first post–Civil War generation of African American medical school graduates. Physicians such as University of Michigan Medical School graduate Dr. Henry Fitzbutler, the founder of Louisville National Medical School, and Dr. Myles V. Lynk, Meharry graduate and founder of the University of West Tennessee, dreamed of solving the Black health crisis by supplying trained African American health professionals to counteract and correct the centuries-old and recently institutionalized Black health status and outcome deficits.

As a result of the proliferation of Black medical schools, Black physicians increased in number from 909 in 1890 to 3,409 by 1910. Nevertheless, this translated into approximate doctor-patient ratios of 1:3,000 Black physicians to Black patients compared to 1:700 White physicians to White patients in the early twentieth century. Even though framing the Black health crisis in terms of manpower shortages represented great professional progress for African Americans, Benjamin Brawley points out it would have required four times this number of Black physicians to equalize these ratios. Moreover, African Americans suffered far more illness and death than Whites. Although these trends suggested that Black participation in the medical, nursing, dental, and pharmaceutical professions in the United States seemed assured by 1900, these figures were also reflections of the huge increases in poorly regulated medical and health professions schools. As Starr observed about the medical school proliferation, "Between 1850 and 1870, the number had grown from 52 to 75; ten years later, it jumped to 100, in another decade to 133, and by 1900 to 160."[212] However, there were other momentous events affecting the medical profession as it entered the new century.[213]

The appearance of a significant cadre of fully trained African American physicians after the Civil War created an entirely new environment in the U.S. health system. Their presence, their numbers, and their performance dictated changed attitudes about Black doctors within and outside the profession. Although White physicians often attempted to discredit them, they were aware of such sterling breakthrough medical performances as Daniel Hale Williams's startling operation on a living human heart in 1893. Henry Fitzbutler's medical competence and brilliant professional performance in Louisville, Kentucky, during the 1870s and 1880s was obvious to both the Black and White communities. Nevertheless, White physicians joined the community in oppressing and discriminating against him in lieu of respecting him professionally. Nathan Frances Mossell's memorable performance, which resulted in his graduating in the upper echelons of his class at the University of Pennsylvania's Medical School in 1882, was well known throughout the medical world. This, however, did not dissipate professional resistance to his acceptance into the Philadelphia Medical Society. White doctors were also aware of Myles Vandahurst Link's publication of the *Medical and Surgical Observer* in 1892, the first African American medical journal, in which he made the first publicly announced call for a national Black medical association. Daniel Hale Williams, along with physicians of both races and influential Chicagoans, opened the first private, racially neutral (which in those days meant Black) hospital in Chicago in 1891—Provident Hospital. All of these major advances for Blacks in the medical professions benefitted African American patients in many ways.[214]

Most Black healers before the Civil War had been either untrained or informally trained providers in the slave health subsystem. With the dismantling of slavery, the basis of practice upon which these caregivers functioned was undercut. As has been revealed, the number of formally trained and apprentice-trained African Americans was tiny due to professional proscription and racism. Thus, the founding and functioning of this growing network of Black medical schools were revolutionary health policy events that forever changed the character of American medicine. No longer would the gentrification of the medical profession, standardization, and medical educational reform that threatened to further depress already abysmal Black health status and outcomes go unquestioned on medical-social grounds.

Unlike many other countries, there were fully trained medical spokesmen for the disadvantaged and underserved in the U.S. health system. Moreover, much of this activity was not dependent upon the good will of the White medical profession or its burgeoning infrastructure. African American medicine would consistently serve as the conscience of American medicine. By taking on this task, it would elevate health care to the level of a civil rights issue in the United

States—something unprecedented and unique in Western culture. Significantly, such an approach would be duplicated later by President Nelson Mandela of South Africa who, immediately following independence, placed reform of that nation's health system near the top of his agenda.[215]

As the cadre of Black physicians grew, their maltreatment at the hands of the White medical establishment intensified. The rejection of the Black Howard faculty by the Medical Society of the District of Columbia, followed by the formulation of the AMA's official policy based on rejection of Black physicians during the early 1870s, set the tone in the profession for nearly a century. Bigotry and discrimination in the medical profession were open and undiluted.

Qualified African American practitioners such as Nathan Frances Mossell created a furor by simply applying to the Philadelphia Medical Society in 1888. He not only had nationally known sponsors such as the famous surgeon D. Hayes Agnew, J. Britton Massey, and the dean of the University of Pennsylvania's medical school James Tyson, but he had also gone beyond the norm by obtaining more than two years of postgraduate training and completing a course at the Philadelphia Polyclinic, now the graduate school of medicine at the University of Pennsylvania. Dean Tyson reminded the Medical Society participants that "Dr. Mossell graduated with an average higher than three fourths of his class."[216] This favorably influenced the discussion on admitting Mossell.

The harsh limitations imposed by White organized medicine translated into severe professional and practice exclusions, isolation, and lost credibility for Black physicians. As the twentieth century approached, Black physicians were increasingly forced to function and interface with many layers of the health system. Admission to medical school was increasingly predicated on strong primary and secondary educational backgrounds, which few Blacks had. By the 1890s, many better schools were requiring a college degree for admission. Few Blacks of that era attended college. If African Americans were admitted to the 10 percent of the medical schools that would consider their applications, they then had to undergo the intense scrutiny and isolation experienced by Blacks in White professional schools of the period. Mossell, after resisting being forced to sit behind a screen during medical school lectures, related "that he attended his early classes at the University of Pennsylvania with a gun in his pocket for protection."[217] Such examples highlight the importance of African American medical schools.

Since few hospitals admitted Blacks for postgraduate hospital training, now known as internships and residencies, acquiring specialty training or hospital expertise was rare unless obtained overseas. After obtaining the requisite training, the physician-candidate then had to take, and pass, the same medical licensing tests taken by Whites. Without the requisite specialty training, academic credentialing, or family connections, most Blacks were automatically excluded from academic medicine and the highly sought-after hospital and faculty appointments. Moreover, membership in local medical societies was required to gain hospital privileges in most communities. With the AMA ban on Black physicians in effect, this was an impossible criterion to meet for all but a few African American physicians. Thus, until the 1960s most Blacks were denied hospital privileges (except at Black hospitals) throughout the United States, primarily because of their lack of local professional organization membership.

Medical society membership was also the key that opened the doors to continuing medical education and subsequent credentialing. It provided professional stimulation, interaction, and collegiality, often in isolated settings and communities. Medical societies were the vehicles for acquiring professional benefits such as malpractice insurance and authoritative and effective representation in medical regulatory and public health matters. As Paul Starr notes, "Professional ostracism carried increasingly serious consequences: denial of hospital privileges, loss of referrals, loss of malpractice insurance, and, in extreme cases, loss of a license to practice."[218] Clearly, there was an inverse relationship between the ability of "outsiders" in the profession to function as physicians and the medical establishment's growth in authority and power throughout the Gilded Age and early Progressive Period. This added untold and increasing burdens to the difficulties encountered by the African American physician during this period.[219]

Based on the evidence provided by the implementation of policies and practices of overt racial segregation and discrimination within the U.S. medical profession, by the late 1880s the growing number of Black physicians saw that separate organization was necessary. Frustrated after repeated attempts to have qualified Black physicians admitted to the Medical Society of the District of Columbia and the AMA, a biracial group of physicians formed the Medico-Chirurgical Society of the District of Columbia. This group, founded in 1884, is usually credited as the nation's first Black medical society. Drs. Purvis and Augusta, although sympathetic to the cause, did not join. The organization lapsed until January 15, 1895, when it was revived and incorporated.

Meanwhile, Dr. J. F. Shadd and Dr. John R. Francis, two highly qualified African American physicians, had been rejected by the Medical Society of the District of Columbia in 1891 and 1894, respectively. Despite these setbacks, organizational efforts were launched outside the nation's major cities. Led by Drs. J. H. Wilkins, Dr. T. E. Speed, Dr. L. M. Wilkins, pharmacist Dr. Cameron, and Dr. Monroe Majors (all but Dr. Speed were Meharry graduates),* a group of 13 African American health professionals formed the Lone Star State Medical, Dental and Pharmaceutical Society in August 1886 in Galveston, Texas. The second state organization, the Old North State Medical Society of North Carolina, was founded one year later. A growing movement for a national African American medical association was first articulated publicly by Dr. Myles V. Lynk in 1892 or 1893. Although it is difficult to tell whether it was planned or not, when Black medical leaders Robert F. Boyd, Daniel Hale Williams, and Lynk converged on Atlanta for the Cotton States Exposition, the opportune moment for

---

*Dr. Speed was a Flint Goodridge Medical School graduate.

forming a national professional organization occurred. They recruited Dr. I. Garland Penn, the chairman of Black exposition activities, and used the occasion of "Doctor's Day" on the evening of November 18, 1895, to form a national medical association. Thus, on that evening in the First Congregational Church at Atlanta, Georgia, Penn presided over the formation of the American Association of Colored Physicians and Surgeons (renamed the National Medical Association [NMA] in 1903), Black medicine's national voice.

Dr. Robert F. Boyd of Nashville, Tennessee, was elected the organization's first president; Daniel Hale Williams served as vice president. Boyd, who incidentally worked as a roving reporter at the Cotton States Exposition for a White newspaper, the *Nashville American*, reported the event, along with other news from the exposition, the following day in the newspaper. Nashville's intense interest was related to preparations for its own exposition in the near future. The medical organization languished for several years. Existing evidence from contemporaneous sources such as *The Washington Bee* in 1896 and *Nashville Banner* in 1905 reflect the organization's inactivity. Its exact founding date was lost to the principals involved and the NMA itself for many years. Dr. Boyd remained titular president for two terms until the next formal meeting of the organization in 1898. The organization did not become active nationally until late in the first decade of the twentieth century. Thus, the AMA's rebirth and reactivation preceded the NMA's by about 10 years. Whether they were fully aware of it or not, African American physicians positioned themselves to take on the struggle of Black people in America for justice and equity in health care in an organized fashion for the first time. American medicine, U.S. health, and the health care system would never be the same again.[220]

Outside the boundaries of the medical mainstream, Black physicians made critical adjustments to the disadvantaged circumstances under which they functioned. Meanwhile, White organized medicine adopted the strategic policy of treating the new African American medical profession as if it did not exist. As far as most of the lay public was concerned during the Gilded Age and Progressive Era, Black medicine was placed behind a veil of invisibility or disdain. Other health issues such as sectarian infighting, the poor state of medical education, and the paucity of truly effective clinical therapies—major preoccupations of the White health professions—were often mentioned under one's breath or with tongue in cheek. Organized medicine kept its problems secret.

As Konold observed about the nineteenth-century White medical profession, "By concealing all issues from lay audiences, physicians created the illusion of authority where there was no authority, and inspired confidence where confidence was not deserved."[221] Often from behind their racial "veil" African American physicians capitalized on the perverse, and often paradoxical, circumstances created by this strategy. For example, many White physicians would not, or preferred not to, treat African Americans. This intensified the need for Black physicians wherever there were large Black populations. In many communities, no hospitals or decent outpatient facilities existed for Blacks. Again, this intensified the need for, and marketing of, African American practitioners and institutions. White physicians often denigrated African Americans and their unique health problems. Black physicians worked to educate, generate public concern about, and correct these same problems. Communications and books written by Black practitioners of the era reflect these realities.

Black physicians, in an effort to adjust to their patients' circumstances, often charged lower fees. Medical ethicist Konold observed that White physicians during this era "carefully guarded their own financial interests."[222] Thus, as Savitt exposes in his work—corroborated by firsthand accounts from Black physicians such as J. Edward Perry and Myles V. Lynk—although Black doctors were relegated to professional caste status, White physicians regarded Negro physicians as economic competitors. This competition was considered "unfair" by White physicians because of their perceptions of Black physician incompetence and lower fee schedules. Clearly, this absolute and discriminatory segregation of the Black medical profession in an environment of exclusion and maltreatment of Black patients ensured the African American profession's survival, despite the negative trappings of racist exclusion. A major theme of this story is how these paradoxical and sometimes pathological relationships evolved and were redefined in the future.[223]

Prejudicial exclusion of Black physicians had another price. Many Black patients doubted the abilities of one of their own race to practice medicine. This often resulted in limiting the availability of vital care to African American patients and further imperiled the viability of an African American medical profession already threatened by the medical establishment. Seeds for doubt were planted by White physicians who publicly questioned the abilities of African American physicians and promoted the traditions of Black dependency and reliance on White physicians for medical care. As Robert F. Boyd, an 1882 Meharry Medical College graduate, observed about Nashville in 1887: "[V]ery few good [Black Nashville] families had ever given colored doctors their practice" because "they did not believe them competent."[224] Moreover, in most places the market had traditionally been dominated by White practitioners.

J. Edward Perry, an 1895 Meharry graduate, was told by a White practitioner he queried about the feasibility of establishing a practice in Columbia, Missouri: "[T]he practice among your people is done by white brethren in the profession and it would be a mighty hard thing for a man of your age and most especially your color to wring it from their hands."[225] Most White physicians wanted to pick and choose among well-to-do Blacks as a back-up supplement to their White practices. But they were glad to refer nonpaying patients, especially Black ones, to African American practitioners. Moreover, Black patients were unethically overutilized as experimental subjects by many members of the White profession and the institutions they supervised. During this inaugural era of the Black medical profession, a growing cadre of Black physicians saw the opportunity to carve out a new niche in American medical practice that would counteract these history-based, often unwholesome, tendencies.[226]

Black physicians, especially from Meharry, which had a Southern base, began to confront these obstacles and disadvantages head-on. Different individuals attacked the situation in different ways. In the Southern urban setting of Nashville, Tennessee, a city with three White medical schools* and a single Black one (usually unmentioned or barely mentioned in the standard histories), the competition was keen. Robert F. Boyd created what was to become the Black prototype for private medical practice in that highly competitive setting. As W. Montague Cobb noted about the 1887 practice environment: "In those days the practice of medicine was considered a very doubtful means of livelihood for a colored man. Dr. Boyd was the first Negro to make the venture in Nashville."[227] One common strategy of the day was earning multiple health professions degrees. Laying such a variegated foundation offered Black doctors some protection from failure in medical practice through broadening their practice base and offering more services. It is understandable why Boyd and the other two members of Meharry's first graduating dental class in 1887 were physicians. Significantly, Boyd's pioneer dental classmate, John Wesley Anderson, also adopted this strategy and built spectacularly successful private practice and philanthropic careers with Meharry and Dallas, Texas, as his focal points. Later, Boyd also earned a pharmacy degree from Meharry—he could thus treat patients, "draw" teeth, and compound and dispense his own medications.

Unacknowledged and unappreciated is the fact that Dr. Boyd and a few of his peers, through these and other actions, created the economic and medical-social milieu that allowed Black doctors to survive on the fringes of a hostile White profession hell-bent on segregating the health system during a period of reaction, Redemption, and Black code legislation in post–Reconstruction America. They accomplished this during a tumultuous period of American medical history when the nation's physicians were in the throes of sectarian, internecine turf wars in a health system already burdened with race, gender, class, and caste problems. Boyd and his colleagues improvised a unique, altruistic medical ethic focused on the underserved that fulfilled pressing medical-social and public health needs and spearheaded a Black hospital movement. These approaches were economically, technologically, and professionally necessary, and Boyd and his African American colleagues largely sidestepped the racial policies of mainstream American medicine, which was busy creating an apartheid-based health delivery system.

Boyd's strategies reflected his character, personal and human qualities, and pride. Their generalizability to African Americans entering the medical profes-

---

*The University of Nashville Medical School, Vanderbilt Medical School (these later merged), and the University of Tennessee Medical School (which later moved to Memphis) were all in Nashville. Shelby Medical College, a prewar medical school opened in 1858, never reopened after the war.

sion in the late nineteenth-century South was crucial. Born a slave in Pulaski, Tennessee, around 1858, he overcame an impoverished background, educational segregation, and social deprivation to earn academic degrees at Central Tennessee College, Fisk University, and Meharry Medical College. Not satisfied with standard medical training, he obtained additional training at the University of Michigan's postgraduate training program at Ann Arbor and at the Post-Graduate Medical School and Hospital in Chicago.

Stamping his personality on Black medical practice patterns, he charted new American medical-social and ethical paths, voluntarily scouring Nashville's jails, alleys, and flop-houses to attend derelicts who needed medical attention. Such actions not only piqued the Nashville professional community's ethical conscience, but also fulfilled vital medical-social and public health needs. His campaign led to an appointment as the city's Jail Physician, and he pushed Nashville to the forefront of Southern cities in public health with his establishment of free clinics and social hygiene programs for the poor. Therefore, Nashville, the South's third largest city behind New Orleans and Richmond at the time, through Boyd's efforts began meeting critical medical-social and public health needs that White physicians chose to ignore. Instead of yielding to stereotypes and public opinion about Black doctors, Boyd led the way in medical, public health, and medical-ethical arenas. He constantly upgraded his clinical and surgical skills at medical centers throughout the country, consulted freely and established professional ties with Nashville's finest physicians regardless of race, and, by virtually "marrying" his practice and his community, was living proof that Black physicians were not just competent, but excellent practitioners.

These developments created a new paradigm, making it possible for Boyd to succeed spectacularly in Nashville's highly competitive medical environment and proving that Black physicians could attract enough private, largely African American, paying patients to allow them to make a living practicing medicine. For African American physicians, by the 1900s, the days of the sundown doctors were over if they took Dr. Boyd's lessons to heart.

These unique experiments in rendering himself essential and virtually irreplaceable in a community's medical-social milieu do not capture all of Robert F. Boyd's contributions. He lectured to church and political groups on sanitation and hygiene and researched and wrote extensively on the scourge of tuberculosis on the Black community. The roots of Black physicians' health promotion and disease prevention activities, planted by James McCune Smith and Martin Robison Delany, were extended and upgraded long before Flexner degraded the concept by suggesting that Black physicians' caste-determined level of capability and role in medicine was as "trained sanitarians." Boyd was not only devoted to public health education; he and others such as John Wesley Anderson were also devoted to Black higher education—especially the institutions that trained them. Boyd was a tireless fundraiser for Fisk and Central Tennessee College, while he and Anderson provided for Meharry. He raised foundation monies for Meharry, spearheaded the drive culminating in the building of Hubbard Hospital, and self-lessly served as chair of several of Meharry's Medical School departments, including anatomy, physiology, and chemistry.

When in the early 1890s Nashville's City Hospital expelled Meharry's medical students, who were there for training purposes (the White medical schools dominated the facility), solely because of their race, Boyd expanded his private hospital operations and threw them open for clinical student training. Meharry's students and administration were allowed to return on a limited basis to Metro Nashville General Hospital, now located on Meharry's campus and serving as its flagship teaching hospital, around 1977 and were granted significant authority by 1990. Boyd was essential in making the Chicago connections necessary to establish the annual Surgical Clinics at Meharry conducted by internationally renowned surgeon Daniel Hale Williams. All of these events, plus his constant pressure on Dr. Hubbard and Meharry's board about the necessity for clinical training in modern medicine, spurred the drive to build Hubbard Hospital, meeting the medical school's vital training needs. Boyd's successful negotiation and mastery of medical practice and the medical education system spilled over into his political and financial endeavors. He became a successful political leader, founded the Peoples Saving Bank and Trust Company (now known as Citizen's Bank of Nashville), and owned the largest Black business in Nashville. These events were all emblematic of Boyd's status as a national Black medical leader and the first president of the American Association of Colored Physicians and Surgeons. At the time of his unexpected death at age 54 of an apparent heart attack on July 20, 1912, he was purportedly one of the wealthiest Black men in the United States.[228]

Post–Civil War Black community leaders, politicians, and civil rights activists observed what Black doctors were doing. They liked what they saw, and embraced and placed Black health high on the community's political and public policy agendas. Health care personnel remained in a privileged position in the African American community until the end of the 1960s' Civil Rights Era. Daniel Hale Williams's medical accomplishments made him a living legend in American medicine. Within the profession he spearheaded the Black hospital movement and made immense contributions to African American medical education. Although his celebrity status generated headlines and shattered White professional and lay assumptions of Black professional inferiority, his inattention to political and certain medical-social matters haunted and eventually limited his career. As Midian O. Bousfield, a contemporary medical leader and personal friend, wrote of him:

> After Dan Williams graduated in medicine, he never had another single interest in life. He saved his money and put it into Provident Hospital. . . . He had great determination and great confidence in himself. He had the natural dexterity to make a surgeon, and he would oper-

*ate all day long on all kinds of cases without exception, pay or no pay.
So single-tracked was his mind that he could not begin to cope with
medical politics. He had no stomach for a fight—he always gave away
before that—twice at Provident and once at Freedmen's. He made few
close friends, if any at all. . . . He was once expelled from a fraternal
organization at the very hey day of his success. He had no admirers in
the Anderson family,* which he seems to have forgotten promptly after
he got out of school. His wife was the one fine thing in his life. . . . Even
Dan would lose much of his preoccupation and boorishness before her.
But he drew more and more within himself and seemed to have no interest in former associates once he moved into new surroundings. No man
ever made less effort to make friends.*[229]*

Certainly, his insular and highly individualistic approach to the practice of medicine could not serve as the example needed by the hundreds of young Black men
Savitt accurately describes in his *Bulletin of the History of Medicine* article, "Entering a White Profession."[230] More than his quiet, behind-the-scenes, dedication and
approach to the African American medical cause was necessary. Men such as
Robert F. Boyd, George Cleveland Hall, and John Wesley Anderson, through both
their leadership and example, served as role models for a generation of African
American physicians entering medical practice in the twentieth century.[231]

A Mixed Legacy

What were the medical and health impacts and legacies of the tumultuous period
from 1861 to 1900 on the African American people? This question is best
answered in a multifaceted fashion. This 39-year period was one of revolutionary
medical progress. Medical and technical advances spurred development of a
belated, but vigorous, U.S. hospital movement. Improvements in medical science and technology mobilized the laboratory in support of clinical medicine
and yielded an expanded range of safe surgical procedures. Many of the health
system's structural components that would evolve into the megacorporate infrastructure appeared. There were improvements in physicians' therapeutic armamentarium. Improvements in medical education that permanently upgraded the
quality of U.S. physicians comprise a list of important and indelible legacies of
this era. All of these advances placed the United States on the threshold of world
medical leadership in the upcoming century.

---

*Almost abandoned during childhood to work-apprenticeships, Williams ended up with a biracial
business-owning family in Janesville, Wisconsin. Throughout his late teens and young adulthood
Williams worked, lived, and was sponsored by the Anderson family. They promoted and sponsored
Williams's high school, academy, medical apprenticeship, and medical educations.

Western clinical medicine made giant strides diagnostically and therapeutically. The incorporation of effective anesthesia, antisepsis and asepsis, and safer surgical techniques rendered surgery effective and essential over a broad range of clinical medicine for the first time. Surgery was no longer confined to operations on the limbs, a few quick and discrete invasive techniques on the eyes and bladder, and operations on the surface of the body. The abdominal and pelvic cavities were now accessible as were lengthy and involved dissections.

Advances in the basic sciences of bacteriology, physiology, and histopathology led to basic public health and therapeutic breakthroughs by the end of the century. Application of the scientific and laboratory methods to biomedical sciences objectified the healing arts and virtually ensured medical progress in the future. The amalgamation of laboratory and clinical medicine created an entire new scientific approach to disease diagnosis and therapy. All of these advances forced modern medicine into hospitals and laid the foundations of the biomedical sciences we see today.

Patients and physicians benefitted from the biomedical progress of the late nineteenth century, depending upon how much access they had to it. The degree of benefit realized by various patient groups in the United States depended on variables in the dynamic and evolving medical-social landscape. Late nineteenth-century U.S. health policy, increasingly poisoned by a racist scientific and medical-social environment, dictated a perverse distribution of health beneficence. In many instances, determination of medical need became subservient to race and class considerations, producing huge and growing access disparities (health care apartheid) in high-quality care between Blacks and Whites. Thus, for African Americans, medical progress was not guaranteed and could not be taken for granted at either patient or provider levels. Professional racial discrimination was extremely damaging to African American practitioners, who for all practical purposes were excluded by their White peers from openly participating in the expanding technical progress. Nevertheless, a few African American physicians such as Dan Williams (who could have passed for White) and Robert F. Boyd (who made himself indispensable to the system) used covert or unconventional techniques to crash professional barriers. But there were also other distressing, longer lasting, and intransigent health and medical-social dysfunctions that were perpetuated and exacerbated by these developments.[232]

Institutionalization of the slave health deficit in the emancipated Black population was a major dysfunctional health and medical-social development. Mediated by health policies incorporating racial exclusion, segregation, and discrimination, differential race- and class-based results and outcomes became the "norm" for the Black population. From an African American perspective, as science-based treatments became more effective, not having them meant that race-based health disparities and outcomes automatically grew. With the notable exceptions of its race and class problems, the Civil War forced the U.S. health system forward materially and structurally from a comparative international perspective. However, seeds were planted in various components of the health system based on race and class that blossomed into flaws that stubbornly persist today. The nationwide policy and acceptance of excluding or segregating Black and socioeconomically disadvantaged patients in separate and unequal facilities was one example. This principle was applied to public and private hospitals, clinics, doctors' offices, mental health facilities, and sanitariums.

The old U.S. almshouse and charity traditions of underfunding and inferiority were carried over into the modern and expanding public and private hospital networks as well as the relatively new public health programs and systems. Moreover, official or *de facto* policies governing most of these institutions and programs dictated that they were either for Whites only or were racially segregated. With few exceptions, Black facilities, when present, were physically inferior. Perhaps as damaging as the normalization and presupposition, followed by the acceptance, of poorer health and health outcomes for Blacks and the poor during the late nineteenth century were professional attitudes about race. As James H. Jones pointed out in *Bad Blood:*

> *Like other intellectuals of the day, late-nineteenth-century physicians were "social Darwinists" who had no difficulty identifying blacks as the race least likely to triumph in the struggle for survival. . . . White physicians of the late nineteenth and early twentieth centuries blamed the decline in black health on self-destructive behavioral traits.*[233]

This train of thought was prominent in the medical literature:

> *A standard feature of the vast majority of medical articles on the health of blacks was a sociomedical profile of a race whose members were rapidly becoming diseased, debilitated, and debauched, and had only themselves to blame. . . . [B]y defining the black health problem in racial terms, physicians absolved themselves of responsibility for what they saw as the Negro's deterioration.*[234]

Clearly, between 1861 and 1900, the U.S. medical profession came to regard African Americans as biologically, mentally, and morally unfit. Their poor health status and outcomes were deemed inevitable and expected. Their disappearance, along with other inferior "races," seemed inevitable as they succumbed in the battle for survival. Another dysfunctional health policy phenomenon was the "blame-the-victim" approach to poor Black health outcome. James Jones noted that White physicians felt that "blacks were solely responsible for the socioeconomic conditions in which they lived, [and] some even suggested that disease held the ultimate solution to the race problem."[235] Held as solely responsible for their plight, African Americans were treated as undeserving of either professional or health system help.[236]

Clarifying these health policy and medical-social dynamics is critical to understanding the legacies of the late nineteenth century that were passed down to America's twentieth-century health system. By 1900, Social Darwinism provided a new rationale for American racism. Moreover, it ideologically justified the new nihilism driving U.S. health policy and medical social attitudes and practices regarding Blacks. Alan M. Brandt portrayed the late-nineteenth-century scientific landscape in a 1978 Hastings Center report:

> *Essentially primitive peoples, it was argued, could not be assimilated into a complex, white civilization. Scientists speculated that in the struggle for survival the Negro in America was doomed. Particularly prone to disease, vice, and crime, black Americans could not be helped by education or philanthropy. Social Darwinists analyzed census data to predict the virtual extinction of the Negro in the 20th century, for they believed the Negro race in America was in the throes of a degenerative evolutionary process.*[237]

Leading supporters of this argument were the White medical and anthropological professions. Physicians in the medical and lay literature, purportedly studying the effects of emancipation on Black health, speculated and almost universally concluded that freedom had caused the physical, moral, and mental degeneration of African Americans. The profession pseudoscientifically "documented" these conclusions with studies on the prevalence and epidemiology of diseases such as syphilis, mental retardation, and tuberculosis in the Black population. Most attempts correlated and compared the rates during slavery and after emancipation.

Studies in medical journals on the sexual nature of African Americans emphasized purported excessive sexuality and observed racial differences. These "scientific" treatises usually contained moral judgments, made unsubstantiated generalizations and stereotypes, and bemoaned the lack of Black morality. As James Jones observed:

> *Few physicians managed to discuss the problem without revealing an inordinate fascination with black sexuality. Their writings both mirrored and augmented the public's stock of sexual stereotypes. They perpetuated the ancient myth that blacks matured physically at early ages and were more sexually active throughout their lives than whites.*

Blacks, they explained, had originated in a warm, tropical climate and were therefore closer on the evolutionary scale to man's bestial ancestors. Physicians pointed also to alleged anatomical and neurological differences. The formidable penis of the black man with its long prepuce offered greater opportunity for venereal infection. Moreover, personal restraints on self-indulgence did not exist, physicians insisted, because the smaller brain of the Negro had failed to develop a center for inhibiting sexual behavior.[238]

Some "medical" studies went so far as to suggest castration instead of lynching as retribution for Black sexual crimes. In the epidemiologically oriented studies, the Civil War was often utilized as the baseline for the prevalence rates on venereal diseases, tuberculosis, and insanity. According to Jones, "From the Civil War to about 1890, physicians discussed syphilis within the general context of the declining health of the black race."[239] Therefore, physicians were opinion leaders in full agreement with the popular and social scientific trends blaming Blacks for their poor health status and outcome. Inferior health access and services, medical abuse, discrimination, racial exclusion, and segregation were never mentioned as responsible for, or even as cofactors explaining, the situation. As Brandt noted in *Sickness and Health in America*, "Doctors generally discounted socioeconomic explanations of the state of black health, arguing that better medical care could not alter the evolutionary scheme."[240] Based on the available evidence, the paradoxical chapter title in John S. Haller, Jr.'s *Outcasts from Evolution: Scientific Attitudes of Racial Inferiority, 1859–1900* — "The Physician versus the Negro" — seems appropriate when speaking of the late nineteenth century.[241]

Physicians, politicians, and other opinion leaders utilized other health-based statistical sources to predict Black extinction. Joseph Camp Kennedy, a statistician and superintendent of the Eighth Census, predicted the slow extinction of the Negro race as an "unerring certainty" as early as 1862. Biased analyses of the Ninth, Tenth, and Eleventh censuses of 1870, 1880, and 1890 corroborated these impressions. Both Black mortality and pre–Civil War population increases were higher. The Eleventh Census also demonstrated that Black birth rates were lower than Whites' for the first time. As Haller pointed out about the growth of the Black extinction myth, "[T]he corroborating beliefs of physicians, the investigations of American insurance companies, the statistical evidence of the United States Army, as well as countless medical reports, precipitated a belief in the Negro's inevitable extinction."[242] These conclusions were reinforced by the interpretation of statistical health care insurance and government data by authorities such as Frederick Hoffmann, who predicted Black extinction by the year 2000 and convinced most insurance companies by 1900 that Blacks were uninsurable. Social scientists, led by luminaries such as Herbert Spencer and William Graham Sumner, who were busy applying Charles Darwin's theories to fields for which they were never intended, also reinforced these racist and nihilistic trends.[243] Finally, as Haller noted in *Outcasts from Evolution:*

> . . . *despite the complexity of the problem and the reservations of many, the belief in the Negro's extinction became one of the most pervasive ideas in American medical and anthropological thought during the late nineteenth century. It was also a fitting culmination to the concept of racial inferiority in American life.*[244]

The concepts of Black biomedical racial inferiority and biological determinism rose to their apogees in the United States during the late nineteenth and early twentieth centuries. As James H. Jones noted in his research and explorations to understand the complex medical professional dynamic leading to the Tuskegee syphilis experiment: "A rare point of agreement among the competing factions was that the health of blacks had to be considered separately from the health of whites."[245] This delineation of "difference" regarding Black and White health in the U.S. was devastating. Physicians were one of the first groups to study Blacks systematically. They also claimed they possessed special and specific scientific knowledge. Therefore, as has been the case in most societies since ancient times, their opinions and declarations carried a disproportionate impact on public opinion. According to Jones, "Physicians did not dissent as a group from white society's pervasive belief in the physical and mental inferiority of blacks. On the contrary, they did a great deal to bolster and elaborate racist attitudes."[246] These unwholesome trends and ideologies buttressed and fed into the concomitant 200-year-old U.S. biomedical tradition of unethically exploiting and overutilizing Blacks and the poor for experimental, demonstration, and research purposes. In fact, for many this veil of inferiority and negativism served as a rationale and justification for these acts. Legacies of this tradition, often in different guises, linger today. All of these phenomena—the medical and scientific assumption of Black racial inferiority and "difference" from the rest of the human family; the assumption of poor and deteriorating Black health status and outcome as normal and inevitable; the belief that Black racial extinction, largely due to health causes, would occur in the twentieth century; the victim-blaming belief that the Black health crisis was the African American's fault; and the belief that a combination of health and social causes working against Blacks would ultimately solve the race problem in America by making the race extinct—hung like a pall over the American health delivery system. There would be no studied, systematic, or concentrated effort to counteract or ameliorate the persistence or the effects these beliefs and policies generated in the health system. This medical-social climate led to outcomes as varied as persistent Black health disparities, discrimination and underrepresentation in the U.S. medical profession, and the continuation of unethical experimentation and scientific overutilization of Blacks in the health system until the late twentieth century.[247]

The most positive and significant health care legacy the late nineteenth century bequeathed African Americans was a Black medical profession and a network of health professions schools. Emergence of legitimate and numerically significant African American medical, dental, nursing, and pharmacy professions during this 39-year period resulted. As Black physicians implemented policies to serve the African American community, they initiated and ensured the founding of Black nursing, dental, pharmacy, and administrative health professions. They also continued and redefined a tradition of placing health concerns on the African American community and national agendas. These developments offered positive, activist alternatives to the racist, nihilistic, and negative health policies and practices offered to Blacks by the mainstream medical establishment on a take-it-or-leave-it basis. While struggling to ensure their permanence and survival, Black physicians assumed the responsibilities for the improvement of the health of African Americans. Their strategies to accomplish this task were varied.[248]

After a fusillade of rejections to their overtures to join the ranks of White organized medicine, Black doctors saw the need for their own organizations. By the 1880s, they began organizing and establishing local and state professional organizations. By 1895 what would become the National Medical Association (the early organization actually included physicians, dentists, and pharmacists), the Black health profession's national voice, was a reality.

During the 1890s, once more in response to exclusion and rejection, Black physicians found it necessary to begin a Black hospital movement. Spearheaded by Black medical leaders such as Daniel Hale Williams, Nathan Francis Mossell, and Robert F. Boyd, Black hospitals, where African American patients could benefit from the latest medical and surgical advances in a positive environment, were realities in a score of Black communities by 1900. These facilities allowed African American physicians to care for their own patients, who were their primary concerns, establish professional credibility, and benefit from the advances offered by hospital training and practice. Another concomitant of this was the beginning of a nurse training movement. Once more, in response to exclusion and racial discrimination, Black health in scientific settings was obviously handicapped without trained nurses to supervise and assist in patient care.

Trained personnel in dentistry and pharmacy were also needed. A new network of health professions training programs, usually headquartered at the Black medical schools, expanded to meet these needs. The Black medical and health professions also mobilized to become community leaders at the local, regional, and national levels. Perpetuating a unique African American tradition initiated in the early nineteenth century by James McCune Smith, Martin Robison Delany, and John Sweat Rock, health considerations became organic components of the Black civil rights and community development movements.[249]

Of all the health system factors that coalesced during the 39-year period leading up to 1900, the emergence of an African American medical profession and the separate infrastructure it created served as the solitary countervailing force designed and tailored to positively influence Black health. African Americans had entered the Civil War with a racially determined health deficit predating their arrival in English North America. Based on the evidence, African American health status deteriorated even further during and after the Civil War due to the dissolution and breakdown of the informal and inferior slave health subsystem.

The temporary positive effect of the Freedmen's Bureau failed to reverse unfavorable Black health trends. Thus, the Reconstruction Era may have been the nadir of Black health in the United States. African Americans were then left in a health care purgatory of neglect and devastation as they were forced to enter a capitalist, market-oriented health system with no health care infrastructure, no money, and a racial stigma. Dependence on charity, self-help, and the creation of a class of formally trained African American health professionals were the health policy strategies adopted by the Black community and their allies. Although the U.S. health system was the beneficiary of many positive technical medical advances during this period, African Americans rarely benefitted because of rampant racial exclusion, segregation, and discrimination in the health system. Therefore, the tide of the slave health deficit was not stemmed—instead, it became an inevitable legacy, ensured by post–Civil War health system policies and practices, that African Americans carried into the twentieth century.[250]

X Conclusion: Laying the Foundations of a Dual and Unequal Health System

Volume One of *An American Health Dilemma: A Medical History of African Americans and the Problem of Race* examines the relationship between race, medicine, and health care in the United States (U.S.) in a systematic and comprehensive manner for the first time. Such an examination helps clarify relationships between anti-Black institutional and individual racism as well as lack of cultural competence that distort the health system in this country. This racial animus, augmented by lingering class problems, contributes to persistent race- and class-based health disparities that have adversely affected African Americans and other disadvantaged populations for almost four hundred years. This study can provide insight into some of the mechanisms and structures that allow the problem to linger stubbornly and that help perpetuate multi-tiered and unequal health delivery in the United States today. Anticipated are explanatory hypotheses leading to research and interventions to correct the system's race and class problems.

Roots of the relationship between racism and bias against non-White people and women in the health professions and biomedical sciences stretch back into the ancient origins of Western culture. From its beginnings, Western science has had a morbid preoccupation with human inequality. Moreover, effects generated by these scientific and medical-social developments and relationships have spilled over into many other areas and dimensions of Western culture. Political and public policy areas were particularly affected. In English North America, rationales justifying permanent Black chattel slavery and the development of a slave health sub-system were two direct results.

Because of the extraordinary scope and complexity of this topic, unique epistemological approaches were indicated and division of the work into two volumes was necessary. The first volume covers the relationship between race, medicine, and health care in Western culture and the United States from antiquity to 1900. An initial chapter provided background on the study of race as an intellectual and scientific discipline over time. The origins of scientific racial classifications and the relationship of race to the history of science from its Greek origins through the Renaissance and Enlightenment to the modern era were detailed. Subsequent chapters covered historical periods from antiquity through the North American English colonial periods up to 1900. Included were explorations of the effects of race- and class-based structuring of the embryonic Colonial health system built around a brutal and socially destructive slave system and a tradition of harsh ideological and religious intolerance toward the poor and dependent.

Chapters covering the Colonial, Republican, Jacksonian and antebellum, Civil War, Reconstruction, and Post-Reconstruction period in the United States relative to African Americans and disadvantaged populations' health experiences were outlined. After the Civil War, the original slave health sub-system was replaced by a racially segregated, substandard system for Blacks erected in the late nineteenth century. Throughout these historical periods in the development of the U.S. health care system, the effects wrought by race-, gender-, and class-based structuring became much more pervasive and influential as the twentieth century approached.

By 1900, an organized and racially segregated medical profession stood on the threshold of total suzerainty over the health system. During the early parts of the new century, White physicians were granted unprecedented authority and power over the entire U.S. health establishment. They created a racially exclusive medical educational and research infrastructure lending scant attention or support to African American health problems or a stubbornly resilient Black physician class. A burgeoning hospital movement, the standard bearer of a new U.S. health infrastructure, was structured along race and class lines. At patient, physician staff, and allied health professional levels, a rigid color line was erected. American medicine remained an individualistic commercial enterprise despite the rise of universal health systems in Europe. During the late nineteenth century, individual fee-for-service medicine formed a strong foundation that grew to dominate the U.S. health system in the twentieth century. Taken as a whole, the twentieth-century foundation and superstructure of a dual and unequal health system based on race, class, institutional configuration, and financing mechanisms was already complete. The direction plotted by these developments will be the subject of *An American Health Dilemma: Race, Medicine, and Health Care in the United States: From 1900 to the Dawn of the New Millennium.*

⤬ *Notes*

Note to the reader: Each reference is given in full the first time it appears in a chapter. Thereafter, a shortened form of the reference, including author(s) and abbreviated title, is given for all other citations within the same chapter.

Preface

1. Blendon RJ, Donelan K. Public opinion and efforts to reform the U.S. health care system: Confronting issues of cost-containment and access to care. *Stanford Law and Policy Review* Fall 1991:146; Summer L, Shapiro I. *Trends in Health Insurance Coverage, 1987 to 1993.* Washington, DC: Center on Budget and Policy Priorities, 1994, pp. 4–6; American Public Health Association. Managed competition: Wonder drug or snake oil? *The Nation's Health* March 1993; 23:1; Blendon RJ, Edwards JN, eds. *System in Crisis: The Case for Health Care Reform* (Vol. 1, *The Future of American Health Care*). New York: Faulkner and Gray, 1991; Stanford University. Health care in America: Armageddon on the horizon? *Stanford Law and Policy Review* Fall 1991; 3:1–260; Lundberg GD. National health care reform: An aura of inevitability is upon us. *Journal of the American Medical Association* 1991; 265:2566–2567.

2. Blendon RJ, Edwards JN, eds. *System in Crisis*; American Public Health Association. Managed competition.

3. Blendon RJ, Edwards JN, eds. *System in Crisis.*

4. Stanford University. Health care in America.

5. Friedman E. The uninsured: From dilemma to crisis. *Journal of the American Medical Association* 1991; 265:2491–2495.

6. Blendon RJ, Edwards JN, eds. *System in Crisis*, American Public Health Association. Managed competition.

7. Starr P. Healthy compromise: Universal coverage and managed competition under a cap. *The American Prospect* Winter 1993; 12:44–52.

8. Johnson H, Broder DS. *The System: The American Way of Politics at the Breaking Point*. Boston: Little, Brown, 1996; Skocpol T. *Boomerang: Health Care Reform and the Turn against Government*. New York: W.W. Norton, 1997.

9. Knox RA. Study sees poor, elderly doing worse in HMO care. *Boston Globe* October 2, 1996:A1, A7; Pear R. Laws won't let H.M.O.s tell doctors what to say. *New York Times* September 17, 1996:A12; Anders G. Who pays the cost of cut-rate heart care? *Wall Street Journal* October 15, 1996:B1, B8; Johannes L. More HMOs order outpatient mastectomies. *Wall Street Journal* November 6, 1996:B1, B8; Kuttner R. Managed-care malpractice. *Boston Globe* November 25, 1996:A15; Broder DS. Candidates skirt the health care issue. *Boston Globe* October 21, 1996:A15. Seger A, et. al. *Boston Sunday Globe*, April 25, 1999: p. C1; Knox RA. HMO's creator urges reform in quality of care. *Boston Sunday Globe*, May 2, 1999: p. A1. Pear R. Insurers ask government to extend health plans. *New York Times*, May 23, 1999, p. A16.

10. Byrd WM, Clayton LA. America's dual health crisis in black and white. Report prepared for the hearings, "Health Care Reform: The African American Agenda," held for the Congressional Black Caucus's Health Brain Trust, 103rd Congress, Special Session, April 13, 1993, Washington, DC; Malone TE, Johnson KW. *Report of the Secretary's Task Force on Black and Minority Health*. Washington, DC: U.S. Department of Health and Human Services, 1986; Byrd WM, Clayton LA. An American health dilemma: A history of blacks in the health system. *Journal of the National Medical Association* 1992; 84:189–200; Feagin JR, Feagin CB. *Racial and Ethnic Relations*, 6th ed. Upper Saddle River, NJ. Prentice Hall, 1999; Byrd WM, Clayton LA. Race, medicine, and health care in the United States: A historical survey, *Journal of the National Medical Association*. In press 2000.

11. Blackwell, A. The impact of health care reform on the African American consumer. Address delivered at "Grassroots Initiative for Health Care Reform," sponsored by Region VI, National Medical Association and "Summit '93: Regional Summit on Health Care Reform," San Francisco, CA, April 30, 1994; Guinier L. *The Tyranny of the Majority: Fundamental Fairness in Representative Democracy*. New York: The Free Press, 1994; Hacker A. *Two Nations: Black and White, Separate, Hostile, Unequal*. New York: Ballantine Books, 1992; expanded and updated edition, 1995.

12. Malone TE, Johnson KW. *Report of the Secretary's Task Force on Black and Minority Health*.

13. Health Policy Advisory Center. The emerging health apartheid in the United States. *Health/PAC Bulletin* 1991; 21:3–4.

14. Byrd WM, Clayton LA. An American health dilemma.

15. Byrd WM, Clayton LA. America's dual health crisis in black and white.

16. Edwards WS. *National Medical Expenditure Survey: Questionnaires and Data Collection Methods for the United States Population*. Rockville, MD: U.S. Department of Health and Human Services, Agency for Health Care Policy and Research, 1989 (DHHS Pub. PHY 89-3440); Cornelius LJ. Limited access to health care continues in minority groups. *National Medical Association News* March/April 1993:1.

17. Byrd WM, Clayton LA. *A Black Health Trilogy* (videotape and 188-page documentary report). Washington, DC: The National Medical Association and the African American Heritage and Education Foundation, 1991.

18. Greenberg DS. Black health: Grim statistics. *The Lancet* 1990; 355:780–781; Thomas VG. Explaining health disparities between African-American and white popula-

tions: Where do we go from here? *Journal of the National Medical Association* 1992; 84:837–840.

19. Byrd WM, Clayton LA. An American health dilemma, Charatz-Litt C. A chronicle of racism: The effects of the white medical community on black health. *Journal of the National Medical Association* 1992; 84:717–725.

20. Charatz-Litt C. A chronicle of racism, Byrd WM, Clayton LA. America's dual health crisis in black and white.

21. Cray E. *In Failing Health: The Medical Crisis and the A.M.A.* Indianapolis: Bobbs-Merrill, 1970; Harmer RM. *American Medical Avarice.* New York: Abelard-Schuman, 1975; Tunley R. *The American Health Scandal.* New York: Harper & Row, 1966; Starr P. *The Social Transformation of American Medicine.* New York: Basic Books, 1982; Cobb WM. The black American in medicine. *Journal of the National Medical Association* 1981; 73 (Suppl 1):1183–1244.

22. Komaromy M, Grumbach K, Drake M. The role of black and Hispanic physicians in providing health care for underserved poulations. *New England Journal of Medicine* 1996; 334:1305–1314; Shea S, Fullilove MT. Entry of black and other minority students in US medical schools: Historical perspectives and recent trends. *New England Journal of Medicine* 1985; 313:933–940; Hanft RS, Fishman LE, Evans W. *Blacks and the Health Professions in the 80s: A National Crisis and a Time for Action.* Prepared for the Association of Minority Health Professions Schools. N.P., 1983; Sullivan LW. The status of blacks in medicine. *New England Journal of Medicine* 1983; 309:807–809.

23. Duster T. *Backdoor to Eugenics.* New York: Routledge, 1990; Brandt AM. Racism and research: The case of the Tuskegee Syphilis Study. In: Leavitt JW, Numbers RL, eds. *Sickness and Health in America: Readings in the History of Medicine and Public Health.* Madison, The University of Wisconsin Press, 1985, pp. 331–343; Reynolds V, Falger V, Vine I, eds. *The Sociobiology of Ethnocentrism: Evolutionary Dimensions of Xenophobia, Discrimination, Racism and Nationalism.* London: Croom Helm, 1987; Herrnstein RJ, Murray C. *The Bell Curve: Intelligence and Class Structure in American Life.* New York: The Free Press, 1994; Fish JM. Mixed blood. *Psychology Today* November/December 1995; 6(28):55; Byne W. Debate: Is homosexuality biologically influenced? The biological evidence challenged. *Scientific American* May 1994; (270):43, 50; LeVay S, Hamer DH. Debate: Is homosexuality biologically influenced? Evidence for a biological influence in male homosexuality. *Scientific American* May 1994; 5(270):43, 44; Chase A. *The Legacy of Malthus: The Social Costs of the New Scientific Racism.* New York: Knopf, 1980; Nelkin D, Tancredi L. *Dangerous Diagnostics: The Social Power of Biological Information.* New York: Basic Books, 1989; Lewontin RC, Rose S, Kamin LJ. *Not in Our Genes: Biology, Ideology, and Human Nature.* New York: Pantheon Books, 1984.

24. Cobb WM. The black American in medicine; Cobb WM. *The First Negro Medical Society: A History of the Medico-Chirurgical Society of the District of Columbia.* Washington, DC: The Associated Publishers, 1939; Charatz-Litt C. A chronicle of racism; Morais HM. *The History of the Negro in Medicine.* New York: Publishers Company, 1967; Byrd WM, Clayton LA. An American health dilemma, Byrd WM. Inquisition, peer review, and black physician survival. *Journal of the National Medical Association* 1987; 79:1027–1029; Wolinsky H. Healing wounds: Lonnie R. Bristow steps up to head the American Medical Association, one of the nation's premier—and most rigidly segregated—professional groups. *Emerge* July/August 1994 10(5):42.

25. Greenberg DS. Black health.

26. Bogdanich W. *The Great White Lie: Dishonesty, Waste, and Incompetence in the Medical Community.* New York: Simon & Schuster, 1991.

27. O'Bannion LC. Are African-American doctors being locked out? The down side of managed care. *National Medical Association News* Winter 1995:1; Byrd WM. Inquisition, peer review, and black physician survival; Byrd WM. *Peer Review: The Perversion of a Process.* Report prepared for the Subcommittee on Civil Rights of the House Committee on the Judiciary, 99th Congress, 2nd Session, 1986; Byrd WM. Inner-city private medical practice: An anachronistic model? Paper prepared for the course Management in Public Health in Industrialized Countries (HPM221), Harvard School of Public Health, October 29, 1991.

28. Starr P. *The Social Transformation of American Medicine*; Byrd WM. Inquisition, peer review, and black physician survival.

29. Byrd WM. *Peer Review: The Perversion of a Process.*

30. Byrd WM, Clayton LA. The history of cancer in blacks in the United States (videotape). Presentation made to the Drew-Meharry-Morehouse Consortium Cancer Center Orientation to Cancer Clinical Trials Program held at Morehouse School of Medicine, Atlanta, GA, November 2, 1990.

31. Byrd WM, Clayton LA. *A Black Health Trilogy.*

Introduction

1. Myrdal G. *An American Dilemma: The Negro Problem in Modern Democracy.* 20th Anniversary Edition. New York: Harper and Row Publishers, 1962, lxix.

2. Myrdal G. *An American Dilemma*, p. lxxii.

3. Smedley A. *Race in North America: Original Evolution of a Worldview.* Second Edition. Boulder, Colorado: Westview Press, 1999, 332–333; Bohennan P, Curtin P. *Africa and Africans.* 4th Edition. Prospect Heights, Illinois: Waveland Press, 1995.

4. Randall VR. Racist health care: Reforming an unjust health care system to meet the needs of African-Americans. *Health Matrix: Journal of Law-Medicine* (Spring, No. 1); 3:127–194, 131; Freund CP. Rhetorical questions: The power of, and behind, a name. *Washington Post*, February 7, 1989, A23; Byrd WM. Race, biology, and health care: Reassessing a relationship. *Journal of Health Care for the Poor and Underserved* 1990; 1:278–292; Morais HM. *The History of the Negro in Medicine.* New York: Publishers Company, 1967, 1. Cobb WM. The black American in medicine. *Journal of the National Medical Association* 1981; 73(Suppl 1):1183–1244; Jaynes GD, Williams RM, eds. *A Common Destiny: Blacks and American Society.* Washington, DC: National Academy Press, 1989, pp. 391–450; Byrd WM, Clayton LA. *A Black Health Trilogy* [videotape and 188-page documentary report]. Washington, DC: The National Medical Association and the African American Heritage and Education Foundation, 1991; Byrd WM, Clayton LA. An American health dilemma: A history of blacks in the health system. *Journal of the National Medical Association* 1992; 84:189–200; Harding V. *There Is a River: The Black Struggle for Freedom in America.* New York: Harcourt Brace Jovanovich, 1981; reprint edition, New York: Vintage Books, 1983.

5. Byrd WM. Race, biology, and health care; Byrd WM, Clayton LA. An American health dilemma; Morais HM. *The History of the Negro in Medicine*; Cobb WM. The black

American in medicine; Numbers RL, ed. *Medicine in the New World: New Spain, New France, and New England.* Knoxville: The University of Tennessee Press, 1987; Blanton WB. *Medicine in Virginia in the Seventeenth Century.* Richmond, VA: The William Byrd Press, Blanton WB. *Medicine in Virginia in the Eighteenth Century.* Richmond, VA: Garrett and Massie, 1931; Sheridan RB. *Doctors and Slaves: A Medical and Demographic History of Slavery in the British West Indies, 1680–1834.* Cambridge: Cambridge University Press, 1985; Savitt TL. *Medicine and Slavery: The Diseases and Health Care of Blacks in Antebellum Virginia.* Urbana: University of Illinois Press, 1987.

6. Brinkley A. *The Unfinished Nation: A Concise History of the American People.* New York: Knopf, 1993; Franklin JH. *From Slavery to Freedom: A History of Negro Americans.* 3rd ed. New York: Knopf, 1967; reprint edition, New York: Vintage Books, 1969; Savitt TL. The use of blacks for medical experimentation and demonstration in the old south. *Journal of Southern History* 1982; 48:331–348; Bullough B, Bullough VL. *Poverty, Ethnic Identity, and Health Care.* New York: Appleton-Century-Crofts, 1972; Dowling HF. *City Hospitals: The Undercare of the Underprivileged.* Cambridge, MA: Harvard University Press, 1982, pp. 1–86; Rosenberg CE. *The Care of Strangers: The Rise of America's Hospital System.* New York: Basic Books, 1987, pp. 1–308; Morais HM. *The History of the Negro in Medicine.* Starr P. *The Social Transformation of American Medicine.* New York: Basic Books, 1982, pp. 1–179; Byrd WM, Clayton LA. An American health dilemma.

7. Cobb WM. The black American in medicine; Rosenberg CE. *The Care of Strangers*; Stevens RA. *American Medicine and the Public Interest.* New Haven, CT: Yale University Press, 1971, pp. 75–541; Bullough B, Bullough VL. *Poverty, Ethnic Identity, and Health Care*; Morais HM. *The History of the Negro in Medicine*, pp. 89–208; Curtis JL. *Blacks, Medical Schools, and Society.* Ann Arbor: The University of Michigan Press, 1971; Dowling HF. *City Hospitals*, pp. 1–83; Ginzberg E. The monetarization of medical care. *New England Journal of Medicine* 1984; 310:1162–1165; Ginzberg E. The destabilization of health care. *New England Journal of Medicine* 1986; 315:757–767; Ginzberg E. *The Medical Triangle: Physicians, Politicians, and the Public.* Cambridge, MA: Harvard University Press, 1990; Starr P. *The Social Transformation of American Medicine*, pp. 145–449; Kongstvedt PR. *The Managed Health Care Handbook.* 2nd ed. Gaithersburg, MD: Aspen Publishers, 1993; Eckholm E. While Congress remains silent health care transforms itself. *New York Times* December 18, 1994:1; Byrd WM, Clayton LA. An American health dilemma; Wolinsky H. Healing wounds: Lonnie R. Bristow steps up to head the American Medical Association, one of the nation's premier—and most rigidly segregated—professional groups. *Emerge* July/August 1994; 10(5):42; Skocpol T. *Boomerang: Health Care Reform and the Turn Against Government.* New York: W.W. Norton and Company, 1997.

8. Starr P. *The Social Transformation of American Medicine*, p. 7.

9. Starr P. *The Social Transformation of American Medicine*, p. 7.

10. Morais HM. *The History of the Negro in Medicine*; Cobb WM. The black American in medicine; Byrd WM. Race, biology, and health care; Byrd WM, Clayton LA. An American health dilemma; Newman DK, Amidei NJ, Carter BL, et al. Second-class medicine. In: *Protest, Politics, and Prosperity: Black Americans and White Institutions, 1940–75.* New York: Pantheon Books, 1978, pp. 187–235. Frankel M. What the poor deserve: Review of *The War Against the Poor*, by Herbert J. Gans. *New York Times Magazine* October 22, 1995: Section 6, 46.

11. Outlaw L. Toward a Critical Theory of Race. In: Goldberg DT, ed. *Anatomy of Racism.* Minneapolis: University of Minnesota Press, 1990, pp. 58–82; quote p. 58.

12. Morais HM. *The History of the Negro in Medicine*; Du Bois WEB. *The Philadelphia Negro: A Social Study*. N.P.: 1899; reprint, New York: Schocken Books, 1967; Du Bois WEB. *Mortality Among Negroes in Cities*. Proceedings of the Conference for Investigation of City Problems. Atlanta: Atlanta University Publications, 1896; Du Bois WEB. *Social and Physical Conditions of Negroes in Cities*. Proceedings of the Second Conference for the Negro City Life. Atlanta: Atlanta University Publications, 1897; Du Bois WEB. *The Health and Physique of the Negro American*. A social study made under the direction of the Eleventh Atlanta Conference. Atlanta: Atlanta University Publications, 1906; U.S. Bureau of the Census. *Negro Population of the United States: 1790–1915* (1918); U.S. Bureau of the Census. *Negroes in the United States 1920–32* (1935); Lewis JH. *The Biology of the Negro*. Chicago: The University of Chicago Press, 1942; Cobb WM. The black American in medicine; Cobb WM. *Medical Care and the Plight of the Negro*. New York: The National Association for the Advancement of Colored People, 1947; Cobb WM. *Progress and Portents for the Negro in Medicine*. New York: The National Association for the Advancement of Colored People, 1948; Ewbank DC. History of black mortality and health before 1940. In: Willis DP, ed. *Health Policies and Black Americans*. New Brunswick, NJ: Transaction Publishers, 1989, pp. 100–128; Byrd WM. Race, biology, and health care; Byrd WM, Clayton LA. An American health dilemma; Byrd WM, Clayton LA. *A Black Health Trilogy*.

13. Cobb WM. *The Black American in Medicine*; Morais HM. *The History of the Negro in Medicine*; Wilson FA, Neuhauser D. *Health Services in the United States*. 2nd ed. Cambridge, MA: Ballinger Publishing Company, 1982; Roberts MJ, Clyde AT. *Your Money or Your Life: The Health Care Crisis Explained*. New York: Doubleday, 1993; Jaynes GD, Williams RM, eds. *A Common Destiny*, pp. 391–450; Du Bois WEB. *Mortality Among Negroes in Cities*; Du Bois WEB. *Social and Physical Conditions of Negroes in Cities*; Byrd WM, Clayton LA. *A Black Health Trilogy*; Du Bois WEB. *The Health and Physique of the Negro American*; Ewbank DC. History of black mortality and health before 1940; Byrd WM, Clayton LA. *Designing a New Health Care System for the United States*. Boston: Harvard School of Public Health, 1992; Byrd WM, Clayton LA. An American health dilemma; Byrd WM, Clayton LA. *A Guide for Health Care Reform* (unpublished document). Rev. ed. Prepared for the "Grassroots Education Initiative for Health Care Reform," sponsored by the Hoosier State Medical Society, National Medical Association and Summit '93: Regional Summit on Health Care Reform, Indianapolis, Indiana, June 18, 1994.

14. Van Sertima I. *They Came Before Columbus*. New York: Random House, 1976; Bernal M. *Black Athena: The Afroasiatic Roots of Classical Civilization* (Vols. 1 and 2, *The Fabrication of Ancient Greece 1785–1985* and *The Archaeological and Documentary Evidence*). New Brunswick, NJ: Rutgers University Press, 1987, 1991; Finch CS. *The African Background to Medical Science: Essays in African History, Science and Civilizations*. London: Karnak House, 1990; Finch CS. *Africa and the Birth of Science and Technology: A Brief Overview*. Decatur, GA: Khenti Publications, 1992; Finch CS. *Echoes of the Old Darkland: Themes From the African Eden*. Decatur, GA: Khenti Publications, 1994; Drake SC. *Black Folk Here and There: An Essay in History and Anthropology* (Vol. 1). Los Angeles: Center for Afro-American Studies, University of California, 1987.

15. Begley S, Chideya F, Wilson L. Out of Egypt, Greece: Seeking the roots of Western civilization on the banks of the Nile. *Newsweek* September 23, 1991; 118:49–50; Asante MK. Putting Africa at the center. *Newsweek* September 23, 1991; 118:46; Gates

HL. Beware of the new pharaohs. *Newsweek* September 23, 1991; 118:47; Lefkowitz M. *Not Out of Africa: How Afrocentrism Became an Excuse to Teach Myth as History.* New York: Basic Books, 1996; Asante MK. Roots of the truth: Repelling attacks on Afrocentrism. *Emerge* July/August 1996; 9(7):66.

16. Haynes MA. The gap in health status between black and white Americans. In: Williams RA, ed. *Textbook of Black-Related Diseases.* New York: McGraw-Hill Book Company, 1975, pp. 1–30; National Center for Health Statistics. Advance report of final mortality statistics, 1989. *Monthly Vital statistics report* 1992:40(8)(Suppl 2). U.S. Department of Health and Human Services. *Report of the Secretary's Task Force on Black and Minority Health* (Vol. 1, *Executive Summary*). Washington, DC: U.S. Government Printing Office, 1985; U.S. Bureau of the Census. *Statistical Abstract of the United States, 1993.* Washington, DC: U.S. Government Printing Office, 1992; Jaynes GD, Williams RM, eds. *A Common Destiny*, pp. 391–450.

17. U.S. Department of Health and Human Services. *Report of the Secretary's Task Force on Black and Minority Health* (Vol. 1); U.S. Department of Health and Human Services. *Report of the Secretary's Task Force on Black and Minority Health* (Vol. 2, *Crosscutting Issues in Minority Health*). Washington, DC: U.S. Government Printing Office, 1985; U.S. Department of Health and Human Services. *Report of the Secretary's Task Force on Black and Minority Health* (Vol. 3, *Cancer*). Washington, DC: U.S. Government Printing Office, 1986; U.S. Department of health and Human Services. *Report of the Secretary's Task Force on Black and Minority Health* (Vol. 4, *Cardiovascular and Cerebrovascular Diseases. Part 1*). Washington, DC: U.S. Government Printing Office, 1986; U.S. Department of Health and Human Services. *Report of the Secretary's Task Force on Black and Minority Health* (Vol. 4, *Cardiovascular and Cerebrovascular Diseases. Part 2*). Washington, DC: U.S. Government Printing Office, 1986; U.S. Department of Health and Human Services. *Report of the Secretary's Task Force on Black and Minority Health* (Vol. 5, *Homicide, Suicide, and Unintentional Injuries*). Washington, DC: U.S. Government Printing Office, 1986; U.S. Department of Health and Human Services. *Report of the Secretary's Task Force on Black and Minority Health* (Vol. 6, *Infant Mortality and Low Birth Weight*). Washington, DC: U.S. Government Printing Office, 1986; U.S. Department of Health and Human Services. *Report of the Secretary's Task Force on Black and Minority Health* (Vol. 7, *Chemical Dependency Diabetes*). Washington, DC: U.S. Government Printing Office, 1986; U.S. Department of Health and Human Services. *Report of the Secretary's Task Force on Black and Minority Health* (Vol. 8, *Hispanic Health Issues: Inventory of DHHS Programs: Survey of Non-Federal Community*). Washington, DC: U.S. Government Printing Office, 1986.

18. Malone TE, Johnson KW. *Report of the Secretary's Task Force on Black and Minority Health.* Washington, DC: U.S. Department of Health and Human Services, 1986; Greenberg DS. Black health: Grim statistics. *The Lancet* 1990; 355:780–781; Byrd WM, Clayton LA. *A Black Health Trilogy*; Jaynes GD, Williams RM, eds. *A Common Destiny*; Clayton LA, Byrd WM. The African American cancer crisis, part 1: The problem. *Journal of Health Care for the Poor and Underserved* 1993; 4: 83–101; Byrd WM, Clayton LA. The African-American cancer crisis, part II: A prescription. *Journal of Health Care for the Poor and Underserved* 1993; 4:102–116; Byrd WM, Clayton LA. An American health dilemma.

19. *Special Health Care Issue: Clinton's Trillion Dollar Cure (And What He Didn't Tell You).* Newsweek October 4, 1993; 14(72):26; U.S. Congress. *Health Security Act.* H.R. 3600/S.1757. *Congressional Record*, November 1993.

20. Malone TE, Johnson KW. *Report of the Secretary's Task Force on Black and Minority Health*; Greenberg DS. Black health.

21. Randall VR. Does Clinton's health care reform proposal ensure (e)qual(ity) of health care for ethnic Americans and the poor? *Brooklyn Law Review* Spring 1994; 1(60):167–237; Byrd WM, Clayton LA. Managed competition: An analysis of consumer concerns. In: Byrd WM, Clayton LA. A *Guide for Health Care Reform* (unpublished manuscript), on file with the National Medical Association, Washington, DC, 1993; U.S. Congress. *Health Security Act*. Eckholm E. While Congress remains silent health care transforms itself.

22. Du Bois WEB. *The Health and Physique of the Negro American*; Cobb WM. *Medical Care and the Plight of the Negro*; Haynes MA. The gap in health status between black and white Americans; Byrd WM, Clayton LA. An American health dilemma; Charatz-Litt C. A chronicle of racism: The effects of the white medical community on black health. *Journal of the National Medical Association* 1992; 84:717–725; Malone TE, Johnson KW. *Report of the Secretary's Task Force on Black and Minority Health*; Greenberg DS. Black health.

23. Roberts MJ, Clyde AT. *Your Money or Your Life: The Health Care Crisis Explained*; Ginzberg E, Ostow M. *The Road to Reform: The Future of Health Care in America*. New York: The Free Press, 1994; Samuelson RJ. Health care: What happens if the best medicine that money can buy is more than we can . . . afford? *Newsweek* October 4, 1993:28.

24. Skocpol T. *Boomerang*, p. 195.

25. Ryan W. *Blaming the Victim*. New York: Vintage Books, 1971; rev. updated ed., New York: Vintage Books, 1976, pp. 142–170; Malone TE, Johnson KW. *Report of the Secretary's Task Force on Black and Minority Health*; Greenberg DS. Black health; Funch DP. A *Report on Cancer Survival in the Economically Disadvantaged*. Report prepared for the American Cancer Society, July 1985.

26. Mangano JJ. Young adults in the 1980s: Why mortality rates are rising. *Health PAC/Bulletin* 1991; 21:19–24; Escarce JJ, Epstein KR, Colby DC, et al. Racial differences in the elderly's use of medical procedures and diagnostic tests. *American Journal of Public Health* 1993; 83:948–954; McCord C, Freeman HP. Excess mortality in Harlem. *New England Journal of Medicine* 1990; 322:173–177.

27. Greenberg DS. Black health; National Center for Health Statistics. *Prevention Profile. Health United States, 1991*. Hyattsville, MD. Public Health Service, 1992; U.S. Department of Health and Human Services. *Health Status of the Disadvantaged Chartbook/1990*. Washington, DC: U.S. Department of Health and Human Services, Public Health Service, Publication No. (HRSA) HRS-P-DV 90-1, 1991; Rosenbaum S, Layton C, Liu J. *The Health of America's Children*. Washington, DC: Children's Defense Fund, 1991.

28. Greenberg DS. Black health; Clayton LA, Byrd WM. Race, a major health status and outcome variable, 1980–1999: With some historical perspectives. *Journal of the National Medical Association*. In press 1999; Morais HM. *The History of the Negro in Medicine*; Byrd WM, Clayton LA. A *Black Health Trilogy*; Mangano JJ. Young adults in the 1980s; National Center for Health Statistics. *Health Status of the Disadvantaged Chartbook/1990*.

29. Lundberg GD. National health care reform: An aura of inevitability is upon us. *Journal of the American Medical Association* 1991; 265:2566–2567; Greenberg DS. Black health; Byrd WM, Clayton LA. A *Black Health Trilogy*. Schulman KA, Berlin JA, Harles

W, et al. *The New England Journal of Medicine* 1999; 340:618–626; Cooper-Petarck L, Gallo JJ, Gonzales JJ, Vu HT, Powe MR, Nelson G, et al. Race, gender, and partnership in the patient-physician relationship. *Journal of the American Medical Association* 1999, 282:583–589.

30. Greenberg DS. Black health; Randall VR. Racist health care: Reforming an unjust health care system to meet the needs of African-Americans. *Health Matrix: Journal of Law-Medicine* Spring 1993 1(3):127–194; Kovner AR, Jonas S, eds. *Jonas and Kovner's Health Care Delivery in the United States*. 6th ed. New York: Springer, 1999; Satcher D. Black access to health care. Presentation for "Black Health: Historical Perspectives and Current Problems" conference, University of Wisconsin Medical School, April 5–7, 1990, Madison, WI; U.S. Department of Health and Human Services. *Cultural Competence for Evaluators: A Guide for Alcohol and Other Drug Abuse Prevention Practitioners Working with Ethnic/Racial Communities*. Rockville, MD: Office for Substance Abuse Prevention, Alcohol, Drug Abuse, and Mental Health Administration, DHHS Publication No. (ADM)92-1884, 1992; Morais HM. *The History of the Negro in Medicine*; Bullough B, Bullough VL. *Poverty, Ethnic Identity, and Health Care*; Ryan W. *Blaming the Victim*, pp. 142–170; Byrd WM, Clayton LA. *A Black Health Trilogy*; Byrd WM. Race, biology, and health care; World Health Organization. *World Health Organization Statistics Annuals* (Vols. 1985–1990, Geneva, 1985–1990); Washington, DC: U.S. Department of Health and Human Services. *Healthy People 2000: National Health Promotion and Disease Prevention Objectives* (summary report). Washington, DC: U.S. Department of Health and Human Services, Public Health Service, Publication No. (PHS) 91-50213, 1990; Samuelson RJ. Health care. Smith DB. *Health Care Divided: Race and Healing a Nation*. Ann Arbor: The University of Michigan Press, 1999.

31. Prothrow-Stith D. *Division of Public Health Practice: Strategic Planning Document*. Boston, MA: Harvard School of Public Health, 1997, p. 8.

32. Ginzberg E. Improving health care for the poor: Lessons from the 1980s. *Journal of the American Medical Association* 1994; 271:464–467; McKenzie N, Bilofsky E. Shredding the safety net: The dismantling of public programs. *Health/PAC Bulletin* 1991; 21:5–11; Sack K. Public hospitals around the country cut basic service. *New York Times* August 20, 1995: 1; Fein EB. Giuliani's plan to lease a hospital is in jeopardy. *New York Times* June 1, 1997: 35; Fialka JJ. Demands on New Orleans's "Big Charity" hospital are symptomatic of U.S. health-care problem. *Wall Street Journal* June 22, 1993: p. A1B; Cornelius LJ. Limited access to health care continues in minority groups. *National Medical Association News* March/April 1993:1; Lasalandra M. Study finds poor elderly are losing out on HMOs. *Boston Herald*, October 2, 1996, p. 19.

33. Sack K. Public hospitals around country cut basic service; Herring HB. Who can heal New York? *New York Times* August 20, 1995:2F.

34. Pear R. HMOs denying more claims for emergency care. *Fort Worth Star-Telegram* July 9, 1995:A7; Public hospitals across nation cutting services under pressure. *Fort Worth Star-Telegram* August 20, 1995: ; McKenzie N, Bilofsky E. Shredding the safety net; Sack K. Public hospitals around the country cut basic service; Fein EB. Giuliani's plan to lease a hospital is in jeopardy; Fialka JJ. Demands on New Orleans's "Big Charity" hospital are symptomatic of U.S. health-care problem; Cornelius LJ. Limited access to health care continues in minority groups. Pollitt K. A Bronx tale. *The Nation*, June 14, 1999, 11.

35. Bradsher K. As 1 million leave ranks of insured, debate heats up. *New York Times* August 27, 1995: 1; Survey: 60 million experience lapses in health coverage. *Physician's*

Financial News January 15, 1995: 2; Lemann N. The structure of success in America. *Atlantic Monthly* August 1995; 2(276):41; Lemann N. The great sorting. *Atlantic Monthly* September 1995; 3(276):84; Kozol J. *Savage Inequalities: Children in America's Schools.* New York: Crown, 1991; Wilson WJ. *The Declining Significance of Race: Blacks and Changing American Institutions.* Chicago: The University of Chicago Press, 1978; 2nd ed., Chicago: The University of Chicago Press, 1980; Wilson WJ. *When Work Disappears: The World of the New Urban Poor.* New York: Knopf, 1996; Massey DS, Denton NA. *American Apartheid: Segregation and the Making of the Underclass.* Cambridge, MA: Harvard University Press, 1993.

36. Konner M. *Medicine at the Crossroads: The Crisis in Health Care.* New York: Pantheon Books, 1993, p. xi; Kongstvedt PR. *The Managed Health Care Handbook.* 2nd ed., pp. 3–4; Johannes L. State probes HMO's denial of some care. *Wall Street Journal* August 16, 1995: T1; Whol S. *The Medical Industrial Complex.* New York: Harmony Books, 1984, p. 95.

37. Fein EB. Teaching hospitals nervous about Medicare overhaul. *Fort Worth Star-Telegram* October 21, 1995:A23; Konner M. *Medicine at the Crossroads: The Crisis in Health Care*; Kongstvedt PR. *The Managed Health Care Handbook.* 2nd ed., pp. 1–11; Whol S. *The Medical Industrial Complex*; Pear R. HMOs denying more claims for emergency care; Public hospitals across nation cutting services under pressure. *Fort Worth Star-Telegram*; McKenzie N, Bilofsky E. Shredding the safety net; Sack K. Public hospitals around the country cut basic service; Fein EB. Giuliani's plan to lease a hospital is in jeopardy; Fialka JJ. Demands on New Orleans's "Big Charity" hospital are symptomatic of U.S. health-care problem; Cornelius LJ. Limited access to health care continues in minority groups.

38. Blendon RJ, Hyams TS, eds. *Reforming the System: Containing Health Care Costs in an Era of Universal Coverage* (Vol. 2, *The Future of American Health Care*). New York: Faulkner and Gray, 1991, p. 66; Randall VR. Does Clinton's health care reform proposal ensure (e)qual(ity) of health care for ethnic Americans and the poor?

39. Blendon RJ, Hyams TS, eds. *Reforming the System: Containing Health Care Costs in an Era of Universal Coverage* (Vol. 2), p. 66; Lundberg GD. National health care reform.

40. Greenberg DS. Black health; Bergner L. Race, health, and health services. *American Journal of Public Health* 1993; 83:939–941; Rowland Hogue CJ, Hargraves MA. Class, race, and infant mortality in the United States. *American Journal of Public Health* 1993; 83:9–12; Polednak AP. Poverty, residential segregation, and black/white mortality ratios in urban areas. *Journal of Health Care of the Poor and Underserved* 1993; 4:363–373; Dula A. Toward an African-American perspective on bioethics. *Journal of Health Care of the Poor and Underserved* 1991; 2:259–269; McCord C, Freeman HP. Excess mortality in Harlem; Smith DB. *Health Care Divided: Race and Healing a Nation.* Ann Arbor: The University of Michigan Press, 1999.

41. Myrdal G. *An American Dilemma: The Negro Problem and Modern Democracy.* New York: Harper & Row, 1944.

42. Myrdal G. *An American Dilemma*; Kovel J. *White Racism: A Psychohistory.* New York: Random House, 1970; reprint ed., New York: Columbia University Press, 1984; Hacker A. *Two Nations: Black and White, Separate, Hostile, Unequal.* New York: Ballantine Books, 1992; Terkel S. *Race: How Blacks and Whites Think and Feel About the American Obsession.* New York: The New Press, 1992.

43. Myrdal G. *An American Dilemma*; p. lxxi.

44. Byrd WM, Clayton LA. *A Black Health Trilogy*; Smith DB. *Health Care Divided: Race and Healing a Nation*. Ann Arbor: The University of Michigan Press, 1999, p. 263.

45. Anderson JD. Secondary school history textbooks and the treatment of black history. In: Hine DC, ed. *The State of Afro-American History: Past, Present, and Future*. Baton Rouge: Louisiana State University Press, 1986, pp. 253–274.

46. Gould SJ. *The Mismeasure of Man*. New York: W.W. Norton and Company, 1981, pp. 19–29; Kragh H. *An Introduction to the Historiography of Science*. Cambridge, England: Cambridge University Press, 1987; paperback ed. 1989, pp. 1–40; Harding S, ed. *The "Racial Economy" of Science: Toward a Democratic Future*. Bloomington: Indiana University Press, 1993; Enthoven AC. The history and principles of managed competition. *Health Affairs* 1993 (Suppl):24–48; Starr P, Zelman WA. Bridge to compromise: Competition under a budget. *Health Affairs* 1993 (Suppl):72–3; U.S. Congress, House of Representatives. *Managed Competition Act of 1992*. 102nd Congress, 2nd session, H.R. 5936. *Congressional Record* September 15, 1992; Honderich T, ed. *The Oxford Companion to Philosophy*. New York: Oxford University Press, 1995, p. 530.

47. Greenberg DS. Black health; Byrd WM. Race, biology, and health care; Byrd WM, Clayton LA. *A Black Health Trilogy*; Clayton LA, Byrd WM. The African American cancer crisis, part 1; Byrd WM, Clayton LA. The African-American cancer crisis, part II; Jaynes GD, Williams RM, eds. *A Common Destiny: Blacks and American Society*. Washington, DC: National Academy Press, 1989; American Cancer Society. *Bridging the Gap in Health Care*. Proceedings from the National Conference on Cancer in the Poor, September 21–23, 1989, Atlanta, GA. American Cancer Society, ed. *Cancer and the Socioeconomically Disadvantaged*. Atlanta, GA. American Cancer Society, 1990; Freeman HP. Cancer in the socioeconomically disadvantaged. In: American Cancer Society, ed. *Cancer and the Socioeconomically Disadvantaged*, pp. 4–26; Patterson JT. *The Dread Disease: Cancer and Modern American Culture*. Cambridge, MA: Harvard University Press, 1987.

48. Byrd WM. Race, biology, and health care; American Cancer Society, ed. *Cancer and the Socioeconomically Disadvantaged*; Jaynes GD, Williams RM, eds. *A Common Destiny*; Blacks seek input in health care proposal. *Jet* May 10, 1993 (84):33; Toner R. Health care wrangle leaves America sour. *International Herald Tribune* September 14, 1994:3; Smith DB. *Health Care Divided: Race and Healing a Nation*. Ann Arbor: The University of Michigan Press, 1999.

49. Jaynes GD, Williams RM, eds. *A Common Destiny: Blacks and American Society*. Manton KG, Patrick CH, Johnson KW. Health differentials between blacks and whites: Recent trends in mortality and morbidity. In: Willis DP, ed. *Health Policies and Black Americans*. New Brunswick, NJ: Transaction Publishers, 1989 pp. 129–199; Davis K, Lillie-Blanton M, Lyons B, et al. Health care for black Americans: The public sector role. In: Willis DP, ed. *Health Policies and Black Americans*, pp. 213–247; Funch DP. *A Report on Cancer Survival in the Economically Disadvantaged*. Report prepared for the American Cancer Society, July 1985; American Cancer Society. *Bridging the Gap in Health Care*; Ryan W. *Blaming the Victim*.

50. Jaynes GD, Williams RM, eds. *A Common Destiny*; Funch DP. *A Report on Cancer Survival in the Economically Disadvantaged*; Byrd WM. Race, biology, and health care; Malone TE, Johnson KW. *Report of the Secretary's Task Force on Black and Minority Health*; Smith DB. *Health Care Divided: Race and Healing a Nation*. Ann Arbor: The University of Michigan Press, 1999.

51. Greenberg DS. Black health; Jones JH. *Bad Blood: The Tuskegee Syphilis Experiment*. New York: The Free Press, 1981; Byrd WM, Clayton LA. An American health dilemma; Lundberg GD. National health care reform; Charatz-Litt C. A chronicle of racism.

52. Sawyer D. "The Tuskegee Study" (videotape segment). *Prime Time Live*, ABC television network, February 6, 1992; Strait G, DiIanni D. "The Deadly Deception" (documentary video segment). *Nova*, Boston, WGBH, 1993; Final report of the Tuskegee Syphilis Study Ad Hoc Advisory Panel. Reiser RJ, Dyck AJ, Curran WJ, eds. In *Ethics in Medicine: Historical Perspectives and Contemporary Concerns*. Cambridge, MA: MIT Press, 1977, pp. 316–321; Thomas SB, Quinn SC. Public health then and now: The Tuskegee syphilis study, 1932 to 1972: Implications for HIV education and AIDS risk education programs in the black community. *American Journal of Public Health* 1991; 81:1498–1504; Byrd WM, Clayton LA. A *Black Health Trilogy*; Robinson LS. Dialogue: Curbing a sick practice: Energy Secretary Hazel O'Leary focuses on government accountability in testing. *Emerge* October 1994; 1(6):20; Washington HA. Of men and mice: Human guinea pigs: Unethical testing targets blacks and the poor. *Emerge* October 1994; 1(6):24; Brandt AM. Racism and research: The case of the Tuskegee Syphilis study. In: Leavitt JW, Numbers RL, eds. *Sickness and Health in America: Readings in the History of Medicine and Public Health*. Madison: The University of Wisconsin Press, 1985, pp. 331–343.

53. Churchill LR. *Rationing Health Care in America: Perceptions and Principles of Justice*. Notre Dame, IN: University of Notre Dame Press, 1987; Ryan W. *Blaming the Victim*; Steinberg S. *The Ethnic Myth: Race, Ethnicity, and Class in America*. N.P.: Atheneum Publishers, 1981; updated and expanded ed., Boston: Beacon Press, 1989; Ryan W. *Equality*. New York: Pantheon Books, 1981; Kaus M. *The End of Equality*. New York: Basic Books, 1992; Sniderman PM, Piazza T. *The Scar of Race*. Cambridge, MA: The Belknap Press of Harvard University Press, 1993, p. 68.

54. Health Policy Advisory Center. The emerging health apartheid in the United States. *Health/PAC Bulletin* 1991; 21:3–4; Ryan W. *Blaming the Victim*; Byrd WM. Race, biology, and health care; Byrd WM, Clayton LA. A *Black Health Trilogy*; Byrd WM, Clayton LA. An American health dilemma; Byrd WM. Race and medicine. Presentation prepared for "Building Bridges: Developing a Culturally Competent Public Health System," a conference sponsored by the State of North Carolina Department of Environment, Health and Natural Resources, Research Triangle Park, June 6, 1995; Smith DB. *Health Care Divided: Race and Healing a Nation*. Ann Arbor: The University of Michigan Press, 1999.

Chapter One

1. Greenberg DS. Black health: Grim statistics. *The Lancet* 1990; 355:780–781; Byrd WM, Clayton LA. America's dual health crisis in black and white. Report prepared for hearings and submitted into the *Congressional Record*. Held for "Health Care Reform: The African American Agenda," Congressional Black Caucus's Health Brain Trust, Congressman Louis Stokes, D-OH, Presiding, 103rd Congress, Special Session, April 13, 1993, Washington, DC; Knowles LL, Prewitt K. *Institutional Racism in America*. Englewood Cliffs, NJ: Prentice-Hall, 1969, pp. 96–114; Kerner O. *Report of the National Advisory Commission on Civil Disorders*. New York: E.P. Dutton, 1968; paperback ed., New

York: Bantam Books, 1968; Randall VR. Racist health care: Reforming an unjust health care system to meet the needs of African-Americans. *Health Matrix: Journal of Law–Medicine* Spring 1993 1(3):127–194; Byrd WM. Race, biology, and health care: Reassessing a relationship. *Journal of Health Care for the Poor and Underserved* 1990; 1:278–292; Byrd WM, Clayton LA. An American health dilemma: A history of blacks in the health system. *Journal of the National Medical Association* 1992; 84:189–200; Hacker A. *Two Nations: Black and White, Separate, Hostile, Unequal.* New York: Ballantine Books, 1992; Farley R, Allen WR. *The Color Line and the Quality of Life in America.* New York: Oxford University Press, 1989; Jaynes GD, Williams RM, eds. *A Common Destiny: Blacks and American Society.* Washington, DC: National Academy Press, 1989; Ginzberg E. Improving health care for the poor: Lessons from the 1980s. *Journal of the American Medical Association* 1994; 271:464–467; Rosenblatt RE. On access to justice, discrimination and health care reform. Testimony before the Health and Environment Subcommittee of the House of Representatives, February 14, 1994; Randall VR. Does Clinton's health care reform proposal ensure (e)qual(ity) of health care for ethnic Americans and the poor? *Brooklyn Law Review* 1994 (Spring, No. 1); 60:167–237.

2. Clayton LA, Byrd WM. Race, a major health status and outcome variable, 1980–1999: With some historical perspectives. *Journal of the National Medical Association.* In press 2000; Health Policy Advisory Center. The emerging health apartheid in the United States. *Health/PAC Bulletin* 1991; 21:3–4; Haynes MA. The gap in health status between black and white Americans. In: Williams RA, ed. *Textbook of Black-Related Diseases.* New York: McGraw-Hill, 1975, pp. 1–30. National Center for Health Statistics. Advance report of final mortality statistics, 1989. *Monthly Vital Statistics Report* 1992:40(8)(Suppl 2); Mangano JJ. Young adults in the 1980s: Why mortality rates are rising. *Health PAC/Bulletin* 1991; 21:19–24; Escarce JJ, Epstein KR, Colby DC, et al. Racial differences in the elderly's use of medical procedures and diagnostic tests. *American Journal of Public Health* 1993; 83:948–954; McCord C, Freeman HP. Excess mortality in Harlem. *New England Journal of Medicine* 1990; 322:173–177; National Center for Health Statistics. *Prevention profile. Health United States, 1991.* Hyattsville, MD: Public Health Service, 1992; U.S. Department of Health and Human Services. *Health Status of the Disadvantaged Chartbook/1990.* Washington, DC: U.S. Department of Health and Human Services, Public Health Service, Publication No. (HRSA) HRS-P-DV 90-1, 1991; Rosenbaum S, Layton C, Liu J. *The Health of America's Children.* Washington, DC: Children's Defense Fund, 1991; U.S. Bureau of the Census. *Statistical Abstract of the United States, 1993.* Washington, DC: U.S. Government Printing Office, 1992; Malone TE, Johnson KW. *Report of the Secretary's Task Force on Black and Minority Health.* Washington, DC: U.S. Department of Health and Human Services, 1986; Greenberg DS. Black health; Clayton LA, Byrd WM. The African American cancer crisis, part 1: The Problem. *Journal of Health Care for the Poor and Underserved* 1993; 4:83–101; Byrd WM, Clayton LA. The African-American cancer crisis, part II: A prescription. *Journal of Health Care for the Poor and Underserved* 1993; 4:102–116; Bergner L. Race, health, and health services. *American Journal of Public Health* 1993; 83:939–941; Rowland Hogue CJ, Hargraves MA. Class, race, and infant mortality in the United States. *American Journal of Public Health* 1993; 83:9–12; Polednak AP. Poverty, residential segregation, and black/white mortality ratios in urban areas. *Journal of Health Care for the Poor and Underserved* 1993; 4:363–373; Byrd WM, Clayton LA. An American health dilemma.

3. West C. *Race Matters.* Boston: Beacon, 1993; Vintage paperback ed., New York: Vintage Books, 1994; Terry RW. *For Whites Only.* Grand Rapids, MI: William B. Eerdmans,

1970; paperback rev. reprint ed., Grand Rapids, MI: William B. Eerdmans, 1992; Sniderman PM, Piazza T. *The Scar of Race*. Cambridge, MA: The Belknap Press of Harvard University Press, 1993; Drake SC. *Black Folk Here and There: An Essay in History and Anthropology* (Vol. 1). Los Angeles: Center for Afro-American Studies, University of California, 1987, pp. 13–114; Feagin JR, Spikes MP. *Living with Racism: The Black Middle-Class Experience*. Boston: Beacon Press, 1994; Massey DS, Denton NA. *American Apartheid: Segregation and the Making of the Underclass*. Cambridge, MA: Harvard University Press, 1993; Wilson WJ. *The Truly Disadvantaged: The Inner City, the Underclass, and Public Policy*. Chicago: The University of Chicago Press, 1987; Simone TM. *About Face: Race in Postmodern America*. Brooklyn, NY: Autonomedia, 1989; Cose E. *The Rage of a Privileged Class*. New York: Harper Collins, 1993; Riggs MT. *Ethnic Notions* (filmstrip). Berkeley, CA: Berkeley Art Center, produced in cooperation with KQED, San Francisco, 1987; Riggs MT. *Color Adjustment* (filmstrip). San Francisco: The American Film Institute and the California Council for the Humanities, produced in cooperation with KQED, San Francisco, 1991; Turner PA. *Ceramic Uncles and Celluloid Mammies: Black Images and Their Influence on Culture*. New York: Anchor Books, 1994; Outlaw L. Toward a critical theory of race. In: Goldberg DT, ed. *Anatomy of Racism*. Minneapolis: University of Minnesota Press, 1990, pp. 58–82. Randall VR. Does Clinton's health care reform proposal ensure (e)qual(ity) of health care for ethnic Americans and the poor? *Brooklyn Law Review* Spring 1994; 1(60):167–237.

4. Banton M, Harwood J. *The Race Concept*. New York: Praeger Publishers, 1975, p. 13.

5. Banton M, Harwood J. *The Race Concept*. New York: Praeger Publishers, 1975; Outlaw L. Toward a critical theory of race. 58–82. In: Goldberg DT, ed. *Anatomy of Racism*. Minneapolis: University of Minnesota Press, 1990, 62; Mish FC, ed. *Webster's Ninth New Collegiate Dictionary*. Springfield, MA: Merriam-Webster, 1990.

6. Banton M, Harwood J. *The Race Concept*; Banton M. *Racial Theories*. Cambridge: Cambridge University Press, 1987, pp. 93–98; Milner R. *The Encyclopedia of Evolution: Humanity's Search for Its Origins*. New York: Facts on File, 1990, pp. 379–380; Pettigrew TF. Prejudice. In: Thernstrom S, Orlov A, Handlin O, eds. *Harvard Encyclopedia of American Ethnic Groups*. Cambridge, MA: The Belknap Press of Harvard University Press, 1980, pp. 820–829. Mish FC, ed. *Webster's Ninth New Collegiate Dictionary*. Springfield, MA: Merriam-Webster, 1990; Terry RW. *For Whites Only*; Sniderman PM, Piazza T. *The Scar of Race*; Montagu A. *Race, Science and Humanity*. New York: Van Nostrand Reinhold, 1963; UNESCO. *The Race Question in Modern Science*. New York: Whiteside and William Morrow, 1956; Kovel J. *White Racism: A Psychohistory*. New York: Random House, 1970; reprint ed., New York: Columbia University Press, 1984; Levin J, Levin W. *The Functions of Discrimination and Prejudice*. 2nd ed. New York: Harper & Row, 1982; Reilly K. *The West and the World: A Topical History of Civilization*. New York: Harper & Row, 1980, pp. 355–383, 449–466; Smith DB. *Health Care Divided: Race and Healing a Nation*. An Arbor: The University of Michigan Press, 1999.

7. Feagin JR, Spikes MP. *Living with Racism*, p. 3.

8. Terry RW. *For Whites Only*, p. 2.

9. Terry RW. *For Whites Only*, p. 2.

10. Terry RW. *For Whites Only*; Feagin JR, Spikes MP. *Living with Racism*; Knowles LL, Prewitt K. *Institutional Racism in America*, pp. 96–114; Steinberg S. *Turning Back:*

The Retreat from Racial Justice in American Thought and Policy, Boston: Beacon Press, 1995; Kerner O. *Report of the National Advisory Commission on Civil Disorders*; Pettigrew TF. Prejudice.

11. Young RJC. *Colonial Desire: Hybridity in Theory, Culture and Race*. London: Routledge, 1995, p. 90.

12. Lévi-Strauss C. Race and history. In: *Race and History*. Paris: United Nations Educational, Scientific and Cultural Organization, 1951, pp. 123–163; quote p. 129.

13. Lévi-Strauss C. Race and history. In: UNESCO, ed. *The Race Question in Modern Science*. New York: Whiteside and William Morrow, pp. 123–163; quote p. 129.

14. Leiris M. Race and culture. In: UNESCO, *The Race Question in Modern Science*, pp. 85–122; quote p. 86.

15. Van den Berghe PL. *Race and Racism: A Comparative Perspective*. New York: Wiley, 1967, p. 27.

16. Reilly K. *The West and the World: A Topical History of Civilization*. New York: Harper & Row, 1980, p. 452.

17. Reilly K. *The West and the World*, p. 452.

18. Van den Berghe PL. *Race and Racism*, p. 30.

19. Lévi-Strauss C. Race and history. In: UNESCO, ed. Reilly K. *The West and the World*; Leiris M. Race and culture; Van den Berghe PL. *Race and Racism*; Kovel J. *White Racism*; Young RJC. *Colonial Desire*; Mazrui AA. *The Africans. A Nine Part Series* (videotapes). Sponsored by the Annenberg/CPB Project, Washington, DC: WETA and BBC, 1986; Mazrui AA. *The Africans: A Triple Heritage*. Boston: Little, Brown, 1986; Davidson B. *The African Slave Trade*. rev. and expanded ed. Boston: Atlantic Monthly Press Book, Little, Brown, 1961.

20. Allport GW. *The Nature of Prejudice*. Reading, MA: Addison-Wesley, 1979; Terry RW. *For Whites Only*; Jones JH. *Bad Blood: The Tuskegee Syphilis Experiment*. New York: The Free Press, 1981; Outlaw L. Toward a critical theory of race; Banton M, Harwood J. *The Race Concept*; Banton M. *Racial Theories*, pp. 93–98; Terry RW. *For Whites Only*; Levin J. *The Foundations of Prejudice*. New York: Harper & Row, 1975. Levin J, Levin W. *The Functions of Discrimination and Prejudice*. 2nd ed. New York: Harper & Row, 1982; Smith DB. *Health Care Divided: Race and Haling a Nation*. Ann Arbor: The University of Michigan Press, 1999.

21. Kovel J. *White Racism*, p. x.

22. Ryan W. *Blaming the Victim*; Reilly K. *The West and the World*; Kovel J. *White Racism*; Terry RW. *For Whites Only*; *About Face*; Feagin JR, Spikes MP. *Living with Racism*; Pettigrew TF. Prejudice.

23. Kovel J. *White Racism*, p. xi.

24. Kovel J. *White Racism*, p. xi.

25. Kozol J. *Savage Inequalities: Children in America's Schools*. New York: Crown, pp. 207–233.

26. Kovel J. *White Racism*, pp. xi, 211–230; Pettigrew TF. Prejudice; Kozol J. *Savage Inequalities*; Orfield, G, Jackson SE. *Dismantling Desegregation: The Quiet Reversal of Brown v. Board of Education*. New York: The New Press, 1996; Lemann N. *The Promised Land: The Great Black Migration and How It Changed America*. New York: Knopf, 1991; Wilson WJ. *The Truly Disadvantaged*; Wilson WJ. *When Work Disappears: The World of the New Urban Poor*. New York: Knopf, 1996.

27. Kovel J. *White Racism*, pp. vi–lv, 211–230; Simone TM. *About Face*; Hacker A. *Two Nations*; Feagin JR, Spikes MP. *Living with Racism*; Lemann N. Taking affirmative action apart. *New York Times Magazine* June 11, 1995; Section 6:36; Kozol J. *Death at an Early Age*. Boston: Houghton Mifflin, 1967; Kozol J. *Savage Inequalities*; Lemann N. The structure of success in America. *Atlantic Monthly* August 1995; 2(276):41; Lemann N. The great sorting. *Atlantic Monthly* September 1995; 3(276):84.

28. Ginzberg E. Improving health care for the poor.

29. Eckholm E. While Congress remains silent health care transforms itself. *New York Times*, December 18, 1994: 1; Kongstvedt PR. *The Managed Health Care Handbook*. 2nd ed. Gaithersburg, MD: Aspen Publishers, 1993; Morais HM. *The History of the Negro in Medicine*. New York: Publishers Company, 1967; Byrd WM, Clayton LA. *A Black Health Trilogy* (videotape and 188-page documentary report). Washington, DC: The National Medical Association and the African American Heritage and Education Foundation; 1991; Newman DK, Amidei NJ, Carter BL, et al. Second-class medicine. In: *Protest, Politics, and Prosperity: Black Americans and White Institutions, 1940–75*. New York: Pantheon Books, 1978, pp. 187–235; Bullough B, Bullough VL. *Poverty, Ethnic Identity, and Health Care*. New York: Appleton-Century-Crofts, 1972; Hanft RS, White CC. Constraining the supply of physicians: Effects on black physicians. In: Willis DP, ed. *Health Policies and Black Americans*. New Brunswick, NJ: Transaction Publishers, 1989, pp. 249–269; Kotelchuck R. Down and out in the "New Calcutta": New York City's health care crisis. *Health/PAC Bulletin* Summer 1989; 19:4–11; Dowling HF. *City Hospitals: The Undercare of the Underprivileged*. Cambridge, MA: Harvard University Press, 1982; Byrd WM, Clayton LA. An American health dilemma; Sack K. Public hospitals around country cut basic service: Some face elimination. *New York Times* August 20, 1995: 1; Public hospitals across nation cutting service under pressure. *Fort Worth Star-Telegram* August 20, 1995:A4; Egyir WK. Harlem Hospital axed. *New York Amsterdam News* April 8, 1995:1; Lewin T. Hospitals serving the poor struggle to retain patients. *New York Times* September 3, 1997:A1.

30. Greenberg DS. Black health; Byrd WM, Clayton LA. An American health dilemma; Starr P. *The Social Transformation of American Medicine*. New York: Basic Books, 1982; Charatz-Litt C. A chronicle of racism: The effects of the white medical community on black health. *Journal of the National Medical Association* 1992; 84:717–725; Sidel VW, Sidel R, eds. *Reforming Medicine: Lessons of the Last Quarter Century*. New York: Pantheon Books, 1984; Ginzberg E. *The Medical Triangle: Physicians, Politicians, and the Public*. Cambridge, MA: Harvard University Press, 1990; Ginzberg E. Improving health care for the poor. Smith DB. *Health Care Divided: Race and Healing a Nation*. Ann Arbor: The University of Michigan Press, 1999.

31. Banton M. *Racial Theories*; Montagu A. *Race, Science and Humanity*; Barzun J. *Race: A Study in Modern Superstition*. N.P., 1937. Barzun J. *Race: A Study in Superstition*. rev. ed. New York: Harper & Row, 1965; Allport GW. *The Nature of Prejudice*; UNESCO, ed. *The Race Question in Modern Science*; Sniderman PM, Piazza T. *The Scar of Race*; Roberts MJ, Clyde AT. *Your Money or Your Life: The Health Care Crisis Explained*. New York: Doubleday, 1993; Mazrui A. Global Africa. Part nine, *The Africans. A Nine-Part Series* (videotapes); Williams J. *Eyes on the Prize: America's Civil Rights Years, 1954–1965*. New York: Viking Penguin, 1987; Kerner O. *Report of the National Advisory Commission on Civil Disorders*; Johnson H, Broder D. *The System: The American Way of Politics at the Breaking Point*. Boston: Little, Brown, 1996.

32. Mayr E. *The Growth of Biological Thought: Diversity, Evolution, and Inheritance.* Cambridge, MA: The Belknap Press of Harvard University Press, 1982, p. 273.

33. Shipman P. *The Evolution of Racism*, p. 269.

34. Milner R. *The Encyclopedia of Evolution*, p. 382.

35. Milner R. *The Encyclopedia of Evolution*, pp. 380–382; King JC. *The Biology of Race.* revised ed. Berkeley: University of California Press, 1981, p. 158; Lewontin RC, Rose S, Kamin LJ. *Not in Our Genes: Biology, Ideology, and Human Nature.* New York: Pantheon Books, 1984, p. 126; Shipman P. *The Evolution of Racism*, pp. 267–271.

36. King JC. *The Biology of Race*, p. 10.

37. Gould SJ. Human equality is a contingent fact of history. In: Gould SJ. *The Flamingo's Smile: Reflections in Natural History.* New York: W.W. Norton, 1985, pp. 185–198; quote p. 194.

38. King JC. *The Biology of Race*; King M, Wilson AC. Evolution at two levels in humans and chimpanzees. *Science* April 11, 1975; 188(4184):107–116. Stringer C, McKie R. *African Exodus: The Origins of Modern Humanity.* New York: Henry Holt and Company, 1996. Lewontin RC, Rose S, Kamin LJ. *Not in Our Genes*; Gould SJ. *The Mismeasure of Man.* New York: W.W. Norton, 1981; Milner R. *The Encyclopedia of Evolution*; Shipman P. *The Evolution of Racism*; Gould SJ. Human equality is a contingent fact of history.

39. Barzun J. *Race: A Study in Modern Superstition*; Barzun J. *Race: A Study in Superstition.* Chase A. *The Legacy of Malthus: The Social Costs of the New Scientific Racism.* New York: Knopf, 1980; King JC. *The Biology of Race*; King M, Wilson AC. Evolution at two levels in humans and chimpanzees. *Science* April 11, 1975; 188(4184):107–116; Montagu A. *Race, Science and Humanity*; UNESCO, ed. *The Race Question in Modern Science*; Hacker A. *Two Nations*; Terkel S. *Race: How Blacks and Whites Think and Feel About the American Obsession.* New York: The New Press, 1992; Tierney J, Wright L, Springen K. The search for Adam and Eve: Scientists claim to have found our common ancestor—a woman who lived 200,000 years ago and left resilient genes that are carried by all of mankind. *Newsweek* January 11, 1988; 61:46; Lewin R. *In the Age of Mankind.* Washington, DC: Smithsonian Books, 1988; Flanagan R. Out of Africa: Out of Africa debate heats up. *Earth: The Science of Our Planet* February 1996; 26. Stringer C, McKie R. *African Exodus: The Origin of Modern Humanity.* New York: Henry Holt and Company, 1996.

40. Montagu A. *Race, Science and Humanity*; Byrd WM. Race, biology, and health care; Drake SC. *Black Folk Here and There: An Essay in History and Anthropology* (Vol. 2). Los Angeles: Center for Afro-American Studies, University of California, 1990; Devisse J. *The Image of the Black in Western Art* (Part 2, From the Early Christian Era to the "Age of Discovery." 1. From the Demonic Threat to the Incarnation of Sainthood). Cambridge, MA: The Minil Foundation, distributed by the Harvard University Press, 1979; Lewis B. The African diaspora and the civilization of Islam. In: Kilson ML, Rothberg RI, eds. *The African Diaspora: Interpretive Essays.* Cambridge, MA: Harvard University Press, 1976, pp. 37–56; Lewis B. *Race and Slavery in the Middle East: An Historical Enquiry.* New York: Oxford University Press, 1990; Sanders R. *Lost Tribes and Promised Lands: The Origins of American Racism.* Boston: Little, Brown, 1978.

41. Lewin R. *In the Age of Mankind*; Gould SJ. *An Urchin in the Storm: Essays about Books and Ideas.* New York: W.W. Norton, 1987, pp. 107–154; Darrough MN, Black RH, eds. *Biological Differences and Social Equality: Implicatins for Social Policy.* Westport,

CT: Greenwood Press, 1983; Fish JM. Mixed blood. *Psychology Today* November/ December 1995; 6(28):55; Chase A. *The Legacy of Malthus*; Wilson EO. *On Human Nature*. Cambridge, MA: Harvard University Press, 1978; Lumsden CJ, Wilson EO. *Genes, Mind, and Culture: The Coevolutionary Process*. Cambridge, MA: Harvard University Press, 1981; Lewontin RC, Rose S, Kamin LJ. *Not in Our Genes*; Duster R. *Backdoor to Eugenics*. New York: Routledge, 1990; Hubbard R, Wald E. *Exploding the Gene Myth: How Genetic Informatin Is Produced and Manipulated by Scientists, Physicians, Employers, Insurance Companies, Educators, and Law Enforcers*. Boston: Beacon Press, 1993; Herrnstein RJ, Murray C. *The Bell Curve: Intelligence and Class Structure in American Life*. New York: The Free Press, 1994.

42. Tierney J, Wright L, Springen K. The search for Adam and Eve; Chandler DL. In shift, many anthropoligsts see race as social construct. *The Boston Sunday Globe* May 11, 1997:A30; Wanniski J. Behind the curve: Journalists who accept the findings of *The Bell Curve* are "benevolent racists." *Forbes MediaCritic* Spring 1995; 3(2):86; Caldwell C. Journalists who dismiss the findings of *The Bell Curve* engage in "intellectual decadence." *Forbes MediaCritic* Spring 1995 3(2):85; Researchers say race isn't base for scientific study. *Fort Worth Star-Telegram* February 20, 1995:A7; Racial characteristics not factors in genetic research. *Jet* March 13, 1995; 18(87):24.

43. King JC. *The Biology of Race*, p. 133.

44. Herrnstein RJ, Murray C. *The Bell Curve*; Coon CS. *The Origin of Races*. New York: Knopf, 1962; Coon CS. *The Living Races of Man*. New York: Knopf, 1965; Baker JR. *Race*. New York: Oxford University Press, 1974; Shipman P. *The Evolution of Racism*; Duster T. *Backdoor to Eugenics*; Nelkin D, Tancredi L. *Dangerous Diagnostics: The Social Power of Biological Information*. New York: Basic Books, 1989; Hubbard R, Wald E. *Exploding the Gene Myth*; Gould SJ. *The Mismeasure of Man*; Lewontin RC, Rose S, Kamin LJ. *Not in Our Genes*; Fish JM. Mixed blood. *Psychology Today* November/ December 1995; 6(28):55.

45. Blendon RJ, Aiken LH, Freeman HE, et al. Access to medical care for black and white Americans: A matter of continuing concern. *Journal of the American Medical Association* 1989; 262:278–281; Ginzberg E. *The Medical Triangle: Physicians, Politicians, and the Public*. Cambridge, MA: Harvard University Press, 1990; Roberts MJ, Clyde AT. *Your Money or Your Life*; Byrd WM, Clayton LA. *A Black Health Trilogy*; Byrd WM, Clayton LA. An American health dilemma; Feagin JR, Spikes MP. *Living with Racism*; Massey DS, Denton NA. *American Apartheid*; Sniderman PM, Piazza T. *The Scar of Race*; Randall VR. Racist health care; Randall VR. Does Clinton's health care reform proposal ensure (e)qual(ity) of health care for ethnic Americans and the poor?

46. Feagin R, Feagin CB. *Racial and Ethnic Relations* 6th ed. Upper Saddle River, NJ: Prentice Hall, 1999; Greenberg DS. Black health; Blendon RJ, Aiken LH, Freeman HE, et al. Access to medical care for black and white Americans; Roberts MJ, Clyde AT. *Your Money or Your Life*; U.S. Department of Health and Human Services. *Health, United States, 1988, and Prevention Profile*. Washington, DC: U.S. Government Printing Office, 1989; U.S. Department of Health and Human Services. *Health Status of the Disadvantaged Chartbook/1990*; U.S. Department of Health and Human Services. *Health, United States, 1991, and Prevention Profile*. Washington, DC: U.S. Government Printing Office, 1992, DHHS Publication No. (PHS) 92-1232; Sniderman PM, Piazza T. *The Scar of Race*; Ryan W. *Blaming the Victim*; Ryan W. *Equality*. New York: Pantheon Books, 1981; Chase A. *The Legacy of Malthus*; West C. *Race Matters*; Cose E. *The Rage of a Privileged*

Class. New York: Harper Collins, Publishers, 1993; paperback ed., New York: Harper Perennial, 1995; Guinier L. *The Tyranny of the Majority: Fundamental Fairness in Representative Democracy*. New York: The Free Press, 1994; Jhally S, Lewis J. *Enlightened Racism:* The Cosby Show, *Audiences, and the Myth of the American Dream*. Boulder, CO: Westview Press, 1992; Ginzberg E, personal interview, July 8, 1995; Auletta K. *The Underclass*. New York: Random House, 1982; paperback ed., New York: Vintage Books, 1983; Gans HJ. *The War Against the Poor: The Underclass and Antipoverty Policy*. New York: Basic Books, 1995; Steinberg S. *Turning Back: The Retreat from Racial Justice in American Thought and Policy*. Boston: Beacon Press, 1995; Fish JM. Mixed blood.

47. Banton M. *Racial Theories*, p. 1.

48. Banton M. *Racial Theories*, p. xi.

49. Wendt H. *From Ape to Adam: The Search for the Ancestry of Man*. Indianapolis: Bobbs-Merrill, 1972, pp. 18–19.

50. Harris JE. *Africans and Their History*. Rev. Ed. New York: New American Library, 1972, p. 16.

51. Milner R. *The Encyclopedia of Evolution: Humanity's Search for Its Origins*. New York: Facts on File, Inc., 1990, p. 201.

52. Banton M. *Racial Theories*, p. xi.

53. Banton M. *Racial Theories*, pp. xi, 1; Gould SJ. *The Mismeasure of Man*, pp. 19–72; Lovejoy AO. *The Great Chain of Being: A Study of the History of an Idea*. Cambridge, MA: Harvard University Press, 1936; reprint paperback ed., 1964; Jordan WD. *White over Black: American Attitudes Toward the Negro, 1550–1812*. New York: W.W. Norton, 1968; Haller Jr. JS. *Outcasts from Evolution: Scientific Attitudes of Racial Inferiority, 1859–1900*. New York: McGraw Hill, 1971, pp. 70–79; Milner R. *The Encyclopedia of Evolution*, p. 201; Sirasi NG. *Medieval and Early Renaissance Medicine: An Introduction to Knowledge and Practice*. Chicago: The University of Chicago Press, 1990; Lyons AS, Petrucelli RJ. *Medicine: An Illustrated History*. New York: Harry N. Abrams, 1978; Stafford BM. *Body Criticism: Imaging the Unseen in Enlightenment Art and Medicine*. Cambridge, MA: The MIT Press, 1991; Gossett TF. *Race: The History of an Idea in America*. New York: Schocken Books, 1965, 3–16; Harris JE. *Africans and Their History*. Rev. ed. New York: New American Library, 1972, 3–28.

54. Gould SJ. *The Mismeasure of Man*, p. 25.

55. Banton M. *Racial Theories*; Banton M, Harwood J. *The Race Concept*. New York: Praeger, 1975; Gould SJ. *The Mismeasure of Man*, pp. 19–112; Milner R. *The Encyclopedia of Evolution*, pp. 360–362, 371, 380–382; Haller JS Jr. *Outcasts from Evolution*; Stanton W. *The Leopard's Spots: Scientific Attitudes Toward Race in America, 1815–1859*. Chicago: The University of Chicago Press, 1960; Gossett TF. *Race: The History of an Idea in America*. Dallas, TX: Southern Methodist University Press, 1963; reprint ed., New York: Schocken Books, 1965, pp. 3–175; Fredrickson GM. *The Black Image in the White Mind: The Debate on Afro-American Character and Destiny, 1871–1914*. New York: Harper & Row, 1971; reprint ed., Middletown, CT: Wesleyan University Press, 1987, pp. 71–96; Jordan WD. *White Over Black*, pp. 43–98; Stannard DE. *American Holocaust: Columbus and the Conquest of the New World*. New York: Oxford University Press, 1992; Shipman P. *The Evolution of Racism*.

56. Banton M, Harwood J. *The Race Concept*, pp. 13–47; Chase A. *The Legacy of Malthus*, pp. 48–200; Gould SJ. *The Mismeasure of Man*; Allan GE. Testing America's intelligence: Eugenics comes to America. 441–475. In: Jacoby R, Glauberman N, eds.

The Bell Curve Debate: History, Documents, Opinions. New York: Times Books, 1995; Milner R. *The Encyclopedia of Evolution*, pp. 360–362, 371, 380–382; Haller JS Jr., Haller RM. *The Physician and Sexuality in Victorian America.* N.P.: University of Illinois Press, 1974; reprint ed., New York: W.W. Norton, 1977, pp. 44–87; Russet CE. *Sexual Science: The Victorian Construction of Womanhood.* Cambridge, MA: Harvard University Press, 1989; Schiebinger L. *The Mind Has No Sex? Women in the Origins of Modern Science.* Cambridge, MA: Harvard University Press, 1989, pp. 16–77; Haller Jr. JS. *Outcasts from Evolution*; Stanton W. *The Leopard's Spots*; Kevles DJ. *In the Name of Eugenics: Genetics and the Uses of Human Heredity.* Berkeley: University of California Press, 1985; Haller MH. *Eugenics: Hereditarian Attitudes in American Thought.* New Brunswick, NJ: Rutgers University Press, 1963; Shipman P. *The Evolution of Racism*, pp. 17–141; Fish JM. Mixed blood.

57. Banton M. *Racial Theories*, pp. 47–154; Banton M, Harwood J. *The Race Concept*; Chase A. *The Legacy of Malthus*; Brinkley A. *The Unfinished Nation: A Concise History of the American People.* New York: Knopf, 1993, pp. 431–441, 471–472, 507–511; Zinn H. *A Peoples History of the United States.* New York: Harper & Row, 1980; paperback ed., New York: Harper Perennial, 1990, pp. 167–246; Gould SJ. *The Mismeasure of Man*; Milner R. *The Encyclopedia of Evolution*, pp. 37, 262–264; Haller Jr. JS. *Outcasts from Evolution*; Stanton W. *The Leopard's Spots*; Gilman SL. *Freud, Race, and Gender.* Princeton, NJ: Princeton University Press, 1993; Proctor RN. *Racial Hygiene: Medicine under the Nazis.* Cambridge, MA: Harvard University Press, 1988; Duster R. *Backdoor to Eugenics*; Shipman P. *The Evolution of Racism*; Herrnstein RJ, Murray C. *The Bell Curve*; Lemann N. The structure of success in America: The untold story of how educational testing became ambition's gateway—and a national obsession. *Atlantic Monthly* August 1995; (276):41; Lemann N. The great sorting: The first mass administrations of a scholastic-aptitude test led with surprising speed to the idea that the nation's leaders would be the people who did well on tests. *Atlantic Monthly* September 1995; 3(276):84.

58. Starr P. *The Social Transformation of American Medicine.* New York: Basic Books, 1982, p. 3.

59. Starr P. *The Social Transformation of American Medicine*, p. 3; Shryock RH. *The Development of Modern Medicine: An Interpretation of the Social and Scientific Factors Involved.* Madison: The University of Wisconsin Press, 1974; Cobb WM. 1981. The black American in medicine. *Journal of the National Medical Association* 73(Suppl 1):1183–1244; Byrd WM. Race, biology, and health care; Byrd WM, Clayton LA. An American health dilemma; Morais HM. *The History of the Negro in Medicine.*

60. Reiser RJ, Dyck AJ, Curran WJ, eds. Final report of the Tuskegee Syphilis Study Ad Hoc Advisory Panel. In Reiser RJ, Dyck AJ, Curran WJ, eds. *Ethics in Medicine: Historical Perspectives and Contemporary Concerns.* Cambridge, MA: MIT Press, 1977, pp. 316–321; Brandt AM. Racism and research: The case of the Tuskegee Syphilis study. In: Leavitt JW, Numbers RL, eds. *Sickness and Health in America: Readings in the History of Medicine and Public Health.* Madison, Wisconsin: The University of Wisconsin Press, 1985, pp. 331–343; Jones JH. *Bad Blood*; Sawyer D. "The Tuskegee Study" (videotape segment). *Prime Time Live*, ABC television network, February 6, 1992.

61. Byrd WM. Race, biology, and health care; Drake SC. *Black Folk Here and There* (Vols. 1 and 2). Byrd WM, Clayton LA. An American health dilemma; Savitt TL. *Medicine and Slavery: The Diseases and Health Care of Blacks in Antebellum Virginia.* Urbana: University of Illinois Press, 1987; Sheridan RB. *Doctors and Slaves: A Medical and Demo-*

graphic History of Slavery in the British West Indies, 1680–1834. Cambridge, England: Cambridge University Press, 1985; Kiple KF, King VH. *Another Dimension to the Black Diaspora: Diet, Disease, and Racism.* Cambridge, England: Cambridge University Press, 1981; Chase A. *The Legacy of Malthus*; Brandt AM. Racism and research; Gould SJ. *Ever Since Darwin: Reflections in Natural History.* New York: W.W. Norton, Gould SJ. *The Mismeasure of Man*; Jones JH. *Bad Blood*; Shipman P. *The Evolution of Racism*; Stanton W. *The Leopard's Spots*; Haller JS, Jr. *Outcasts from Evolution*; Dula A. Toward an African-American perspective on bioethics. *Journal of Health Care for the Poor and Underserved* 1991; 2:259–269; Hearnshaw LS. *Cyril Burt Psychologist.* Ithaca, NY: Cornell University Press, 1979; Ginzberg E, Dutka AB. *The Financing of Biomedical Research.* Baltimore: The Johns Hopkins University Press, 1989.

62. Kragh H. *An Introduction to the Historiography of Science.* Cambridge, England: Cambridge University Press, 1987; paperback ed. 1989, p. 41.

63. Kragh H. *An Introduction to the Historiography of Science*, p. 42.

64. Kragh H. *An Introduction to the Historiography of Science*, p. 18.

65. Chase A. *The Legacy of Malthus*, pp. 5, 17–19; Jones JH. *Bad Blood*; Fineberg KS, Peters JD, Willson JR, et al. *Obstetrics/Gynecology and the Law.* Ann Arbor: Health Administration Press, 1984, pp. 233–234; Beecher HK. Ethics and clinical research. *New England Journal of Medicine* 1966; 274;1354–1360; Breitman R. *The Architect of Genocide: Himmler and the Final Solution.* New York: Knopf, 1991, pp. 139–140, 152–153, 181, 201; Lifton RJ. *The Nazi Doctors: Medical Killing and the Psychology of Genocide.* New York: Basic Books, 1986; Annas GJ, Grodin MA, eds. *The Nazi Doctors and the Nuremberg Code: Human Rights in Human Experimentation.* New York: Oxford University Press, 1992; Caplen AL, ed. *When Medicine Went Mad: Bioethics and the Holocaust.* Totowa, NJ: Humane Press, 1992; Aly G, Chroust P, Pross C. *Cleansing the Fatherland: Nazi Medicine and Racial Hygiene.* Baltimore: The Johns Hopkins University Press, 1994. Arad Y, ed. *The Pictorial History of the Holocaust.* New York: Macmillan, 1990, pp. 204, 206–207, 263, 310–311; McGregor DK. *Sexual Surgery and the Origins of Gynecology; J. Marion Sims, His Hospital, and His Patients.* New York: Garland, 1989, pp. 29, 35, 42–47, 52–55, 59–68, 76–77; Veatch RM. Benefiting mentally retarded children by giving them hepatitis. In: Veatch RM. *Case Studies in Medical Ethics.* Cambridge, Massachusetts: Harvard University Press, 1977, pp. 274–277.

66. Kragh H. *An Introduction to the Historiography of Science*; Byrd WM. Race, biology, and health care; Byrd WM, Clayton LA. An American health dilemma; Dula A. Toward an African-American perspective on bioethics; Hearnshaw LS. *Cyril Burt Psychologist*; Lurie E. *Louis Agassiz: A Life in Science.* Chicago: The University of Chicago Press, 1960; McGregor DK. *Sexual Surgery and the Origins of Gynecology*; Horsman R. *Josiah Nott of Mobile: Southerner, Physician, and Racial Theorist.* Baton Rouge: Louisiana State University Press, 1987. Chase A. *The Legacy of Malthus: The Social Costs of the New Scientific Racism.* New York: Alfred A. Knopf, 1980; Shipman P. *The Evolution of Racism: Human Differences and the Use and Abuse of Science.* New York: Simon and Schuster, 1994; Katz J. *Experimentation with Human Beings.* New York: Russel Sage Foundation, 1972; Tucker WH. *The Science and Politics of Racial Research.* Urbana: University of Illinois Press, 1994.

67. Jones JH. *Bad Blood*; Byrd WM. Race, biology, and health care; Byrd WM, Clayton LA. The "slave health deficit": Racism and health outcomes. *Health/PAC Bulletin* 1991; 21:25–28; Byrd WM, Clayton LA. An American health dilemma; Morais HM. *The*

History of the Negro in Medicine; Savitt TL. *Medicine and Slavery*; Sidel VW, Sidel R, eds. *Reforming Medicine*; Bullough B, Bullough VL. *Poverty, Ethnic Identity, and Health Care*; Newman DK, Amidei NJ, Carter BL, et al. Second-class medicine.

68. Greenberg DS. Black health; Chase A. *The Legacy of Malthus*; Bagdikian BH. *The Media Monopoly*. Boston: Beacon Press, 1983; Malone TE, Johnson KW. *Report of the Secretary's Task Force on Black and Minority Health*; Byrd WM, Clayton LA. An American health dilemma; Konner M. *Medicine at the Crossroads: The Crisis in Health Care*. New York: Pantheon Books, 1993, pp. ix–xxii.

69. Devisse J. *The Image of the Black in Western Art* (Part 2, *From the Early Christian Era to the "Age of Discovery"*. 1. *From the Demonic Threat to the Incarnation of Sainthood*), pp. 50–52; Vercoutter J, Leclant J, Snowden FM, Jr, et al. *The Image of the Black in Western Art* (Part 1, *From the Pharaohs to the Fall of the Roman Empire*). Cambridge, MA: The Minil Foundation, distributed by the Harvard University Press, 1976; Pieterse JN. White on Black: Images of Africa and Blacks in Western Popular Culture. New Haven: Yale University Press, 1992; Drake SC. *Black Folk Here and There* (Vol. 2); Harris JE. *Africans and Their History.* revised and updated ed. New York: New American Library, 1972, pp. 13–17; Sanders R. *Lost Tribes and Promised Lands: The Origins of American Racism*. Boston: Little, Brown and Company 1978; Byrd WM. Race, biology, and health care; Morais HM. *The History of the Negro in Medicine*; Gossett TF. *Race: The History of an Idea in America*, pp. 3–8; Davis DB. *Slavery and Human Progress*. New York: Oxford University Press, 1984; Drake SC. *Black Folk Here and There* (Vol. 1); Snowden Jr. FM. *Blacks in Antiquity: Ethiopians in the Greco-Roman Experience*. Cambridge, MA: The Belknap Press of Harvard University Press, 1970.

70. Finley M. *Ancient Slavery and Modern Ideology*. Great Britain: Chatto and Windus, 1980; paperback ed., New York: Pelican Books, 1983, p. 119.

71. Finley M. *Ancient Slavery and Modern Ideology*, p. 118; Drake SC. *Black Folk Here and There: An Essay in History and Anthropology* (Vol. 2), pp. 71–72.

72. Harris JE. *Africans and Their History*, p. 15.

73. Harris JE. *Africans and Their History*, p. 15.

74. Harris JE. *Africans and Their History*, p. 16.

75. Harris JE. *Africans and Their History*, p. 16.

76. Goldberg DT. The social formation of racist discourse. In: Goldberg DT, ed. *Anatomy of Racism*. Minneapolis: University of Minnesota Press, 1990, pp. 295–318; Harris JE. *Africans and Their History*, pp. 13–28; Wassermann HP. *Ethnic Pigmentation: Historical, Psychological, and Clinical Aspects*. New York: American Elsevier, 1974, pp. 13–21; Devisse J. *The Image of the Black in Western Art* (Part 2, *From the Early Christian Era to the "Age of Discovery."* 1. *From the Demonic Threat to the Incarnation of Sainthood*), pp. 37–80; Drake SC. *Black Folk Here and There* (Vols. 1 and 2); Pietërse JN. *White on Black: Images of Africa and Blacks in Western Popular Culture*. New Haven: Yale University Press, 1992; Lewin R. *In the Age of Mankind*; Snowden FM Jr. *Blacks in Antiquity*; Finley M. *Ancient Slavery and Modern Ideology*, McEvedy C. *The World History Factfinder*. N.P.: Grisewood and Dempsy, 1984; rev. and updated ed., New York: Gallery Books, 1989.

77. Goldberg DT. The social formation of racist discourse, p. 301.

78. Goldberg DT. The social formation of racist discourse, p. 301.

79. Outlaw L. Toward a critical theory of race, pp. 58–63.

80. Goldberg DT. The social formation of racist discourse, p. 301.

81. Goldberg DT. The social formation of racist discourse, p. 301.

82. Goldberg DT. The social formation of racist discourse, p. 302.

83. Goldberg DT. The social formation of racist discourse, p. 301; Outlaw L. Toward a critical theory of race, pp. 58–82; Drake SC. *Black Folk Here and There* (Vol. 2); Devisse J. *The Image of the Black in Western Art* (Part 2, *From the Early Christian Era to the "Age of Discovery."* 1. *From the Demonic Threat to the Incarnation of Sainthood*); Finley M. *Ancient Slavery and Modern Ideology*; Nisbet R. *Prejudices: A Philosophical Dictionary.* Cambridge, MA: Harvard University Press, 1982, pp. 35–40; Snowden FM Jr. *Blacks in Antiquity*; Lovejoy AO. *The Great Chain of Being.*

84. Wassermann HP. *Ethnic Pigmentation*; p. 18.

85. Drake SC. *Black Folk Here and There* (Vol. 2), p. 42.

86. Drake SC. *Black Folk Here and There* (Vol. 2), pp. 71–72.

87. Wassermann HP. *Ethnic Pigmentation*, pp. 17–19; Drake SC. *Black Folk Here and There: An Essay in History and Anthropology* (Vol. 2), pp. 70–76; Snowden FM, Jr. *Blacks in Antiquity*; Lovejoy AO. *The Great Chain of Being*, pp. 93–98.

88. Davis DB. *The Problem of Slavery in Western Culture.* Ithaca, NJ: Cornell University Press, 1966, p. 67.

89. Davis DB. *The Problem of Slavery in Western Culture*, p. 67.

90. Finley M. *Ancient Slavery and Modern Ideology*, p. 118.

91. Drake SC. *Black Folk Here and There: An Essay in History and Anthropology* (Vol. 2); Snowden FM Jr. *Blacks in Antiquity.*

92. Devisse J. *The Image of the Black in Western Art* (Part 2, *From the Early Christian Era to the "Age of Discovery."* 1. *From the Demonic Threat to the Incarnation of Sainthood*), pp. 50–51.

93. Davis DB. *The Problem of Slavery in Western Culture*, pp. 66–90; Devisse J. *The Image of the Black in Western Art* (Part 2, *From the Early Christian Era to the "Age of Discovery."* 1. *From the Demonic Threat to the Incarnation of Sainthood*), pp. 50–51; Wassermann HP. *Ethnic Pigmentation*, p. 18; Patterson O. *Slavery and Social Death: A Comparative Study.* Cambridge, MA: Harvard University Press, 1982, pp. 86–94.

94. Bender GA. *Great Moments in Medicine.* Detroit: Northwood Institute Press, 1966, pp. 56–61.

95. Bender GA. *Great Moments in Medicine*, p. 57.

96. Guthrie D. *A History of Medicine.* Philadelphia: J.B. Lippincott, 1946, p. 74.

97. Bender GA. *Great Moments in Medicine*, pp. 34–39, 50–61; Nuland SB. *Doctors: The Biography of Medicine.* New York: Knopf, 1988, pp. 3–60; Lyons AS, Petrucelli RJ. *Medicine: An Illustrated History.* New York: Harry N. Abrams, 1978, pp. 153–264; Sigerist HE. *The Great Doctors: A Biographical History of Medicine.* New York: W.W. Norton, 1933; reprint ed., New York: Dover Publications, 1971, pp. 29–37, 68–77; Haeger K. *The Illustrated History of Surgery.* New York: Bell, 1988, pp. 34–67; Guthrie D. *A History of Medicine*, pp. 39–83.

98. Drake SC. *Black Folk Here and There: An Essay in History and Anthropology* (Vol. 2), p. 56.

99. Davis DB. *Slavery and Human Progress*, p. 42.

100. Drake SC. *Black Folk Here and There* (Vol. 2), p. 45.

101. Davis DB. *Slavery and Human Progress*, p. 328, n. 58; Drake SC. *Black Folk Here and There* (Vol. 2), p. 57.

102. Davis DB. *Slavery and Human Progress*, p. 328 n. 58; Drake SC. *Black Folk Here and There* (Vol. 2), p. 57; Lewis B. *Race and Slavery in the Middle East: An Historical Enquiry.* New York: Oxford University Press, 1990, p. 52.

103. Drake SC. *Black Folk Here and There* (Vol. 2), pp. 45, 56–58; Davis DB. *Slavery and Human Progress*, p. 42; Nuland SB. *Doctors: The Biography of Medicine*, pp. 31–60; Lewis B. *Race and Slavery in the Middle East*, p. 52.

104. Drake SC. *Black Folk Here and There* (Vol. 2), p. 72.

105. Davis DB. *Slavery and Human Progress*, p. 42.

106. Finley M. *Ancient Slavery and Modern Ideology*, pp. 71–72.

107. Drake SC. *Black Folk Here and There* (Vol. 2), p. 58.

108. Devisse J. *The Image of the Black in Western Art* (Part 2, *From the Early Christian Era to the "Age of Discovery."* 1. *From the Demonic Threat to the Incarnation of Sainthood*), p. 52.

109. Drake SC. *Black Folk Here and There* (Vol. 2); Davis DB. *Slavery and Human Progress*; Devisse J. *The Image of the Black in Western Art* (Part 2, *From the Early Christian Era to the "Age of Discovery."* 1. *From the Demonic Threat to the Incarnation of Sainthood*); Lewis B. *Race and Slavery in the Middle East*, p. 52; Byrd WM. Race, biology, and health care; Finley M. *Ancient Slavery and Modern Ideology*, pp. 105–107.

110. Drake SC. *Black Folk Here and There* (Vol. 2), pp. 37–76; Devisse J. *The Image of the Black in Western Art* (Part 2, *From the Early Christian Era to the "Age of Discovery."* 1. *From the Demonic Threat to the Incarnation of Sainthood*), pp. 19–22, 46; Davis DB. *Slavery and Human Progress*, p. 42.

111. Drake SC. *Black Folk Here and There* (Vol. 2), pp. 44–58; Davis DB. *The Problem of Slavery in Western Culture*, pp. 83–88, 451; Devisse J. *The Image of the Black in Western Art* (Part 2, *From the Early Christian Era to the "Age of Discovery."* 1. *From the Demonic Threat to the Incarnation of Sainthood*), pp. 52–57; Harris JE. *Africans and Their History*, pp. 13–18; Sanders R. *Lost Tribes and Promised Lands*, p. 49; Pieterse JN. *White on Black: Images of Africa and Blacks in Western Popular Culture.* New Haven: Yale University Press, 1992.

112. Guthrie D. *A History of Medicine*, p. 80.

113. Guthrie D. *A History of Medicine*, pp. 79–80; Sirasi NG. *Medieval and Early Renaissance Medicine*; Byrd WM. Race, biology, and health care.

114. Lyons AS, Petrucelli RJ. *Medicine: An Illustrated History*, pp. 278–365; Bullough VL. *The Development of Medicine as a Profession: The Contribution of the Medieval University to Modern Medicine.* New York: Hafner, 1966; Luce HR. *Life's Picture History of Western Man.* New York: Time Incorporated, 1951, pp. 11–70; McEvedy C. *The World History Factfinder*, pp. 40–72; Byrd WM. Race, biology, and health care.

115. Lyons AS, Petrucelli RJ. *Medicine: An Illustrated History*, p. 265.

116. Roberts JM. *The Penguin History of the World.* London: Penguin, 1990, pp. 277–395, 458–507; Lyons AS, Petrucelli RJ. *Medicine: An Illustrated History*, pp. 265–365; Stone N, ed. *The Times Atlas of World History.* 3rd ed. Maplewood, NJ: Hammond, 1989, pp. 104–107, 110–113, 116–125, 134–145.

117. Majno G. *The Healing Hand: Man and Wound in the Ancient World.* Cambridge, MA: Harvard University Press, 1975, pp. 420–421.

118. Majno G. *The Healing Hand*, pp. 420–422; Lyons AS, Petrucelli RJ. *Medicine: An Illustrated History*, pp. 294–317; Guthrie D. *A History of Medicine*, pp. 84–88.

119. Lyons AS, Petrucelli RJ. *Medicine: An Illustrated History*, p. 283.

120. Lyons As, Petrucelli RJ. *Medicine: An Illustrated History*, p. 283.

121. Lyons AS, Petrucelli RJ. *Medicine: An Illustrated History*, pp. 276–291; Sirasi NG. *Medieval and Early Renaissance Medicine*; Byrd WM. Race, biology, and health care; Guthrie D. *A History of Medicine*, pp. 84–85, 96–102.

122. Pimienta-Bey JV. Moorish Spain: Academic source and foundation for the rise and success of western European universities in the middle ages. In: Van Sertima I, ed. *Golden Age of the Moor*. New Brunswick, NJ: Transaction Publishers, 1992, pp. 182–247; quote p. 182.

123. Pimienta-Bey JV. Moorish Spain, p. 182.

124. Majno G. *The Healing Hand*, p. 420.

125. Sirasi NG. *Medieval and Early Renaissance Medicine*, p. 11.

126. Pimienta-Bey JV. Moorish Spain, p. 211.

127. Chandler WB. The Moor: Light of Europe's Dark Age. In: Van Sertima I, ed. *African Presence in Early Europe*. New Brunswick, NJ: Transaction Publishers, 1990, pp. 144–175; Pimienta-Bey JV. Moorish Spain; Brend B. *Islamic Art*. Cambridge, MA: Harvard University Press, 1991, pp. 46–50; Lyons AS, Petrucelli RJ. *Medicine: An Illustrated History*, pp. 294–365; Guthrie D. *A History of Medicine*, pp. 84–102; Sirasi NG. *Medieval and Early Renaissance Medicine*; Bullough VL. *The Development of Medicine as a Profession*.

128. Murray G. *Slavery in the Arab World*. New York: New Amsterdam Books, 1989, p. 99.

129. Lewis B. The African diaspora and the civilization of Islam. In: Kilson ML, Rothberg RI, eds. *The African Diaspora: Interpretive Essays*. Cambridge, MA: Harvard University Press, 1976, pp. 37–56; quote p. 49.

130. Devisse J. *The Image of the Black in Western Art* (Part 2, *From the Early Christian Era to the "Age of Discovery."* 1. *From the Demonic Threat to the Incarnation of Sainthood*), pp. 50–57, 52; Lewis B. The African diaspora and the civilization of Islam; Lewis B. *Race and Slavery in the Middle East*; Veatch RM. *A Theory of Medical Ethics*, p. 55; Gordon M. *Slavery in the Arab World*, pp. 98–104.

131. Lyons AS, Petrucelli RJ. *Medicine: An Illustrated History*, p. 298.

132. Pimienta-Bey JV. Moorish Spain, p. 216.

133. Drake SC. *Black Folk Here and There* (Vol. 2), p. 42.

134. Sirasi NG. *Medieval and Early Renaissance Medicine*, pp. 10–13; Lyons AS, Petrucelli RJ. *Medicine: An Illustrated History*, pp. 294–317; Sigerist HE. *The Great Doctors*, pp. 68–87; Guthrie D. *A History of Medicine*, pp. 84–107; Pimienta-Bey JV. Moorish Spain.

135. Lewis B. *Race and Slavery in the Middle East*, p. 55; Sanders R. *Lost Tribes and Promised Lands*, pp. 55–58.

136. Devisse J. *The Image of the Black in Western Art* (Part 2, *From the Early Christian Era to the "Age of Discovery."* 1. *From the Demonic Threat to the Incarnation of Sainthood*), p. 46.

137. Lewis B. The African diaspora and the civilization of Islam, pp. 37–56; Lewis B. *Race and Slavery in the Middle East*; Sanders R. *Lost Tribes and Promised Lands*; Davis DB. *The Problem of Slavery in Western Culture*, pp. 40–52; Davis DB. *Slavery and Human Progress*, pp. 35–70; Byrd WM. Race, biology, and health care.

138. Sirasi NG. *Medieval and Early Renaissance Medicine*, p. 13.

139. Sirasi NG. *Medieval and Early Renaissance Medicine*; Pimienta-Bey JV. Moorish Spain; Lyons AS, Petrucelli RJ. *Medicine: An Illustrated History*, pp. 294–365; Sigerist HE. *The Great Doctors*, pp. 78–94.

140. Davis DB. *The Problem of Slavery in Western Culture*, p. 41.

141. Lewis B. The African diaspora and the civilization of Islam, pp. 37–56; Lewis B. *Race and Slavery in the Middle East*, pp. 28–61, 99–102; Sanders R. *Lost Tribes and Promised Lands*; Davis DB. *The Problem of Slavery in Western Culture*, pp. 40–52; Davis DB. *Slavery and Human Progress*, pp. 35–70; Byrd WM. Race, biology, and health care; Devisse J. *The Image of the Black in Western Art* (Part 2, *From the Early Christian Era to the "Age of Discovery."* 1. *From the Demonic Threat to the Incarnation of Sainthood*), pp. 35, 50–119; Pieterse JN. *White on Black: Images of Africa and Blacks in Western Popular Culture*. New Haven: Yale University Press, 1992.

142. Lyons AS, Petrucelli RJ. *Medicine: An Illustrated History*, p. 369.

143. Reed J. Scientific racism. In Wilson CR, Ferris W, eds. *Encyclopedia of Southern Culture*. Chapel Hill: The University of North Carolina Press, 1989, pp. 1358–1360; quote p. 1358.

144. Roberts J. *The Triumph of the West*. Boston: Little, Brown, 1985, pp. 95–172; Roberts JM. *The Penguin History of the World*, pp. 458–530; Lyons AS, Petrucelli RJ. *Medicine: An Illustrated History*, pp. 368–463; Rabb TK, Jersey B. *Renaissance* (videotape). A five-part series produced by Vision Quest in cooperation with the Annenberg/CPB Project, South Carolina Public Television, 1993; Sirasi NG. *Medieval and Early Renaissance Medicine*, pp. 1–47; Chase A. *The Legacy of Malthus*, pp. xv–xxii, 1–12; Byrd WM. Race, biology, and health care; Levin J, Levin W. *The Functions of Discrimination and Prejudice*. 2nd ed.; Banton M, Harwood J. *The Race Concept*.

145. Roberts J. *The Triumph of the West*; Roberts JM. *The Penguin History of the World*. pp. 489–530; Burke J. Fit to rule. In: Burke J. *The Day the Universe Changed*. Boston: Little, Brown, 1985, pp. 239–273; Lyons AS, Petrucelli RJ. *Medicine: An Illustrated History*, pp. 368–463; Rabb TK, Jersey B. *Renaissance* (videotape); Jonas G. *The Circuit Riders: Rockefeller Money and the Rise of Modern Science*. New York: W.W. Norton, 1989, pp. 43–50; Kragh H. *An Introduction to the Historiography of Science*; Levin J, Levin W. *The Functions of Discrimination and Prejudice*; Stannard DE. *American Holocaust: Columbus and the Conquest of the New World*. New York: Oxford University Press, 1992; Wassermann HP. *Ethnic Pigmentation*, pp. 22–41; Davis DB. *The Problem of Slavery in the Age of Revolution, 1770–1823*. Ithaca, NY: Cornell University Press, 1975.

146. Roberts J. *The Triumph of the West*, pp. 117–172; Sanders R. *Lost Tribes and Promised Lands*; Du Bois WEB. *The Suppression of the African Slave Trade to the United States of America, 1638–1870*. N.P., 1896; reprint, Baton Rouge: Louisiana State University Press, 1969; Davidson B. *The African Slave Trade*; Thomas H. *The Slave Trade: The Story of the Atlantic Slave Trade: 1440–1870*. New York: Simon and Schuster, 1997.

147. Savitt T. Black health on the plantation: Masters, slaves, and physicians. In: Leavitt JW, Numbers RL, eds. *Sickness and Health in America: Readings in the History of Medicine and Public Health*. Madison: The University of Wisconsin Press, 1985, pp. 313–330; Savitt TL. *Medicine and Slavery*; Stampp KM. *The Peculiar Institution: Slavery in the Ante-Bellum South*. New York: Knopf, 1956; reprint ed., New York: Vintage Books, 1956; Mellon J, ed. *Bullwhip Days: The Slaves Remember*. New York: Weidenfeld and Nicolson, 1988; Huggins NI. *Black Odyssey: The Afro-American Ordeal in Slavery*. New

York: Pantheon Books, 1977; reprint ed., New York: Vintage Books, 1979; David PA, Gutman HG, Sutch R, et al. *Reckoning with Slavery: A Critical Study in the Quantitative History of American Negro Slavery.* New York: Oxford University Press, 1976.

148. Davidson B. *The African Slave Trade;* Thomas H. *The Slave Trade: The Story of the Atlantic Slave Trade: 1440–1870.* New York: Simon and Schuster, 1997; Davis DB. *The Problem of Slavery in Western Culture;* Klein HS. *The Middle Passage: Comparative Studies in the Atlantic Slave Trade.* Princeton, NJ: Princeton University Press, 1978; Curtain PD. *The Atlantic Slave Trade: A Census.* Madison: The University of Wisconsin Press, 1969; Du Bois WEB. *The Negro.* New York: Henry Holt, 1915; reprint ed., London: Oxford University Press, 1970; Mannix DP, Cowley M. *Cargoes: The Atlantic Slave Trade, 1518–1865.* New York: Viking Press, 1962; Roberts J. *The Triumph of the West;* Byrd WM, Clayton LA. The "slave health deficit": Racism and health outcomes. *Health/PAC Bulletin* 1991; 21:25–28; Byrd WM, Clayton LA. *A Black Health Trilogy;* Bancroft F. *Slave Trading in the Old South.* New York: Frederick Ungar Publishing Company, 1959.

149. Shryock RH. *The Development of Modern Medicine,* pp. 3–16; Guthrie D. *A History of Medicine,* pp. 134–175; Meadows J. *The Great Scientists.* New York: Oxford University Press, 1987, pp. 29–68; Ackerknecht EH. *A Short History of Medicine.* rev. ed. Baltimore: The Johns Hopkins University Press, 1982, pp. 94–127; Davis DB. *The Problem of Slavery in Western Culture,* p. 454; Wassermann HP. *Ethnic Pigmentation,* pp. 27, 35, 39; Jordan WD. *White Over Black,* p. 246; Byrd WM. Race, biology, and health care; Rabb TK, Jersey B. *The Scientists.* Segment one, *Renaissance* (videotape). A five-part series produced by Vision Quest in cooperation with the Annenberg/CPB Project, South Carolina Public Television, 1993.

150. Guthrie D. *A History of Medicine,* pp. 156–161; Bender GA. *Great Moments in Medicine.* Detroit: Northwood Institute Press, 1966, pp. 76–83; Lyons AS, Petrucelli RJ. *Medicine: An Illustrated History,* pp. 368–423; Rabb TK, Jersey B. *The Scientists.* Segment one, *Renaissance* (videotape); Stannard DE. *American Holocaust,* p. 209; Rogers JA. *Nature Knows No Color Line: Research into the Negro Ancestry in the White Race.* 3rd ed. St. Petersburg, FL: Helga M. Rogers, 1980, p. 20; Muir H, ed. *Larousse Dictionary of Scientists.* New York: Larousse, 1994, p. 396.

151. Chase A. *The Legacy of Malthus,* p. 72.

152. Chase A. *The Legacy of Malthus,* p. 72.

153. Chase A. *The Legacy of Malthus,* pp. xv–xxii, 2–23; Byrd WM, Clayton LA. Race, medicine, and health care in the United States: A historical survey. *Journal of the National Medical Association.* In press 1999; Nuland SB. *Doctors: The Biography of Medicine.* New York: Alfred A. Knopf, 1988, pp. 61–119; Lyons AS, Petrucelli RJ. *Medicine: An Illustrated History,* pp. 368–423; Bender GA. *Great Moments in Medicine,* pp. 84–98; Gould SJ. *The Mismeasure of Man,* pp. 19–233; Gilman SL. *Freud, Race, and Gender,* p. 18; Kosa J, Zola IK, eds. *Poverty and Health: A Sociological Analysis.* rev. ed. Cambridge, MA: Harvard University Press, 1975; Fredrickson GM, Knobel DT. History of prejudice and discrimination. In: Thernstrom S, Orlov A, Handlin O, eds. *Harvard Encyclopedia of American Ethnic Groups.* Cambridge, MA: The Belknap Press of Harvard University Press, 1980, pp. 829–847.

154. Lyons AS, Petrucelli RJ. *Medicine: An Illustrated History,* p. 427.

155. Chase A. *The Legacy of Malthus,* pp. 68–110; Milner R. *The Encyclopedia of Evolution,* pp. 380–382; Lyons AS, Petrucelli RJ. *Medicine: An Illustrated History,* pp.

368–423; Gould SJ. *The Mismeasure of Man;* Stanton W. *The Leopard's Spots,* pp. 1–14; Haller JS, Jr. *Outcasts from Evolution,* pp. 1–11.

156. Lyons AS, Petrucelli RJ. *Medicine: An Illustrated History,* p. 427.

157. Milner R. *The Encyclopedia of Evolution,* p. 236.

158. Jordan WD. *White Over Black,* pp. 29–32.

159. Lyons AS, Petrucelli RJ. *Medicine: An Illustrated History,* pp. 427–466; Jordan WD. *White Over Black,* pp. 3–43, 216–265, 482–511; Marshall PJ, Williams G. *The Great Map of Mankind: Perceptions of New Worlds in the Age of Enlightenment.* Cambridge, MA: Harvard University Press, 1982, pp. 33–40, 227–257; Milner R. *The Encyclopedia of Evolution.*

160. Lyons AS, Petrucelli RJ. *Medicine: An Illustrated History,* pp. 427–466; Milner R. *The Encyclopedia of Evolution;* Gould SJ. *The Mismeasure of Man.*

161. Shipman P. *The Evolution of Racism: Human Differences and the Use and Abuse of Science.* New York: Simon and Schuster, 1994; Duster R. *Backdoor to Eugenics.* New York: Routledge, 1990; Chase A[llan]. *The Legacy of Malthus: The Social Costs of the New Scientific Racism;* Hubbard R, Wald E. *Exploding the Gene Myth: How Genetic Information Is Produced and Manipulated by Scientists, Physicians, Employers, Insurance Companies, Educators, and Law Enforcers.* Boston: Beacon Press, 1993; Gould SJ. *The Mismeasure of Man.*

162. Jordan WD. *White Over Black: American Attitudes Toward the Negro, 1550–1812.* Gould SJ. Wide hats and narrow minds. Pp. 145–151. In: Gould SJ. *The Panda's Thumb: More Reflections in Natural History.* New York: W.W. Norton, 1980; Gould SJ. *The Mismeasure of Man.* New York: Gilman SL. *Freud, Race, and Gender.*

163. Milner R. *The Encyclopedia of Evolution: Humanity's Search for Its Origins.* New York: Facts on File, 1990; Gould SJ. *The Mismeasure of Man.* New York: W.W. Norton, 1981; Gilman SL. *Freud, Race, and Gender.* Princeton, NJ: Princeton University Press, 1993, p. 18. Jordan WD. *White Over Black;* Chase A. *The Legacy of Malthus;* Herrnstein RJ, Murray C. *The Bell Curve: Intelligence and Class Structure in American Life.* New York: The Free Press, 1994; Stannard DE. *American Holocaust: Columbus and the Conquest of the New World.* New York: Oxford University Press, 1992; Shipman P. *The Evolution of Racism: Human Differences and the Use and Abuse of Science.* New York: Simon and Schuster, 1994; Haller JS Jr. *Outcasts from Evolution: Scientific Attitudes of Racial Inferiority, 1859–1900.* New York: McGraw-Hill, 1971; Stanton W. *The Leopard's Spots: Scientific Attitudes toward Race in America, 1815–1859.* Chicago: The University of Chicago Press, 1960; Gould SJ. Curveball. In: Fraser S, ed. *The Bell Curve Wars: Race, Intelligence, and the Future of America.* New York: Basic Books, 1995, pp. 11–22; *National Digest.* Researchers say race isn't base for scientific study. *Fort Worth Star-Telegram,* Monday, February 20, 1995, Section A-7; *Education. Jet* (March 13, 1995, No. 18); 87:24.

164. Chase A. *The Legacy of Malthus,* pp. 86–87; Nuland SB. *Doctors: The Biography of Medicine,* pp. 120–144; Meadows J. *The Great Scientists,* pp. 49–68; Bender GA. *Great Moments in Medicine,* pp. 100–107; Lyons AS, Petrucelli RJ. *Medicine: An Illustrated History;* Davis DB. *The Problem of Slavery in Western Culture,* p. 454; Sigerist HE. *The Great Doctors,* pp. 138–149.

165. Lyons AS, Petrucelli RJ. *Medicine: An Illustrated History,* pp. 427–468; Sigerist HE. *The Great Doctors,* pp. 138–149; Bender GA. *Great Moments in Medicine,* pp. 100–115; Davis DB. *The Problem of Slavery in Western Culture,* p. 454; Jordan WD. *White*

Over Black, pp. 246, 585; Wassermann HP. *Ethnic Pigmentation*, pp. 27–29, 45; Chase A. *The Legacy of Malthus*, pp. 86–87.

166. Jordan WD. *White Over Black*, fn 217–218.

167. Marshall PJ, Williams G. *The Great Map of Mankind*, pp. 242–243.

168. Gould SJ. *The Mismeasure of Man*; Lyons AS, Petrucelli RJ. *Medicine: An Illustrated History*; Marshall PJ, Williams G. *The Great Map of Mankind*, pp. 33–40, 227–257; Gossett TF. *Race: The History of an Idea in America*, pp. 32–34; Davis DB. *The Problem of Slavery in Western Culture*, pp. 454–455; Bender GA. *Great Moments in Medicine*; Jordan WD. *White Over Black*, pp. 217–218, 246; Milner R. *The Encyclopedia of Evolution*, p. 371; Chase A. *The Legacy of Malthus*, p. 88.

169. Magnusson M., ed. *Cambridge Biographical Dictionary*. Cambridge, England: Cambridge University Press, 1900, p. 900.

170. Marshall PJ, Williams G. *The Great Map of Mankind*, p. 245.

171. Gould SJ. *The Mismeasure of Man*, p. 35.

172. Honour H. *The Image of the Black in Western Art. Part IV. From the American Revolution to World War I. 2. Black Models and White Myths*. Cambridge, MA: Menil Foundation, Distributed by Harvard University Press, 1989, p. 13.

173. Jordan WD. *White Over Black*, p. 230.

174. Jordan WD. *White Over Black*, p. 236.

175. Jordan WD. *White Over Black*, pp. 216–263, 483–511; Byrd WM, Clayton LA. Meharry Medical Archive-NMA Slide Collection. Nashville and Boston: Meharry Medical Library, Countway Medical Library of Harvard Medical School, 1991–1996; Haller JS. *Outcasts from Evolution*, pp. 1–14; Magnusson M., ed. *Cambridge Biographical Dictionary*, pp. 225–226, 900; Marshall PJ, Williams G. *The Great Map of Mankind*, p. 245; Pieterse JN. *White on Black: Images of Africa and Blacks in Western Popular Culture*. Pp. 30–51; Davis DB. *The Problem of Slavery in Western Culture*, pp. 454–455; Honour H. *The Image of the Black in Western Art. Part IV. From the American Revolution to World War I. 2. Black Models and White Myths*, pp. 13–14; Cohen IB. *Album of Science: From Leonardo to Lavoisier, 1450–1800*. New York: Charles Scribner's Sons, 1980, p. 228; Gould SJ. *The Mismeasure of Man*, p. 35; Stanton W. *The Leopard's Spots*; Muir H, ed. *Larousse Dictionary of Scientists*, pp. 83, 321.

176. Cogan T. *The Works of the Late Professor Camper on the Connexion Between the Science of Anatomy and the Arts of Drawing, Painting, Statuary: Containing a Treatise on the Natural Difference of Features in Persons of Different Countries and Periods of Life; And on Beauty, with a New Method of Sketching Heads, National Features, and Portraits of Individuals, with Accuracy, Illustrated with Seventeen Plates, Explanatory of the Professor's Leading Principles*. Two Books. A New Edition. London: J. Hearne, 1821, p. 9.

177. Haller JS, Jr. *Outcasts from Evolution*, p. 9.

178. Haller JS, Jr. *Outcasts from Evolution*, p. 5.

179. Blumenbach JF. *A manual of the elements of natural history*. London: W. Simpkin and R. Marshall, 1825, p. 37.

180. Magnusson M., ed. *Cambridge Biographical Dictionary*, p. 167.

181. Banton M, Harwood J. *The Race Concept*; Banton M. *Racial Theories*, pp. 1–32; Jordan WD. *White Over Black*; Byrd WM, Clayton LA. Meharry Medical Archive-NMA Slide Collection; Horsman R. *Race and Manifest Destiny: The Origins of American Racial Anglo-Saxonism*. Cambridge, MA: Harvard University Press, 1981, pp. 43–61;

Chase A. *The Legacy of Malthus*, pp. 85–110; Haller JS. *Outcasts from Evolution*, pp. 3–14; Magnusson M., ed. *Cambridge Biographical Dictionary*, pp. 167, 225–226, 376, 900; Marshall PJ, Williams G. *The Great Map of Mankind*, p. 245; Honour H. *The Image of the Black in Western Art. Part IV. From the American Revolution to World War I. 2. Black Models and White Myths*, p. 13; Peck SR. *Atlas of Human Anatomy for the Artist*. New York: Oxford University Press, 1979, iv, pp. 236–241; Byrd WM, Clayton LA. The "slave health deficit"; David PA, Gutman HG, Sutch R, et al. *Reckoning with Slavery: A Critical Study in the Quantitative History of American Negro Slavery*. New York: Oxford University Press, 1976; Fogel RW. *Without Consent or Contract: The Rise and Fall of American Slavery*. New York: W.W. Norton and Company, 1989; Savitt TL. *Medicine and Slavery*; Boorstin DJ. *The Discoverers*. (two-volume illustrated deluxe ed.). New York: Harry Abrams, 1991, pp. 652–665; Cohen IB. *Album of Science: From Leonardo to Lavoisier, 1450–1800*. New York: Charles Scribner's Sons, 1980, p. 228; Gould SJ. *The Mismeasure of Man*, p. 35; Stanton W. *The Leopard's Spots*; Boorstin DJ. The equality of the human species. In: Boorstin DJ. *Hidden History: Exploring Our Secret Past*. New York: Harper & Row, 1987; paperback ed., New York: Vintage Books, 1989, pp. 111–123; Milner R. *The Encyclopedia of Evolution*, pp. 242–243; Muir H, ed. *Larousse Dictionary of Scientists*, pp. 124–125; Pieterse JN. White on Black: Images of Africa and Blacks in Western Popular Culture. Pp. 30–51.

182. Berkowitz JS. *The College of Physicians of Philadelphia Portrait Catalogue*. Philadelphia: College of Physicians of Philadelphia, 1984, p. 29.

183. Gould SJ. *The Mismeasure of Man*, p. 36.

184. Gould SJ. *The Mismeasure of Man*; Banton M, Harwood J. *The Race Concept*; Banton M. *Racial Theories*, pp. 28–32; Gould SJ. The Hottentot Venus. In: Gould SJ. *The Flamingo's Smile: Reflections in Natural History*. New York: W.W. Norton, 1985, pp. 291–305; Stocking Jr. GW. French anthropology in 1800. In: Stocking GW. *Race, Culture, and Evolution: Essays in the History of Anthropology*. Chicago: The University of Chicago press, 1982, pp. 13–40; quotes pp. 16, 29–40; Nott JC, Gliddon GR, Maurey A, et al. *Indigenous Races of the Earth or, New Chapters of Ethnological Inquiry*. Philadelphia: J.B. Lippincott, 1857, p. 628; Berkowitz JS. *The College of Physicians of Philadelphia Portrait Catalogue*, pp. 29–31; Honour H. *The Image of the Black in Western Art. Part IV. From the American Revolution to World War I. 2. Black Models and White Myths*, pp. 17–19, 52–55.

185. Gould SJ. *The Mismeasure of Man*, p. 36.

186. Hutchins RM, ed. *Great Books of the Western World* (Vol. 49, *Darwin. The Descent of Man and Selection in Relation to Sex*, by Charles Darwin). Chicago: University of Chicago Press, 1952, p. 336.

187. Gould SJ. *The Mismeasure of Man*, pp. 35–38; Banton M, Harwood J. *The Race Concept*, p. 36; Banton M. *Racial Theories*; Jordan WD. *White Over Black*; Muir H, ed. *Larousse Dictionary of Scientists*, pp. 124–125, 130–131, 333–334.

188. Gould SJ. Bound by the great chain. In: Gould SJ. *The Flamingo's Smile: Reflections in Natural History*, pp. 281–291; quote pp. 285–286.

189. Gould SJ. Bound by the great chain, pp. 285–286.

190. Gould SJ. Bound by the great chain, p. 288.

191. Jordan WD. *White Over Black*, p. 498.

192. Jordan WD. *White Over Black*, p. 498.

193. Banton M. *Racial Theories*, p. 53.

194. Banton M. *Racial Theories*, p. 54.

195. Banton M, Harwood J. *The Race Concept*, pp. 25–30; Banton M. *Racial Theories*; Jordan WD. *White Over Black*, pp. 498, 505; Byrd WM, Clayton LA. Meharry Medical Archive-NMA Slide Collection; Horsman R. *Race and Manifest Destiny*; Fredrickson GM. *The Black Image in the White Mind*; Bender GA. *Great Moments in Medicine*; Chase A. *The Legacy of Malthus*; Shipman P. *The Evolution of Racism*; Haller JS. *Outcasts from Evolution*.

196. Gould SJ. *The Mismeasure of Man*, p. 39.

197. Jordan WD. *White Over Black*, p. 514.

198. Horsman R. *Race and Manifest Destiny: The Origins of American Racial Anglo-Saxonism*. Cambridge, MA: Harvard University Press, 1981, pp. 116–120.

199. Gould SJ. *The Mismeasure of Man*, p. 39; Horsman R. *Race and Manifest Destiny*, pp. 116–120; Smith SS; Jordan WD, ed. *An Essay on the Causes of the Variety of Complexion and Figure in the Human Species*. Cambridge, MA: The Belknap Press of Harvard University Press, 1965, pp. xxxi–liii; Jordan WD. *White Over Black*, pp. 482–541; Banton M. *Racial Theories*, pp. 12–15, 32–45; Fredrickson GM. *The Black Image in the White Mind*, pp. 71–74.

200. Horsman R. *Race and Manifest Destiny*, pp. 116–120; Byrd WM, Clayton LA. The "slave health deficit"; Fogel RW. *Without Consent or Contract*, pp. 114–153; Ewbank DC. History of black mortality and health before 1940. In: Willis DP, ed. *Health Policies and Black Americans*. New Brunswick, NJ: Transaction Publishers, 1989, pp. 100–128; Stampp KM. *The Peculiar Institution: Slavery in the Ante-Bellum South*; Savitt TL. *Medicine and Slavery*; Gould SJ. *The Mismeasure of Man*; Fredrickson GM. *The Black Image in the White Mind*, pp. 43–98.

201. Beider RE. *Science Encounters the Indian, 1820–1880: The Early Years of American Ethnology*. Norman: University of Oklahoma Press, 1986, pp. 55–103; Banton M, Harwood J. *The Race Concept*, pp. 27–29; Banton M. *Racial Theories*, pp. 32–46; Gould SJ. *The Mismeasure of Man*, pp. 32–72; Stanton W. *The Leopard's Spots*, pp. 15–53; Haller JS Jr. *Outcasts from Evolution*, pp. 3–39, 69–86; Stigler SM. *The History of Statistics: The Measurement of Uncertainty before 1900*. Cambridge, MA. The Belknap Press of Harvard University Press, 1986, pp. 161–194.

202. Gould SJ. *The Mismeasure of Man*, p. 51.

203. Beider RE. *Science Encounters the Indian, 1820–1880*, pp. 55–103; Banton M. *Racial Theories*, pp. 32–46; Gould SJ. *The Mismeasure of Man*, pp. 32–72; Dunglison R. *Human Physiology with Three Hundred and Sixty-Eight Illustrations* (two vols., 6th ed.). Philadelphia: Lea and Blanchard, 1846, p. 631; Berkowitz JS. *The College of Physicians of Philadelphia Portrait Catalogue*, pp. 18–19, 29–31, 137; Stanton W. *The Leopard's Spots*, pp. 15–53; Horsman R. *Race and Manifest Destiny*, pp. 56–57, 116–120; Croskey JW. *History of Blockley: A History of the Philadelphia General Hospital from Its Inception, 1731–1928*. Philadelphia: F.A. Davis Company, 1929; Haller JS Jr. *Outcasts from Evolution*, pp. 3–39, 69–86; Stigler SM. *The History of Statistics*, pp. 161–194; Gay P. *Age of Enlightenment. Great Ages of Man: A History of the World's Cultures*. New York: Time, 1965, p. 68; Gossett TF. *Race: The History of an Idea in America*, pp. 71–83.

204. Gould SJ. *The Mismeasure of Man*, pp. 44–45.

205. Stanton W. *The Leopard's Spots*; Gould SJ. *The Mismeasure of Man*, pp. 39–72; Horsman R. *Race and Manifest Destiny*, pp. 125–157; Gould SJ. Flaws in the Victorian veil. 169–176. In: Gould SJ. *The Panda's Thumb: More Reflections in Natural History*.

New York: W.W. Norton and Company, 1980; Horsman R. *Josiah Nott of Mobile*; Duffy J. State's rights medicine. In: Wilson CR, Ferris W, eds. *The Encyclopedia of Southern Culture*. Chapel Hill: The University of North Carolina Press, 1989, pp. 1355–1356; Kaufman M, Galishoff S, Savitt TL, eds. *Dictionary of American Medical Biography* (two vols.). Westport, CT: Greenwood Press, pp. 125–126, 539–540, 556–557.

206. Beider RE. *Science Encounters the Indian, 1820–1880*, pp. 55–103; Gould SJ. *The Mismeasure of Man*; Stanton W. *The Leopard's Spots*; Haller Jr. JS. *Outcasts from Evolution*; Gossett TF. *Race: The History of an Idea in America*; Horsman R. *Josiah Nott of Mobile*; Lurie E. *Louis Agassiz: A Life in Science*; Fredrickson GM. *The Black Image in the White Mind*, pp. 43–57, 58–70, 71–98.

207. Chase A. *The Legacy of Malthus*, p. 97.

208. Chase A. *The Legacy of Malthus*, p. 71.

209. Chase A. *The Legacy of Malthus*, pp. 71, 97–107, 517–518; Horsman R. *Josiah Nott of Mobile*, pp. 171–200, 216; Stigler SM. *The History of Statistics*, pp. 265–299; Milner R. *The Encyclopedia of Evolution*, pp. 183–185, 414–415, 421–422; Gould SJ. *The Mismeasure of Man*, pp. 75–77, 117; Hearnshaw LS. *Cyril Burt Psychologist*.

210. Banton M. *Racial Theories*, pp. 65–169; Stringer C, McKie R. *African Exodus: The Origins of Modern Humanity*. New York: Henry Holt and Company, 1996; Shipman P. *The Evolution of Racism*; Chase A. *The Legacy of Malthus*, pp. 2–175, 191; Degler CN. *In Search of Human Nature: The Decline and Revival of Darwinism in American Social Thought*. New York: Oxford University Press, 1991; Haller JS, Jr. *Outcasts from Evolution*; Haller MH. *Eugenics: Hereditarian Attitudes in American Thought*. New Brunswick, NJ: Rutgers University Press, 1963; Lewontin RC, Rose S, Kamin LJ. *Not in Our Genes*; Outlaw L. Toward a critical theory of race, pp. 58–82; Stigler SM. *The History of Statistics*; Kevles DJ. *In the Name of Eugenics*.

211. Outlaw L. Toward a critical theory of race, p. 65.

212. Banton M, Harwood J. *The Race Concept*, pp. 30–91; Banton M. *Racial Theories*, pp. 99–169; Allport GW. *The Nature of Prejudice*; Adorno TW, Else F, Levinson DJ, et al. *The Authoritarian Personality*. Abr. ed. New York: W.W. Norton, 1982; Gould SJ. *The Mismeasure of Man*; Shipman P. *The Evolution of Racism*; Myrdal G. *An American Dilemma: The Negro Problem and Modern Democracy*. New York: Harper & Row, 1944; Herskovits MJ. *The Myth of the Negro Past*. New York: Harper & Brothers, 1941; reprint ed., Boston: Beacon Press, 1958; Herskovits MJ. *Franz Boas: The Science of Men in the Making*. New York: Charles Scribner's Sons, 1953; Chase A. *The Legacy of Malthus*, pp. 176–200, 323–341, 528–624; Frazier EF. *The Negro in the United States*. rev. ed. New York: Macmillan, 1957; Jencks C. *Rethinking Social Policy: Race, Poverty, and the Underclass*. Cambridge, MA. Harvard University Press, 1992; Hacker A. *Two Nations: Black and White, Separate, Hostile, Unequal*; Wilson WJ. *The Truly Disadvantaged*; Jones JH. *Bad Blood*; Takaki RY. *Iron Cages: Race and Culture in Nineteenth-Century America*. New York: Knopf, 1979; Sniderman PM, Piazza T. *The Scar of Race*; Massey DS, Denton NA. *American Apartheid*; Outlaw L. Toward a critical theory of race; Researchers say race isn't base for scientific study. *Fort Worth Star-Telegram* February 20, 1995:A7; Racial characteristics not factors in genetic research. *Jet* March 13, 1995; 18(87):24.

213. Barker M. Biology and the new racism. In: Goldberg DT, ed. *Anatomy of Racism*, pp. 18–37; quote p. 19.

214. Lewontin RC, Rose S, Kamin LJ. *Not in Our Genes*, p. 234.

215. Goldberg DT. Introduction. In: Goldberg DT, ed. *Anatomy of Racism*, pp. xi–xxiii; quote p. xvi.

216. Goldberg DT. Introduction. In: Goldberg DT, ed. *Anatomy of Racism.*

217. Count EW. The biological basis of human sociality. *American Anthropologist* 1958; 60: 1049–1085; Lorenz K. *Evolution and Modification of Behavior.* Chicago: University of Chicago Press, 1965; Wilson EO. *Sociobiology: The New Synthesis.* Cambridge, MA: Harvard University Press, 1975; Dawkins R. *The Selfish Gene.* Oxford: Oxford University Press, 1976; Tiger L, Fox R. *The Imperial Animal.* New York: Holt, Rinehart and Winston, 1971; Gould SJ The nonscience of human nature, pp. 237–242. In: Gould SJ. *Ever Since Darwin: Reflections in Natural History.* New York: W.W. Norton and Company, 1977; Lewontin RC, Rose S, Kamin LJ. *Not in Our Genes*; Barker M. Biology and the new racism; Gould SJ. Biological potentiality vs. biological determinism. In: Gould SJ. *Ever Since Darwin: Reflections in Natural History.* New York: W.W. Norton and Company, 1977, pp. 251–259; Reynolds V, Falger V, Vine I, eds. *The Sociobiology of Ethnocentrism: Evolutionary Dimensions of Xenophobia, Discrimination, Racism and Nationalism.* London: Croom Helm, 1987; Milner R. *The Encyclopedia of Evolution*, pp. 96–97, 156, 254–255, 401–402, 403–404; Shipman P. *The Evolution of Racism*, pp. 229–261; Herrnstein RJ, Murray C. *The Bell Curve*; Chase A. *The Legacy of Malthus*; LeVay S, Hamer DH. Evidence for a biological influence in male homosexuality. *Scientific American* May 1994; 5(270):44–49; Byne W. The biological evidence challenged. *Scientific American* May 1994; 5(270):50–55.

218. Hacker A. *Two Nations: Black and White, Separate, Hostile, Unequal*; Sniderman PM, Piazza T. *The Scar of Race*; Simone TM. *About Face*; Feagin JR, Spikes MP. *Living with Racism: The Black Middle-Class Experience.* Boston: Beacon Press, 1994; Wilson WJ. *The Declining Significance of Race: Blacks and Changing American Institutions.* 2nd ed. Chicago: The University of Chicago Press, 1980; Wilson WJ. *The Truly Disadvantaged*; Auletta K. *The Underclass*; Gans HJ. *The War Against the Poor: The Underclass and Antipoverty Policy.* New York: Basic Books, 1995; Fukuyama F. *Trust: The Social Virtues and the Creation of Prosperity.* New York: The Free Press, 1995; Jhally S, Lewis J. *Enlightened Racism: The Cosby Show, Audiences, and the Myth of the American Dream*; Kozol J. *Savage Inequalities*; Swinton DH. The economic status of African Americans: "Permanent" poverty and inequality. In: Dewart J, ed. *The State of Black America 1991.* New York: National Urban League, Inc., 1991, pp. ; Kovel J. *White Racism: A Psychohistory*; Feagin JR, Feagin CB. Racial and Ethnic Relations. 6th ed. Upper Saddle River, NJ: Prentice Hall, 1999; Steinberg S. *Turning Back: The Retreat from Racial Justice in American Thought and Policy.* Boston: Beacon Press, 1995.

219. Kovel J. *White Racism: A Psychohistory*, p. 34.

220. Kovel J. *White Racism: A Psychohistory*, pp. 36–37.

221. Kovel J. *White Racism: A Psychohistory*, p. 37.

222. Kovel J. *White Racism: A Psychohistory*, p. 37.

223. Edelman MW. *The State of America's Children Yearbook 1995.* Washington, DC: Children's Defense Fund, 1995; Barksdale JM, Kilcourse T. Children's Defense Fund—Putting children first: The world's imperiled children. *Political Trend Letter.* Washington, DC: Joint Center for Political and Economic Studies. *Focus* June 1995; 6(23):1–3; Edelman MW. *Families in Peril: An Agenda for Social Change.* Cambridge, MA: Harvard University Press, 1987; Sidel R. *Keeping Women and Children Last: Amer-*

ica's War on the Poor. Rev. ed. New York: Penguin Books, 1998; Dowling CG, Atwood JE. The way we live: Women and children behind bars. *Life* October 1997: 76.

224. Steinberg S. *The Ethnic Myth*; Pettigrew TF. Prejudice; Feagin JR, Spikes MP. *Living with Racism: The Black Middle-Class Experience*. Boston: Beacon Press, 1994; Wilson WJ. *The Declining Significance of Race*; Wilson WJ. *The Truly Disadvantaged*; Auletta K. *The Underclass*; Gans HJ. *The War Against the Poor*; Hacker A. *Two Nations: Black and White, Separate, Hostile, Unequal*. New York: Ballantine Books, 1992. Enlarged and Updated ed. 1995; Feagin JR, Vera H. *White Racism: The Basics*. New York: Routledge, 1995; Fukuyama F. *Trust: The Social Virtues and the Creation of Prosperity*. New York: The Free Press, 1995; Marable M. *How Capitalism Underdeveloped Black America: Problems in Race, Political Economy and Society*. Boston: South End Press, 1983; Marable M. *Race, Reform, and Rebellion: The Second Reconstruction in Black America, 1945–1990*. rev. 2nd ed. Jackson: University Press of Mississippi, 1991; Jhally S, Lewis J. *Enlightened Racism*; Kovel J. *White Racism: A Psychohistory*; Herman ES, Chomsky N. *Manufacturing Consent: The Political Economy of the Mass Media*. New York: Pantheon Books, 1988; Bagdikian BH. *The Media Monopoly*. Boston: Beacon Press, 1983; Lee MA, Solomon N. *Unreliable Sources: A Guide to Detecting Bias in News Media*. New York: Carol Publishing Group, 1990; Steinberg S. *Turning Back: The Retreat from Racial Justice in American Thought and Policy*. Boston: Beacon Press, 1995.

225. Omni M, Winant H. *Racial Formation in the United States: From the 1960s to the 1980s*. London: Routledge and Kegan Paul, 1986; Byrd WM, Clayton LA. *A Black Health Trilogy*; Kovel J. *White Racism: A Psychohistory*; Outlaw L. Toward a critical theory of race; Pettigrew TF. Prejudice. Steinberg S. *Turning Back: The Retreat from Racial Justice in American Thought and Policy*. Boston: Beacon Press, 1995.

226. Horkheimer M. Traditional and critical theory. In: Horkheimer M. *Critical Theory*. New York: Herder and Herder, 1972, pp. 188–243.

227. Outlaw L. Toward a critical theory of Race, p. 58.

228. Adorno TW, Else F, Levinson DJ, et al. *The Authoritarian Personality*, p. xi.

229. Adorno TW, Else F, Levinson DJ, et al. *The Authoritarian Personality*; Arato A, Gebhardt E, eds. *The Essential Frankfurt School Reader*. New York: Continuum, 1982; Myrdal G. *An American Dilemma*; Allport GW. *The Nature of Prejudice*; Outlaw L. Toward a critical theory of race; Levin J, Levin W. *The Functions of Discrimination and Prejudice*. 2nd ed., UNESCO, ed. *The Race Question in Modern Science*; Montagu A. *Race, Science and Humanity*; Audi R, ed. *The Cambridge Dictionary of Philosophy*. Cambridge: Cambridge University Press, pp. 170; Steinberg S. *Turning Back: The Retreat from Racial Justice in American Thought and Policy*. Boston: Beacon Press, 1995.

230. Outlaw L. Toward a critical theory of race; Newman DK, Amidei NJ, Carter BL, et al. Second-class medicine, pp. 187–235. In: *Protest, Politics, and Prosperity: Black Americans and White Institutions, 1940–75*; Marable M. *Race, Reform, and Rebellion*; Savitt DB. *Health Care Divided: Race and Healing a Nation*. Ann Arbor: The University of Michigan Press, 1999; Williams J. *Eyes on the Prize*; Mazrui AA. *The Africans*, pp. 274–293; Mazrui AA. *Global Africa*. Part 9, *The Africans*. A *Nine-Part Series* (videotapes); Davidson B. *The Rise of Nationalism*. Episode 7, *Africa. An Eight-Part Series* (videotapes). Produced by Mitchell Beazley Television, RM Arts/Channel Four co-production in association with the Nigerian Television Authority, 1984; Byrd WM, Clayton LA. An American health dilemma; Morais HM. *The History of the Negro in Medicine*; Cobb WM. The Black American in Medicine; Byrd WM, Clayton LA. *A Black Health Trilogy*; Wilson FA,

Neuhauser D. *Health Services in the United States.* 2d ed. Cambridge, MA: Ballinger Publishing Company, 1982, pp. 193–197.

231. Outlaw L. Toward a critical theory of race; Schroyer T. *The Critique of Domination: The Origins and Development of Critical Theory.* Boston: Beacon Press, 1973; Brinkley A. *The Unfinished Nation: A Concise History of the American People.* New York: Knopf, 1993, pp. 831–911; Zinn H. *A Peoples History of the United States;* Marable M. *Race, Reform, and Rebellion,* pp. 149–230; Morais HM. *The History of the Negro in Medicine;* Newman DK, Amidei NJ, Carter BL, et al. Second-class medicine; Byrd WM, Clayton LA. An American health dilemma; Byrd WM, Clayton LA. *A Black Health Trilogy;* UNESCO, ed. *The Race Question in Modern Science;* Fineman H. Special report: The revenge of the Right. *Newsweek* November 21, 1994:36; Fineman H. Newt Gingrich: Can he lead? *Newseek* November 21, 1994:40; Feagin JR, Spikes MP. *Living with Racism: The Black Middle-Class Experience.* Boston: Beacon Press, 1994; Steinberg S. *Turning Back: The Retreat from Racial Justice in American Thought and Policy.* Boston: Beacon Press, 1995; Chomsky N. *Deferring Democracy.* New York: Hill and Wong, 1992; Chomsky N. *Profit Over People: Neoliberalism and Global Order.* New York: Seven Stories Press, 1999. Simone TM. *About Face;* Sniderman PM, Piazza T. *The Scar of Race;* Montagu A. *Race, Science and Humanity;* Williams J. *Eyes on the Prize;* Mazrui AA. *The Africans. A Nine-Part Series* (videotapes). Mazrui AA. *The Africans: A Triple Heritage.*

232. Banton M. *The Idea of Race.*

233. Adorno TW, Else F, Levinson DJ, et al. *The Authoritarian Personality,* p. 102; Outlaw L. Toward a critical theory of race.

234. Adorno TW, Else F, Levinson DJ, et al. *The Authoritarian Personality,* p. 103; Outlaw L. Toward a critical theory of race.

235. Steinberg S. *The Ethnic Myth,* p. 42.

236. Adorno TW, Else F, Levinson DJ, et al. *The Authoritarian Personality;* Outlaw L. Toward a critical theory of Race; Montagu A. *Race, Science and Humanity,* pp. iii–71; UNESCO, ed. *The Race Question in Modern Science;* Shipman P. *The Evolution of Racism,* pp. 156–170; Steinberg S. *Turning Back: The Retreat from Racial Justice in American Thought and Policy.* Steinberg S. *The Ethnic Myth;* Hacker A. *Two Nations: Black and White, Separate, Hostile, Unequal;* Farley R, Allen WR. *The Color Line and the Quality of Life in America.* New York: Oxford University Press, 1989; Zweigenhaft RL, Domhoff GW. *Blacks in the White Establishment? A Study of Race and Class in America.* New Haven, CT: Yale University Press, 1991; Massey DS, Denton NA. *American Apartheid;* Feagin JR, Spikes MP. *Living with Racism;* Fredrickson GM, Knobel DT. History of prejudice and discrimination; Kovel J. *White Racism: A Psychohistory;* Simone TM. *About Face;* Gans HJ. *The War Against the Poor.*

237. Steinberg S. *The Ethnic Myth,* p. 43.

238. Kovel J. *White Racism: A Psychohistory,* pp. xxi, xxv, xxviii–xxxii; Hacker A. *Two Nations: Black and White, Separate, Hostile, Unequal;* Feagin JR, Feagin CB. *Racial and Ethnic Relations.* 6th ed. Upper Saddle River, NJ: Prentice Hall, 1999; Steinberg S. *Turning Back: The Retreat from Racial Justice in American Thought and Policy.* Boston: Beacon Press, 1995; Auletta K. *The Underclass;* Fukuyama F. *Trust: The Social Virtues and the Creation of Prosperity;* Gans HJ. *The War Against the Poor.*

239. King G, Bendel. A statistical model estimating the number of African American physicians in the United States. *Journal of the National Medical Association* 1995; 84:264–272.

240. Kovel J. *White Racism: A Psychohistory,* pp. ix–41; Fredrickson GM, Knobel DT. History of prejudice and discrimination; Pettigrew TF. Prejudice; Outlaw L. Toward a critical theory of race; Steinberg S. *The Ethnic Myth;* Greenberg DS. Black health; Byrd WM, Clayton LA. An American health dilemma; Shea S, Fullilove MT. Entry of black and other minority students in US medical schools: Historical perspectives and recent trends. *New England Journal of Medicine* 1985; 313:933–940; Sindler AP. *Bakke, DeFunis, and Minority Admissions: The Quest for Equal Opportunity.* New York: Longman, 1978; Dreyfuss J, Lawrence C. *The Bakke Case: The Politics of Inequality.* New York: Harcourt, Brace, Jovanovich, 1979; Lemann N. Taking affirmative action apart. *New York Times Magazine* June 11, 1995; Section 6:36; Morais HM. *The History of the Negro in Medicine;* Robert Wood Johnson Foundation. Special Report Number One, The Foundation's Minority Medical Training Programs, "Minority Applicants to Medical School Are Better Qualified Today Than in Mid-70s, Yet Less Likely to Be Accepted." Princeton, NJ: Robert Wood Johnson Foundation, 1987.

241. Kovel J. *White Racism: A Psychohistory,* p. xii.

242. Kovel J. *White Racism: A Psychohistory,* pp. ix–41; Feagin JR, Spikes MP. *Living with Racism: The Black Middle-Class Experience.* Boston: Beacon Press, 1994; Steinberg S. *Turning Back;* Cose E. *Color-Blind: Seeing Beyond Race in a Race-Obsessed World.* New York: HarperCollins, 1997; Glazer N, Ueda R. Policy against prejudice and discrimination. In: Thernstrom S, Orlov A, Handlin O, eds. *Harvard Encyclopedia of American Ethnic Groups;* Hacker A. *Two Nations: Black and White, Separate, Hostile, Unequal;* Williams J. *Eyes on the Prize;* Hampton H. *Eyes on the Prize II.* (videotape). An eight-part documentary video produced by Blackside, Inc., WGBH, Boston, and the Corporation for Public Broadcasting, 1990; Marable M. *Race, Reform, and Rebellion;* Swinton DH. The economic status of African Americans: "Permanent" poverty and inequality. In: Dewart J, ed. *The State of Black America 1991.* New York: National Urban League, Inc., 1991; Swinton DH. The economic status of African Americans: Limited ownership and persistent inequality. In: Tidwell BJ, ed. *The State of Black America 1992.* New York: National Urban League, Inc., 1992, pp. ; Swinton DH. The economic status of African Americans during the Reagan-Bush era: Withered opportunities, limited outcomes, and uncertain outlook. In: Tidwell BJ, ed. *The State of Black America 1993.* New York: National Urban League, Inc., 1993, pp. 135–200; Farley R, Allen WR. *The Color Line and the Quality of Life in America;* Wolff EN. *Top Heavy: A Study of the Increasing Inequality of Wealth in America.* New York: The Twentieth-Century Fund Press, 1995; Willis DP, ed. *Health Policies and Black Americans;* Woody B. *Managing Crisis Cities: The New Black Leadership and the Politics of Resource Allocation.* Westport, CT: Greenwood Press, 1982.

243. Kovel J. *White Racism: A Psychohistory,* p. xii.

244. Swinton DH. The economic status of African Americans during the Reagan-Bush era, p. 135.

245. Wolff EN. *Top Heavy,* p. 2.

246. Farley R, Allen WR. *The Color Line and the Quality of Life in America;* Kovel J. *White Racism: A Psychohistory,* pp. ix–41; Hacker A. *Two Nations: Black and White, Separate, Hostile, Unequal;* Swinton DH. The economic status of African Americans: "Permanent" poverty and inequality; Swinton DH. The economic status of African Americans: Limited ownership and persistent inequality; Swinton DH. The economic status of African Americans during the Reagan-Bush era; Wolff EN. *Top Heavy;* Feagin JR, Vera H. *White Racism: The Basics.* New York: Routledge, 1995; Byrd WM, Clayton LA. An Ameri-

can health dilemma; Wilson WJ. *The Truly Disadvantaged*; Auletta K. *The Underclass*; Gans HJ. *The War Against the Poor*; Wilson FA, Neuhauser D. *Health Services in the United States.* 2nd ed.; Cose E. The good news about Black Americans. *Newsweek,* June 7, 1999, 28.

247. Farley R, Allen WR. *The Color Line and the Quality of Life in America,* p. 250.

248. Robinson LS. Dialogue: Economist David H. Swinton: Inequities of the past block progress. *Emerge* October 1993; 1(5):18.

249. Kovel J. *White Racism: A Psychohistory,* p. xiv.

250. Wilson WJ. *The Truly Disadvantaged,* pp. 138–139.

251. Farley R, Allen WR. *The Color Line and the Quality of Life in America*; Hacker A. *Two Nations: Black and White, Separate, Hostile, Unequal*; Swinton DH. The economic status of African Americans: "Permanent" poverty and inequality; Swinton DH. The economic status of African Americans: Limited ownership and persistent inequality; Swinton DH. The economic status of African Americans during the Reagan-Bush era; Auletta K. *The Underclass*; Gans HJ. *The War Against the Poor*; Byrd WM, Clayton LA. An American health dilemma; Kovel J. *White Racism: A Psychohistory,* pp. ix–41; Wilson WJ. *The Truly Disadvantaged*; Kaus M. *The End of Equality*; Neuhauser D. *Health Services in the United States.* 2nd ed.

252. Clayton LA, Byrd WM. Race, a major health outcome variable, 1980–1999: With some historical perspectives. *Journal of the National Medical Association.* In press 2000.

253. Washington H. Managing men's health. *Emerge,* October 1995:16.

254. National Center for Health Statistics. *Health United States, 1995.* Hyattsville, MD: Public Health Service, 1996; National Center for Health Statistics. *Health United States, 1994.* Hyattsville, MD: Public Health Service, 1995; National Center for Health Statistics. *Prevention Profile. Health United States, 1991.* Hyattsville, MD: Public Health Service, 1992; Clayton LA, Byrd WM. Race, a major health status and outcome variable, 1980–1999: With some historical perspectives. *Journal of the National Medical Association.* In press 2000; Kochanek KD, Jeffrey DM, Rosenberg HM. Why did black life expectancy decline from 1984 through 1989 in the United States? *American Journal of Public Health* 1994; 84:938–944; Haynes MA. The gap in health status between black and white Americans; Byrd WM, Clayton LA. An American health dilemma; Greenberg DS. Black health; Kovel J. *White Racism: A Psychohistory*; Ginzberg E. Improving health care for the poor; Walinsky A. The crisis of public order. *Atlantic Monthly* July 1995; 1(276):39; Hacker A. *Two Nations: Black and White, Separate, Hostile, Unequal*; Auletta K. *The Underclass*; Gans HJ. *The War Against the Poor*; Farley R, Allen WR. *The Color Line and the Quality of Life in America*; New York Times October 24, 1982, 255.

255. Wilson WJ. *The Declining Significance of Race*; Wilson WJ. *The Truly Disadvantaged*; Wilson WJ. *When Work Disappears*; Lemann N. *The Promised Land*; Auletta K. *The Underclass*; Gans HJ. *The War Against the Poor*; Chicago Tribune. *The American Millstone: An Examination of the Nation's Permanent Underclass.* Chicago: Contemporary Books, Glasgow DG. *The Black Underclass: Poverty, Unemployment, and Entrapment of Ghetto Youth.* London: Jossey-Bass Limited, 1980; paperback ed., New York: Vintage Books, 1981; Moynihan DP. *The Negro Family: The Case for National Action.* Washington, DC: Department of Labor, 1965; Washington H. The widening gap in race-based pollution. *Emerge* July/August 1995; 19; Kozol J. *Savage Inequalities*; pp. 10–11.

256. Walinsky A. The crisis of public order.

257. Schlosser E. The prison-industrial complex. *The Atlantic Monthly*, December, 1998, 51, 52.

258. Kovel J. *White Racism: A Psychohistory*, p. xvii.

259. Pinkney A. *The Myth of Black Progress*. Cambridge, England: Cambridge University Press, 1984; Wilson WJ. *The Truly Disadvantaged;* Swinton DH. The economic status of African Americans during the Reagan-Bush era; Hacker A. *Two Nations: Black and White, Separate, Hostile, Unequal;* Auletta K. *The Underclass;* Gans HJ. *The War Against the Poor;* Fukuyama F. *Trust: The Social Virtues and the Creation of Prosperity;* Farley R, Allen WR. *The Color Line and the Quality of Life in America;* Massey DS, Denton NA. *American Apartheid;* Ryan W. *Blaming the Victim;* U.S. Department of Health and Human Services. *Health, United States, 1991, and Prevention Profile;* Kochanek KD, Jeffrey DM, Rosenberg HM. Why did black life expectancy decline from 1984 through 1989 in the United States? Haynes MA. The gap in health status between black and white Americans; Byrd WM, Clayton LA. An American health dilemma; Greenberg DS. Black health; Kovel J. *White Racism: A Psychohistory;* Ginzberg E. Improving health care for the poor; Walinsky A. The crisis of public order; Schlosser E. The prison-industrial complex. *The Atlantic Monthly*, December 1998, 51; Egyir WK. Harlem Hospital axed; Kotelchuk R. Down and out in the "New Calcutta": New York City's health care crisis. *Health/PAC Bulletin* Summer 1989; 19:4–11.

260. Kovel J. *White Racism: A Psychohistory*, p. xix.

261. Feagin JR, Spikes MP. *Living with Racism;* Hacker A. *Two Nations: Black and White, Separate, Hostile, Unequal;* Simone TM. *About Face;* Sniderman PM, Piazza T. *The Scar of Race;* Glazer N, Ueda R. Policy against prejudice and discrimination; Auletta K. *The Underclass;* Gans HJ. *The War Against the Poor;* Fukuyama F. *Trust: The Social Virtues and the Creation of Prosperity;* Malone TE, Johnson KW. *Report of the Secretary's Task Force on Black and Minority Health;* Cose E. *The Rage of a Privileged Class;* West C. *Race Matters;* Pinkney A. *The Myth of Black Progress;* Massey DS, Denton NA. *American Apartheid;* Kovel J. *White Racism: A Psychohistory*, p. xix; Simonte TM. *About Face.*

262. O'Hear A. Conservatism. In: Honderich T, ed. *The Oxford Companion to Philosophy.* Oxford: Oxford University Press, 1995, pp. 156–158; quote p. 157.

263. Higginbotham Jr. AL. Fifty years of civil rights. *Ebony* November 1995; 1;(51):148; Savage, David G. Lone justice: Silent, aloof and frquently dogmatic, Clarence Thomas' judicial persona emerges. *The Dallas Morning News* October 16, 1994:8J; Coleman TW. Doubting Thomas: Some of Clarence Thomas' former supporters feel betrayed. *Emerge* November 1993; 2;(5):38.

264. Glazer N, Ueda R. Policy against prejudice and discrimination; Nevin D, Bills RE. *The Schools That Fear Built: Segregationist Academies in the South.* Washington, DC: Acropolis Books Ltd., 1976; Shearer J, Stekler P. *The Keys to the Kingdom (1974–1980).* Episode 7, *Eyes on the Prize II.* (videotape). Kozol J. *Savage Inequalities;* Auletta K. *The Underclass;* Gans HJ. *The War Against the Poor;* Fukuyama F. *Trust: The Social Virtues and the Creation of Prosperity;* Morais HM. *The History of the Negro in Medicine;* Byrd WM, Clayton LA. An American health dilemma; Dreyfuss J, Lawrence C. *The Bakke Case: The Politics of Inequality;* Sindler AP. *Bakke, DeFunis, and Minority Admissions;* Wing KR, Rose MG. Health facilities and the enforcement of civil rights. In: Roemer R, McKray G, eds. *Legal Aspects of Health Policy: Issues and Trends.* Westport, CT: Greenwood Press, 1980, pp. 243–267; Rice MF, Jones W. Public policy compliance/enforcement and black American health: Title VI of the civil rights act of 1964. In: Jones Jr W,

Rice MF, eds. *Health Care Issues in Black America: Policies, Problems, and Prospects.* New York: Greenwood Press, 1987, pp. 98–115; Sardell A. *The U.S. Experiment in Social Medicine: The Community Health Center Program, 1956–1986.* Pittsburgh: The University of Pittsburgh Press, 1988.

265. Kovel J. *White Racism: A Psychohistory*; Simone TM. *About Face*; Steinberg S. *Turning Back: The Retreat from Racial Justice in American Thought and Policy.* Boston: Beacon Press, 1995; Smith DB. *Health Care Divided: Race and Healing a Nation.* Ann Arbor: The University of Michigan Press, 1999. Sniderman PM, Piazza T. *The Scar of Race*; Auletta K. *The Underclass*; Gans HJ. *The War Against the Poor*; Fukuyama F. *Trust: The Social Virtues and the Creation of Prosperity*; Marable M. *Race, Reform, and Rebellion*; Honderich T, ed. *The Oxford Companion to Philosophy*; Nisbet R. Conservatism; Lemann N. Taking affirmative action apart. *New York Times Magazine* June 11, 1995; Section 6: 36; Feagin JR, Spikes MP. *Living with Racism*; Newman DK, Amidei NJ, Carter BL, et al. Second-class medicine; Nevin D, Bills RE. *The Schools That Fear Built*; Morais HM. *The History of the Negro in Medicine*; Byrd WM, Clayton LA. An American health dilemma; Byrd WM, Clayton LA. *A Black Health Trilogy*; Rice MF, Jones W. Public policy compliance/enforcement and black American health: Title VI of the Civil Rights Act of 1964. In: Jones W Jr, Rice MF, eds. *Health Care Issues in Black America: Policies, Problems, and Prospects.* New York: Greenwood Press, 1987, pp. 99–117; Wing KR, Rose MG. Health facilities and the enforcement of civil rights; Minerbrook S. Home ownership anchors the middle class: But lending game sinks many prospective owners. *Emerge* October 1993; 1(5):42; Williams J. *Eyes on the Prize*; Wiley E, III. Black America's quest for education: The euphoria of the "Brown" decision has faded to reveal recurring problems of access and inequality. *Emerge* May 1994; 8(5):30; Curry GE, ed. Separate and unequal: The education of blacks forty years after Brown. *Emerge* May 1994 (Special Issue); 8(5):2–72; Orfield E, Eaton SE. *Dismantling Desegregation: The Quick Reversal of Brown v. Board of Education.* New York: The New Press, 1996; A new divide between Black and White. *Newsweek*, June 21, 1999, 64; Yemma J. Schools resegregating, study says. *Boston Sunday Globe*, April 6, 1997. Gaines AA, Hicks RA. Black year in revue. *Emerge* December/January, 1995; 3(6):45; Hampton H. *Eyes on the Prize* (videotape). A six-part documentary video produced by Blackside, Inc., WGBH, Boston, and the Corporation for Public Broadcasting, 1987; Hampton H. *Eyes on the Prize II* (videotape).

266. Kovel J. *White Racism: A Psychohistory*, p. x.

267. Simone TM. *About Face*, pp. 27–28.

268. MacLeod GK. An overview of managed health care. In: Kongstvedt PR. *The Managed Health Care Handbook.* 2nd ed., pp. 3–28; quote pg. 3.

269. Drucker PF. *Management Tasks, Responsibilities, Practices.* New York: Harper & Row, 1974, p. 3.

270. Drucker PF. *Management Tasks, Responsibilities, Practices.* New York: Harper & Row, 1974, p. 3.

271. Kovel J. *White Racism: A Psychohistory*, p. xx.

272. Hacker A. *Two Nations: Black and White, Separate, Hostile, Unequal*; Marable M. *Race, Reform, and Rebellion*; Auletta K. *The Underclass*; Gans HJ. *The War Against the Poor*; Fukuyama F. *Trust: The Social Virtues and the Creation of Prosperity*; Cannon L. *Official Negligence: How Rodney King and the Riots Changed Los Angeles and the LAPD*, New York: Times Books, 1997; Orfield G, Eaton SE. *Dismantling Desegregation: The Quiet Reversal of Brown v. Board of Education.* New York: The New Press, 1996; Hamp-

ton H. *Eyes on the Prize* (videotape); Hampton H. *Eyes on the Prize II* (videotape); National Medical Association. A collaborative effort of the Summit '93 Health Coalition. *Grass Roots Education Initiative for Health Care Reform.* Washington, DC: National Medical Association in association with the Robert Wood Johnson Foundation, 1994; Smith DB. *Health Care Divided: Race and Healing a Nation.* Ann Arbor: The University of Michigan Press, 1999. Kovel J. *White Racism: A Psychohistory;* Merida K. Politics or economics: Has the search for black empowerment gone astray? *Emerge* November 1993; 2(5):52; Cooper KJ. Black caucus flexes muscle, independence. *Emerge* October 1993; 1(5):24; Cooper KJ. New congress foils black caucus gains. *Emerge* February 1995; 4(6):18; Williams J. *Eyes on the Prize;* Low WA, Clift VA. eds. *Encyclopedia of Black America.* New York: McGraw-Hill; reprint ed., New York: Da Capo Press, 1981, pp. 422–423, 467, 679–684; Woody B. *Managing Crisis Cities: The New Black Leadership and the Politics of Resource Allocation.* Westport, CT: Greenwood Press, 1982; Steinberg S. *Turning Back: The Retreat from Racial Justice in American Thought and Policy.* Boston: Beacon Press, 1995; Feagin JR, Spikes MP. *Living with Racism: The Black Middle-Class Experience.* Boston: Beacon Press, 1994; Cose E. *Color-Blind: Seeing Beyond Race in a Race-Obsessed World.* New York: HarperCollins Publishers, 1997.

273. Kovel J. *White Racism: A Psychohistory,* pp. ix–lviii, 34–41; Allport GW. *The Nature of Prejudice;* Steinberg S. *Turning Back: The Retreat From Racial Justice in American Thought and Policy.* Boston: Beacon Press, 1995; Feagin JR, Spikes MP. *Living with Racism: The Black Middle-Class Experience.* Boston: Beacon Press, 1994; Cose E. *Color-Blind: Seeing beyond Race in a Race-Obsessed World.* New York: HarperCollins Publishers, 1997. Simone TM. *About Face;* Smith DB. *Health Care Divided: Race and Healing a Nation.* Ann Arbor: The University of Michigan Press, 1999. Eckholm E. While Congress remains silent health care transforms itself. *New York Times* December 18, 1994: 1; Kongstvedt PR. *The Managed Health Care Handbook.* 2nd ed.; Drucker PF. *Management Tasks, Responsibilities, Practices;* Whol S. *The Medical Industrial Complex.* New York: Harmony Books, 1984; Cose E. *The Rage of a Privileged Class;* Jhally, S, Lewis J. Enlightened Racism; Curry GE. The black man distorted: A gallery of twisted images. *Emerge* October 1995; 7(7):42; West c. *Race Matters;* Feagin JR, Spikes MP. *Living with Racism;* Massey DS, Denton NA. *American Apartheid;* Gross B. *Friendly Fascism.* Boston: South End, 1982; Auletta K. *The Underclass;* Gans HJ. *The War Against the Poor;* Fukuyama F. *Trust: The Social Virtues and the Creation of Prosperity;* Gaines AA, Hicks RA. Black year in revue. *Emerge* December/January 1995; 3(6):45; Coleman T. Doubting Thomas: Some of Clarence Thomas' former supporters feel betrayed; Lemann N. Taking affirmative action apart; Berry MF. Affirmative action: Political opportunists exploit racial fears. *Emerge* May 1995; 7(6):28; Minerbrook S. Home ownership anchors the middle class; Williams J. *Eyes on the Prize;* Byrd WM, Clayton LA. An American health dilemma; Byrd WM. Race, biology, and health care; Farley R, Allen WR. *The Color Line and the Quality of Life in America;* Updegrave WL. Race and money. *Money* December 1989; 152; Woody B. *Managing Crisis Cities;* Hampton H. *Eyes on the Prize* (videotape); Hampton H. *Eyes on the Prize II* (videotape).

274. Mazrui AA. *The Africans: A Triple Heritage,* p. 302; Mazrui AA. *Global Africa.* Part 9, *The Africans.*

275. Sniderman PM, Piazza T. *The Scar of Race;* Feagin JR, Spikes MP. *Living with Racism;* Marable M. *Race, Reform, and Rebellion;* Pettigrew TF. Prejudice; Fredrickson GM, Knobel DT. History of prejudice and discrimination; Glazer N, Ueda R. Policy

against prejudice and discrimination; Kozol J. *Savage Inequalities*; Kovel J. *White Racism: A Psychohistory*; Levin J, Levin W. *The Functions of Discrimination and Prejudice.* 2nd ed.; Auletta K. *The Underclass*; Gans HJ. *The War Against the Poor*; Fukuyama F. *Trust: The Social Virtues and the Creation of Prosperity*; Jhally S, Lewis J. *Enlightened Racism*; Riggs MT. *Ethnic Notions* (filmstrip); Riggs MT. *Color Adjustment* (filmstrip); Turner PA. *Ceramic Uncles and Celluloid Mammies*; Hacker A. *Two Nations: Black and White, Separate, Hostile, Unequal.* Steinberg S. *Turning Back: The Retreat from Racial Justice in American Thought and Policy.* Boston: Beacon Press, 1996; Cose E. *Color-Blind: Seing Beyond Race in a Race-Obsessed World.* New York: HarperCollins Publishers, 1997; Smith DB. Orfield G, Eaton SE. *Dismantling Desegretation: The Quiet Reversal of Brown v. Board of Education.* New York: The New Press, 1996; Feagin JR, Feagin CB. *Racial and Ethnic Relations.* 6th ed. Upper Saddle River, NJ: Prentice Hall Publishers, 1999. Kinder DR, Sanders LM. *Divided by Color: Racial Politics and Democratic Ideals.* Chicago: The University of Chicago Press, 1996; Sniderman PM, Carmines EG. *Reaching Beyond Race.* Cambridge, Massachusetts: Harvard University Press, 1997; Schuman H, Steeh C, Bobo L, Krysan M. *Racial Attitudes in America: Trends and Interpretations.* Revised Edition. Cambridge, Massachusetts: Harvard University Press, 1997.

276. Kovel J. *White Racism: A Psychohistory,* pp. ix–x.

277. Omi M, Winant H. *Racial Formation in the United States: From the 1960s to the 1980s.* London: Routledge and Kegan Paul, 1986, pp. 68–69.

278. Omi M, Winant H. *Racial Formation in the United States,* p. 54.

279. Outlaw L. Toward a critical theory of race, p. 77.

280. Kovel J. *White Racism: A Psychohistory*; Outlaw L. Toward a critical theory of race; Omi M, Winant H. *Racial Formation in the United States.*

281. Fredrickson GM. *The Black Image in the White Mind.*

282. Young RJC. *Colonial Desire: Hybridity in Theory, Culture and Race.* London: Routledge, 1995, p. 91.

283. Fredrickson GM. *The Black Image in the White Mind*; Outlaw L. Toward a critical theory of race; Omi M, Winant H. *Racial Formation in the United States*; Williams E. *Capitalism and Slavery.* Chapel Hill: The University of North Carolina Press, 1944; paperback ed., Chapel Hill: University of North Carolina Press, 1994; Du Bois WEB. *The Suppression of the African Slave Trade to the United States of America, 1638–1870.* N.P., 1896; reprint, Baton Rouge: Louisiana State University Press, 1969; Williams E. *From Columbus to Castro: The History of the Caribbean, 1492–1969.* London: Andre Deutsche Limited, 1970; paperback ed., New York: Vintage Books, 1984; Marable M. *How Capitalism Underdeveloped Black America*; Marable M. *Race, Reform, and Rebellion*; Auletta K. *The Underclass*; Gans HJ. *The War Against the Poor*; Fukuyama F. *Trust: The Social Virtues and the Creation of Prosperity*; Stannard DE. *American Holocaust*; Kongstvedt PR. *The Managed Health Care Handbook.* 2nd ed., pp. xvii–xviii, 1–27; Eckholm E. While Congress remains silent health care transforms itself; Starr P. *The Social Transformation of American Medicine.*

284. Stannard DE. *American Holocaust*; Du Bois WEB. *The Negro.* New York: Henry Holt, 1915; reprint ed., London: Oxford University Press, 1970; Du Bois WEB. *The Suppression of the African Slave Trade to the United States of America, 1638–1870*; Davidson B. *The African Slave Trade.*

285. Outlaw L. Toward a critical theory of race; Omi M, Winant H. *Racial Formation in the United States*; Pettigrew TF. Prejudice; Hacker A. *Two Nations: Black and*

White, Separate, Hostile, Unequal; Kongstvedt PR. The Managed Health Care Handbook. 2nd ed., pp. xvii–xviii, 1–27; Eckholm E. While Congress remains silent health care transforms itself; Terry RW. For Whites Only, Feagin JR, Spikes MP. Living with Racism; Simone TM. About Face; Young RJC. Colonial Desire; Weisbord RG. Genocide? Birth Control and the Black American. Westport, CT: Greenwood Press, 1975; Parsons T. The Social System. Glencoe, IL. The Free Press, 1951; Jaco EG. Patients, Physicians, and Illness: A Sourcebook in Behavioral Science and Health. 3rd ed. New York: The Free Press, 1979; Starr P. The Social Transformation of American Medicine; Tosteson DC. An open letter from the Dean to the Harvard community: Letter from second-year students: Letter from HMS Third World Caucus. Harvard Medical Area Focus January 9, 1992: 8–13.

286. Devisse J. The Image of the Black in Western Art (Part 2, From the Early Christian Era to the "Age of Discovery." 1. From the Demonic Threat to the Incarnation of Sainthood), p. 8.

287. Outlaw L. Toward a critical theory of race, p. 77.

288. Outlaw L. Toward a critical theory of race; Winant O, Winant H. Racial Formation in the United States; Two Nations: Black and White, Separate, Hostile, Unequal; Feagin JR, Spikes MP. Living with Racism; Simone TM. About Face; Auletta K. The Underclass; Gans HJ. The War Against the Poor; Fukuyama F. Trust: The Social Virtues and the Creation of Prosperity; Young RJC. Colonial Desire; Jaco EG. Patients, Physicians, and Illness; Starr P. The Social Transformation of American Medicine; Morais HM. The History of the Negro in Medicine; Du Bois WEB. The Souls of Black Folk: Essays and Sketches. Chicago: A. C. McClurg, 1903; unabridged reprint ed., New York: Dodd, Mead, 1979.

Chapter Two

1. Bender GA. Great Moments in Medicine. Detroit: Northwood Institute Press, 1966, pp. 8–33; Lyons AS, Petrucelli RJ. Medicine: An Illustrated History. New York: Harry N. Abrams, 1978, pp. 30–41, 57–103; Wood M. Legacy (videotapes). Six-part series produced in cooperation with Maryland Public Television and Central Independent Television, 1991; Gardner JL. Reader's Digest Atlas of the World. Pleasantville, NY: The Reader's Digest Association, 1987, pp. 20–21.

2. Ackerknecht EH. A Short History of Medicine. rev. ed. Baltimore: The Johns Hopkins University Press, 1982, pp. 3–63; Bender GA. Great Moments in Medicine, pp. 8–33; Lyons AS, Petrucelli RJ. Medicine: An Illustrated History, pp. 30–41, 57–293; Thorwald J. Science and Secrets of Early Medicine: Egypt, Babylonia, India, China, Mexico, Peru. New York: Harcourt, Brace and World, 1962; Finch CS. The African Background to Medical Science: Essays in African History, Science and Civilizations. London: Karnak House, 1990; Finch CS. Science and symbol in Egyptian medicine: Commentaries on the Edwin Smith papyrus. In: Van Sertima I, ed. Egypt Revisited: Journal of African Civilizations. New Brunswick, NJ: Transaction Publishers, 1989, pp. 325–351; Sirasi NG. Medieval and Early Renaissance Medicine: An Introduction to Knowledge and Practice. Chicago: The University of Chicago Press, 1990.

3. Ackerknecht EH. A Short History of Medicine; Bender GA. Great Moments in Medicine; Lyons AS, Petrucelli RJ. Medicine: An Illustrated History, pp. 67, 57–103; Thorwald J. Science and Secrets of Early Medicine, pp. 14–176.

4. Ackerknecht EH. A *Short History of Medicine,* pp. 19–34; Bender GA. *Great Moments in Medicine,* pp. 14–19; Lyons AS, Petrucelli RJ. *Medicine: An Illustrated History,* pp. 58–69; Thorwald J. *Science and Secrets of Early Medicine,* pp. 105–176.

5. Thorwald J. *Science and Secrets of Early Medicine,* p. 49.

6. Newsome F. Black contributions to the early history of Western medicine. *Journal of the National Medical Association* 1979; 71:189–193; Finch CS. The African background of medical science. In: Van Sertima I, ed. *Blacks in Science: Ancient and Modern.* New Brunswick, NJ: Transaction Publishers, 1983, pp. 140–156; Finch CS. Science and symbol in Egyptian medicine; Ackerknecht EH. A *Short History of Medicine,* pp. 19–34; Lyons AS, Petrucelli RJ. *Medicine: An Illustrated History,* pp. 76–103; Thorwald J. *Science and Secrets of Early Medicine,* pp. 13–104.

7. Osler Sir W. *Evolution of Modern Medicine.* New Haven, CT: London and London, 1921, p. 10.

8. Ackerknecht EH. A *Short History of Medicine,* pp. 19–34; Estes JW. *The Medical Skills of Ancient Egypt.* Canton, MA: Science History Publications/USA, 1989; Lyons AS, Petrucelli RJ. *Medicine: An Illustrated History,* pp. 76–103; Newsome F. Black contributions to the early history of Western medicine; Thorwald J. *Science and Secrets of Early Medicine;* pp. 13–104.

9. Lyons AS, Petrucelli RJ. *Medicine: An Illustrated History,* p. 101; Estes JW. *The Medical Skills of Ancient Egypt;* Thorwald J. *Science and Secrets of Early Medicine,* pp. 13–104.

10. Lyons AS, Petrucelli RJ. *Medicine: An Illustrated History,* p. 101; Sigerist HE. *The Great Doctors: A Biographical History of Medicine.* New York: W.W. Norton, 1933; reprint ed., New York: Dover Publications, 1971, pp. 21–28; Estes JW. *The Medical Skills of Ancient Egypt,* pp. 114, 117, 119–133; Thorwald J. *Science and Secrets of Early Medicine,* pp. 49, 94–97, 102–104.

11. Ackerknecht EH. A *Short History of Medicine,* pp. 19–34; Bender GA. *Great Moments in Medicine,* pp. 8–13; Estes JW. *The Medical Skills of Ancient Egypt,* pp. 13–104; Newsome F. Black contributions to the early history of Western medicine; Finch CS. The African background of medical science; Finch CS. Science and symbol in Egyptian medicine; Lyons AS, Petrucelli RJ. *Medicine: An Illustrated History,* pp. 76–103; Thorwald J. *Science and Secrets of Early Medicine,* pp. 13–104.

12. Finch CS. The African background of medical science; Lyons AS, Petrucelli RJ. *Medicine: An Illustrated History,* pp. 76–103; Ransford O. *Bid the Sickness Cease: Disease in the History of Black Africa.* London: John Murray, 1983.

13. Bender GA. *Great Moments in Medicine,* pp. 8–13; Newsome F. Black contributions to the early history of Western medicine; Finch CS. The African background of medical science; Finch CS. Science and symbol in Egyptian medicine; Lyons AS, Petrucelli RJ. *Medicine: An Illustrated History,* pp. 92–103; Thorwald J. *Science and Secrets of Early Medicine,* pp. 60–93.

14. Sigerist HE. *The Great Doctors,* pp. 21–28; Cobb WM. 1981. The black American in medicine. *Journal of the National Medical Association* 73(Suppl 1):1183–1244; Bender GA. *Great Moments in Medicine,* pp. 8–13; Newsome F. Black contributions to the early history of Western medicine; Finch CS. The African background of medical science; Finch CS. Science and symbol in Egyptian medicine; Lyons AS, Petrucelli RJ. *Medicine: An Illustrated History,* pp. 90–92, 101–103; Thorwald J. *Science and Secrets of Early Medicine,* pp. 94–97, 101–104; Asante MK. Roots of the truth, *Emerge* July/August 1996 9(7):66.

15. Asante MK. Roots of the truth; James GGM. *Stolen Legacy: Greek Philosophy Is Stolen Egyptian Philosophy*. New York: Philosophical Library, 1954; reprint ed., Newport News, VA: United Brothers Communication Systems, 1989; Van Sertima I. *They Came Before Columbus*. New York: Random House, 1976; Bernal M. *Black Athena: The Afroasiatic Roots of Classical Civilization* (Vol. 1, *The Fabrication of Ancient Greece 1785–1985*). New Brunswick, NJ: Rutgers University Press, 1987; Bernal M. *Black Athena: The Afroasiatic Roots of Classical Civilization* (Vol. 2, *The Archaeological and Documentary Evidence*). New Brunswick, NJ: Rutgers University Press, 1991; Diop CA. Origin of the ancient Egyptians. In: Mokhtar G, ed. *General History of Africa. II: Ancient Civilizations of Africa*. Berkeley: University of California Press, 1981, pp. 27–57; Diop CA. *The African Origin of Civilization: Myth or Reality*, ed. and trans. Cook M. Westport, CT: Lawrence Hill and Company, 1974; Diop CA. *Civilization or Barbarism: An Authentic Anthropology*, trans. Ngemi YM, ed. Salemson HJ, de Jager M. Westport, CT: Lawrence Hill Books, 1991; Davidson B. The ancient world and Africa: Whose roots? pp. 39–52. In: Van Sertima I, ed. *Egypt Revisited: Journal of African Civilizations*. New Brunswick: Translation Publishers, 1989; Drake SC. *Black Folk Here and There: An Essay in History and Anthropology* (Vol. 1). Los Angeles: Center for Afro-American Studies, University of California, 1987; Drake SC. *Black Folk Here and There: An Essay in History and Anthropology* (Vol. 2). Los Angeles: Center for Afro-American Studies, University of California, 1990; Finch CS. The African background of medical science; Finch CS. The black roots of Egypt's glory. In: Van Sertima I, ed. *Great Black Leaders: Ancient and Modern*. New Brunswick, NJ: Transaction Publishers, 1988, pp. 138–143; Finch CS. Imhotep the physician: Archetype of the great man. In: Van Sertima I, ed. *Great Black Leaders: Ancient and Modern*, pp. 213–231; Finch CS. Science and symbol in Egyptian medicine; Finch CS. Nile genesis: Continuity of culture from the great lakes to the delta. In: Van Sertima I, ed. *Egypt Child of Africa*. New Brunswick, NJ: Transaction Publishers, 1994, pp. 34–54; Finch CS. *Africa and the Birth of Science and Technology: A Brief Overview*. Decatur, GA: Khenti Publications, 1992; Finch CS. *Echoes of the Old Darkland: Themes from the African Eden*. Decatur, GA: Khenti Publications, 1994; Van Sertima I. Race and origin of the Egyptians. In: Van Sertima I, ed. *Egypt Revisited*, pp. 2–8; Asante MK. *The Afrocentric Idea*. Philadelphia: Temple University Press, 1987; Asante MK. *Afrocentricity*. Trenton, NJ: Africa World Press, 1988; Asante MK. *Kemet, Afrocentricity and Knowledge*. Trenton, NJ: Africa World Press, 1990.

16. Rogers JA. *World's Great Men of Color* (Vol. 1). New York: Collier Macmillan, 1972, pp. 1–24, 38–42.

17. Bernal M. *Black Athena* (Vols. 1 and 2); Diop CA. Origin of the ancient Egyptians; Davidson B. The ancient world and Africa: Whose roots?; Drake SC. *Black Folk Here and There* (Vol. 1); Finch CS. The African background of medical science; Van Sertima I. Race and origin of the Egyptians; Asante MK. Roots of the truth.

18. Bernal M. *Black Athena* (Vols. 1 and 2); Diop CA. Origin of the ancient Egyptians; Davidson B. The ancient world and Africa: Whose roots?; Drake SC. *Black Folk Here and There* (Vol. 1); Chandler, WB. Of gods and men: Egypt's old kingdom. In: Van Sertima I. *Egypt Revisited*, pp. 117–182; Newsome F. Black contributions to the early history of Western medicine; Finch CS. The African background of medical science; Finch CS. The Black roots of Egypt's glory; Finch CS. Imhotep the physician; Finch CS. Science and symbol in Egyptian medicine; Finch CS. Nile genesis; Finch CS. *Africa and the Birth of Science and Technology*; Finch CS. *Echoes of the Old Darkland*; Van Sertima I.

Race and origin of the Egyptians; Lyons AS, Petrucelli RJ. *Medicine: An Illustrated History*, p. 101; Sigerist HE. *The Great Doctors*, pp. 21–28; Estes JW. *The Medical Skills of Ancient Egypt*, pp. 114, 117, 119–133; Thorwald J. *Science and Secrets of Early Medicine*, pp. 49, 94–97, 102–104; Van Sertima I. Race and origin of the Egyptians.

19. Veatch RM. *A Theory of Medical Ethics*. New York: Basic Books, 1981; Health Policy Advisory Center. The emerging health apartheid in the United States. *Health/PAC Bulletin* 1991; 21:3–4; Byrd WM, Clayton LA. An American health dilemma: A history of blacks in the health system. *Journal of the National Medical Association* 1992; 84:189–200; Charatz-Litt C. A chronicle of racism: The effects of the white medical com-
- munity on black health. *Journal of the National Medical Association* 1992; 84:717–725.

20. Lyons AS, Petrucelli RJ. *Medicine: An Illustrated History*, pp. 58–69; Thorwald J. *Science and Secrets of Early Medicine*, pp. 13–176; Bender GA. *Great Moments in Medicine*, pp. 8–25.

21. Mazrui AA. *The Africans* (videotapes). A nine-part series sponsored by the Annenberg/CPB Project, Washington, DC: WETA and BBC, 1986; Mazrui AA. *The Africans: A Triple Heritage*. Boston: Little, Brown, 1986; Davidson B. *Let Freedom Come: Africa in Modern History*. Boston: Little, Brown, 1978, pp. 53–58; Davidson B. *Africa* (videotapes). An eight-part series produced by Mitchell Beazley Television, RM Arts/Channel Four co-production in association with the Nigerian Television Authority, 1984; Bender GA. *Great Moments in Medicine*. Detroit: Northwood Institute Press, 1966; Thorwald J. *Science and Secrets of Early Medicine: Egypt, Babylonia, India, China, Mexico, Peru*. New York: Harcourt, Brace and World, 1962.

22. Sigerist HE. *The Great Doctors*, pp. 21–77; Nuland SB. *Doctors: The Biography of Medicine*, pp. 3–60; Lyons AS, Petrucelli RJ. *Medicine: An Illustrated History*, pp. 153–229.

23. Finch CS. The African background of medical science; Newsome F. Black contributions to the early history of Western medicine; Estes JW. *The Medical Skills of Ancient Egypt*, pp. 114, 117, 119–133; Lyons AS, Petrucelli RJ. *Medicine: An Illustrated History*, pp. 152–261; Sigerist HE. *The Great Doctors*, pp. 29–77.

24. Bernal M. *Black Athena* (Vols. 1 and 2); Van Sertima I. Race and origin of the Egyptians; Diop CA. Origin of the ancient Egyptians; Davidson B. The ancient world and Africa: Whose roots?; Chandler WB. Of Gods and men: Egypt's old kingdom.

25. Harris JE. *Africans and Their History*, pp. 13–28; Wassermann HP. *Ethnic Pigmentation: Historical, Psychological, and Clinical Aspects*. New York: American Elsevier, 1974, pp. 13–20; Jordan WD. *White Over Black: American Attitudes Toward the Negro, 1550–1812*. New York: W. W. Norton, 1968, pp. 11–12, 60.

26. Drake SC. *Black Folk Here and There*. (Vol. 1), p. 249; Harris JE. *Africans and Their History*, pp. 14–15; Patterson O. *Slavery and Social Death: A Comparative Study*. Cambridge, MA: Harvard University Press, 1982, pp. 177–178.

27. Sigerist HE. *The Great Doctors*, p. 33.

28. Finley MI. *Ancient Slavery and Modern Ideology*. New York: Penguin Books, 1980, p. 106.

29. Finley MI. *Ancient Slavery and Modern Ideology*, pp. 93–122; Bullough VL. *The Development of Medicine as a Profession: The Contribution of the Medieval University to Modern Medicine*. New York: Hafner Publishing, 1966, pp. 6–31; Lyons AS, Petrucelli RJ. *Medicine: An Illustrated History*, pp. 76–103, 152–261; Veatch RM. *A Theory of Medical Ethics*, pp. 18–26, 147–162.

30. Veatch RM. A *Theory of Medical Ethics*, pp. 154–159; Finley MI. *Ancient Slavery and Modern Ideology*, pp. 93–122; Bullough VL. *The Development of Medicine as a Profession*, pp. 6–31; Lyons AS, Petrucelli RJ. *Medicine: An Illustrated History*, pp. 76–103, 152–261; Churchill LR. *Rationing Health Care in America: Perceptions and Principles of Justice*. Notre Dame, IN: University of Notre Dame Press, 1987, pp. 27–57.

31. Sigerist HE. *The Great Doctors*, pp. 43–44; Haeger K. *The Illustrated History of Surgery*, pp. 45–46.

32. Majno G. *The Healing Hand: Man and Wound in the Ancient World*. Cambridge, MA: Harvard University Press, 1975, p. 354.

33. Savitt TL. The use of blacks for medical experimentation and demonstration in the old south. *Journal of Southern History* 1982; 48:331–348; Walker HE. *The Negro in the Medical Profession*. Publications of the University of Virginia Phelps-Stokes Fellowship Papers. University of Virginia, 1949, p. 7; Heaton CE. Medicine in New York during the English colonial period, 1664–1775. *Bulletin of the History of Medicine* 1945; 17:9–37.

34. Majno G. *The Healing Hand*, p. 339.

35. Majno G. *The Healing Hand*, p. 339.

36. Majno G. *The Healing Hand*, p. 339.

37. Majno G. *The Healing Hand*, pp. 339–394; Bullough VL. *The Development of Medicine as a Profession*, pp. 6–31; Lyons AS, Petrucelli RJ. *Medicine: An Illustrated History*, pp. 230–261.

38. Lyons AS, Petrucelli RJ. *Medicine: An Illustrated History*, p. 231.

39. Majno G. *The Healing Hand*, pp. 339–422; Lyons AS, Petrucelli RJ. *Medicine: An Illustrated History*, pp. 151–261; Bullough VL. *The Development of Medicine as a Profession*, pp. 6–31.

40. Guthrie D. A *History of Medicine*. Philadelphia: J.B. Lippincott, 1946, pp. 81–83.

41. Majno G. *The Healing Hand*, pp. 339–422; Lyons AS, Petrucelli RJ. *Medicine: An Illustrated History*, pp. 230–249; Bullough VL. *The Development of Medicine as a Profession*, pp. 6–31.

42. Sigerist HE. *The Great Doctors*, pp. 56–77; Majno G. *The Healing Hand*, pp. 389–392; Bullough VL. *The Development of Medicine as a Profession*, pp. 6–31.

43. Guthrie D. A *History of Medicine*, p. 81.

44. Guthrie D. A *History of Medicine*, pp. 81–82.

45. Guthrie D. A *History of Medicine*, pp. 81–83; Lyons AS, Petrucelli RJ. *Medicine: An Illustrated History*, pp. 230–261; Sirasi NG. *Medieval and Early Renaissance Medicine*, pp. 1–10; Bullough VL. *The Development of Medicine as a Profession*, pp. 23–31; Majno G. *The Healing Hand*, pp. 381–394.

46. Bullough VL. *The Development of Medicine as a Profession*, p. 24.

47. Bullough VL. *The Development of Medicine as a Profession*, p. 24.

48. Bender GA. *Great Moments in Medicine*, pp. 50–61; Lyons AS, Petrucelli RJ. *Medicine: An Illustrated History*, pp. 230–261; Majno G. *The Healing Hand*, pp. 390–393; Nuland SB, *Doctors: The Biography of Medicine*, pp. 3–60; Sigerist HE. *The Great Doctors*, pp. 29–77; Bullough VL. *The Development of Medicine as a Profession*, pp. 6–31.

49. Drake SC. *Black Folk Here and There* (Vol. 2), p. 72.

50. Davis DB. *Slavery and Human Progress*. New York: Oxford University Press, 1984, pp. 42, 328 n. 58; Lewis B. *Race and Slavery in the Middle East: An Historical Enquiry*. New York: Oxford University Press, 1990, p. 52.

51. Lewis B. The African diaspora and the civilization of Islam. In: Kilson ML, Rotberg RI, eds. *The African Diaspora: Interpretive Essays.* Cambridge, MA: Harvard University Press, 1976, pp. 37–56; Sanders R. *Lost Tribes and Promised Lands: The Origins of American Racism.* Boston: Little, Brown, 1978, pp. 49–64; Davis DB. *Slavery and Human Progress,* pp. 42, 328 n. 58; Lewis B. *Race and Slavery in the Middle East,* p. 52; Devisse J. *The Image of the Black in Western Art* (Part 2, From the Early Christian Era to the "Age of Discovery." 1. From the Demonic Threat to the Incarnation of Sainthood. Cambridge, MA: The Menil Foundation, distributed by the Harvard University Press, 1979, pp. 52, 50–119, 216 n. 70, 218 (n. 114, 117, 118, 122), 219 (n. 124, 125, 132).

52. Banton M, Harwood J. *The Race Concept.* New York: Praeger, 1975; Banton M. *Racial Theories.* Cambridge: Cambridge University Press, 1987; Barzun J. *Race: A Study in Modern Superstition.* N.P., 1937. *Race: A Study in Superstition.* revised ed., New York: Harper & Row, 1965; Beider RE. *Science Encounters the Indian, 1820–1880: The Early Years of American Ethnology.* Norman: University of Oklahoma Press, 1986; Byrd WM. Race, biology, and health care: Reassessing a relationship. *Journal of Health Care for the Poor and Underserved* 1990; 1:278–292; Chase A. *The Legacy of Malthus: The Social Costs of the New Scientific Racism.* New York: Knopf, 1980; Cogan T. *The Works of the Late Professor Camper of the Connexion Between the Science of Anatomy and the Arts of Drawing, Painting, Statuary in Two Books.* London: J. Hearne, 1821; Gould SJ. *The Mismeasure of Man.* New York: W.W. Norton, 1981; Haller JS. *Outcasts from Evolution: Scientific Attitudes of Racial Inferiority, 1859–1900.* New York: McGraw Hill, 1971; Honour H. *The Image of the Black in Western Art.* (Part IV, From the American Revolution to World War I. 2. Black Models and White Myths). Cambridge: The Menil Foundation, distributed by Harvard University Press, 1989; Jones JH. *Bad Blood: The Tuskegee Syphilis Experiment.* New York: The Free Press, 1981; Jordan WD. *White Over Black: American Attitudes Toward the Negro, 1550–1812.* New York: W. W. Norton, Inc., 1968; Morton SG. *Crania Americana or a Comparative View of the Skulls of Various Aboriginal Nations of North and South America to Which is prefixed An Essay on the Varieties of the Human Species.* Philadelphia: J. Dobson, 1839; Nott JC, Gliddon GR. *Types of Mankind or, Ethnological Researches.* Philadelphia: Lippincott, Grambo and Company, 1854; Stanton W. *The Leopard's Spots: Scientific Attitudes Toward Race in America, 1815–1859.* Chicago: The University of Chicago Press, 1960.

53. Morais HM. *The History of the Negro in Medicine.* New York: Publishers Company, 1967; Jones JH. *Bad Blood;* Byrd WM, Clayton LA. The "slave health deficit": Racism and health outcomes. *Health/PAC Bulletin* 1991; 21:25–28; Byrd WM. Race, biology, and health care.

54. Harris JE. *Africans and Their History,* pp. 16–28; Sanders R. *Lost Tribes and Promised Lands,* pp. 39–64, 152–165; Davis DB. *The Problem of Slavery in Western Culture.* Ithaca: Cornell University Press, 1966, pp. 62–121.

55. Wetterau B. *The New York Public Library Book of Chronologies.* 1st ed. New York: Stonesong Press, 1990, pp. 98–101; Luce HR. *Life's Picture History of Western Man.* New York: Time, 1951, pp. 7–70; Lyons AS, Petrucelli RJ. *Medicine: An Illustrated History;* Roberts JM. *The Triumph of the West,* pp. 35–77.

56. Wetterau B. *The New York Public Library Book of Chronologies.* 1st ed. pp. 98–101; Luce HR. *Life's Picture History of Western Man,* pp. 7–70; Lyons AS, Petrucelli RJ. *Medicine: An Illustrated History;* Roberts JM. *The Triumph of the West,* pp. 35–77; Lloyd GER, ed. *Hippocratic Writings.* Middlesex, England: Penguin Books, 1978, p. 57.

57. Ackerknecht EH. *A Short History of Medicine*, pp. 73–93; Bender GA. *Great Moments in Medicine*, pp. 62–75; Haeger K. *The Illustrated History of Surgery*, pp. 63–93; Bullough VL. *The Development of Medicine as a Profession*, pp. 32–45; Lyons AS, Petrucelli RJ. *Medicine: An Illustrated History*, pp. 264–317; Majno G. *The Healing Hand*, pp. 417–422; Sirasi NG. *Medieval and Early Renaissance Medicine*, pp. 6–16; Bergonzoni F, Fanti M. *L' Archiginnasio Di Bologna*. Bologna: Lions Club Bologna-Archignnasio, 1986–1987; Drake SC. *Black Folk Here and There: An Essay in History and Anthropology*. Vol. 2. Los Angeles: Center for Afro-American Studies, University of California, 1990; Sigerist HE. *The Great Doctors: A Biographical History of Medicine*. Rev. Edition. Baltomore: The Johns Hopkins University Press, 1982; Guthrie D. *A History of Medicine*. Philadelphia: JB Lippincott Company, 1946.

58. Bender GA. *Great Moments in Medicine*, pp. 56–75; Haeger K. *The Illustrated History of Surgery*, pp. 59–93; Lyons AS, Petrucelli RJ. *Medicine: An Illustrated History*, pp. 264–317; Sirasi NG. *Medieval and Early Renaissance Medicine*, pp. 6–16; Bergonzoni F, Fanti M. *L' Archiginnasion Di Bologna*.

59. Devisse J. *The Image of the Black in Western Art* (Part 2. *From the Early Christian Era to the "Age of Discovery."* 1. *From the Demonic Threat to the Incarnation of Sainthood*), p. 47.

60. Ackerknecht EH. *A Short History of Medicine*, pp. 73–93; Bender GA. *Great Moments in Medicine*, pp. 62–107; Haeger K. *The Illustrated History of Surgery*, pp. 63–122; Bullough VL. *The Development of Medicine as a Profession*; Starr P. *The Social Transformation of American Medicine*, pp. 3–144; Byrd WM, Clayton LA. An American health dilemma; Lyons AS, Petrucelli RJ. *Medicine: An Illustrated History*, pp. 264–365; Majno G. *The Healing Hand*, pp. 417–422; Sirasi NG. *Medieval and Early Renaissance Medicine*; Drake SC. *Black Folk Here and There* (Vol. 2), pp. 1–226; Sanders R. *Lost Tribes and Promised Lands*, pp. 39–64; Devisse J. *The Image of the Black in Western Art* (Part 2. *From the Early Christian Era to the "Age of Discovery."* 1. *From the Demonic Threat to the Incarnation of Sainthood*); Devisse J, Mollat M. *The Image of the Black in Western Art* (Part 2. *From the Early Christian Era to the "Age of Discovery."* 2. *Africans in the Christian Ordinance of the World* [*Fourteenth to the Sixteenth Century*]). Cambridge, MA: The Menil Foundation, distributed by Harvard University Press, 1979.

61. Drake SC. *Black Folk Here and There* (Vol. 2); Sanders R. *Lost Tribes and Promised Lands*, pp. 39–64, 152–188, 211–225; Chappell W. *A Short History of the Printed Word*. New York: Dorset Press, 1970; Devisse J. *The Image of the Black in Western Art* (Part 2. *From the Early Christian Era to the "Age of Discovery."* 1. *From the Demonic Threat to the Incarnation of Sainthood*); Devisse J, Mollat M. *The Image of the Black in Western Art* (Part 2. *From the Early Christian Era to the "Age of Discovery."* 2. *Africans in the Christian Ordinance of the World* [*Fourteenth to the Sixteenth Century*]); Sanders R. *Lost Tribes and Promised Lands*.

62. Brandt AM. Racism and research: The case of the Tuskegee Syphilis Study. In: Leavitt JW, Numbers RL, eds. *Sickness and Health in America: Readings in the History of Medicine and Public Health*. Madison: The University of Wisconsin Press, 1985, pp. 331–343; Byrd WM. Race, biology, and health care; Charatz-Litt C. A chronicle of racism; Morais HM. *The History of the Negro in Medicine*; Reed J. Scientific racism. In: Wilson CR, Ferris W, eds. *Encyclopedia of Southern Culture*. Chapel Hill: The University of North Carolina Press, 1989, pp. 1358–1360; Veatch RM. *A Theory of Medical Ethics*.

63. Drake SC. *Black Folk Here and There* (Vol. 2), pp. 45, 56–57; Davis DB. *Slavery and Human Progress*, p. 42; Devisse J. Christians and black. In: Devisse J. *The Image of the*

Black in Western Art (Part 2. *From the Early Christian Era to the "Age of Discovery."* 1. *From the Demonic Threat to the Incarnation of Sainthood*), pp. 37–64; Davis DB. *Slavery and Human Progress*, pp. 42, 328 n. 58.

64. Abercrombie TJ, Barbey B. When the Moors ruled Spain. *National Geographic* July 1988; 86–119; Dor-Ner Z, Sheller WG. *Columbus and the Age of Discovery.* New York: William Morrow, 1991, pp. 17–24; Roberts J. *The Triumph of the West*, pp. 79–98, 117–132; Chandler WB. The Moor: Light of Europe's Dark Age. In: Van Sertima I, ed. *African Presence in Early Europe*, pp. 144–175; Lane-Poole S. *The Story of the Moors in Spain*. N.P. 1886; reprint ed., Baltimore: Black Classic Press, 1990; Lewis B. The African diaspora and the civilization of Islam; Lewis B. *Race and Slavery in the Middle East*; Sanders Sr. *Lost Tribes and Promised Lands*; Davidson B. *Africa*. An Eight-Part Series [video-tapes]. Produced by Mitchell Beazley Television, RM Arts/Channel Four co-production in association with the Nigerian Television Authority, 1984; Dor-Ner Z. Chidd G. *Columbus and the Age of Discovery* [videotape]. A documentary video series produced by the National Endowment for the Humanities, and the Corporation for Public Broadcasting, 1991; Roberts J. "New Worlds," segment of *Triumph of the West*. [videotape]. A multi-part documentary produced by the BBC, 1985.

65. Cox GO. *African Empires and Civilizations.* New York: African Heritage Studies Publishers, 1974, p. 146.

66. Chandler WB. The Moor: Light of Europe's Dark Age, p. 161.

67. Abercrombie TJ, Barbey B. When the Moors ruled Spain; Chandler WB. The Moor: Light of Europe's Dark Age; Cox GO. *African Empires and Civilizations*; Lane-Pool S. *The Story of the Moors in Spain*; Lewis B. The African diaspora and the civilization of Islam; Lewis B. *Race and Slavery in the Middle East*, pp. 3–61; Sanders R. *Lost Tribes and Promised Lands*.

68. Davis DB. *Slavery and Human Progress*, pp. 42, 48; Devisse J. *The Image of the Black in Western Art* (Part 2. *From the Early Christian Era to the "Age of Discovery."* 1. *From the Demonic Threat to the Incarnation of Sainthood*), pp. 52, 50–119, 216 n. 70, 218 (n. 114, 117, 118, 122), 219 (n. 124, 125, 132); Lewis B. The African diaspora and the civilization of Islam; Lewis B. *Race and Slavery in the Middle East*, pp. 10, 52–53; Sanders R. *Lost Tribes and Promised Lands*.

69. Lewis B. The African diaspora and the civilization of Islam; Lewis B. *Race and Slavery in the Middle East*; Gordon M. *Slavery in the Arab World*, pp. 98–100; Drake SC. *Black Folk Here and There* (Vol. 2); Lyons AS, Petrucelli RJ. *Medicine: An Illustrated History*, pp. 264–317; Sigerist HE. *The Great Doctors*, pp. 78–94; Ackerknecht EH. *A Short History of Medicine*, pp. 79–93; Guthrie D. *A History of Medicine*, pp. 84–110.

70. Roberts JM. *The Penguin History of the World.* London: Penguin Books, 1990, pp. 498–507, 628–636, 521–530; Boorstin DJ. *The Discoverers.* New York: Random House, Inc., 1983; Two-volume illustrated deluxe edition, New York: Harry N. Abrams, 1991; Cohen IB. *Album of Science: From Leonardo to Lavoisier, 1450–1800.* New York: Charles Scribner's Sons, 1980; Luce HR. *Life's Picture History of Western Man*, pp. 71–100; Meadows J. *The Great Scientists.* New York: Oxford University Press, 1987, pp. 29–68; Wetterau B. *The New York Public Library Book of Chronologies*; Wood M. *The Barbarian West*. Part six, *Legacy*. A six-part Series (videotape). A production of Maryland Public Television and Central Independent Television, 1991.

71. Majno G. *The Healing Hand*, pp. 420–422; Sirasi NG. *Medieval and Early Renaissance Medicine*; Haeger K. *The Illustrated History of Surgery*, pp. 75–141; Rossetti L. *The University of Padua: An Outline of Its History*. Trieste, Italy: Edizioni LINT Trieste,

1983; Bullough VL. *The Development of Medicine as a Profession*; Lyons AS, Petrucelli RJ. *Medicine: An Illustrated History*, pp. 318–365; Finch CS. The African background of medical science.

72. Gould SJ. *The Mismeasure of Man*; Chase A. *The Legacy of Malthus*; Barzun J. *Race: A Study in Modern Superstition*. N.P., 1937. Barzun J. *Race: A Study in Superstition*. revised ed. New York: Harper & Row, 1965; Reed J. Scientific racism;" Brandt AM. Racism and research; Jones JH. *Bad Blood*; Thomas SB, Quinn SC. Public health then and now: The Tuskegee syphilis study, 1932 to 1972: Implications for HIV education and AIDS risk education programs in the black community. *American Journal of Public Health* 1991; 81:1498–1504.

73. Stannard DE. *American Holocaust: Columbus and the Conquest of the New World*. New York: Oxford University Press, 1992, p. 209.

74. Lyons AS, Petrucelli RJ. *Medicine: An Illustrated History*, pp. 368–423; Sirasi NG. *Medieval and Early Renaissance Medicine; Doctors and Slaves: A Medical and Demographic History of Slavery in the British West Indies, 1680–1834*. Cambridge: Cambridge University Press, 1985; Sigerist HE. *The Great Doctors*, pp. 95–137; Bender GA. *Great Moments in Medicine*, pp. 76–91; Rogers JA. *Nature Knows No Color Line: Research into the Negro Ancestry in the White Race*. 3rd ed. St. Petersburg, FL: Helga M. Rogers, 1980. p. 20; Stannard DE. *American Holocaust*.

75. Sanders R. *Lost Tribes and Promised Lands*; Du Bois WEB. *The Suppression of the African Slave Trade to the United States of America, 1638–1870*. N.P., 1896; reprint, Baton Rouge: Louisiana State University Press, 1969; Davidson B. *The African Slave Trade*; Numbers RL, ed. *Medicine in the New World*; Sheridan RB. *Doctors and Slaves*.

76. Scobie E. African women in early Europe. In: Van Sertima, I, ed. *African Presence in Early Europe*, pp. 203–222; quote p. 203.

77. Scobie E. African women in early Europe; Scobie E. The black in Western Europe. In: Van Sertima, I, ed. *African Presence in Early Europe*, pp. 190–202; Honour H. *The Image of the Black in Western Art* (Part IV. *From the American Revolution to World War I. 1. Slaves and Liberators*). Cambridge: The Menil Foundation, distributed by Harvard University Press, 1989; Honour H. *The Image of the Black in Western Art* (Part IV. *From the American Revolution to World War I. 2. Black Models and White Myths*). Cambridge: The Menil Foundation, distributed by Harvard University Pres, 1989.

78. Stannard DE. *American Holocaust*; Sanders R. *Lost Tribes and Promised Lands*.

79. Viola HJ, Margolis C. *Seeds of Change: A Quincentennial Commemoration*. Washington: Smithsonian Institution Press, 1991; Thomas H. The Slave Trade: *The Story of the Atlantic Slave Trade: 1440–1870*. New York: Simon and Schuster, 1997. Dor-Ner Z, Sheller WG. *Columbus and the Age of Discovery*. New York: William Morrow and Company, 1991; Everett S. *The Slaves: An Illustrated History of the Monstrous Evil*. New York: G.P. Putnam's Sons, 1978; Stannard DE. *American Holocaust*; Sanders R. *Lost Tribes and Promised Lands*; Freyre G. *The Masters and the Slaves: A Study in the Development of Brazilian Civilization*. New York: Knopf, 1956.

80. Kiple KF, King VH. *Another Dimension to the Black Diaspora: Diet, Disease, and Racism*. Cambridge, England: Cambridge University Press, 1981; Savitt TL. *Medicine and Slavery: The Diseases and Health Care of Blacks in Antebellum Virginia*. Urbana: University of Illinois Press, 1987; Savitt T. Black health on the plantation: Masters, slaves, and physicians. In: Leavitt JW, Numbers RL, eds. *Sickness and Health in America: Readings in the History of Medicine and Public Health*, pp. 313–330; Davidson B. *The African*

Slave Trade; Du Bois WEB. *The Negro.* New York: Henry Holt, 1915; reprint ed., London: Oxford University Press, 1970; Sheridan RB. *Doctors and Slaves.*

81. Ransford O. *Bid the Sicness Cease*, p. 7.

82. Ransford O. *Bid the Sickness Cease*, pp. 1–53; Savitt TL. *Medicine and Slavery*; Sheridan RB. *Doctors and Slaves.*

83. Davidson B. *The African Slave Trade*, pp. 95–101, 271–283; Klein HS. *The Middle Passage: Comparative Studies in the Atlantic Slave Trade.* Princeton, NJ: Princeton University Press, 1978, pp. 228–251; Curtin PD. *The Atlantic Slave Trade: A Census.* Madison: The University of Wisconsin Press, 1969, pp. 265–273, 275–286.

84. Dow GF. *Slave Ships and Slaving.* Salem, MA: Marine Research Society, 1927; reprint ed., Toronto: Coles Publishing Company, 1980; Ransford O. *Bid the Sickness Cease*, p. 7; Everett S. *The Slaves: An Illustrated History of the Monstrous Evil*; Davidson B. *The African Slave Trade*; Davidson B. *Africa* (videotapes); Kiple KF, King VH. *Another Dimension to the Black Diaspora*; Mannix DP, Cowley M. *Cargoes: The Atlantic Slave Trade, 1518–1865.* New York: Viking Press, 1962; Mazrui AA. *The Africans* (videotapes); Mazrui AA. *The Africans: A Triple Heritage*; Sheridan RB. *Doctors and Slaves*; Viola HJ, Margolis C. *Seeds of Change.*

85. Sheridan RB. *Doctors and Slaves*, p. 132.

86. Sheridan RB. *Doctors and Slaves*, p. 132.

87. Sheridan RB. *Doctors and Slaves*, p. 109.

88. Dow GF. *Slave Ships and Slaving*, pp. 6, 108–109, 140–141, 167; Mannix DP, Cowley M. *Cargoes: The Atlantic Slave Trade, 1518–1865*; Sheridan RB. *Doctors and Slaves*, pp. 109–114; Viola HJ, Margolis C. *Seeds of Change*; Pope-Hennessy J. *Sins of the Fathers: A Study of the Atlantic Slave Traders, 1441–1807.* New York: Knopf, 1967; reprint ed., New York: Capricorn Books, 1969, p. 78.

89. Ransford O. *Bid the Sickness Cease*, pp. 27–35; Sheridan RB. *Doctors and Slaves*, pp. 72–75, 82–96, 227, 314; Savitt TL. *Medicine and Slavery*, pp. 171–184; Jordan WC. Voodoo medicine. In: RA Williams, ed. *Textbook of Black-Related Diseases*, pp. 715–738; Diop CA. *Precolonial Black Africa: A Comparative Study of the Political and Social Systems of Europe and Black Africa, from Antiquity to the Formation of Modern States.* Westport, CT: Lawrence Hill and Company, 1987; Byrd WM, Clayton LA. The "slave health deficit"; Finch CS. The African background of medical science.

90. Viola HJ, Margolis C. *Seeds of Change*; Gratus J. *The Great White Lie: Slavery, Emancipation, and Changing Racial Attitudes.* New York: Monthly Review Press, 1973; Sheridan RB. *Doctors and Slaves*; Savitt TL. *Medicine and Slavery.*

91. Sheridan RB. *Doctors and Slaves*; Gratus J. *The Great White Lie*; Dow GF. *Slave Ships and Slaving*; Katz WL. *Black People Who Made the Old West.* New York: Thomas Y. Crowell Company, 1977; reprint ed., Trenton, NJ: Africa World Press, 1992, pp. 3–9.

Chapter Three

1. Risse GB. Medicine in New Spain. In: Numbers RL, ed. *Medicine in the New World: New Spain, New France, and New England.* Knoxville: The University of Tennessee Press, 1987, pp. 12–63; quote p. 29.

2. Numbers RL, ed. *Medicine in the New World*; Stannard DE. *American Holocaust: Columbus and the Conquest of the New World*. New York: Oxford University Press, 1992; Burns R, Ades L. *The Way West: The Way the West Was Lost and Won, 1845–1893* (videotape). A six-hour documentary series for *The American Experience*, Boston: WGBH Educational Foundation, WGBH, Boston, 1995; Williams E. *From Columbus to Castro: The History of the Caribbean, 1492–1969*. London: Andre Deutsche Limited, 1970; paperback ed., New York: Vintage Books, 1984; Bender GA. *Great Moments in Medicine*. Detroit: Northwood Institute Press, 1966, p. 208; Field Enterprises. *The World Book Encyclopedia*. Chicago: Field Enterprises, 1957; Grolier Electronic Publishing. *The New Grolier Multimedia Encyclopedia* (Release 6, MPC Version). Novato, CA: The Software Toolworks, 1993; Sheridan RB. *Doctors and Slaves: A Medical and Demographic History of Slavery in the British West Indies, 1680–1834*. Cambridge: Cambridge University Press, 1985.

3. Risse GB. Medicine in New Spain; Stannard DE. *American Holocaust*; Thomas H. *The Slave Trade: The Story of the Atlantic Slave Trade: 1440–1870*. New York: Simon and Schuster, 1997; Williams E. From Columbus to Castro; Numbers R, ed. *Medicine in the New World*; Field Enterprises. *The World Book Encyclopedia*; Grolier Electronic Publishing. *The New Grolier Multimedia Encyclopedia* (Release 6, MPC Version); Sheridan RB. *Doctors and Slaves*; August I. *A Pictorial History of the Slave Trade*. Geneva: Minerva, 1971.

4. Risse GB. Medicine in New Spain; Stannard DE. *American Holocaust*; Thomas H. *The Slave Trade: The Story of the Atlantic Slave Trade: 1440–1870*. New York: Simon and Schuster, 1997; Williams E. *From Columbus to Castro*; Numbers R, ed. *Medicine in the New World*; Field Enterprises. *The World Book Encyclopedia*; Grolier Electronic Publishing. *The New Grolier Multimedia Encyclopedia* (Release 6, MPC Version); Sheridan RB. *Doctors and Slaves*.

5. Stannard DE. *American Holocaust*, p. 204.

6. Williams E. *From Columbus to Castro*; Numbers R, ed. *Medicine in the New World*; Thomas H. *The Slave Trade: The Story of the Atlantic Slave Trade: 1440–1870*. New York: Simon and Schuster, 1997; Davis DB. *The Problem of Slavery in Western Culture*. Ithaca, NY: Cornell University Press, 1966, pp. 165–223; Davis DB. *Slavery and Human Progress*. New York: Oxford University Press, 1984, pp. 51–82; Sanders R. *Lost Tribes and Promised Lands: The Origins of American Racism*. Boston: Little, Brown, 1978, pp. 112–165; Field Enterprises. *The World Book Encyclopedia*; Grolier Electronic Publishing. *The New Grolier Multimedia Encyclopedia* (Release 6, MPC Version); Sheridan RB. *Doctors and Slaves*; Stannard DE. *American Holocaust*.

7. August I. *A Pictorial History of the Slave Trade*, p. 7.

8. Stannard DE. *American Holocaust*; Williams E. *From Columbus to Castro*; Numbers R, ed. *Medicine in the New World*; Thomas H. *The Slave Trade: The Story of the Atlantic Slave Trade: 1440–1870*. New York: Simon and Schuster, 1997; Davis DB. *The Problem of Slavery in Western Culture*, pp. 165–223; Sanders R. *Lost Tribes and Promised Lands*, pp. 112–165; Field Enterprises. *The World Book Encyclopedia*; Grolier Electronic Publishing. *The New Grolier Multimedia Encyclopedia* (Release 6, MPC Version); Sheridan RB. *Doctors and Slaves*.

9. Jordan WD. *White over Black: American Attitudes toward the Negro, 1550–1812*. N.P.: University of North Carolina Press, 1968; Norton Library ed., New York: W.W. Norton, 1977.

10. Higginbotham AL. *In the Matter of Color: Race and the American Legal Process, the Colonial Period*. New York: Oxford University Press, 1978, p. 53.

11. Higginbotham AL. *In the Matter of Color,* p. 54.

12. Higginbotham AL. *In the Matter of Color: Race and the American Legal Process, The Colonial Period.* New York: Oxford University Press, 1978; Reed J. "Scientific Racism." 1358–1360. In Wilson CR, Ferris W, eds. *Encyclopedia of Southern Culture.* Chapel Hill: The University of North Carolina Press, 1989; Lauber AW. *Indian Slavery in Colonial Times Within the Present Limits of the United States.* New York, 1913. reprint ed. Williamstown, MA: Corner House Publishers, 1979; Jones JH. *Bad Blood: The Tuskegee Syphilis Experiment.* New York: The Free Press, 1981, pp. 1–29; Thomas H. *The Slave Trade: The Story of the Atlantic Slave Trade: 1440–1870.* New York: Simon and Schuster, 1997; Johnson C, Smith P. *Africans in America: America's Journey through Slavery.* New York: Harcourt, Brace, 1998; Morgan ES. *American Slavery American Freedom: The Ordeal of Colonial Virginia.* New York: W.W. Norton and Company, 1975.

13. Jones JH. *Bad Blood: The Tuskegee Syphilis Experiment.* New York: The Free Press, 1981, pp. 14, 28.

14. Devisse J. *The Image of the Black in Western Art* (Part 2, *From the Early Christian Era to the "Age of Discovery."* 1. *From the Demonic Threat to the Incarnation of Sainthood*). Cambridge, MA: The Menil Foundation, distributed by the Harvard University Press, 1979; Leiris M. Race and culture, pp. 85–122. In: UNESCO. *The Race Question in Modern Science.* New York: Whiteside Inc., and William Morrow Company, 1956; United Nations Educational, Scientific and Cultural Organization; Gossett TF. *Race: The History of an Idea in America.* Dallas, TX: Southern Methodist University Press, 1963; reprint ed., New York: Schocken Books, 1965, pp. 14–16; Marshall PJ, Williams G. *The Great Map of Mankind: Perceptions of New Worlds in the Age of Enlightenment.* Cambridge, MA: Harvard University Press, 1982, p. 228; Lévi-Strauss C. Race and history, pp. 123–163. In: UNESCO. *The Race Question in Modern Science.* New York: Whiteside Inc., and William Morrow Company, 1956; Davis DB. *The Problem of Slavery in Western Culture.*

15. Sevitt TL. *Medicine and Slavery: The Diseases and Health Care of Blacks in Antebellum Virginia.* Urbana: University of Illinois Press, 1987; Sheridan RB. *Doctors and Slaves: A Medical and Demographic History of Slavery in the British West Indies.* Cambridge: Cambridge University Press, 1985; Thomas H. *The Slave Trade: The Story of the Atlantic Slave Trade: 1440–1870.* New York: Simon and Schuster, 1997; Bell E. Slaves in the Family. New York: Ballantine Books, 1998; Rosenberg CE. *The Care of Strangers: The Rise of America's Hospital System.* New York: Basic Books, 1987; Rosenberg CE. Community and communities: The evolution of the American hospital. In: Long DE, Golden J, eds. *The American General Hospital: Communities and Social Contexts.* Ithaca, NY: Cornell University Press, 1989, pp. 3–17; Gossett, TF. *Race: The History of an Idea in America,* pp. 14–16; Lovejoy AO. *The Great Chain of Being: A Study of the History of an Idea.* Cambridge, MA: Harvard University Press, 1936; reprint paperback ed., 1964.

16. Ransford O. *Bid the Sickness Cease: Disease in the History of Black Africa.* London: John Murray (Publishers), 1983; Savitt TL. *Medicine and Slavery: The Diseases and Health Care of Blacks in Antebellum Virginia.* Urbana: University of Illinois Press, 1987; Sheridan RB. *Doctors and Slaves;* Kiple KF, King VH. *Another Dimension to the Black Diaspora: Diet, Disease, and Racism.* Cambridge, England: Cambridge University Press, 1981; August I. *A Pictorial History of the Slave Trade.*

17. Coles R. *The Nation* June 20, 1966.

18. Bullough B, Bullough VL. *Poverty, Ethnic Identity, and Health Care.* New York: Appleton-Century-Crofts, 1972; Dula A. Toward an African American perspective on

bioethics. *Journal of Health Care for the Poor and Underserved* 1991; 2:259–269; Jones JH. *Bad Blood: The Tuskegee Syphilis Experiment.* New York: The Free Press, 1981; Byrd WM. "Widening Racial Health Disparities: A Continuum." A presentation in Turning Back the Clock: Widening Health Differentials in Urban Areas, sponsored by Medical Care Forum on Bioethics, American Public Health Association, 120th Annual Meeting and Exhibition, Washington, D.C., November 9, 1992; Byrd WM, Clayton LA. An American health dilemma: A history of blacks in the health system. *Journal of the National Medical Association* 1992; 84:189–200; Morais HM. *The History of the Negro in Medicine.* Under auspices of The Association for the Study of Negro Life and History. New York: Publishers Company, Inc., 1967, pp. 154–158; Veatch RM. *A Theory of Medical Ethics.* New York: Basic Books, 1981.

19. Blanton WB. *Medicine in Virginia in the Eighteenth Century.* Richmond: Garrett and Massie, 1931, p. 157.

20. Sheridan RB. *Doctors and Slaves,* p. 115.

21. Klein HS. *The Middle Passage: Comparative Studies in the Atlantic Slave Trade.* Princeton, NJ: Princeton University Press, 1978; Sheridan RB. *Doctors and Slaves;* Ransford O. *Bid the Sickness Cease;* Huggins NI. *Black Odyssey: The Afro-American Ordeal in Slavery.* New York: Pantheon Books, 1977; reprint ed., New York: Vintage Books, 1979; Byrd WM. *The Color Line: Race and Medicine in America.* Unpublished manuscript, Fort Worth, Texas, Summer 1985.

22. Blanton WB. *Medicine in Virginia in the Seventeenth Century.* Richmond: The William Byrd Press, 1930, p. 74.

23. Blanton WB. *Medicine in Virginia in the Seventeenth Century;* Savitt T. Black health on the plantation: Masters, slaves, and physicians. In: Leavitt JW, Numbers RL, eds. *Sickness and Health in America: Readings in the History of Medicine and Public Health.* Madison: The University of Wisconsin Press, 1985, pp. 313–330; Savitt TL. *Medicine and Slavery;* August I. *A Pictorial History of the Slave Trade.*

24. Starr P. *The Social Transformation of American Medicine.* New York: Basic Books, 1982, p. 7.

25. Starr P. *The Social Transformation of American Medicine,* p. 7.

26. Blanton WB. *Medicine in Virginia in the Seventeenth Century;* Savitt T. Black health on the plantation; Savitt TL. *Medicine and Slavery.*

27. Elkins SM. *Slavery: A Problem in American Institutional and Intellectual Life.* 3rd ed. Chicago: The University of Chicago Press, 1976, p. 1.

28. Higginbotham AL. *In the Matter of Color,* pp. 155–156.

29. Curtis JL. *Blacks, Medical Schools, and Society.* Ann Arbor: The University of Michigan Press, 1971; Dowling HF. *City Hospitals: The Undercare of the Underprivileged.* Cambridge, MA: Harvard University Press, 1982; Ginzberg E. *The Medical Triangle: Physicians, Politicians, and the Public.* Cambridge, MA: Harvard University Press, 1990; Byrd WM, Clayton LA. An American health dilemma: A history of blacks in the health system. *Journal of the National Medical Association* 1992; 84:189–200; Higginbotham AL. *In the Matter of Color: Race and the American Legal Process, the Colonial Period.* New York: Oxford University Press, 1978, pp. 54–55, 121, 177–178, 198–199, 249–250, 253–254, 258, 263, 279, 282; Health Policy Advisory Center. The emerging health apartheid in the United States. *Health/PAC Bulletin* 1991; 21:3–4; Kotelchuck R. Down and out in the "New Calcutta": New York City's health care crisis. *Health/PAC Bulletin* 1989 (Summer); 19:4–11; Kurtis B. *Slavery's Buried Past.* Documentary video segment for

The New Explorers, Boston, WGBH, December 18, 1996; Sheridan RB. *Doctors and Slaves: A Medical and Demographic History of Slavery in the British West Indies, 1680–1834*. Cambridge: Cambridge University Press, 1985.

30. Rosenberg CE. *The Care of Strangers*, p. 301.

31. Rosenberg CE. *The Care of Strangers*, p. 302.

32. Starr P. *The Social Transformation of American Medicine*, pp. 30–59.

33. Starr P. *The Social Transformation of American Medicine*, pp. 30–59; Savitt TL. *Medicine and Slavery*: Manning KR. Health and health care providers. In: Salzman J, Smith DL, West C. eds. *Encyclopedia of African-American Culture and History*. 5 Vols. New York: Macmillan Library Reference USA, Simon and Schuster Macmillan, 1996, pp. 1247–1255; Morais HM. *The History of the Negro in Medicine*. Under auspices of The Association for the Study of Negro Life and History. New York: Publishers Company, 1967.

34. Manning KR. Folk medicine. In: Salzman J, Smith DL, West C, eds. *Encyclopedia of African American Culture and History*. New York: Macmillan Library Reference USA, 1996, pp. 1002–1003; Jones JH. *Bad Blood: The Tuskegee Syphilis Experiment*. New York: The Free Press, 1981; Byrd WM. Race, biology, and health care: Reassessing a relationship. *Journal of Health Care for the Poor and Underserved* 1990; 1:278–292; Reed J. Scientific racism. In Wilson CR, Ferris W, eds. *Encyclopedia of Southern Culture*. Chapel Hill: The University of North Carolina Press, 1989, pp. 1358–1360; Brandt AM. Racism and research: The case of the Tuskegee Syphilis Study. In: Leavitt JW, Numbers RL, eds. *Sickness and Health in America: Readings in the History of Medicine and Public Health*. Madison: The University of Wisconsin Press, 1985, pp. 331–343; Duffy J. States' rights medicine. In Wilson CR, W Ferris, eds. *Encyclopedia of Southern Culture*. Chapel Hill: The University of North Carolina Press, 1989; pp. 1355–1356.

35. Blanton WB. *Medicine in Virginia in the Seventeenth Century*. Richmond: The William Byrd Press, 1930, p. 3; Cray E. *In Failing Health: The Medical Crisis and the A.M.A*. Indianapolis: Bobbs-Merrill, 1970; Numbers RL. *Almost Persuaded: American Physicians and Compulsory Health Insurance, 1912–1920*. Baltimore: The Johns Hopkins University Press, 1978; Brown ER. *Rockefeller Medicine Men: Medicine and Capitalism in America*. Berkeley: University of California Press, 1979; Newman DK, Amidei NJ, Carter BL, et al. Second class medicine. In: *Protest, Politics, and Prosperity: Black Americans and White Institutions, 1940–75*. New York: Pantheon Books, 1978, pp. 187–235.

36. Davidson B. *Black Mother: The African Slave Trade*. Boston: Little, Brown. *The African Slave Trade*. Boston: Little, Brown, 1980, p. 284.

37. Davidson B. *The African Slave Trade*; Savitt T. Black health on the plantation: Masters, slaves, and physicians. In: Leavitt JW, Numbers RL, eds. *Sickness and Health in America*, pp. 313–330; Savitt TL. *Medicine and Slavery*; Owens LH. *This Species of Property: Slave Life and Culture in the Old South*. Oxford: Oxford University Press, 1976; Kurtis B. *Slavery's Buried Past*.

38. Bousefield MO. An account of physicians of color in the United States. *Bulletin of the History of Medicine* 1945; 17:61–84; Cobb WM. The black American in medicine. *Journal of the National Medical Association* 1981; 73 (Suppl 1):1183–1244; Byrd WM, Clayton LA. The "slave health deficit": Racism and health outcomes. *Health/PAC Bulletin* 1991; 21:25–28; Curtis JL. *Blacks, Medical Schools, and Society*. Ann Arbor: The University of Michigan Press, 1971; Savitt TL. *Medicine and Slavery*; Sheridan RB. *Doctors and Slaves*; Morais HM. *The History of the Negro in Medicine*. New York: Publishers Company, 1967.

39. Morais HM. *The History of the Negro in Medicine*; Byrd WM. Race, biology, and health care; Byrd WM, Clayton LA. The "slave health deficit"; Sutch R. The care and feeding of slaves. In: David PA, Gutman HG, Sutch R, et al. *Reckoning with Slavery: A Critical Study in the Quantitative History of American Negro Slavery*. New York: Oxford University Press, 1976, pp. 231–301; Blanton WB. *Medicine in Virginia in the Seventeenth Century*; Blanton WB. *Medicine in Virginia in the Eighteenth Century*; Bousefield MO. An account of physicians of color in the United States; Cobb WM. 1981. The black American in medicine; Savitt TL. *Medicine and Slavery*; Manson-Bahr PEC, Bell DR. *Manson's Tropical Diseases*. 19th ed. London: Baillière Tindall, 1987; Sheridan RB. *Doctors and Slaves*.

Chapter Four

1. Ackerknecht EH. *A Short History of Medicine*. Rev. ed. Baltimore: The Johns Hopkins University Press, 1982; Sanders R. *Lost Tribes and Promised Lands: The Origins of American Racism*. Boston: Little, Brown, 1978; Stannard DE. *American Holocaust: Columbus and the Conquest of the New World*. New York: Oxford University Press, 1992; Viola HJ, Margolis C. *Seeds of Change: A Quincentennial Commemoration*. Washington, DC: Smithsonian Institution Press, 1991; Grolier Electronic Publishing. United States history. In: *The New Grolier Multimedia Encyclopedia*. Release 6, MPC Version. Novato, CA: The Software Toolworks, 1993; Field Enterprises. United States, history of. In: *The World Book Encyclopedia: In Eighteen Volumes and Reading and Study Guide* (Vol. 17). Chicago: Field Enterprises, 1957, pp. 8328–8358.

2. Ackerknecht EH. *A Short History of Medicine*; Numbers RL, ed. *Medicine in the New World: New Spain, New France, and New England*. Knoxville: The University of Tennessee Press, 1987; Stevens R. *American Medicine and the Public Interest*. New Haven, CT: Yale University Press, 1971; Grolier Electronic Publishing United States history; Field Enterprises. United States, history of.

3. Ackerknecht EH. *A Short History of Medicine*. Rev. ed., pp. 218–219.

4. Ackerknecht EH. *A Short History of Medicine*. Rev. ed., pp. 218–226.

5. Ackerknecht EH. *A Short History of Medicine*. Rev. Ed.; Numbers RL, ed. *Medicine in the New World*; Byrd WM, Clayton LA. An American health dilemma: A history of blacks in the health system. *Journal of the National Medical Association*, 1992; 84:189–200; Morais HM. *The History of the Negro in Medicine*. New York: Publishers Company, 1967; Savitt TL. *Medicine and Slavery: The Diseases and Health Care of Blacks in Antebellum Virginia*. Urbana: University of Illinois Press, 1987; Bernstein RB, Rice KS. *Are We To Be a Nation? The Making of the Constitution*. Cambridge, MA: Harvard University Press, 1987; Grolier Electronic Publishing. United States history; Field Enterprises. United States, history of.

6. Elkins SM. *Slavery: A Problem in American Institutional and Intellectual Life*. 3rd ed. Chicago: The University of Chicago Press, 1976, p. 47.

7. Bennett L. *Before the Mayflower: A History of the Negro in America, 1619–1964*. Rev. ed. Chicago: Johnson Publishing Company, 1961; paperback ed., Baltimore: Penguin Books, 1966; Davis DB. *The Problem of Slavery in Western Culture*. Ithaca, NY: Cornell University Press, 1966, p. 340; Davis DB. *The Problem of Slavery in the Age of*

Revolution, 1770–1823. Ithaca, NY: Cornell University Press, 1975; Wilson CR, W Ferris, eds. *Encyclopedia of Southern Culture.* Chapel Hill: The University of North Carolina Press, 1989; Elkins SM. *Slavery: A Problem in American Institutional and Intellectual Life.* 3rd ed.; Genovese ED. *The Political Economy of Slavery: Studies in the Economy and Society of the Slave South.* New York: Vintage Books, 1965; Genovese ED. *The World the Slaveholders Made: Two Essays in Interpretation.* New York: Pantheon Books, 1969; paperback ed., Middletown, CT: Wesleyan University Press, 1988; Tannenbaum F. *Slave and Citizen: The Negro in the Americas.* New York: Knopf, 1946; paperback ed., New York: Vintage Books, N.D.; Huggins NI. *Black Odyssey: The Afro-American Ordeal in Slavery.* New York: Pantheon Books, 1977; reprint ed., New York: Vintage Books, 1979; Williams E. *From Columbus to Castro: The History of the Caribbean, 1492–1969.* London: Andre Deutsche Limited, 1970; paperback ed., New York: Vintage Books, 1984; Takaki RY. *Iron Cages: Race and Culture in Nineteenth-Century America.* New York: Knopf, 1979; Grolier Electronic Publishing. United States history; Field Enterprises. United States, history of; Starr P. *The Social Transformation of American Medicine.* New York: Basic Books, 1982.

8. Novotny A, Smith C, eds. *Images of Healing: A Portfolio of American Medical and Pharmaceutical Practice in the 18th, 19th, and Early 20th Centuries.* New York: Macmillan, 1980; Rosenberg CE. *The Care of Strangers: The Rise of America's Hospital System.* New York: Basic Books, 1987; Dowling HF. *City Hospitals: The Undercare of the Underprivileged.* Cambridge, MA: Harvard University Press, 1982; Davis DB. *The Problem of Slavery in the Age of Revolution, 1770–1823;* Stampp KM. *The Peculiar Institution: Slavery in the Ante-Bellum South.* New York: Knopf, 1956, reprint ed., New York: Vintage Books, 1956; Grolier Electronic Publishing. United States history; Field Enterprises. United States, history of.

9. Postell WD. *The Health of Slaves on Southern Plantations.* Baton Rouge: Louisiana State University Press, 1951. Reprinted Gloucester, MA: Peter Smith, 1970; Bennett L. *Before the Mayflower;* Davis DB. *The Problem of Slavery in Westrn Culture,* p. 340; Davis DB. *The Problem of Slavery in the Age of Revolution, 1770–1823;* Wilson CR, W Ferris, eds. *Encyclopedia of Southern Culture;* Elkins SM. *Slavery: A Problem in American Institutional and Intellectual Life.* 3rd ed.; Genovese ED. *The Political Economy of Slavery;* Genovese ED. *The World the Slaveholders Made;* Tannenbaum F. *Slave and Citizen;* Huggins NI. *Black Odyssey;* Williams E. *From Columbus to Castro;* Takaki RY. *Iron Cages;* Grolier Electronic Publishing. United States history; Field Enterprises. United States, history of; Starr P. *The Social Transformation of American Medicine.*

10. Fitzhugh G. *A Sociology for the South; or, The Failure of Free Society.* Richmond, VA: A. Morris, 1854; Fitzhugh G. *Cannibals All! or, Slaves without Masters.* Richmond, VA: A. Morris, 1857; Genovese ED. *The World the Slaveholders Made;* Elkins SM. *Slavery: A Problem in American Institutional and Intellectual Life.* 3rd ed.; Gossett TF. *Race: The History of an Idea in America.* Dallas, TX: Southern Methodist University Press, 1963, reprint ed., New York: Schocken Books, 1965; Fredrickson GM. *The Black Image in the White Mind;* Takaki RY. *Iron Cages;* Roberts J. *The Triumph of the West.* Boston: Little, Brown, 1985.

11. Gossett TF. *Race: The History of an Idea in America;* Davis DB. *The Problem of Slavery in the Age of Revolution, 1770–1823.* Bilstein RE. Technology. In: Wilson CR, W Ferris, eds. *Encyclopedia of Southern Culture,* pp. 1363–1364; Elkins SM. *Slavery: A Problem in American Institutional and Intellectual Life.* 3rd ed.; Genovese ED. *The Political*

Economy of Slavery; Genovese ED. *The World the Slaveholders Made*; Takaki RY. *Iron Cages*.

12. Ransford O. *Bid the Sickness Cease: Disease in the History of Black Africa*. London: John Murray Publishers, 1983, pp. 138–139; Parkinson W. *This Gilded African: Toussaint L'Overture*. London: Quartet Books, 1980; James CLR. *The Black Jacobins: Toussaint L'Ouverture and and the San Domingo Revolution*. 2nd rev. ed. New York: Vintage Books, 1963.

13. Ransford O. *Bid the Sickness Cease*, pp. 138–139.

14. Bernstein RB, Rice KS. *Are We To Be a Nation?*, pp. 161–171, 175–178; Davis DB. *The Problem of Slavery in the Age of Revolution, 1770–1823*; Grolier Electronic Publishing. United States history; Field Enterprises. United States, history of.

15. Smillie WG. The period of great epidemics in the United States (1800–1875). In: Winslow CEA, et al., eds., *The History of American Epidemiology*. St. Louis: Mosby, 1952, p. 69.

16. Rothstein WG. *American Physicians in the 19th Century: From Sects to Science*. Baltimore, Maryland: The Johns Hopkins University Press, 1972, p. 55.

17. Sigerist HE. An outline of the development of the hospital. *Bulletin of the Institute of the History of Medicine*. 1936; 4:573–581; Vogel MJ. *The Invention of the Modern Hospital: Boston 1870–1930*. Chicago: University of Chicago Press, 1980, pp. 1–2.

18. Dowling HF. *City Hospitals: The Undercare of the Underprivileged*, p. 12.

19. Novotny A, Smith C, eds. *Images of Healing*, p. 13.

20. Rosenberg CE. *The Care of Strangers*; Novotny A, Smith C, eds. *Images of Healing*; Vogel MJ. *The Invention of the Modern Hospital*; Sigerist HE. An outline of the development of the hospital, pp. 573–581.

21. Dowling HF. *City Hospitals*; Shryock RH. *Medicine in America: Historical Essays*. Baltimore: The Johns Hopkins Press, 1966; Vogel MJ. *The Invention of the Modern Hospital: Boston 1870–1930*; Novotny A, Smith C, eds. *Images of Healing*; Lyons AS, Petrucelli RJ. *Medicine: An Illustrated History*. New York: Harry N. Abrams, 1978; Savitt TL. *Medicine and Slavery*; Starr P. *The Social Transformation of American Medicine*; Rosenberg CE. *The Care of Strangers*.

22. Dowling HF. *City Hospitals*; Shryock RH. *Medicine in America*; Vogel MJ. *The Invention of the Modern Hospital: Boston 1870–1930*; Novotny A, Smith C, eds. *Images of Healing*; Lyons AS, Petrucelli RJ. *Medicine: An Illustrated History*; Savitt TL. *Medicine and Slavery*; Starr P. *The Social Transformation of American Medicine*; Rosenberg CE. *The Care of Strangers*.

23. Nuland SB. *Doctors: The Biography of Medicine*. New York: Knopf, 1988; Jordan WD. *White over Black: American Attitudes toward the Negro, 1550–1812*. New York: W. W. Norton, 1968, pp. 218–223, 227, 246; Gould SJ. *The Mismeasure of Man*. New York: W.W. Norton, 1981, p. 35; Davis DB. *The Problem of Slavery in Western Culture*, pp. 453–455; Wassermann HP. *Ethnic Pigmentation: Historical, Psychological, and Clinical Aspects*. New York: American Elsevier Publishing Company, 1974, 26–38; Stannard DE. *American Holocaust: Columbus and the Conquest of the New World*. New York: Oxford University Press, 1992. 209.

24. Gossett TF. *Race: The History of an Idea in America*, p. 33.

25. Jordan WD. *White over Black*, p. 217.

26. Lewin R. *In the Age of Mankind*. Washington, DC: Smithsonian Books, 1988, pp. 18–22.

27. Jordan WD. *White over Black*, p. 32.

28. Jordan WD. *White over Black*, p. 217; Lewin R. *In the Age of Mankind*; Marshall PJ, Williams G. *The Great Map of Mankind: Perceptions of New Worlds in the Age of Enlightenment*. Cambridge, MA: Harvard University Press, 1982.

29. Gossett TF. *Race: The History of an Idea in America*, p. 32.

30. Jordan WD. *White over Black*, p. 217.

31. Jordan WD. *White over Black*, p. 218.

32. Jordan WD. *White over Black*, p. 217; Barzun J. *Race: A Study in Modern Superstition*. New York: Harper & Row, 1937. Barzun J. *Race: A Study in Superstition*. Rev. ed. New York: Harper & Row, 1965, pp. 34–35; Gossett TF. *Race: The History of an Idea in America*; Horsman R. *Race and Manifest Destiny: The Origins of American Racial Anglo-Saxonism*. Cambridge, MA: Harvard University Press, 1981.

33. Cohen IB. *Album of Science: From Leonardo to Lavoisier, 1450–1800*. New York: Charles Scribner's Sons, 1980, esp. Figure 311, p. 228.

34. Jordan WD. *White over Black*, pp. 226–227.

35. Boorstin DJ. The equality of the human species. In: Boorstin DJ, *Hidden History: Exploring Our Secret Past*. New York: Harper & Row, 1987, paperback ed., New York: Vintage Books, 1989, pp. 111–123; Gossett TF. *Race: The History of an Idea in America*, pp. 42–43, 51–53; Jordan WD. *White over Black*, pp. 430–481.

36. Boorstin DJ. The equality of the human species. 111–123. In: Boorstin DJ. *Hidden History: Exploring our Secret Past*. New York: Harper and Row Publishers, Inc., 1987. Paperback Edition. New York: Vintage Books, 1989; Haller JS. *Outcasts from Evolution: Scientific Attitudes of Racial Inferiority, 1859–1900*. New York: McGraw Hill Book Company, 1971; Haller JS, Haller RM. *The Physician and Sexuality in Victorian America*. N.P.: University of Illinois Press, 1974. Reprint Edition. New York: W.W. Norton, 1977; Reed J. "Scientific Racism." 1358–1360. In Wilson CR, Ferris W, eds. *Encyclopedia of Southern Culture*. Chapel Hill: The University of North Carolina Press, 1989; Jordan WD. *White Over Black: American Attitudes Toward the Negro, 1550–1812*. New York: W. W. Norton, 1968, p. 530.

37. Barzun J. *Race: A Study in Modern Superstition*; Barzun J. *Race: A Study in Superstition*; Gay P. *Age of Enlightenment. Great Ages of Man: A History of the World's Cultures*. New York: Time, 1965; Gossett TF. *Race: The History of an Idea in America*, p. 71; Haller JS. *Outcasts from Evolution*; Horsman R. *Race and Manifest Destiny*, pp. 54–55; Lyons AS, Petrucelli RJ. *Medicine: An Illustrated History*, p. 485; Magnusson M ed. *Cambridge Biographical Dictionary*. Cambridge: Cambridge University Press, 1990, p. 867; Stafford BM. *Body Criticism: Imaging the Unseen in Enlightenment Art and Medicine*. Cambridge, MA: MIT Press, 1991.

38. Haller JS Jr. *Outcasts from Evolution*, p. 4.

39. Haller JS Jr. *Outcasts from Evolution*, p. 5.

40. Haller JS Jr. *Outcasts from Evolution*, p. 5.

41. Haller JS Jr. *Outcasts from Evolution*, p. 5.

42. Jordan WD. *White over Black*, pp. 230, 236.

43. Beider RE. *Science Encounters the Indian, 1820–1880: The Early Years of American Ethnology*. Norman: University of Oklahoma Press, 1986; Boorstin DJ. *The Discoverers*. New York: Random House, 1983, two-volume illustrated deluxe ed. New York: Harry Abrams, 1991, pp. 666–679; Honour H. *The Image of the Black in Western Art (Part IV, From the American Revolution to World War I. 2. Black Models and White Myths)*. Cam-

bridge: The Menil Foundation, 1989; Jordon WD. *White over Black*; Magnusson M, ed. *Cambridge Biographical Dictionary*, pp. 225–226; Marshall PJ, Williams G. *The Great Map of Mankind*, pp. 244–246; Wendt H. *From Ape to Adam: The Search for the Ancestry of Man*. Indianapolis: Bobbs-Merrill, 1972.

44. Horsman R. *Race and Manifest Destiny*, p. 55.

45. Gossett TF. *Race: The History of an Idea in America*, p. 70.

46. Fredrickson GM. *The Black Image in the White Mind: The Debate on Afro-American Character and Destiny, 1871–1914*. New York: Harper & Row Publishers, 1971, reprint ed., Middletown, CT: Wesleyan University Press, 1987; Dunglison R. *Human Physiology with Three Hundred and Sixty-Eight Illustrations* (two vols., 6th ed.). Philadelphia: Lea and Blanchard, 1846; Beider RE. *Science Encounters the Indian, 1820–1880*, p. 61; Gossett TF. *Race: The History of an Idea in America*, pp. 69–70; Cogan T. *The Works of the Late Professor Camper on the Connexion Between the Science of Anatomy and the Arts of Drawing, Painting, Statuary: Containing a Treatise on the Natural Difference of Features in Persons of Different Countries and Periods of Life; And on Beauty, With a New Method of Sketching Heads, National Features, and Portraits of Individuals, with Accuracy, Illustrated with Seventeen Plates, Explanatory of the Professor's Leading Principles*. Two Books. A New Edition. London: J. Hearne, 1821; Honour H. *The Image of the Black in Western Art (Part IV. From the American Revolution to World War I. 2. Black Models and White Myths)*; Haller JS. *Outcasts from Evolution*, pp. 9–13; Horsman R. *Race and Manifest Destiny*, p. 55; Magnusson M., ed. *Cambridge Biographical Dictionary*, p. 254; Peck SR. *Atlas of Human Anatomy for the Artist*. Oxford: Oxford University Press, 1951, reprint ed., 1979, pp. 238–241; *Stedman's Medical Dictionary*, 21st ed., s.v. "Camper."

47. Winchell A. *Preadamites; or A Demonstration of the Existence of Men Before Adam; together with A Study of Their Condition, Antiquity, Racial Affinities, and Progressive Dispersion over the Earth*. Chicago: S. C. Griggs, 1880, pp. 71–73, 253–254; Berkowitz JS. *The College of Physicians of Philadelphia Portrait Catalogue*. Philadelphia: College of Physicians of Philadelphia, 1984, pp. 29–31; Byrd WM. Race, biology, and health care: Reassessing a relationship. *Journal of Health Care for the Poor and Underserved* 1990; 1:278–292; Gould SJ. *The Mismeasure of Man*; Gould SJ. The Hottentot Venus. In: Gould SJ, *The Flamingo's Smile: Reflections in Natural History*. New York: W. W. Norton, 1985, pp. 291–305; Honour H. *The Image of the Black in Western Art (Part IV, From the American Revolution to World War I. 2, Black Models and White Myths)*; Cambridge: Menil Foundation, Inc., Distributed by Harvard University Press, 1989; Jordon WD. *White over Black*; Magnusson M, ed. *Cambridge Biographical Dictionary*, p. 376. Nott JC, et al., *Indigenous Races of the Earth or, New Chapters of Ethnological Inquiry*. Philadelphia: J. B. Lippincott, 1857, p. 628; Stocking GW. French anthropology in 1800. In: *Race, Culture, and Evolution: Essays in the History of Anthropology*. New York: The Free Press, 1968, reprint ed. Chicago: The University of Chicago Press, 1982, pp. 30, 35, 39; Wendt H. *From Ape to Adam*.

48. Gould SJ. Bound by the great chain. In: *The Flamingo's Smile*, pp. 281–291.

49. Gould SJ. Bound by the great chain; Jordan WD. *White over Black*, pp. 499–502; Stanton W. *The Leopard's Spots: Scientific Attitudes toward Race in America, 1815–1859*. Chicago: The University of Chicago Press, 1960, pp. 16–18; Gossett TF. *Race: The History of an Idea in America*, pp. 47–51.

50. Jordan WD. *White over Black*, p. 518.

51. Bender GA. *Great Moments in Medicine*. Detroit: Northwood Institute Press, 1966; Gossett TF. *Race: The History of an Idea in America*, pp. 40–41; Jordon WD. *White over Black*, pp. 517–521; Stafford BM. *Body Criticism*, pp. 306–324; Proctor RN. *Racial Hygiene: Medicine under the Nazis*. Cambridge, MA: Harvard University Press, 1988, p. 10; Stanton W. *The Leopard's Spots*, pp. 6–7; Takaki RY. *Iron Cages*, pp. 30–34.

52. Boorstin DJ. The equality of the human species; Fredrickson GM. *The Black Image in the White Mind*, pp. 82–96; Gould SJ. *The Mismeasure of Man*, pp. 30–72; Chase A. *The Legacy of Malthus: The Social Costs of the New Scientific Racism*. New York: Knopf, 1980, pp. 2–322; Haller JS. *Outcasts from Evolution*; Haller JS, Haller RM. *The Physician and Sexuality in Victorian America*. Reprint ed. New York: W. W. Norton, 1977, pp. x, 52, 58; Jones JH. *Bad Blood: The Tuskegee Syphilis Experiment*. New York: The Free Press, 1981; Jordan WD. *White over Black*, p. 530.

53. Byrd WM, Clayton LA. Segment 2, *A History of Blacks in the Health System*. Segment 3, *Blacks in the Health Professions: Historical and Contemporary Issues*. From *A Black Health Trilogy* (videotape and 188-page documentary report). Washington, D.C.: The National Medical Association and the African American Heritage and Education Foundation; 1991; Byrd WM. *Documentary Report: Negro Diseases and Physiological Peculiarities*. Nashville: Cancer Control Research Unit, Meharry Medical College, July 12, 1990. In: Byrd WM, Clayton LA. *A Black Health Trilogy* (videotape and 188-page documentary report). Washington, DC: The National Medical Association and the African American Heritage and Education Foundation; 1991. Revised Edition. Washington, DC: The National Medical Association, 1994; Stampp KM. *The Peculiar Institution: Slavery in the Ante-Bellum South*. New York: Alfred A. Knopf, 1956. Reprint Edition. New York: Vintage Books, 1956; Byrd WM. Race, biology, and health care: Reassessing a relationship. *Journal of Health Care for the Poor and Underserved* 1990; 1:278–292; Byrd WM, Clayton LA. An American health dilemma: A history of blacks in the health system. *Journal of the National Medical Association* 1992; 84:189–200; Duffy J. States' Rights Medicine, pp. 1355–1356. In Wilson CR, W Ferris, eds. *Encyclopedia of Southern Culture*. Chapel Hill: The University of North Carolina Press, 1989; Byrd WM, Clayton LA. The "slave health deficit": Racism and health outcomes. *Health/PAC Bulletin* 1991; 21:25–28; Reed J. "Scientific Racism," pp. 1358–1360. In Wilson CR, Ferris W, eds. *Encyclopedia of Southern Culture*. Chapel Hill: The University of North Carolina Press, 1989; Brinkley A. *The Unfinished Nation: A Concise History of the American People*. New York: Alfred A. Knopf, 1993, pp. 302–303.

54. Ewbank DC. History of black mortality and health before 1940. In: Willis DP, ed., *Health Policies and Black Americans*. New Brunswick, NJ: Transaction Publishers, 1989, pp. 100–128; esp. pp. 125–126.

55. Ewbank DC. History of black mortality and health before 1940.

56. Reuter EB. *The American Race Problem*. Rev. 3rd ed. New York: Thomas Y. Crowell Company, 1970, p. 157.

57. Reuter EB. *The American Race Problem*, p. 157.

58. Reuter EB. *The American Race Problem*, p. 157.

59. Fogel RW. *Without Consent or Contract: The Rise and Fall of American Slavery*. New York: W. W. Norton, 1989, p. 128.

60. David PA, et al., eds. *Reckoning with Slavery: A Critical Study in the Quantitative History of American Negro Slavery*. New York: Oxford University Press, 1976, p. 284.

61. Ewbank DC. History of black mortality and health before 1940, p. 116.

62. Phillips UB. *American Negro Slavery: A Survey of the Supply, Employment and Control of Negro Labor As Determined by the Plantation Regime.* Paperback ed. Baton Rouge: Louisiana State University Press, 1966; Reuter EB. *The American Race Problem*; Ewbank DC. History of black mortality and health before 1940; Fogel RW. *Without Consent or Contract*, pp. 116–153; Steckel RH. Slave mortality: Analysis of evidence from plantation records. *Social Science History* 1979; 3:86–114; Farley R, Allen WR. *The Color Line and the Quality of Life in America.* New York: Oxford University Press, 1989; Farley R. *Growth of the Black Population: A Study of Demographic Trends.* Chicago: Markham, 1970; Sutch R. The care and feeding of slaves. In: David PA, et al., eds., *Reckoning with Slavery*, pp. 231–301; Savitt TL. *Medicine and Slavery*; Postell WD. *The Health of Slaves on Southern Plantations.*

63. Owens LH. *This Species of Property: Slave Life and Culture in the Old South.* Oxford: Oxford University Press, 1976; Savitt TL. Black health on the plantation: Masters, slaves, and physicians. In: Numbers RL, Savitt TL, eds. *Science and Medicine in the Old South.* Baton Rouge: Louisiana State University Press, 1989, pp. 327–355; Boles JB. *Black Southerners 1619–1869.* Lexington: The University of Kentucky Press, 1984; Reuter EB. *The American Race Problem*; Ewbank DC. History of black mortality and health before 1940; Fogel RW. *Without Consent or Contract*, pp. 116–153; Sutch R. The care and feeding of slaves; 1976; Savitt TL. *Medicine and Slavery*; Postell WD. *The Health of Slaves on Southern Plantations*; Manson-Bahr PEC, Bell DR. *Manson's Tropical Diseases.* 19th ed. London: Baillière Tindall, 1987.

64. Sutch R. The care and feeding of slaves, p. 278.

65. Owens LH. *This Species of Property*; Savitt TL. Black health on the Plantation; Boles JB. *Black Southerners 1619–1869*; Fogel RW. *Without Consent or Contract*, pp. 116–153; Sutch R. The care and feeding of slaves; Savitt TL. *Medicine and Slavery*; Postell WD. *The Health of Slaves on Southern Plantations.*

66. Owens LH. *This Species of Property*; Savitt TL. Black health on the Plantation; Boles JB. *Black Southerners 1619–1869*; Fogel RW. *Without Consent or Contract*, pp. 116–153; Sutch R. The care and feeding of slaves; Savitt TL. *Medicine and Slavery*; Postell WD. *The Health of Slaves on Southern Plantations.*

67. Savitt TL. Black health on the plantation, p. 343.

68. Genovese ED. *The Political Economy of Slavery*, pp. 159–167.

69. Owens LH. *This Species of Property*; Savitt TL. Black health on the plantation; Boles JB. *Black Southerners 1619–1869*; Fogel RW. *Without Consent or Contract*, pp. 116–153; Sutch R. The care and feeding of slaves; Savitt TL. *Medicine and Slavery*; Postell WD. *The Health of Slaves on Southern Plantations*; Thomas H. *The Slave Trade: The Story of the Atlantic Slave Trade: 1440–1870.* New York: Simon and Schuster, 1997. Isselbacher KJ, et al., eds. *Harrison's Principles of Internal Medicine.* 13th ed. New York: McGraw-Hill, 1994, pp. 628–630, 685–687, 740–743, 2474–2478.

70. Bancroft F. *Slave Trading in the Old South.* New York: Frederick Ungar Publishing, 1959; Tyler RC, Murphy LR, eds. *The Slave Narratives of Texas.* Austin: The Encino Press, 1974; Owens LH. *This Species of Property*; Savitt TL. Black health on the plantation; Boles JB. *Black Southerners 1619–1869*; Fogel RW. *Without Consent or Contract*, pp. 116–153; Sutch R. The care and feeding of slaves; Savitt TL. *Medicine and Slavery*; Postell WD. *The Health of Slaves on Southern Plantations.*

71. Savitt TL. Black health on the plantation, p. 343.

72. Owens LH. *This Species of Property*; Savitt TL. Black health on the plantation, pp. 327–355; Boles JB. *Black Southerners 1619–1869*; Fogel RW. *Without Consent or Contract*, pp. 116–153; Sutch R. The care and feeding of slaves; Savitt TL. *Medicine and Slavery*; Postell WD. *The Health of Slaves on Southern Plantations*.

73. Shryock RH. Medical sources and the social historian. In: Shryock RH, *Medicine in America: Historical Essays*, pp. 275–297.

74. Owens LH. *This Species of Property*; Savitt TL. Black health on the plantation; Boles JB. *Black Southerners 1619–1869*; Fogel RW. *Without Consent or Contract: The Rise and Fall of American Slavery*, pp. 116–153; Sutch R. The care and feeding of slaves; Savitt TL. *Medicine and Slavery*; Postell WD. *The Health of Slaves on Southern Plantations*; Tyler RC, Murphy LR, eds. *The Slave Narratives of Texas*, p. xxxi.

75. Mellon J, ed. *Bullwhip Days: The Slaves Remember*. New York: Weidenfeld and Nicolson, 1988, pp. 146–149; Owens LH. *This Species of Property*; Savitt TL. Black health on the plantation; Boles JB. *Black Southerners 1619–1869*; Fogel RW. *Without Consent or Contract*, pp. 116–153; Sutch R. The care and feeding of slaves; Savitt TL. *Medicine and Slavery*; Postell WD. *The Health of Slaves on Southern Plantations*.

76. Genovese ED. *From Rebellion to Revolution: Afro-American Slave Revolts in the Making of The New World*. Baton Rouge: Louisiana State University Press, 1979, paperback ed., New York: Vintage Books, 1981, p. 38.

77. Katz WL. *Breaking the Chains: African-American Slave Resistance*. New York: Atheneum, 1990, p. 101.

78. McManus EJ. *A History of Negro Slavery in New York*. Syracuse, NY: Syracuse University Press, 1966, p. 136.

79. Wood PH. *Black Majority: Negroes in Colonial South Carolina from 1670 through the Stono Rebellion*. New York: Knopf, 1974, paperback ed., New York: W. W. Norton, 1975, p. 278.

80. Wood PH. *Black Majority*, pp. 236–238; Weisbord RG. *Genocide? Birth Control and the Black American*. Westport, CT: Greenwood Press, 1975; Kovel J. *White Racism: A Psychohistory*. New York: Random House, 1970, reprint ed., New York: Columbia University Press, 1984; Genovese ED. *From Rebellion to Revolution*; Parker SG. Lynching as human sacrifice. *Harvard Magazine* November–December 1996, 2:23; Patterson O. *Rituals of Blood: Consequences of Slavery in Two American Centuries*. Washington: Civitas/Counterpoint, 1999, pp. 169–232.

81. Savitt T. Black health on the plantation, p. 344.

82. Savitt T. Black health on the plantation, p. 344.

83. Owens LH. *This Species of Property*; Savitt TL. Black health on the plantation; Boles JB. *Black Southerners 1619–1869*; Fogel RW. *Without Consent or Contract*, pp. 116–153; Sutch R. The care and feeding of slaves; Savitt TL. *Medicine and Slavery*; Postell WD. *The Health of Slaves on Southern Plantations*.

84. Roberts MJ. *Your Money or Your Life: The Health Care Crisis Explained*. New York: Doubleday, 1993; Byrd WM, Clayton LA. *Designing a New Health Care System for the United States*. Boston: Harvard School of Public Health, 1992; Banton M, Harwood J. *The Race Concept*. New York: Praeger Publishers, 1975; Banton M. *Racial Theories*. Cambridge: Cambridge University Press, 1987, pp. 93–98; Outlaw L. Toward a critical theory of race. In: Goldberg DT, ed. *Anatomy of Racism*. Minneapolis: University of Minnesota Press, 1990, pp. 58–82; Terry RW. *For Whites Only*. Grand Rapids, MI: Erdmans, 1970; Levin J. *The Functions of Prejudice*. New York: Harper & Row, 1975. Levin J, Levin W.

The Functions of Discrimination and Prejudice. 2nd Edition. New York: Harper & Row, Publishers, 1982.

85. Numbers RL, ed. *Medicine in the New World*; Cobb WM. 1981. The black American in Medicine. *Journal of the National Medical Association* 73 (Suppl 1):1183–1244; Starr P. *The Social Transformation of American Medicine*; Morais HM. *The History of the Negro in Medicine*; Stevens R. *American Medicine and the Public Interest.* New Haven, CT: Yale University Press, 1971; Rosenberg CE. *The Care of Strangers*; Shryock RH. *The Development of Modern Medicine: An Interpretation of the Social and Scientific Factors Involved.* Madison: The University of Wisconsin Press, 1974; Haller JS, Jr. *American Medicine in Transition 1840–1910.* Urbana: University of Illinois Press, 1981, pp. 36–99.

86. Curry LP. *The Free Black in Urban America, 1800–1850: The Shadow of the Dream.* Chicago: The University of Chicago Press, 1981, p. 132.

87. Wade RC. *Slavery in the Cities: The South, 1820–1860.* New York: Oxford University Press, 1964, paperback, reprint ed., New York: Oxford University Press, 1970, pp. 138–141; Savitt TL. *Medicine and Slavery*; Curry LP. *The Free Black in Urban America, 1800–1850: The Shadow of the Dream.* Chicago: The University of Chicago Press, 1981; Dowling HF. *City Hospitals: The Undercare of the Underprivileged*; Novotny A, Smith C. eds. *Images of Healing: A Portfolio of American Medical and Pharmaceutical Practice in the 18th, 19th, and early 20th Centuries.* New York: Macmillan, 1980.

88. Curry LP. *The Free Black in Urban America, 1800–1850*, p. 132.

89. Curry LP. *The Free Black in Urban America, 1800–1850*, p. 132.

90. Wade RC. *Slavery in the Cities: The South 1820–1860*, p. 138.

91. Wade RC. *Slavery in the Cities: The South, 1820–1860*, pp. 138–141; Savitt TL. *Medicine and Slavery*; Curry LP. *The Free Black in Urban America, 1800–1850*; Dowling HF. *City Hospitals: The Undercare of the Underprivileged*; Novotny A, Smith C. eds. *Images of Healing.*

92. Phillips UB. *American Negro Slavery: A Survey of the Supply, Employment and Control of Negro Labor As Determined by the Plantation Regime.* N.P.: D. Appleton and Company, 1918, paperback ed., Baton Rouge: Louisiana State University Press, 1966; Postell WD. *The Health of Slaves on Southern Plantations*; Savitt TL. *Medicine and Slavery*; Sheridan RB. *Doctors and Slaves: A Medical and Demographic History of Slavery in the British West Indies, 1680–1834.* Cambridge: Cambridge University Press, 1985; Horsman R. *Josiah Nott of Mobile: Southerner, Physician, and Racial Theorist.* Baton Rouge: Louisiana State University Press, 1987.

93. Lyons AS, Petrucelli RJ. *Medicine: An Illustrated History*, p. 489.

94. Rosenberg CE. *The Care of Strangers*, p. 317.

95. Rosenberg CE. *The Care of Strangers*, pp. 316–322; Lyons AS, Petrucelli RJ. *Medicine: An Illustrated History*, pp. 489–493; Savitt TL. *Medicine and Slavery*, pp. 213–217; Novotny A, Smith C. eds. *Images of Healing*, p. 30; Starr P. *The Social Transformation of American Medicine*; Sardell A. *The U.S. Experiment in Social Medicine: The Community Health Center Program, 1956–1986.* Pittsburgh, PA: The University of Pittsburgh Press, 1988.

96. Ludmerer KM. *Learning to Heal: The Development of American Medical Education.* New York: Basic Books, 1985; Rosenberg CE. *The Care of Strangers*; Rothstein WG. *American Medical Schools and the Practice of Medicine*; Savitt TL. The use of blacks for medical experimentation and demonstration in the old south. *Journal of Southern History*

1982; 48:331–348; Savitt TL. *Medicine and Slavery*, pp. 280–307; McGregor DK. *Sexual Surgery and the Origins of Gynecology: J. Marion Sims, His Hospital, and His Patients.* New York: Garland 1989.

97. Myrdal G. *An American Dilemma: The Negro Problem and Modern Democracy.* New York: Harper & Row, 1944, pp. 167–171.

98. Myrdal G. *An American Dilemma*; Byrd WM. Race, biology, and health care; Byrd WM, Clayton LA. An American health dilemma; Byrd WM, Clayton LA. The "slave health deficit": Racism and health outcomes. *Health/PAC Bulletin* 1991; 21:25–28; Savitt TL. *Medicine and Slavery*; Charatz-Litt C. A chronicle of racism: The effects of the white medical community on black health. *Journal of the National Medical Association* 1992; 84:717–725.

99. Savitt TL. *Medicine and Slavery*, p. 46.

100. Ransford O. *Bid the Sickness Cease*; Kiple KF, King VH. *Another Dimension to the Black Diaspora: Diet, Disease, and Racism.* Cambridge, England: Cambridge University Press, 1981; Savitt T. Black health on the plantation; Savitt TL. *Medicine and Slavery*; Sheridan RB. *Doctors and Slaves*; Manson-Bahr PEC, Bell DR. *Manson's Tropical Diseases.*

101. Gould SJ. *The Mismeasure of Man*; Jordan WD. *White over Black*; Byrd WM. Documentary report: Negro diseases and physiological peculiarities. Nashville, TN: Cancer Control Research Unit, Meharry Medical College, July 12, 1990. In: Byrd WM, Clayton LA. *A Black Health Trilogy* (videotape and 188-page documentary report). Washington, DC: The National Medical Association and the African American Heritage and Education Foundation, 1991, revised ed., Washington, DC: The National Medical Association, 1994.

102. Ludmerer KM. *Learning to Heal: The Development of American Medical Education.* New York: Basic Books, 1985; Byrd WM, Clayton LA. The "slave health deficit"; Ransford O. *Bid the Sickness Cease*; Kiple KF, King VH. *Another Dimension to the Black Diaspora*; Savitt T. Black health on the plantation; Savitt TL. *Medicine and Slavery.*

103. Morais HM. *The History of the Negro in Medicine*, p. 12.

104. Bousfield MO. An account of physicians of color in the United States. *Bulletin of the History of Medicine* 1945; 17:61–84, esp. 63.

105. Ludmerer KM. *Learning to Heal*, p. 14.

106. Bousfield MO. An account of physicians of color in the United States, p. 62.

107. Bousfield MO. An account of physicians of color in the United States; Morais HM. *The History of the Negro in Medicine*; Kenney JA. *The Negro in Medicine.* Tuskegee: Tuskegee Institute Press, 1912; Curtis JL. *Blacks, Medical Schools, and Society.* Ann Arbor: The University of Michigan Press, 1971; The black American in medicine. *Journal of the National Medical Association* 1981; 73 (Suppl 1):1183–1244; Falk LA. Black abolitionist doctors and healers, 1810–1885. *Bulletin of the History of Medicine* 1980; 54:253–272; Numbers RL, ed. *Medicine in the New World*; Kiple KF, King VH. *Another Dimension to the Black Diaspora*; Savitt TL. *Medicine and Slavery*; Sheridan RB. *Doctors and Slaves.*

108. Bousfield MO. An account of physicians of color in the United States; Morais HM. *The History of the Negro in Medicine*, pp. 7–10; Kenney JA. *The Negro in Medicine*; Curtis JL. *Blacks, Medical Schools, and Society*; Kenney JA. *The Negro in Medicine*; Cobb WM. The black American in medicine; Falk LA. Black abolitionist doctors and healers, 1810–1885; Numbers RL, ed. *Medicine in the New World*; Kiple KF, King VH. *Another*

Dimension to the Black Diaspora; Savitt TL. *Medicine and Slavery*; Sheridan RB. *Doctors and Slaves*.

109. Morais HM. *The History of the Negro in Medicine*, p. 8.

110. Bousfield MO. An account of physicians of color in the United States; Morais HM. *The History of the Negro in Medicine*; Cobb WM. The black American in medicine; Wolinsky H. Healing wounds: Lonnie R. Bristow steps up to head the American Medical Association, one of the nation's premier—and most rigidly segregated—professional groups. *Emerge* July/August 1994; 10(5):42.

111. Ackerknecht EH. *A Short History of Medicine*, pp. 128–156; Bender GA. *Great Moments in Medicine*, pp. 124–175; Dowling HF. *City Hospitals*; Shryock RH. *Medicine in America: Historical Essays*; Shryock RH. *The Development of Modern Medicine*, pp. 17–108; Vogel MJ. *The Invention of the Modern Hospital*; Novotny A, Smith C, eds. *Images of Healing*; Lyons AS, Petrucelli RJ. *Medicine: An Illustrated History*; Savitt TL. *Medicine and Slavery*; Starr P. *The Social Transformation of American Medicine*.

112. Dowling HF. *City Hospitals*; Shryock RH. *Medicine in America: Historical Essays*; Vogel MJ. *The Invention of the Modern Hospital*; Novotny A, Smith C, eds. *Images of Healing*; Lyons AS, Petrucelli RJ. *Medicine: An Illustrated History*; Savitt TL. *Medicine and Slavery*; Starr P. *The Social Transformation of American Medicine*.

113. Dowling HF. *City Hospitals*; Shryock RH. *Medicine in America*; Vogel MJ. *The Invention of the Modern Hospital*; Novotny A, Smith C, eds. *Images of Healing*; Lyons AS, Petrucelli RJ. *Medicine: An Illustrated History*; Savitt TL. *Medicine and Slavery*; Starr P. *The Social Transformation of American Medicine*.

114. Rosenberg CE. *The Care of Strangers*, p. 19.

115. Stevens R. *American Medicine and the Public Interest*; Ackerknecht EH. *A Short History of Medicine*; Lyons AS, Petrucelli RJ. *Medicine: An Illustrated History*; Novotny A, Smith C, eds. *Images of Healing*; Shryock RH. Medical perspectives on the Civil War. In: *Medicine in America: Historical Essays*, pp. 90–108; Dowling HF. *City Hospitals*; Rosenberg CE. *The Care of Strangers*; Starr P. *The Social Transformation of American Medicine*; Kaufman M, Galishoff S, Savitt TL, eds. *Dictionary of American Medical Biography* (2 Vols.). Westport, CT: Greenwood Press, 1984.

116. Stevens R. *American Medicine and the Public Interest*; Ackerknecht EH. *A Short History of Medicine*; Lyons AS, Petrucelli RJ. *Medicine: An Illustrated History*; Novotny A, Smith C, eds. *Images of Healing*; Shryock RH. Medical perspectives on the Civil War; Dowling HF. *City Hospitals*; The American Anti-Slavery Society. *American Slavery As It Is: Testimony of a Thousand Witnesses. The Anti-Slavery Examiner*, 1839 (No. 6), New York: The American Anti-Slavery Society, 1839, pp. 44–45, 55, 169–171, 175–176; Savitt TL. *Medicine and Slavery*, pp. 280–307; Rosenberg CE. *The Care of Strangers*.

117. Stevens R. *American Medicine and the Public Interest*; Starr P. *The Social Transformation of American Medicine*, pp. 37–47; Numbers RL, ed. *Medicine in the New World*; Ackerknecht EH. *A Short History of Medicine*; Lyons AS, Petrucelli RJ. *Medicine: An Illustrated History*; Novotny A, Smith C, eds. *Images of Healing*; Shryock RH. Medical perspectives on the Civil War; Dowling HF. *City Hospitals*; Rosenberg CE. *The Care of Strangers*.

118. Rosenberg CF. *The Care of Strangers*, p. 176.

119. Byrd WM, Clayton LA. The "slave health deficit"; Byrd WM, Clayton LA. An American health dilemma; Starr P. *The Social Transformation of American Medicine*, pp. 3–78; Stevens R. *American Medicine and the Public Interest*, pp. 9–33; Ackerknecht EH. *A*

Short History of Medicine, pp. 128–156; Haller JS, Jr. *American Medicine in Transition 1840–1910.* Urbana: University of Illinois Press, 1981; Lyons AS, Petrucelli RJ. *Medicine: An Illustrated History;* Novotny A, Smith C, eds. *Images of Healing;* Shryock RH. Medical perspectives on the Civil War; Charatz-Litt C. A chronicle of racism; Dowling HF. *City Hospitals;* Rosenberg CE. *The Care of Strangers,* pp. 15–68, 168–200.

120. Byrd WM. Race, biology, and health care; Roberts J. *The Triumph of the West;* Burke J. *The Day the Universe Changed.* Boston: Little, Brown, 1985, pp. 179, 239–273; Young RJC. *Colonial Desire: Hybridity in Theory, Culture and Race.* London: Routledge, 1995, pp. 121–123; King JC. *The Biology of Race.* Rev. ed. Berkeley: University of California Press, 1981; King M, Wilson AC. Evolution at two levels in humans and chimpanzees. *Science* April 11, 1975; 188(4184);107–116; Chase A. *The Legacy of Malthus: The Social Costs of the New Scientific Racism.* New York: Knopf, 1980; Comas J. *Racial Myths* (United Nations Education, Scientific and Cultural Organization, The Race Question in Modern Science Series). Paris: UNESCO, 1958; Lewontin RC, Rose S, Kamin LJ. *Not in Our Genes: Biology, Ideology, and Human Nature.* New York: Pantheon Books, 1984; Reynolds V, Falger V, Vine I, eds. *The Sociobiology of Ethnocentrism: Evolutionary Dimensions of Xenophobia, Discrimination, Racism and Nationalism.* London: Croom Helm, 1987.

121. Smith JA. A lecture introductory to the second course of anatomical instruction in the College of Physicians and Surgeons for the State of New York . . . *New-York Medical and Philosophical Journal and Review* 1809; 1:32–48; Stanton W. *The Leopard's Spots,* pp. 18–19; Horsman R. *Race and Manifest Destiny,* pp. 116–117; Jordan WD. *White over Black,* pp. 505–506; Banton M. *Racial Theories,* pp. 32, 39.

122. Stanton W. *The Leopard's Spots,* p. 19.

123. Stanton W. *The Leopard's Spots,* pp. 19–22; Fredrickson GM. *The Black Image in the White Mind,* p. 73; Horsman R. *Race and Manifest Destiny,* pp. 117–120; Jordan WD. *White over Black,* pp. 521, 523, 533–534.

124. Gould SJ. *The Mismeasure of Man,* p. 31.

125. Gould SJ. *The Mismeasure of Man,* p. 35.

126. Reed J. Scientific racism. In Wilson CR, Ferris W, eds. *Encyclopedia of Southern Culture.* Chapel Hill: The University of North Carolina Press, 1989, pp. 1358–1360.

127. Gould SJ. *The Mismeasure of Man,* p. 31.

128. Chang K. UM professor questions lack of diversity in genome project. *The Baltimore Sun* (Maryland section) February 22, 1997.

129. Gould SJ. *The Mismeasure of Man,* pp. 30–39; Banton M, Harwood J. *The Race Concept;* Banton M. *Racial Theories;* Young RJC. *Colonial Desire,* pp. 118–141; Lifton RJ. *The Nazi Doctors: Medical Killing and the Psychology of Genocide.* New York: Basic Books, 1986; Lifton RJ, Markusen E. *The Genocidal Mentality: Nazi Holocaust and Nuclear Threat.* New York: Basic Books, 1990; Proctor RN. *Racial Hygiene;* Stannard DE. *American Holocaust;* Gilman SL. *Freud, Race, and Gender.* Princeton, NJ: Princeton University Press, 1993; Reynolds V, Falger V, Vine I, eds. *The Sociobiology of Ethnocentrism: Evolutionary Dimensions of Xenophobia, Discrimination, Racism and Nationalism.* London: Croom Helm, 1987; Ryan W. *Blaming the Victim;* Chase A. *The Legacy of Malthus;* Haller MH. *Eugenics: Hereditarian Attitudes in American Thought.* New Brunswick, NJ: Rutgers University Press, 1963; Kevles DJ. *In the Name of Eugenics: Genetics and the Uses of Human Heredity.* Berkeley: University of California Press, 1985; Duster R. *Backdoor to Eugenics.* New York: Routledge, 1990.

130. Rush B. Observations intended to favour a supposition that the black color (as it is called) of the Negroes is derived from the leprosy. *American Philosophical Society, Transactions* 1799; 4:289–297.

131. Jordan WD. *White over Black*, p. 517.

132. Jordan WD. *White over Black*, pp. 517–521, 530; Owens LH. *This Species of Property*, pp. 31, 84; Postell WD. *The Health of Slaves on Southern Plantations*, pp. 81–82; Stampp KM. *The Peculiar Institution*, pp. 109, 302–304, 308–309; Takaki RT. *Iron Cages*, pp. 28–35.

133. Warner JH. The idea of Southern medical distinctiveness: Medical knowledge and practices in the Old South. In: Numbers RL, Savitt TL, eds. *Science and Medicine in the Old South*. Baton Rouge: Louisiana State University Press, 1989, pp. 179–205; Franklin JH. *A Southern Odyssey: Travelers in the Antebellum North*. Baton Rouge: Louisiana State University Press, 1976; Warner JH. A Southern medical reform: The meaning of the Antebellum argument for Southern medical education. In: Numbers RL, Savitt TL, eds. *Science and Medicine in the Old South*, pp. 206–225; Byrd WM. *Documentary Report: Negro Diseases and Physiological Peculiarities*; Jordan WD. *White over Black*, pp. 517–521, 530; Owens LH. *This Species of Property*, pp. 31, 84; Postell WD. *The Health of Slaves on Southern Plantations*, pp. 81–82; Stampp KM. *The Peculiar Institution*, pp. 109, 302–304, 308–309; Takaki RT. *Iron Cages*, pp. 28–35.

Chapter Five

1. O'Reilly K. *Nixon's Piano: Presidents and Racial Politics from Washington to Clinton*. New York: The Free Press, 1995, pp. 31–51; Takaki RY. *Iron Cages: Race and Culture in Nineteenth-Century America*. New York: Knopf, 1979, pp. 69–144; Wilson V. *The Book of the Presidents*. Brookeville, MD: American History Research Associates, 1962, pp. 8–41.

2. Brinkley A. *The Unfinished Nation: A Concise History of the American People*. New York: Knopf, 1993, pp. 192–362; Takaki RY. *Iron Cages*; Ewbank DC. History of Black mortality and health before 1940. In: Willis DP, ed. *Health Policies and Black Americans*. New Brunswick, NJ: Transaction Publishers, 1989, pp. 100–128; Savitt TL. *Medicine and Slavery: The Diseases and Health Care of Blacks in Antebellum Virginia*. Urbana: University of Illinois Press, 1987; Farley R. *Growth of the Black Population: A Study of Demographic Trends*. Chicago: Markham Publishing, 1970; Fogel RW. *Without Consent or Contract: The Rise and Fall of American Slavery*. New York: W. W. Norton, 1989, pp. 127–132; Roberts JM. *History of the World*. New York: Knopf, 1976; revised reprint paperback ed., *The Penguin History of the World*. London: Penguin Books, 1990; McEvedy C. *World History Factfinder*. N.P.: Grisewood and Dempsey, 1984; revised and updated ed., New York: Gallery Books, 1989, pp. 129–136; *The New Grolier Multimedia Encyclopedia*, MPC Version, Release 6, s.v. United States history; *The World Book Encyclopedia*, 39th ed., s.v. History of the United States; *The World Book Encyclopedia*, 39th ed., s.v. War of 1812; Watkins TH. A low comedy for high stakes: The taking of California. *American Heritage* February 1973; 2(24):4.

3. Morais HM. *The History of the Negro in Medicine*. New York: Publishers Company, 1967; Farley R. *Growth of the Black Population*, pp. 20–21; Starr P. *The Social Trans-*

formation of American Medicine. New York: Basic Books, 1982; Stevens RA. *American Medicine and the Public Interest.* New Haven, CT: Yale University Press, 1971; Rothstein WG. *American Physicians in the Nineteenth Century: From Sects to Science.* Baltimore: The Johns Hopkins University Press, 1972, pp. 55, 249–250; Ackerknecht EH. *A Short History of Medicine.* revised ed. Baltimore, MD: The Johns Hopkins University Press, 1982, pp. 218–226.

4. Takaki RY. *Iron Cages,* p. 78.

5. Takaki RY. *Iron Cages,* p. 77.

6. Du Bois WEB. *Black Reconstruction in America: An Essay Toward a History of the Part Which Black Folk Played in the Attempt to Reconstruct Democracy in America, 1860–1880.* N.P.: Harcourt, Brace and Company, 1935; reprint ed., Cleveland, OH: Meridian Books, The World Publishing Company, 1964, p. 4.

7. Brinkley A. *The Unfinished Nation,* pp. 271–362; Takaki RY. *Iron Cages,* pp. 69–170; Roberts JM. *History of the World;* Ward GC, Burns R, Burns K. *The Civil War.* New York: Knopf, 1990; Campbell RB. *An Empire for Slavery: The Peculiar Institution in Texas, 1821–1865.* Baton Rouge: Louisiana State University Press, 1989, pp. 67–95; Genovese ED. *The Political Economy of Slavery: Studies in the Economy and Society of the Slave South.* New York: Vintage Books, 1965; Genovese ED. *The World the Slaveholders Made: Two Essays in Interpretation.* New York: Pantheon Books, 1969; paperback ed., Middletown, CT: Wesleyan University Press, 1988; Du Bois WEB. *Black Reconstruction in America;* Wetterau B. *The New York Public Library Book of Chronologies.* New York: Stonesong Press, 1990; McEvedy C. *World History Factfinder; The New Grolier Multimedia Encyclopedia,* MPC Version, Release 6, s.v. United States history; *The World Book Encyclopedia,* 39th ed., s.v. History of the United States; *The World Book Encyclopedia,* 39th ed., s.v. War of 1812; Watkins TH. A low comedy for high stakes.

8. Roberts J. *The Triumph of the West.* Boston: Little, Brown, 1985, p. 203.

9. Farley R, Allen WR. *The Color Line and the Quality of Life in America.* New York: Oxford University Press, 1989, pp. 7–11; Faust DG. Slavery in the American experience. In: Campbell EDC, Jr., Rice K., eds. *Before Freedom Came: African-American Life in the Antebellum South.* Charlottesville: The Museum of the Confederacy, Richmond and the University Press of Virginia, 1991 pp. 1–19, quote p. 11; Roberts JM. *History of the World,* pp. 710–713; Takaki RY. *Iron Cages,* pp. 3–144; Oates SB. Children of darkness. *American Heritage* October 1973; 6(24):42; U.S. Bureau of the Census. *Negro Population of the United States: 1790–1915* (1918), p. 53.

10. Roberts JM. *History of the World,* p. 712.

11. O'Reilly K. *Nixon's Piano,* p. 10.

12. Brinkley A. *The Unfinished Nation;* Takaki RY. *Iron Cages;* Roberts JM. *History of the World,* pp. 710–713; Byrd WM, Clayton LA. The "slave health deficit": Racism and health outcomes. *Health/PAC Bulletin* 1991; 21:25–28; Sanders R. *Lost Tribes and Promised Lands: The Origins of American Racism.* Boston: Little, Brown, 1978; Stannard DE. *American Holocaust: Columbus and the Conquest of the New World.* New York: Oxford University Press, 1992; *The New Grolier Multimedia Encyclopedia,* MPC Version, Release 6, s.v. United States history; Oates SB. Children of darkness.

13. Takaki RY. *Iron Cages,* p. 112.

14. Fitzhugh G. *Cannibals All! or, Slaves Without Masters.* Cambridge, MA: The Belknap Press of Harvard University Press, 1960.

15. Fredrickson GM. *The Black Image in the White Mind: The Debate on Afro-American Character and Destiny, 1871–1914*. New York: Harper & Row, 1971; reprint ed., Middletown, CT: Wesleyan University Press, 1987, pp. 66–67.

16. Oates SB. Children of darkness, p. 91.

17. Fredrickson GM. *The Black Image in the White Mind*, pp. 63–64.

18. Brinkley A. *The Unfinished Nation*, pp. 304–362; Takaki RY. *Iron Cages*, pp. 80–154; Faust DG. Slavery in the American experience, p. 11; Kovel J. *White Racism: A Psychohistory*. New York: Random House, 1970, reprint ed., New York: Columbia University Press, 1984; Roberts JM. *History of the World*, pp. 710–713; Sanders R. *Lost Tribes and Promised Lands*; Stannard DE. *American Holocaust*; *The New Grolier Multimedia Encyclopedia*, MPC Version, Release 6, s.v. United States history; Oates SB. Children of darkness.

19. Tocqueville A de. *Democracy in America* (two vols.). Ed. JP Mayer, Trans. G Lawrence. New York: Harper & Row, 1966; paperback ed., New York: Harper Perennial, 1988, p. 669.

20. Tocqueville A de. *Democracy in America*, p. 508.

21. Brinkley A. *The Unfinished Nation*; Takaki RY. *Iron Cages*; Roberts JM. *History of the World*; *The New Grolier Multimedia Encyclopedia*, MPC Version, Release 6, s.v. United States history; *The World Book Encyclopedia*, 39th ed., s.v. History of the United States; *The World Book Encyclopedia*, 39th ed., s.v. War of 1812; Tocqueville A de. *Democracy in America*, p. 508; Dowling HF. *City Hospitals: The Undercare of the Underprivileged*. Cambridge, MA: Harvard University Press, 1982; Stevens RA. *American Medicine and the Public Interest*; Byrd WM, Clayton LA. The "slave health deficit"; Sanders R. *Lost Tribes and Promised Lands*; Stannard DE. *American Holocaust: Columbus and the Conquest of the New World*.

22. Brinkley A. *The Unfinished Nation*, p. 351.

23. Brinkley A. *The Unfinished Nation*, pp. 325–362; Watkins TH. A Low comedy for high stakes.

24. Takaki RY. *Iron Cages*; Cobb WM. The Black American in medicine. *Journal of the National Medical Association* 1981; 73(Suppl 1):1183–1244; Byrd WM, Clayton LA. An American health dilemma: A history of blacks in the health system. *Journal of the National Medical Association* 1992; 84:189–200; Byrd WM. Race, biology, and health care: Reassessing a relationship. *Journal of Health Care for the Poor and Underserved* 1990; 1:278–292.

25. Roberts JM. *History of the World*, p. 711.

26. *The New Grolier Multimedia Encyclopedia*, MPC Version, Release 6, s.v. United States history.

27. Roberts JM. *History of the World*; Morais HM. *The History of the Negro in Medicine*; Byrd WM, Clayton LA. The "slave health deficit"; Cobb WM. The Black American in medicine; Byrd WM, Clayton LA. *A Black Health Trilogy* (videotape and 188-page documentary report). Washington, DC: The National Medical Association and the African American Heritage and Education Foundation, 1991; Hughes L, Meltzer M, Lincoln CE. *A Pictorial History of Black Americans*. rev. 5th ed. New York: Crown Publishers, 1983, pp. 40–51; O'Reilly K. *Nixon's Piano*, p. 41.

28. Rosenberg CE. *The Care of Strangers: The Rise of America's Hospital System*. New York: Basic Books, 1987, p. 4.

29. Rosenberg CE. *The Care of Strangers*; Rothman DJ. Our brother's keepers. *American Heritage* December 1972; 1(24):38; Shryock RH. *The Development of Modern Medicine: An Interpretation of the Social and Scientific Factors Involved.* Madison: The University of Wisconsin Press, 1974; Starr P. *The Social Transformation of American Medicine.*

30. Rosenberg CE. *The Care of Strangers*; Rothman DJ. Our brother's keepers; Shryock RH. *The Development of Modern Medicine*; Starr P. *The Social Transformation of American Medicine.*

31. McNeill WH. *Plagues and Peoples.* New York: Doubleday, 1976, paperback ed., New York: Anchor Books, 1989, p. 151; Ziegler P. *The Black Death*, N.P.: John Day Company, 1969. Paperback Edition. New York: Harper Torchbooks, 1971, pp. 53–54; Rosenberg CE. *The Care of Strangers.*

32. Rosenberg CE. *The Care of Strangers*, p. 15.

33. Rosenberg CE. *The Care of Strangers*; Rothman DJ. Our brother's keepers; Savitt TL. *Medicine and Slavery.*

34. Rosenberg CE. *The Care of Strangers*; Rothman DJ. Our brother's keepers; Dowling HF. *City Hospitals*; Savitt TL. *Medicine and Slavery.*

35. The American Anti-Slavery Society. American slavery as it is: Testimony of a thousand witnesses. *The Anti-Slavery Examiner* 1839; 6:44–45, 55, 167–171; Savitt TL. The use of blacks for medical experimentation and demonstration in the old south. *Journal of Southern History* 1982; 48:331–348; Brandt AM. Racism and research: The case of the Tuskegee syphilis study. In: Leavitt JW, Numbers RL, eds. *Sickness and Health in America: Readings in the History of Medicine and Public Health.* Madison: The University of Wisconsin Press, 1985, pp. 331–343; Kenney JA. Second annual oration on surgery. *Journal of the National Medical Association* 1941; 33:203–214; Savitt TL. *Medicine and Slavery*, pp. 257–258.

36. Wade RC. *Slavery in the Cities: The South 1820–1860.* London: Oxford University Press, 1964, p. 138.

37. Wade RC. *Slavery in the Cities*, pp. 138–141; Savitt TL. *Medicine and Slavery*; Curry LP. *The Free Black in Urban America, 1800–1850: The Shadow of the Dream.* Chicago: The University of Chicago Press, 1981; Dowling HF. *City Hospitals*; Novotny A, Smith C, eds. *Images and Healing: A Portfolio of American Medical and Pharmaceutical Practice in the Eighteenth, Nineteenth, and early Twentieth Centuries.* New York: Macmillan, 1980; Horsman R. *Josiah Nott of Mobile: Southerner, Physician, and Racial Theorist.* Baton Rouge: Louisiana State University Press, 1987.

38. Rosenberg CE. *The Care of Strangers*, p. 5.

39. Rosenberg CE. *The Care of Strangers*; Novotny A, Smith C. eds. *Images of Healing*; Rothman DJ. Our brother's keepers; Savitt TL. *Medicine and Slavery.*

40. Cray E. *In Failing Health: The Medical Crisis and the A.M.A.* Indianapolis: Bobbs-Merrill, 1970; Novotny A, Smith C, eds. *Images of Healing*; Cobb WM. *The First Negro Medical Society: A History of the Medico-Chirurgical Society of the District of Columbia.* Washington, DC: The Associated Publishers, 1939; Bender GA. *Great Moments in Medicine.* Detroit: Northwood Institute Press, 1966; Wolinsky H. Healing wounds: Lonnie R. Bristow steps up to head the American Medical Association, one of the nation's premier—and most rigidly segregated—professional groups. *Emerge* July–August 1994; 10(5):42.

41. Bender GA. *Great Moments in Medicine*, p. 236.

42. Bender GA. *Great Moments in Medicine*; Shryock RH. *Medicine in America: Historical Essays*. Baltimore: The Johns Hopkins Press, 1966; Ackerknecht EH. *A Short History of Medicine*. revised ed., Baltimore: The Johns Hopkins University Press, 1982; Morais HM. *The History of the Negro in Medicine*; Cobb WM. 1981. The Black American in medicine; The American Anti-Slavery Society. American slavery as it is.

43. Ryan W. *Blaming the Victim*. New York: Vintage Books, 1971, rev. updated ed., New York: Vintage Books, 1976; Rothman DJ. Our brother's keepers; Churchill LR. *Rationing Health Care in America: Perceptions and Principles of Justice*. Notre Dame, IN: University of Notre Dame Press, 1987; Rosenberg CE. *The Care of Strangers*; Dula A. Toward an African-American perspective on bioethics. *Journal of Health Care for the Poor and Underserved* 1991; 2:259–269; Randall VR. Slavery, segregation and racism: Trusting the health care system ain't always easy! An African American perspective on bioethics. *Saint Louis University Public Law Review* 1996 2(15):191–235; Starr P. *The Social Transformation of American Medicine*; Morais HM. *The History of the Negro in Medicine*; Bullough B, Bullough VL. *Poverty, Ethnic Identity, and Health Care*. New York: Appleton-Century-Crofts, 1972; McGregor DK. *Sexual Surgery and the Origins of Gynecology: J. Marion Sims, His Hospital, and His Patients*. New York: Garland, 1989; Shryock RH. *Medicine in America*, p. 131; Lewis JH. Contribution of an unknown Negro to anesthesia. *Journal of the National Medical Association* 1931; 23:23–24; Kosa J, Zola IK, eds. *Poverty and Health: A Sociological Analysis*. rev. ed. Cambridge, MA: Harvard University Press, 1975.

44. Walker HE. *The Negro in the Medical Profession*. N.P.: University of Virginia, 1949, p. 7; Shryock RH. *The Development of Modern Medicine*, p. 177.

45. McGregor DK. *Sexual Surgery and the Origins of Gynecology*, p. 244.

46. McGregor DK. *Sexual Surgery and the Origins of Gynecology*, p. 304.

47. Bender GA. *Great Moments in Medicine*, p. 190.

48. Morais HM. *The History of the Negro in Medicine*; Bullough B, Bullough VL. *Poverty, Ethnic Identity, and Health Care*; Walker HE. *The Negro in the Medical Profession*; Cobb WM. Integration in medicine: A national need. *Journal of the National Medical Association* 1957; 49:4; Novotny A, Smith C, eds. *Images of Healing*, pp. 43–47; McGregor DK. *Sexual Surgery and the Origins of Gynecology*; Fausto-Sterling A. Anatomy. In: *Encyclopedia of African American Culture and History*. Eds. Salzman J, Smith DL, West C. New York: Macmillan Library Reference USA, 1996; Shryock RH. *Medicine in America*, p. 131; Lyons AS, Petrucelli RJ. *Medicine: An Illustrated History*. New York: Harry N. Abrams, 1978, pp. 504, 523–524, 553–554; Lewis JH. Contribution of an unknown Negro to anesthesia; Bender GA. *Great Moments in Medicine*, pp. 184–197; Nuland SB. *Doctors: The Biography of Medicine*. New York: Knopf, 1988, pp. 263–303; Kosa J, Zola IK, eds. *Poverty and Health*.

49. Rosenberg CE. *The Care of Strangers*; Starr P. *The Social Transformation of American Medicine*; Morais HM. *The History of the Negro in Medicine*; Bullough B, Bullough VL. *Poverty, Ethnic Identity, and Health Care*; Novotny A, Smith C, eds. *Images of Healing*, pp. 43–47; McGregor DK. *Sexual Surgery and the Origins of Gynecology*; Shryock RH. *Medicine in America*, p. 131; Lyons AS, Petrucelli RJ. *Medicine: An Illustrated History*, pp. 504, 523–524, 553–554; Lewis JH. Contribution of an unknown Negro to anesthesia; Bender GA. *Great Moments in Medicine*, pp. 184–197; Nuland SB. *Doctors:*

The Biography of Medicine, pp. 263–303; Stampp KM. *The Peculiar Institution*; Faust DG. Slavery in the American experience; Kosa J, Zola IK, eds. *Poverty and Health*.

50. Dula A. Toward an African-American perspective on bioethics; Randall VR. Slavery, segregation and racism.

51. Dula A. Toward an African-American perspective on bioethics; Randall VR. Slavery, segregation and racism; Veatch RM. *A Theory of Medical Ethics*. New York: Basic Books, 1981; Walker HE. *The Negro in the Medical Profession*; Byrd WM. Race, biology, and health care; Cobb WM. Integration in medicine; Nuland SB. *Doctors: The Biography of Medicine*, pp. 31–93; Bullough VL. *The Development of Medicine As a Profession: The Contribution of the Medieval University to Modern Medicine*. New York: Hafner Publishing, pp. 22–23, 26–27, 59, 62–65; Lyons AS, Petrucelli RJ. *Medicine: An Illustrated History*, p. 229; The American Anti-Slavery Society. American slavery as it is; Novotny A, Smith C, eds. *Images of Healing*, pp. 14, 121; Rosenberg CE. *The Care of Strangers*; Churchill LR. *Rationing Health Care in America*; Numbers RL, ed. *Medicine in the New World: New Spain, New France, and New England*. Knoxville: The University of Tennessee Press, 1987, pp. 17, 119; Savitt TL. The use of blacks for medical experimentation and demonstration in the old south; Savitt TL. *Medicine and Slavery*; Sirasi NG. *Medieval and Early Renaissance Medicine: An Introduction to Knowledge and Practice*. Chicago: The University of Chicago Press, 1990, p. 86; McGregor DK. *Sexual Surgery and the Origins of Gynecology*, pp. 52–57; Haeger K. *The Illustrated History of Surgery*. New York: Bell Publishing, 1988, p. 45.

52. Shryock RH. *The Development of Modern Medicine*, p. 39.

53. Charatz-Litt C. A chronicle of racism: The effects of the white medical community on black health. *Journal of the National Medical Association* 1992; 84:717–725; Savitt TL. *Medicine and Slavery*; Bullough B, Bullough VL. *Poverty, Ethnic Identity, and Health Care*; Savitt TL. The use of blacks for medical experimentation and demonstration in the old south; McGregor DK. *Sexual Surgery and the Origins of Gynecology*, pp. 8–81; Lewis JH. Contribution of an unknown Negro to anesthesia; Kenney JA. Second annual oration on surgery; Walker HE. *The Negro in the Medical Profession*; Cobb WM. Integration in medicine: A national need; Fausto-Sterling A. Anatomy.

54. Lyons AS, Petrucelli RJ. *Medicine: An Illustrated History*, p. 504.

55. Lewis JH. Contribution of an unknown Negro to anesthesia.

56. Dula A. Toward an African-American perspective on bioethics; Reiser RJ, Dyck AJ, Curran WJ, eds. Final report of the Tuskegee Syphilis Study Ad Hoc Advisory Panel. In: *Ethics in Medicine: Historical Perspectives and Contemporary Concerns*. Cambridge, MA: MIT Press, 1977, pp. 316–321; Randall VR. Slavery, segregation and racism; Veatch RM. *A Theory of Medical Ethics*; Jones JH. *Bad Blood: The Tuskegee Syphilis Experiment*; Nuland SB. *Doctors: The Biography of Medicine*; Savitt TL. The use of blacks for medical experimentation and demonstration in the old south; Savitt TL. *Medicine and Slavery*; Sirasi NG. *Medieval and Early Renaissance Medicine*; Lyons AS, Petrucelli RJ. *Medicine: An Illustrated History*.

57. Stampp KM. *The Peculiar Institution*; Kiple KF, King VH. *Another Dimension to the Black Diaspora: Diet, Disease, and Racism*. Cambridge, England: Cambridge University Press, 1981; Savitt TL. *Medicine and Slavery*; Owens LH. *This Species of Property: Slave Life and Culture in the Old South*. Oxford: Oxford University Press, 1976; Boles JB. *Black Southerners 1619–1869*. Lexington: The University of Kentucky Press, 1984; David

PA, et al. *Reckoning with Slavery: A Critical Study in the Quantitative History of American Negro Slavery.* New York: Oxford University Press, 1976; Roberts JM. *History of the World;* p. 711.

58. Katz WL. *Breaking the Chains: African-American Slave Resistance.* New York: Atheneum, 1990; Nichols CH. *Many Thousands Gone: The Ex-Slaves Account of their Bondage and Freedom.* Leiden, Netherlands: E.J. Brill, 1963, paperback ed., Blooming-ton: Indiana University Press, p. 51; David PA, et al. *Reckoning with Slavery;* Campbell EDC, Jr., Rice K., eds. *Before Freedom Came: African-American Life in the Antebellum South.*

59. Stampp KM. *The Peculiar Institution,* pp. 245–251; Fogel RW. *Without Consent or Contract,* pp. 119–123; Tyler RC, Murphy LR, eds. *The Slave Narratives of Texas.* Austin: The Encino Press, 1974, pp. xxvi, 20–21, 36; Mellon J, ed. *Bullwhip Days: The Slaves Remember.* New York: Weidenfeld and Nicolson, 1988, pp. 147–149; Owens LH. *This Species of Property,* pp. 184–185, 277; Magee MJ. The old slave house. In: Magee MJ. *Cavern of Crime,* Smithland, KY: The Livingston Ledger, 1973, pp. 49–54; Nichols CH. *Many Thousands Gone,* p. 21; Oakes J. *The Ruling Race: A History of American Slave-holders.* New York: Knopf, 1982, reprint ed., New York: Vintage Books, 1983, pp. 172–173; Bancroft F. *Slave Trading in the Old South.* New York: Frederick Ungar Publish-ing, 1959; Gutman H, Sutch R. Victorians all? The sexual mores and conduct of slaves and their masters. In: David PA, et al., eds. *Reckoning with Slavery,* pp. 134–162; Sutch R. The care and feeding of slaves. In: David PA, et al., eds. *Reckoning with Slavery,* pp. 231–301; Savitt TL. *Medicine and Slavery;* Sheridan RB. *Doctors and Slaves;* Ewbank DC. History of Black mortality and health before 1940. In: Willis DP, ed. *Health Policies and Black Americans.* New Brunswick, NJ: Transaction Publishers, 1989, pp. 100–128; Ryan KJ, Berkowitz R, Barbieri RL. *Kistner's Gynecology: Principles and Practice.* 5th ed. Chicago: Year Book Medical Publishers, 1990, p. 349; Isselbacher K, Braunwald E, Wilson JD, et al., eds. *Harrison's Principles of Internal Medicine.* 13th ed. New York: McGraw-Hill, 1994, p. 2029.

60. Savitt TL. *Medicine and Slavery;* Rosenberg CE. *The Care of Strangers;* Sheri-dan RB. *Doctors and Slaves;* Ewbank DC. History of Black mortality and health before 1940; Christianson EH. Medicine in New England. In: Numbers RL, ed. *Medicine in the New World,* pp. 101–153; Stampp KM. *The Peculiar Institution,* pp. 245–251; Fogel RW. *Without Consent or Contract;* Tyler RC, Murphy LR, eds. *The Slave Narratives of Texas;* Mellon J, ed. *Bullwhip Days;* Owens LH. *This Species of Property;* Nichols CH. *Many Thousands Gone;* Oakes J. *The Ruling Race;* Sutch R. The care and feeding of slaves.

61. Genovese ED. *From Rebellion to Revolution,* p. 4.

62. Harding V. *There Is a River: The Black Struggle for Freedom in America.* New York: Harcourt Brace Jovanovich, 1981, reprint ed., New York: Vintage Books, 1983, p. 61.

63. Oates SB. Children of darkness, p. 42.

64. Savitt TL. *Medicine and Slavery;* Stampp KM. *The Peculiar Institution;* Byrd WM, Clayton LA. The "slave health deficit"; Byrd WM, Clayton LA. An American health dilemma; Genovese ED. *From Rebellion to Revolution;* Harding V. *There Is a River;* Katz WL. *Breaking the Chains: African-American Slave Resistance.* New York: Atheneum, 1990; Byrd WM, Clayton LA. *A Black Health Trilogy;* Weisbord RG. *Genocide? Birth Con-trol and the Black American.* Westport, CT: Greenwood Press, 1975; Kovel J. *White Racism: A Psychohistory.* New York: Random House, 1970, reprint ed., New York: Colum-bia University Press, 1984; Wood PH. *Black Majority: Negroes in Colonial South Carolina*

from 1670 through the Stono Rebellion. New York: Knopf, 1974, paperback ed., New York: W. W. Norton, 1975, pp. 221–223, 271–284; Katz WL. *Breaking the Chains: African American Slave Resistance*. New York: Atheneum, 1990, 52–53; McManus EJ. *A History of Negro Slavery in New York*. Syracuse, NY: Syracuse University Press, 1966, p. 136; Oates SB. Children of darkness.

65. Oates SB. Children of darkness; Genovese ED. *From Rebellion to Revolution*; Harding V. *There Is a River*; Wood PH. *Black Majority*, pp. 135–136, 236–238n; Katz WL. *Breaking the Chains*.

66. Katz WL. *Breaking the Chains*, pp. 24–25.

67. Stampp KM. *The Peculiar Institution*, pp. 245–251; Fogel RW. *Without Consent or Contract*, pp. 119–123; Tyler RC, Murphy LR, eds. *The Slave Narratives of Texas*, pp. xxvi, 20–21, 36; Mellon J, ed. *Bullwhip Days*, pp. 147–149; Owens LH. *This Species of Property*, pp. 184–185, 277; Magee MJ. The old slave house; Nichols CH. *Many Thousands Gone*, p. 21; Oakes J. *The Ruling Race*, pp. 172–173; Bancroft F. *Slave Trading in the Old South*; Gutman H, Sutch R. Victorians all?; Joyner C. The world of the plantation slaves. In: Campbell EDC Jr, Rice K., eds. *Before Freedom Came*, pp. 50–99; White DG. Female slaves in the plantation South. In: Campbell EDC Jr, Rice K., eds. *Before Freedom Came*, pp. 101–121; Phillips UB. *American Negro Slavery: A Survey of the Supply, Employment and Control of Negro Labor As Determined by the Plantation Regime*. N.P.: D. Appleton and Company, 1918; paperback ed., Baton Rouge: Louisiana State University Press, 1966; Sutch R. The care and feeding of slaves; Savitt TL. *Medicine and Slavery*; Sheridan RB. *Doctors and Slaves*; Ewbank DC. History of Black mortality and health before 1940.

68. Ewbank DC. History of Black mortality and health before 1940; Farley R. *Growth of the Black Population*; Farley R, Allen WR. *The Color Line and the Quality of Life in America*. New York: Oxford University Press, 1989; Fogel RW. *Without Consent or Contract*.

69. Farley R, Allen WR. *The Color Line and the Quality of Life in America*, p. 14.

70. Curry LP. *The Free Black in Urban America, 1800–1850: The Shadow of the Dream*. Chicago: The University of Chicago Press, 1981, p. 138.

71. Savitt TL. *Medicine and Slavery*, pp. 140–141.

72. Ewbank DC. History of Black mortality and health before 1940; Savitt TL. *Medicine and Slavery*; Farley R, Allen WR. *The Color Line and the Quality of Life in America*, pp. 14–15; David PA, et al. *Reckoning with Slavery*, p. 285; Farley R. *Growth of the Black Population*; Curry LP. *The Free Black in Urban America, 1800–1850*; Fogel RW. *Without Consent or Contract*.

73. Bousfield MO. An account of physicians of color in the United States. *Bulletin of the History of Medicine* 1945; 17:61–84, quote p. 63.

74. Bousfield MO. An account of physicians of color in the United States; Morais HM. *The History of the Negro in Medicine*, pp. 154–155; Cobb WM. The Black American in medicine; Byrd WM. Race, biology, and health care; Byrd WM, Clayton LA. An American health dilemma; Moeller DW. *Environmental Health*. Cambridge, MA: Harvard University Press, 1992, pp. 6–7; Sidel VW, Sidel R, eds. *Reforming Medicine: Lessons of the Last Quarter Century*. New York: Pantheon Books, 1984; Bullough B, Bullough VL. *Poverty, Ethnic Identity, and Health Care*. New York: Appelton-Century-Crofts, 1972; Schulman KA, Berlin JA, Harless W, Karner JF, Sistrunk S, Gersh BJ, et al. *New England Journal of Medicine* 1999; 340:618–626; Cooper Patrick L, Gallo JJ, Gonzales JJ, Vu HT,

Powe Neil R, Nelson C. *Journal of the American Medical Association* 1999; 282:583–589; Clayton LA, Byrd WM. Race, a major health status and outcome variable, 1980–1999: With some historical perspectives. *Journal of the National Medical Association.* In press 2000.

75. Katz WL. *Breaking the Chains,* p. 24.

76. Katz WL. *Breaking the Chains,* p. 22.

77. Savitt TL. *Medicine and Slavery;* Sutch R. The care and feeding of slaves; Genovese ED. *Roll Jordan Roll: The World the Slaves Made.* New York: Pantheon Books, 1972, paperback ed., New York: Vintage Books, 1976, pp. 524–535, 550–561; Fogel RW. *Without Consent or Contract;* Genovese ED. *The Political Economy of Slavery;* Katz WL. *Breaking the Chains;* Nichols CH. *Many Thousands Gone,* pp. 51–70; Campbell EDC, Jr., Rice K., eds. *Before Freedom Came;* Moeller DW. *Environmental Health;* Kurtis B. "Slavery's Buried Past," *The New Explorers* (videotape), WGBH, Boston, Bill Kurtis Productions, December 18, 1996.

78. Savitt TL. *Medicine and Slavery;* Stampp KM. *The Peculiar Institution;* Byrd WM, Clayton LA. The :slave health deficit"; Byrd WM, Clayton LA. An American health dilemma; Genovese ED. *From Rebellion to Revolution;* Harding V. *There Is a River;* Katz WL. *Breaking the Chains;* Byrd WM, Clayton LA. *A Black Health Trilogy;* Weisbord RG. *Genocide? Birth Control and the Black American;* Kovel J. *White Racism: A Psychohistory;* Wood PH. *Black Majority,* pp. 221–223, 271–284; Katz WL. *Breaking the Chains: African-American Slave Resistance.* New York: Atheneum, 1990, pp. 52–53, 100–101; McManus EJ. *A History of Negro Slavery in New York;* Oates B. Children of darkness.

79. Shryock RH. Medical perspectives on the Civil War, pp. 90–108. In: Shryock RH. *Medicine in America: Historical Essays.* Baltimore: The Johns Hopkins Press, 1966; Lyons AS, Petrucelli RJ. *Medicine: An Illustrated History;* Bender GA. *Great Moments in Medicine.*

80. Starr P. *The Social Transformation of American Medicine;* Shryock RH. *The Development of Modern Medicine;* Stevens R. *American Medicine and the Public Interest;* Lyons AS, Petrucelli RJ. *Medicine: An Illustrated History.*

81. Cobb WM. James McCune Smith. *Journal of the National Medical Association* 1952; 44:160–162; Bousfield MO. An account of physicians of color in the United States. *Bulletin of the History of Medicine* 1945; 17:61–84; Novotny A, Smith C. eds. *Images of Healing;* Takaki RY. *Iron Cages;* Morais HM. *The History of the Negro in Medicine;* Walsh MR. *Doctors Wanted No Women Need Apply: Sexual Barriers in the Medical Profession, 1835–1975.* New Haven, CT: Yale University Press, 1977.

82. Stevens R. *American Medicine and the Public Interest,* p. 13.

83. Stevens R. *American Medicine and the Public Interest,* p. 13.

84. Novotny A, Smith C, eds. *Images of Healing;* Stevens R. *American Medicine and the Public Interest;* Starr P. *The Social Transformation of American Medicine;* Armstrong D, Armstrong EM. *The Great American Medicine Show: Being an Illustrated History of Hucksters, Healers, Health Evangelists, and Heroes from Plymouth Rock to the Present.* New York: Prentice Hall, 1991.

85. Stevens RA. *American Medicine and the Public Interest,* pp. 26–27.

86. Starr P. *The Social Transformation of American Medicine,* pp. 37–47; Stevens R. *American Medicine and the Public Interest;* Numbers RL, ed. *Medicine in the New World;* Brinkley A. *The Unfinished Nation: A Concise History of the American People.* New York: Knopf, 1993, pp. 241–270; Takaki RY. *Iron Cages,* pp. 80–107.

87. Haller JS Jr. *American Medicine in Transition 1840–1910.* Urbana: University of Illinois Press, 1981, p. 212.

88. Haller JS Jr. *American Medicine in Transition 1840–1910,* p. 212.

89. Haller JS Jr. *American Medicine in Transition 1840–1910;* Takaki RY. *Iron Cages,* pp. 80–107, 96; Lyons AS, Petrucelli RJ. *Medicine: An Illustrated History;* Morais HM. *The History of the Negro in Medicine;* Cobb WM. The Black American in medicine; Ludmerer KM. *Learning to Heal: The Development of American Medical Education.* New York: Basic Books, 1985; Novotny A, Smith C, eds. *Images of Healing;* Byrd WM, Clayton LA. *A Black Health Trilogy;* Starr P. *The Social Transformation of American Medicine.*

90. Bender GA. *Great Moments in Medicine,* p. 215.

91. Haller JS Jr. *American Medicine in Transition 1840–1910;* Lyons AS, Petrucelli RJ. *Medicine: An Illustrated History;* Morais HM. *The History of the Negro in Medicine;* Bullough VL. *The Development of Medicine As a Profession;* Veatch RM. *A Theory of Medical Ethics;* Bender GA. *Great Moments in Medicine,* pp. 208–219; Cobb WM. The Black American in medicine; Ludmerer KM. *Learning to Heal;* Byrd WM, Clayton LA. *A Black Health Trilogy;* Starr P. *The Social Transformation of American Medicine;* Walsh MR. *Doctors Wanted No Women Need Apply: Sexual Barriers in the Medical Profession, 1835–1975.* New Haven, CT: Yale University Press, 1977; Newman DK, et al. *Protest, Politics, and Prosperity: Black Americans and White Institutions, 1940–75.* New York: Pantheon Books, 1978, pp. 187–235.

92. Lyons AS, Petrucelli RJ. *Medicine: An Illustrated History;* Morais HM. *The History of the Negro in Medicine;* Cobb WM. The Black American in medicine; Ludmerer KM. *Learning to Heal;* Novotny A, Smith C, eds. *Images of Healing;* Byrd WM, Clayton LA. *A Black Health Trilogy.*

93. Starr P. *The Social Transformation of American Medicine,* p. 41.

94. Starr P. *The Social Transformation of American Medicine,* pp. 37–47; Stevens R. *American Medicine and the Public Interest;* Christianson EH. Medicine in New England.

95. Starr P. *The Social Transformation of American Medicine;* Lyons AS, Petrucelli RJ. *Medicine: An Illustrated History;* Shryock RH. *The Development of Modern Medicine;* Walsh MR. *"Doctors Wanted: No Women Need Apply": Sexual Barriers in the Medical Profession, 1835–1975;* Armstrong D, Armstrong EM. *The Great American Medicine Show,* pp. 1–38.

96. Gould SJ. Bound by the great chain. In: Gould SJ. *The Flamingo's Smile: Reflections in Natural History.* New York: W. W. Norton, 1985, pp. 281–290; Stanton W. *The Leopard's Spots: Scientific Attitudes Toward Race in America, 1815–1859.* Chicago: The University of Chicago Press, 1960; Gould SJ. *The Mismeasure of Man.* New York: W. W. Norton, 1981; Burns R, Ades L. "The Way West: The Way the West Was Lost and Won, 1845–1893" (six-hour documentary series on videotape), *The American Experience,* WGBH Educational Foundation, WGBH, Boston, 1995.

97. Beider RE. *Science Encounters the Indian, 1820–1880: The Early Years of American Ethnology.* Norman: University of Oklahoma Press, 1986, pp. 55–103; Gould SJ. *The Mismeasure of Man,* pp. 19–72; Stanton W. *The Leopard's Spots;* Horsman R. *Race and Manifest Destiny: The Origins of American Racial Anglo-Saxonism.* Cambridge, MA: Harvard University Press, 1981, pp. 116–157.

98. Gould SJ. *The Mismeasure of Man,* p. 44.

99. Gould SJ. *The Mismeasure of Man,* p. 46.

100. Gould SJ. *The Mismeasure of Man,* p. 46.

101. Gould SJ. *The Mismeasure of Man*, p. 47.

102. Gould SJ. *The Mismeasure of Man*, p. 50.

103. Gould SJ. *The Mismeasure of Man*, pp. 19–72; Gossett TF. *Race: The History of an Idea in America*, pp. 59–60; Haller Jr. JS. *Outcasts from Evolution*, pp. 76–77, 84–86.

104. Beider RE. *Science Encounters the Indian, 1820–1880*, pp. 55–103; Gould SJ. *The Mismeasure of Man*; Dunglison R. *Human Physiology with Three Hundred and Sixty-Eight Illustrations* (two vols., 6th ed.). Philadelphia: Lea and Blanchard, 1846; Berkowitz JS. *The College of Physicians of Philadelphia Portrait Catalogue*. Philadelphia: College of Physicians of Philadelphia, 1984; Stanton W. *The Leopard's Spots*; Horsman R. *Race and Manifest Destiny*; Jordan WD. *White over Black: American Attitudes toward the Negro, 1550–1812*. New York: W. W. Norton, 1968; Banton M. *Racial Theories*. Cambridge: Cambridge University Press, 1987; Jones JH. *Bad Blood: The Tuskegee Syphilis Experiment*. New York: The Free Press, 1981; Reiser RJ, Dyck AJ, Curran WJ, eds. Final report of the Tuskegee Syphilis Study Ad Hoc Advisory Panel; Thomas SB, Quinn SC. Public health then and now: The Tuskegee syphilis study, 1932 to 1972: Implications for HIV education and AIDS risk education programs in the Black community. *American Journal of Public Health* 1991; 81:1498–1504.

105. Byrd WM. Race, biology, and health care; Duffy J. States' rights medicine. In: Wilson CR, W Ferris, eds. *Encyclopedia of Southern Culture*. Chapel Hill: The University of North Carolina Press, 1989, pp. 1355–1356; Haller Jr. JS. *Outcasts from Evolution*; Horsman R. *Josiah Nott of Mobile*; Jordan WD. *White over Black*; Nott JC, Gliddon GR. *Types of Mankind or, Ethnological Researches*. Philadelphia: Lippincott, Grambo and Company, 1854; Nott JC, et al. *Indigenous Races of the Earth or, New Chapters of Ethnological Inquiry*. Philadelphia: J.B. Lippincott and Company, 1857; Proctor RN. *Racial Hygiene: Medicine under the Nazis*. Cambridge, MA: Harvard University Press, 1988; Reed J. Scientific racism. In Wilson CR, Ferris W, eds. *Encyclopedia of Southern Culture*, pp. 1358–1360.

106. Byrd WM. Documentary Report: Negro Diseases and Physiological Peculiarities. Nashville: Cancer Control Research Unit, Meharry Medical College, July 12, 1990. In: Byrd WM, Clayton LA. *A Black Health Trilogy*. Duffy J. States' rights medicine; Gossett TF. *Race: The History of an Idea in America*, pp. 40–41, 48–49, 57; Gould SJ. *The Mismeasure of Man*, pp. 34–35, 70–71; Gould SJ. Bound by the great chain; Jones JH. *Bad Blood*, pp. 11, 17, 24; Jordan WD. *White over Black*, pp. 505–506, 517–521, 523, 526, 530; Postell WD. *The Health of Slaves on Southern Plantations*. Baton Rouge: Louisiana State University Press, 1951, pp. 81–82; Reed J. Scientific racism; Savitt TL. *Medicine and Slavery*, p. 42; Shryock RH. *Medicine in America*, pp. 49, 96–97; Stampp KM. *The Peculiar Institution*, pp. 109, 302–304, 308–309; Stanton W. *The Leopard's Spots*, pp. 18–19; Numbers RL, Savitt TL, eds. *Science and Medicine in the Old South*.

107. Dunglison R. *Human Physiology with Three Hundred and Sixty-Eight Illustrations*, p. 631.

108. Takaki RY. *Iron Cages*, p. 138.

109. Takaki RY. *Iron Cages*, p. 138.

110. Takaki RY. *Iron Cages*, pp. 136–147; Beider RE. *Science Encounters the Indian, 1820–1880*, pp. 55–103; Gould SJ. *The Mismeasure of Man*; Dunglison R. *Human Physiology with Three Hundred and Sixty-Eight Illustrations*; Berkowitz JS. *The College of Physicians of Philadelphia Portrait Catalogue*; Stanton W. *The Leopard's Spots*; Horsman R. *Race and Manifest Destiny*; Jordan WD. *White over Black*; Banton M. *Racial Theories*;

Young RJC. *Colonial Desire: Hybridity in Theory, Culture and Race.* London: Routledge, 1995, p. 122; Kaufman M, Galishoff S, Savitt TL, eds. *Dictionary of American Medical Biography* (two vols.). Westport, CT: Greenwood Press, 1984, pp. 113–114, 219, 357–358.

111. Takaki RY. *Iron Cages*, pp. 109–110.

112. Takaki RY. *Iron Cages*, p. 110.

113. Bousfield MO. An account of physicians of color in the United States; Takaki RY. *Iron Cages*, pp. 136–147; Morais HM. *The History of the Negro in Medicine*, pp. 7–38; Cobb WM. 1981. The Black American in medicine; Brinkley A. *The Unfinished Nation: A Concise History of the American People.* New York: Knopf, 1993, pp. 200–362.

114. Morais HM. *The History of the Negro in Medicine*; Cobb WM. 1981. The Black American in medicine; Ludmerer KM. *Learning to Heal*; Byrd WM, Clayton LA. An American health dilemma; Bullough B, Bullough VL. *Poverty, Ethnic Identity, and Health Care*; Stevens R. *American Medicine and the Public Interest*; Ackerknecht EH. *A Short History of Medicine*; Lyons AS, Petrucelli RJ. *Medicine: An Illustrated History*; Novotny A, Smith C, eds. *Images of Healing*; Shryock RH. Medical perspectives on the Civil War. In: *Medicine in America: Historical Essays*, pp. 90–108; Dowling HF. *City Hospitals*; Rosenberg CE. *The Care of Strangers.*

115. Bousfield MO. An account of physicians of color in the United States; Morais HM. *The History of the Negro in Medicine*; Cobb WM. The Black American in medicine.

116. Bousfield MO. An account of physicians of color in the United States.

117. Bousfield MO. An account of physicians of color in the United States, p. 64.

118. Cobb WM. James McCune Smith; Bousfield MO. An account of physicians of color in the United States; Falk LA. Black abolitionist doctors and healers, 1810–1885. *Bulletin of the History of Medicine* 1980; 54:253–272; Dickerson DC. The Black physician. A paper presented at the "Black Health: Historical Perspectives and Current Issues Conference." Department of the History of Medicine, University of Wisconsin-Madison, April 6, 1990; Beardsley EH. *A History of Neglect: Health Care for Blacks and Mill Workers in the Twentieth-Century South.* Knoxville: The University of Tennessee Press, 1987; Byrd WM, Clayton LA. *A Black Health Trilogy*; Cobb WM. The Black American in medicine; Woodson, CG. *The Negro Professional Man and the Community.* Washington, DC: The Association for the Study of Negro Life and History, 1934; Wolinsky H. Healing wounds; Morais HM. *The History of the Negro in Medicine*; Bousfield MO. An account of physicians of color in the United States.

119. Ullman V. *Martin R. Delany: The Beginnings of Black Nationalism.* Boston: Beacon Press, 1971, pp. 87–88.

120. Ullman V. *Martin R. Delany*, p. 138.

121. Ullman V. *Martin R. Delany*; Cobb WM. Dr. David J. Peck: First Negro to graduate from an American medical school. *Bulletin of the Medico-Chirurgical Society of the District of Columbia* 1949; 6(2):3; Sterling D. *The Making of an Afro-American: Martin Robison Delany, 1812–1885.* Garden City, NY: Doubleday and Company, 1971; Morais HM. *The History of the Negro in Medicine.*

122. Hughes L, et al. *A Pictorial History of Black Americans*, p. 95.

123. Hughes L, et al. *A Pictorial History of Black Americans*; Walsh MR. *"Doctors Wanted: No Women Need Apply"*; Takaki RY. *Iron Cages.*

124. Takaki RY. *Iron Cages*, p. 137.

125. Cobb WM. 1981. The Black American in medicine; Takaki RY. *Iron Cages*, pp. 108–144; Afro-American Asclepius. *MD Magazine* April 1963; 202–205; Bousfield MO.

An account of physicians of color in the United States; Morais HM. *The History of the Negro in Medicine*; Cobb WM. The Black American in medicine; Sterling D. *The Making of an Afro-American*; Ullman V. *Martin R. Delany: The Beginnings of Black Nationalism*. Boston: Beacon Press, 1971; Walsh MR. *Doctors Wanted No Women Need Apply*.

126. Contee CG. John Sweat Rock, M.D., Esq., 1825–1866. *Journal of the National Medical Association* 1976; 68:237–242; Morais HM. *The History of the Negro in Medicine*; Bousfield MO. An account of physicians of color in the United States; Logan RW, Winston MR, eds. *Dictionary of American Negro Biography*. New York: W.W. Norton, 1982.

127. Kenney JA. *The Negro in Medicine*. Tuskegee: Tuskegee Institute Press, 1912, p. 7.

128. Morais HM. *The History of the Negro in Medicine*, pp. 5, 13, 84, 216; Afro-American Asclepias. *MD Magazine*; Kenney JA. *The Negro in Medicine*, pp. 32–33; Bousfield MO. An account of physicians of color in the United States.

129. Afro-American Asclepias. *MD Magazine*; Morais HM. *The History of the Negro in Medicine*, p. 37; Cobb WM. Alexander Thomas Augusta. *Journal of the National Medical Association* 1952; 44:327–329; Bousfield MO. An account of physicians of color in the United States; Epps CH Jr., Johnson DG, Vaughan AL. Black medical pioneers: African-American "firsts" in academic and organized medicine: Part two. *Journal of the National Medical Association* 1993; 85:703–720, 706; Kenney JA. *The Negro in Medicine*.

130. Morais HM. *The History of the Negro in Medicine*, p. 28.

131. Curtis JL. *Blacks, Medical Schools, and Society*. Ann Arbor: The University of Michigan Press, 1971, p. 11; Kaufman M, Galishoff S, Savitt TL, eds. *Dictionary of American Medical Biography*, pp. 193–194; Logan RW, Winston MR, eds. *Dictionary of American Negro Biography*, pp. 169–172; Morais HM. *The History of the Negro in Medicine*, pp. 27–29; Sterling D. *The Making of an Afro-American*; Takaki RY. *Iron Cages*; Ullman V. *Martin R. Delany*.

132. Falk LA. Black abolitionist doctors and healers, 1810–1885. *Bulletin of the History of Medicine* 1980; 54:253–272, 259.

133. Bousfield MO. An account of physicians of color in the United States; Morais HM. *The History of the Negro In Medicine*, pp. 26–28; Kenney JA. *The Negro in Medicine*, p. 7.

134. Morais HM. *The History of the Negro in Medicine*, p. 26.

135. Morais HM. *The History of the Negro in Medicine*, pp. 7–38; Cobb WM. William Wells Brown, M.D. (1816–1884). *Journal of the National Medical Association* 1955; 47:207–211.

136. Boles JB. *Black Southerners 1619–1869*, p. 107.

137. Boles JB. *Black Southerners 1619–1869*, p. 107.

138. Boles JB. *Black Southerners 1619–1869*, p. 107.

139. Postell WD. *The Health of Slaves on Southern Plantations*. Baton Rouge: Louisiana State University Press, 1951 reprint ed. Gloucester, MA: Peter Smith, 1970; Savitt TL. *Medicine and Slavery*; Vlach JM. Plantation landscapes of the antebellum South. In: Campbell EDC Jr., Rice K., eds. *Before Freedom Came: African-American Lives in the Antebellum South*, pp. 21–49; Sheridan RB. *Doctors and Slaves*; Horsman R. *Josiah Nott of Mobile*; McGregor DK. *Sexual Surgery and the Origins of Gynecology*; Jordan WC. Voodoo medicine. In: RA Williams, ed. *Textbook of Black-Related Diseases*. New York: McGraw-Hill, 1975, pp. 715–738.

140. Postell WD. *The Health of Slaves on Southern Plantations*; Savitt TL. *Medicine and Slavery*; Vlach JM. Plantation landscapes of the antebellum south; Sheridan RB. *Doctors and Slaves*; Farley R. *Growth of the Black Population*; Farley R, Allen WR. *The Color Line and the Quality of Life in America*. New York: Oxford University Press, 1989; Fogel RW. *Without Consent or Contract*; Savitt TL. Black health on the plantation. In: Numbers RL, Savitt TL, eds. *Science and Medicine in the Old South*. Baton Rouge: Louisiana State University Press, 1989, pp. 327–355.

141. Falk LA. Black abolitionist doctors and healers, 1810–1885; Hine DC. Tubman, Harriet Ross (c. 1821–1913). In: Hine DC, ed. *Black Women in America: An Historical Encyclopedia* (two vols.). Brooklyn, NY: Carlson Publishing, 1993, pp. 1176–1180; Mellon J, ed. *Bullwhip Days*, p. 64; Taylor MW. *Harriet Tubman: Antislavery Activist*. New York: Chelsea House Publishers, 1991, pp. 10, 84–86; Painter NI. Truth, Sojourner (c. 1799–1883). In: Hine DC, ed. *Black Women in America*, pp. 1172–1180.

142. Still J. *Early Recollections and Life of Dr. James Still, 1812–1885*. facsimile ed. Medford, NJ: Medford Historical Society, 1971; Cobb WM. "Dr." James Still—New Jersey pioneer. *Journal of the National Medical Association* 1963; 55:196–199; Cobb WM. The Black American in medicine; Kaufman M, Galishoff S, Savitt TL, eds. *Dictionary of American Medical Biography*, p. 720; Low WA, Clift VA, eds. *Encyclopedia of Black America*. New York: McGraw-Hill, reprint ed., New York: Da Capo Press, 1981, p. 809; Morais HM. *The History of the Negro in Medicine*, p. 22.

143. Falk LA. Black abolitionist doctors and healers, 1810–1885; Cobb WM. The Black American in medicine; Kaufman M, Galishoff S, Savitt TL, eds. *Dictionary of American Medical Biography*, p. 656; Low WA, Clift VA, eds. *Encyclopedia of Black America*, p. 736; Morais HM. *The History of the Negro in Medicine*, p. 24; Porter DB. David Ruggles, 1810–1849; Hydropathic practitioner. Parts 1, 2. *Journal of the National Medical Association* 1957; 49:67–72, 130–134; Porter DB. Ruggles, David. In Logan RW, Winston MR, eds. *Dictionary of American Negro Biography*, pp. 536–538.

144. Morais HM. *The History of the Negro in Medicine*, p. 23.

Chapter Six

1. Ward GC, Burns R, Burns K. *The Civil War*. New York: Knopf, 1990.

2. Morais HM. *The History of the Negro in Medicine*. New York: Publishers Company, 1967; White HA. *The Freedmen's Bureau in Louisiana*. Baton Rouge: Louisiana State University Press, 1970; Shryock RH. *The Development of Modern Medicine: An Interpretation of the Social and Scientific Factors Involved*. Madison: The University of Wisconsin Press, 1974; Rosenberg CE. *The Care of Strangers: The Rise of America's Hospital System*. New York: Basic Books, 1987; Bennett L Jr. *Black Power U.S.A.: The Human Side of Reconstruction*. Chicago: Johnson Publishing, 1967, paperback ed., Baltimore: Penguin Books, 1969, p. 71.

3. Hughes L, Meltzer M, Lincoln CE. *A Pictorial History of Black Americans*. Rev. 5th ed. New York: Crown Publishers, 1983, p. 197.

4. Ward GC, Burns R, Burns K. *The Civil War*; Du Bois WEB. *Black Reconstruction in America: An Essay Toward a History of the Part Which Black Folk Played in the Attempt*

to *Reconstruct Democracy in America, 1860–1880.* N.P.: Harcourt, Brace and Company, 1935, reprint ed., Cleveland, OH: Meridian Books, The World Publishing Company, 1964; Bennett L. *Black Power U.S.A.*; Frazier EF. *The Negro in the United States.* rev. ed. New York: The Macmillan Company, 1957; *The World Book Encyclopedia,* 39th ed., War of 1812; *The World Book Encyclopedia,* 39th ed., History of the United States; *The World Book Encyclopedia,* 39th ed., Reconstruction; *The New Grolier Multimedia Encyclopedia,* MPC Version, Release 6, s.v. United States history.

   5. Breeden JO. Science and medicine. In: Wilson CR, Ferris W, eds. *Encyclopedia of Southern Culture.* Chapel Hill: The University of North Carolina Press, 1989, pp. 1337–1343, note p. 1340.

   6. Hughes L, Meltzer M, Lincoln CE. *A Pictorial History of Black Americans,* p. 188.

   7. Bennett L. *Black Power U.S.A.,* p. 71.

   8. White HA. *The Freedmen's Bureau in Louisiana,* pp. 41–63; Bennett Jr. L. *Black Power U.S.A.,* p. 71; Du Bois WEB. *Black Reconstruction in America; The World Book Encyclopedia,* 39th ed., War of 1812; *The World Book Encyclopedia,* 39th ed., History of the United States; *The World Book Encyclopedia,* 39th ed., Reconstruction; *The New Grolier Multimedia Encyclopedia,* MPC Version, Release 6, s.v. United States history.

   9. Morais HM. *The History of the Negro in Medicine;* White HA. *The Freedmen's Bureau in Louisiana;* Shryock RH. *The Development of Modern Medicine;* Bennett L Jr. *Black Power U.S.A.;* U.S. Department of Health and Human Services. *Health in America: 1776–1976.* Washington, DC: U.S. Health Resources Administration, DHEW Pub. No. (HRA) 76-616, 1976.

   10. Morais HM. *The History of the Negro in Medicine;* White HA. *The Freedmen's Bureau in Louisiana;* Degler CN. *In Search of Human Nature: The Decline and Revival of Darwinism in American Social Thought.* New York: Oxford University Press, 1991; Shryock RH. *The Development of Modern Medicine; The World Book Encyclopedia,* 39th ed., s.v. Reconstruction; *The New Grolier Multimedia Encyclopedia,* MPC Version, Release 6, s.v. United States history; Bennett L Jr. *Black Power U.S.A.;* Burke J. Fit to rule. In: *The Day the Universe Changed.* Boston: Little, Brown, 1985, pp. 239–273; McEvedy C. *The World History Factfinder.* N.P.: Grisewood and Dempsy Ltd., 1984, rev. and updated ed., New York: Gallery Books, 1989.

   11. Beardsley EH. *A History of Neglect: Health Care for Blacks and Mill Workers in the Twentieth-Century South.* Knoxville: The University of Tennessee Press, 1987, p. 12.

   12. Beardsley EH. *A History of Neglect,* p. 12.

   13. Morais HM. *The History of the Negro in Medicine;* White HA. *The Freedmen's Bureau in Louisiana;* Bremner RH. *The Public Good: Philanthropy and Welfare in the Civil War Era.* New York: Knopf, 1980; Shryock RH; Woodson, Carter Godwin. *The Negro Professional Man and the Community.* Washington, DC: The Association for the Study of Negro Life and History, 1934; Shryock RH. *The Development of Modern Medicine;* Ward GC, Burns R, Burns K. *The Civil War;* Du Bois WEB. *Black Reconstruction in America;* Bennett L. *Black Power U.S.A.;* Wade WC. *The Fiery Cross: The Ku Klux Klan in America.* New York: Simon & Schuster, 1987, pp. 9–116; Frazier EF. *The Negro in the United States; The World Book Encyclopedia,* 39th ed., War of 1812; *The World Book Encyclopedia,* 39th ed., History of the United States; *The World Book Encyclopedia,* 39th ed., Reconstruction; *The New Grolier Multimedia Encyclopedia,* MPC Version, Release 6, s.v. United States history; Beardsley EH. *A History of Neglect.*

   14. Ewbank DC. History of Black mortality and health before 1940. In: Willis DP,

ed. *Health Policies and Black Americans.* New Brunswick, NJ: Transaction Publishers, 1989, pp. 100–128; Shryock RH. *Medicine in America*; Morais HM. *The History of the Negro in Medicine*; Farley R. *Growth of the Black Population: A Study of Demographic Trends.* Chicago: Markham Publishing, 1970; Farley R, Allen WR. *The Color Line and the Quality of Life in America.* New York: Oxford University Press, 1989; Reuter EB. *The American Race Problem.* rev. 3rd ed. New York: Thomas Y. Crowell Company, 1970; Bremner RH. *The Public Good*; White HA. *The Freedmen's Bureau in Louisiana.*

    15. Breeden JO. Science and medicine, p. 134.

    16. Du Bois WEB. *Black Reconstruction in America*; Frazier EF. *The Negro in the United States*; White HA. *The Freedmen's Bureau in Louisiana*; Blassingame JW. *Black New Orleans, 1860–1880*; Morais HM. *The History of the Negro in Medicine*; Genovese ED. *The Political Economy of Slavery: Studies in the Economy and Society of the Slave South.* New York: Vintage Books, 1965; David PA, et al., eds. *Reckoning with Slavery: A Critical Study in the Quantitative History of American Negro Slavery.* New York: Oxford University Press, 1976; Harwood M. Better for us to be separated. *American Heritage* December 1972; 1(24):54.

    17. Morais HM. *The History of the Negro in Medicine*; Perry JE. *Forty Cords of Wood: Memoirs of a Medical Doctor.* Jefferson City, MO: Lincoln University Press, 1947; Organ CH, Kosiba MM, eds. *A Century of Black Surgeons: The U.S.A. Experience.* Norman, Oklahoma: Transcript Press; Kenney JA. *The Negro in Medicine.* Tuskegee: Tuskegee Institute Press, 1912; Cobb WM. *The First Negro Medical Society: A History of the Medico-Chirurgical Society of the District of Columbia.* Washington, DC: The Associated Publishers, 1939; Du Bois WEB. *The Health and Physique of the Negro American.* Atlanta: Atlanta University Publications, 1906; Byrd WM. Race, biology, and health care: Reassessing a relationship. *Journal of Health Care for the Poor and Underserved* 1990; 1:278–292.

    18. Cornish DT. *The Sable Arm: Negro Troops in the Union Army, 1861–1865.* New York: W. W. Norton, 1966, p. 288.

    19. Bremner RH. *The Public Good*; Russell JH. *The Free Negro in Virginia, 1619–1865.* Baltimore: Johns Hopkins Press, 1913, reprint paperback ed., New York: Dover Publications, 1969; White HA. *The Freedmen's Bureau in Louisiana*; Du Bois WEB. *Black Reconstruction in America*; Mohr CL. *On the Threshold of Freedom: Masters and Slaves in Civil War Georgia.* Athens: The University of Georgia Press, 1986; Frazier EF. *The Negro in the United States.*

    20. Cornish DT. *The Sable Arm*, p. xi.

    21. Cornish DT. *The Sable Arm*, p. 288.

    22. Barbeau AE, Henri F. *The Unknown Soldiers: Black American Troops in World War I.* Philadelphia: Temple University Press, 1974, p. 15.

    23. Cornish DT. *The Sable Arm*, p. 269.

    24. Barbeau AE, Henri F. *The Unknown Soldiers*, p. 15.

    25. Barbeau AE, Henri F. *The Unknown Soldiers*, p. 15.

    26. Cornish DT. *The Sable Arm*; Hughes L, Meltzer M, Lincoln CE. *A Pictorial History of Black Americans*; Barbeau AE, Henri F. *The Unknown Soldiers*; Morais HM. *The History of the Negro in Medicine*; Low WA, Clift VA, eds. *Encyclopedia of Black America.* New York: McGraw-Hill, reprint ed., New York: Da Capo Press, 1981.

    27. Fredrickson GM. *The Inner Civil War: Northern Intellectuals and the Crisis of the Union.* New York: N.P., 1965, p. 100; Haller Jr. JS. *Outcasts from Evolution: Scientific Attitudes of Racial Inferiority, 1859–1900.* New York: McGraw Hill, 1971, p. 19.

28. Haller JS Jr. *Outcasts from Evolution;* Shryock RH. A medical perspective on the Civil War. In: Shryock RH. *Medicine in America: Historical Essays.* Baltimore: The Johns Hopkins Press, 1966, pp. 90–108; Horsman R. *Race and Manifest Destiny: The Origins of American Racial Anglo-Saxonism.* Cambridge, MA: Harvard University Press, 1981; Kevles DJ. *In the Name of Eugenics: Genetics and the Uses of Human Heredity.* Berkeley: University of California Press, 1985, p. 305; Gould SJ. *The Mismeasure of Man.* New York: W. W. Norton, 1981; Berry LH. *I Wouldn't Take Nothin' for My Journey: Two Centuries of an Afro-American Minister's Family.* Chicago: Johnson Publishing, 1981.

29. Haller JS Jr. *Outcasts from Evolution;* Horsman R. *Race and Manifest Destiny,* pp. 55–56; Kevles DJ. *In the Name of Eugenics,* p. 305; Gould SJ. *The Mismeasure of Man;* Magnusson M., ed. *Cambridge Biographical Dictionary.* Cambridge: Cambridge University Press, 1990, p. 1204; Stanton W. *The Leopard's Spots: Scientific Attitudes Toward Race in America, 1815–1859.* Chicago: The University of Chicago Press, 1960, p. 25; Stigler SM. *The History of Statistics: The Measurement of Uncertainty before 1900.* Cambridge, MA: The Belknap Press of Harvard University Press, 1986, pp. 161–194; Du Bois WEB. *Black Reconstruction in America.*

30. Haller JS Jr. *Outcasts from Evolution,* p. 26.

31. Haller JS Jr. *Outcasts from Evolution,* p. 23.

32. Haller JS Jr. *Outcasts from Evolution;* Horsman R. *Race and Manifest Destiny,* pp. 55–56; Kevles DJ. *In the Name of Eugenics,* p. 305; Gould SJ. *The Mismeasure of Man;* Magnusson M., ed. *Cambridge Biographical Dictionary,* p. 1204; Stanton W. *The Leopard's Spots,* p. 25; Stigler SM. *The History of Statistics,* pp. 161–194; Du Bois WEB. *Black Reconstruction in America,* p. 3; Thernstrom S, Orlov A, Handlin O, eds. *Harvard Encyclopedia of American Ethnic Groups.* Cambridge, MA: The Belknap Press of Harvard University Press, 1980.

33. Haller JS Jr. *Outcasts from Evolution,* p. 28.

34. Haller JS Jr. *Outcasts from Evolution,* pp. 29–30.

35. Haller JS Jr. *Outcasts from Evolution,* pp. 19–34; Gould SJ. Bound by the great chain. In: Gould SJ. *The Flamingo's Smile: Reflections in Natural History.* New York: W. W. Norton, 1985, pp. 281–291; Jordan WD. *White over Black: American Attitudes Toward the Negro, 1550–1812.* New York: W. W. Norton, 1968, pp. 499–502; Stanton W. *The Leopard's Spots,* pp. 16–18; Fredrickson GM. *The Black Image in the White Mind: The Debate on Afro-American Character and Destiny, 1871–1914.* New York: Harper & Row, 1971, reprint ed., Middletown, CT: Wesleyan University Press, 1987; Chase A. *The Legacy of Malthus: The Social Costs of the New Scientific Racism.* New York: Knopf, 1980; Harrison DD, Cooke CW. An elucidation of factors influencing physicians' willingness to perform elective female sterilization. *Obstetrics and Gynecology* 1988; 72:565–569; Weisbord RG. *Genocide? Birth Control and the Black American.* Westport, CT: Greenwood Press, 1975; Bullough B, Bullough VL. *Poverty, Ethnic Identity, and Health Care.* New York: Appleton-Century-Crofts, 1972; Baxter JH. *Statistics, Medical and Anthropological, of the Provost Marshal-General's Bureau, Derived from Records of the Examination for Military Service in the Armies of the United States during the Late War of the Rebellion, of over a Million Recruits, Drafted Men, Substitutes, and Enrolled Men.* Washington, DC: N.P., 1875; Proctor RN. *Racial Hygiene: Medicine under the Nazis.* Cambridge, MA: Harvard University Press, 1988; Lifton RJ. *The Nazi Doctors: Medical Killing and the Psychology of Genocide.* New York: Basic Books, 1986; Lifton RJ, Eric Markusen. *The Genocidal Men-*

tality: Nazi Holocaust and Nuclear Threat. New York: Basic Books, 1990; U.S. Department of Health and Human Services. *Cultural Competence for Evaluators: A Guide for Alcohol and Other Drug Abuse Prevention Practitioners Working with Ethnic/Racial Communities.* Rockville, MD: Office for Substance Abuse Prevention, Alcohol, Drug Abuse, and Mental Health Administration, DHHS Publication No. (ADM)92-1884, 1992.

36. Haller Jr. JS. *Outcasts from Evolution*; Hunt SB. The Negro as a soldier. *Quarterly Journal of Psychological Medicine* October 1867; 1:175; Hunt SB. The Negro as a soldier. *London Anthropological Review* 1869, 42–43; Russett CE. *Sexual Science: The Victorian Construction of Womanhood.* Cambridge, MA: Harvard University Press, 1989, p. 29; Gould SJ. Wide hats and narrow minds. In: Gould SJ. *The Panda's Thumb: More Reflections in Natural History.* New York: W. W. Norton, 1980, pp. 145–151; Gould SJ. *The Mismeasure of Man.*

37. Low WA, Clift VA, eds. *Encyclopedia of Black America*, p. 834.

38. Shryock RH. A medical perspective on the civil war. In: Shryock RH. *Medicine in America: Historical Essays*, pp. 90–108.

39. Cobb WM. Alexander Thomas August. *Journal of the National Medical Association* 1952; 44:327–329, note p. 328.

40. Cobb WM. Alexander Thomas Augusta, note p. 328.

41. Cobb WM. Alexander Thomas Augusta; Clift VA. eds. *Encyclopedia of Black America*; Morais HM. *The History of the Negro in Medicine*; Ward GC, Burns R, Burns K. *The Civil War*, p. 253; Shryock RH. A medical perspective on the civil war; Pettigrew TF. Prejudice. In: Thernstrom S, Orlov A, Handlin O, eds. *Harvard Encyclopedia of American Ethnic Groups.* Cambridge, MA: The Belknap Press of Harvard University Press, 1980, pp. 820–829.

42. Ullman V. *Martin R. Delany: The Beginnings of Black Nationalism.* Boston: Beacon, 1971, pp. 283–284; Cobb WM. Alexander Thomas Augusta.

43. Morais HM. *The History of the Negro in Medicine*, pp. 20–38; Cobb WM. Martin Robison Delany. *Journal of the National Medical Association* 1952; 44:232–238; Barbeau AE, Henri F. *The Unknown Soldiers: Black American Troops in World War I.* Philadelphia: Temple University Press, 1974; Cobb WM. Alexander Thomas Augusta; Ullman V. *Martin R. Delany.*

44. Cornish DT. *The Sable Arm*, p. 101.

45. Cornish DT. *The Sable Arm*, p. 101.

46. Morh CL. *On the Threshold of Freedom: Masters and Slaves in Civil War Georgia.* Athens: The University of Georgia Press, 1986, p. 210.

47. Ward GC, Burns R, Burns K. *The Civil War*; Mohr CL. *On the Threshold of Freedom.*

48. Mohr CL. *On the Threshold of Freedom*, p. 178.

49. Ward GC, Burns R, Burns K. *The Civil War*; Mohr CL. *On the Threshold of Freedom*; Shryock RH. A medical perspective on the Civil War. In: Shryock RH. *Medicine in America: Historical Essays*, pp. 90–108.

50. Bremner RH. *The Public Good: Philanthropy and Welfare in the Civil War Era.* New York: Knopf, 1980, p. 98.

51. Mohr CL. *On the Threshold of Freedom*, p. 94.

52. Bremner RH. *The Public Good*, p. 98.

53. Bremner RH. *The Public Good*, p. 98.

54. Bremner RH. *The Public Good,* p. 98.

55. Ward GC, Burns R, Burns K. *The Civil War;* Mohr CL. *On the Threshold of Freedom;* Hughes L, Meltzer M, Lincoln CE. *A Pictorial History of Black Americans;* Bremner RH. *The Public Good.*

56. Bremner RH. *The Public Good,* p. 98.

57. Bremner RH. *The Public Good,* p. 99.

58. Bremner RH. *The Public Good,* p. 99.

59. Ward GC, Burns R, Burns K. *The Civil War;* Mohr CL. *On the Threshold of Freedom;* Hughes L, Meltzer M, Lincoln CE. *A Pictorial History of Black Americans;* Bremner RH. *The Public Good,* p. 99.

60. Harwood M. Better for us to be separated.

61. Ward GC, Burns R, Burns K. *The Civil War,* p. 253.

62. Bremner RH. *The Public Good;* Harwood M. Better for us to be separated; Du Bois WEB. *Black Reconstruction in America,* pp. 6–9; Russell JH. *The Free Negro in Virginia, 1619–1865.* Baltimore: Johns Hopkins Press, 1913, reprint paperback ed., New York: Dover Publications, 1969.

63. Bremner RH. *The Public Good,* p. 115.

64. Bremner RH. *The Public Good,* p. 115.

65. Bremner RH. *The Public Good,* p. 119.

66. Bremner RH. *The Public Good,* p. 119.

67. Bremner RH. *The Public Good,* p. 119.

68. Bremner RH. *The Public Good;* Du Bois WEB. *Black Reconstruction in America;* Hughes L, Meltzer M, Lincoln CE. *A Pictorial History of Black Americans; The World Book Encyclopedia,* 39th ed., s.v. Reconstruction.

69. Hughes L, Meltzer M, Lincoln CE. *A Pictorial History of Black Americans,* p. 186.

70. Mohr CL. *On the Threshold of Freedom: Masters and Slaves in Civil War Georgia.* Athens: The University of Georgia Press, 1986, p. 168.

71. Bremner RH. *The Public Good,* p. 116.

72. Bremner RH. *The Public Good,* p. 116.

73. Morais HM. *The History of the Negro in Medicine,* p. 49.

74. Morais HM. *The History of the Negro in Medicine,* p. 50.

75. White HA. *The Freedmen's Bureau in Louisiana.* Baton Rouge: Louisiana State University Press, 1970, p. 70.

76. White HA. *The Freedmen's Bureau in Louisiana;* Blassingame JW. *Black New Orleans, 1860–1880;* Bremner RH. *The Public Good;* Morais HM. *The History of the Negro in Medicine.*

77. White HA. *The Freedmen's Bureau in Louisiana;* Blassingame JW. *Black New Orleans, 1860–1880;* Bremner RH. *The Public Good;* Morais HM. *The History of the Negro in Medicine.*

78. Higginbotham AL, Jr. *Shades of Freedom: Racial Politics and Presumptions of the American Legal Process.* New York: Oxford University Press, 1996, pp. 88–91, 235 (n. 47).

79. Higginbotham AL, Jr. *Shades of Freedom,* pp. 108–118.

80. Du Bois WEB. *Black Reconstruction in America,* p. 694.

81. Du Bois WEB. *Black Reconstruction in America,* pp. 670–710; Hughes L, Meltzer M, Lincoln CE. *A Pictorial History of Black Americans; The New Grolier Multimedia Encyclopedia,* MPC Version, Release 6, s.v. United States history; Kluger R. *Simple Justice: The History of* Brown v. Board of Education *and Black America's Struggle for*

Equality. New York: Knopf, 1976, paperback ed., New York: Vintage Books, 1977; Higginbotham AL, Jr. *Shades of Freedom.*

82. Blassingame JW. *The Slave Community: Plantation Life in the Antebellum South.* New York: Oxford University Press, 1972; Bremner RH. *The Public Good;* Summerville J. *Educating Black Doctors: A History of Meharry Medical College.* University: The University of Alabama Press, 1983; Rabinowitz HN. *Race Relations in the Urban South, 1865–1890.* New York: Oxford University Press, 1978; White HA. *The Freedmen's Bureau in Louisiana;* Morais HM. *The History of the Negro in Medicine,* p. 50.

83. Summerville J. *Educating Black Doctors,* p. 12.

84. Summerville J. *Educating Black Doctors,* p. 10.

85. Doyle DH. *Nashville in the New South, 1880–1930,* p. 83; Byrd WM. *A Black Health Trilogy* (videotape). Nashville, TN: African American Heritage and Education Foundation; 1991; Hubbard GW. Yesterday, today and tomorrow. *Journal of the National Medical Association* 1909; 1:133–135; Hubbard GW. Meharry Medical College—Dean Hubbard. *Journal of the National Medical Association* 1915; 7:324–325; Kaufman M, Galishoff S, Savitt TL, eds. *Dictionary of American Medical Biography,* pp. 372–373; Meharry Medical College. Black Medical History Archive Collection. Meharry Medical College Library, Kresge Learning Resources Center, Meharry Medical College, Nashville, TN; Morais HM. *The History of the Negro in Medicine;* Roman CV. *Meharry Medical College: A History.* Nashville, TN: Sunday School Publishing Board of the National Baptist Convention, 1934; Summerville J. *Educating Black Doctors.*

86. Bremner RH. *The Public Good,* p. 119.

87. Bremner RH. *The Public Good;* Churchill LR. *Rationing Health Care in America: Perceptions and Principles of Justice.* Notre Dame, IN: University of Notre Dame Press, 1987; Ryan W. *Blaming the Victim.* New York: Vintage Books, 1971, revised, updated ed., New York: Vintage Books, 1976; Veatch RM. *A Theory of Medical Ethics.* New York: Basic Books, 1981; Morais HM. *The History of the Negro in Medicine;* Summerville J. *Educating Black Doctors.*

88. Manning KR. *Black Apollo of Science: The Life of Ernest Everett Just.* New York: Oxford University Press, 1983, pp. 10–11.

89. Manning KR. *Black Apollo of Science,* p. 10.

90. Manning KR. *Black Apollo of Science,* p. 10.

91. Morais HM. *The History of the Negro in Medicine;* Cobb WM. The Black American in medicine. *Journal of the National Medical Association* 1981; 73 (Suppl 1):1183–1244; Bousfield MO. An account of physicians of color in the United States. *Bulletin of the History of Medicine* 1945; 17:61–84; Byrd WM. Robert F. Boyd: A Life of Triumph. *Meharry Alumni Magazine* 1988; 9:17; Hine DC. *Black Women in White: Racial Conflict and Cooperation in the Nursing Profession, 1890–1950.* Bloomington: Indiana University Press, 1989, p. 205; Byrd WM. Race, biology, and health care: Reassessing a relationship. *Journal of Health Care for the Poor and Underserved* 1990; 1:278–292.

92. Brawley B. *A Social History of the American Negro: Being A History of the Negro Problem in the United States Including a History and Study of the Republic of Liberia.* New York: Macmillan, 1921, paperback ed., London: Collier-Macmillan, 1970, p. 301.

93. Logan RW. *The Negro in American Life and Thought: The Nadir, 1877–1901.* New York: Macmillan, 1954. *The Betrayal of the Negro: From Rutherford B. Hayes to Woodrow Wilson.* Enlarged, revised, paperback ed., London: Collier-Macmillan, 1965, p. 276.

94. Brawley B. A *Social History of the American Negro*; Logan RW. *The Negro in American Life and Thought*; *The Betrayal of the Negro*; Hughes L, Meltzer M, Lincoln CE. *A Pictorial History of Black Americans*; Kluger R. *Simple Justice*; Higginbotham AL, Jr. *Shades of Freedom*, pp. 169–182.

95. Brawley B. A *Social History of the American Negro*, p. 298.

96. Morais HM. *The History of the Negro in Medicine*; Cobb WM. The Black American in medicine; Bousfield MO. An account of physicians of color in the United States; Byrd WM. R.F. Boyd: To serve this present age. A paper read before the R.F. Boyd Medical Society, Nashville, Tennessee, June 8, 1988; Brawley B. A *Social History of the American Negro*.

97. Morais HM. *The History of the Negro in Medicine*; Cobb WM. The Black American in medicine; Bousfield MO. An account of physicians of color in the United States; Byrd WM. Robert F. Boyd: A life of triumph. *Meharry Alumni Magazine* 1988; 9:17; Hine DC. *Black Women in White*, p. 205; Byrd WM. Race, biology, and health care.

98. Novotny A, Smith C, eds. *Images of Healing: A Porfolio of American Medical and Pharmaceutical Practice in the Eighteenth, Nineteenth, and Early Twentieth Centuries*. New York: Macmillan, 1980, p. 69.

99. Shryock RH. *The Development of Modern Medicine*, pp. 181–182.

100. Shryock RH. A medical perspective on the Civil War; Shryock RH. *The Development of Modern Medicine*; Morais HM. *The History of the Negro in Medicine*; Novotny A, Smith C, eds. *Images of Healing*; Mohr CL. *On the Threshold of Freedom*; Bremner RH. *The Public Good*; White HA. *The Freedmen's Bureau in Louisiana*; Breeden JO. Science and medicine; Riley HD. Moore, Samuel P. (1813–1889) Confederate surgeon. In: Wilson CR, Ferris W, eds. *Encyclopedia of Southern Culture*, pp. 1374–1375.

101. Morais HM. *The History of the Negro in Medicine*; Cobb WM. The Black American in medicine; Byrd WM, Clayton LA. *A Black Health Trilogy* (videotape and 188-page documentary report). Washington, DC: The National Medical Association and the African American Heritage and Education Foundation; 1991; Byrd WM, Clayton LA. An American health dilemma; Byrd WM. Race, biology, and health care; Bremner RH. *The Public Good*; White HA. *The Freedmen's Bureau in Louisiana*; Breeden JO. Science and medicine; Warner JH. Education, medical. In: Wilson CR, Ferris W, eds. *Encyclopedia of Southern Culture*, pp. 1349–1350.

102. Nelkin D, Tancredi L. *Dangerous Diagnostics: The Social Power of Biological Information*. New York: Basic Books, 1989; Illich I. *Medical Nemesis: The Expropriation of Health*. New York: Pantheon Books, 1976, paperback ed., Toronto: Bantam Books, 1977; Fuchs VR. *The Health Economy*. Cambridge, MA: Harvard University Press, 1986; Whol S. *The Medical Industrial Complex*. New York: Harmony Books, 1984; Sidel VW, Sidel R, eds. *Reforming Medicine: Lessons of the Last Quarter Century*. New York: Pantheon Books, 1984; Brown ER. *Rockefeller Medicine Men: Medicine and Capitalism in America*. Berkeley: University of California Press, 1979; Rosenberg CE. *The Care of Strangers: The Rise of America's Hospital System*. New York: Basic Books, 1987; Starr P. *The Social Transformation of American Medicine*. New York: Basic Books, 1982; Stevens R. *American Medicine and the Public Interest*. New Haven, CT: Yale University Press, 1971; Ginzberg E. *The Medical Triangle: Physicians, Politicians, and the Public*. Cambridge, MA: Harvard University Press, 1990; Roberts MJ, Clyde AT. *Your Money or Your Life: The Health Care Crisis Explained*. New York: Main Street Books, 1993.

103. Byrd WM, Clayton LA. "Health System Component Analysis: A Health Policy Analytic Tool." A documentary report prepared for Summit '93: Regional Summits on Health Care Reform, Department HPM, Harvard School of Public Health, November 1993; Wilson FA, Neuhauser D. *Health Services in the United States*. 2nd ed. Cambridge, MA: Ballinger Publishing, 1982.

104. Byrd WM, Clayton LA. "Designing a New Health Care System for the United States" (unpublished document). Boston: Harvard School of Public Health, 1992; Wilson FA, Neuhauser D. *Health Services in the United States*.

105. Rosenberg CE. *The Care of Strangers*, p. 5.

106. Rosenberg CE. *The Care of Strangers*; Shryock RH. *The Development of Modern Medicine*; Morais HM. *The History of the Negro in Medicine*; Charatz-Litt C. A chronicle of racism: The effects of the White medical community on black health. *Journal of the National Medical Association* 1992; 84:717–725; Byrd WM, Clayton LA. An American health dilemma.

107. Vogel MJ. *The Invention of the Modern Hospital: Boston 1870–1930*. Chicago: The University of Chicago Press, 1980, p. 109.

108. Vogel MJ. *The Invention of the Moder Hospital*, p. 99.

109. Vogel MJ. *The Invention of the Modern Hospital*; Starr P. *The Social Transformation of American Medicine*.

110. Starr P. *The Social Transformation of American Medicine*, pp. 62–63.

111. Starr P. *The Social Transformation of American Medicine*; Rosenberg CE. *The Care of Strangers*; Dowling HF. *City Hospitals: The Undercare of the Underprivileged*; Morais HM. *The History of the Negro in Medicine*; Cobb WM. *Medical Care and the Plight of the Negro*. New York: The National Association for the Advancement of Colored People, 1947; Cobb WM. *Progress and Portents for the Negro in Medicine*. New York: The National Association for the Advancement of Colored People, 1948.

112. Christianson EH. Medicine in New England. In: Numbers RL, ed. *Medicine in the New World: New Spain, New France, and New England*. Knoxville: The University of Tennessee Press, 1987, pp. 101–153; quote p. 130.

113. Starr P. *The Social Transformation of American Medicine*, p. 62.

114. Christianson EH. Medicine in New England; Starr P. *The Social Transformation of American Medicine*, p. 62; Stevens R. *American Medicine and the Public Interest*, pp. 22–33.

115. Rabinowitz HN. *Race Relations in the Urban South, 1865–1890*. New York: Oxford University Press, 1978, p. 128.

116. Rabinowitz HN. *Race Relations in the Urban South, 1865–1890*; Breeden JO. Science and medicine 1337–1343. In: Wilson CR, Fermis W, eds. *Encyclopedia of Southern Culture*. Chapel Hill: The University of North Carolina Press, 1989; Kosa J, Zola IK, eds. *Poverty and Health: A Sociological Analysis*. Rev. ed. Cambridge, MA: Harvard University Press, 1975; Dowling HF. *City Hospitals: The Undercare of the Underprivileged*; Rosenberg CE. *The Care of Strangers*; Bremner RH. *The Public Good*; White HA. *The Freedmen's Bureau in Louisiana*; U.S. Department of Health and Human Services. *Health in America: 1776–1976*. Washington, DC: U.S. Health Resources Administration, DHEW Pub. No. (HRA) 76-616, 1976; White HA. *The Freedmen's Bureau in Louisiana*; Fee E. The origins and development of public health in the United States, pp. 35–72. In: Detels R, Holland WW, McEwen J, Omesin GS, eds. *Oxford Textbook of Public Health*. Volume

1. *The Scope of Public Health.* 3rd ed. New York: Oxford University Press, 1997; Fee E. History and development of public health. 10–30. In: Sutchfield ED, Keck CW. *Principles of Public Health Practice.* Albany, NY: Delmar Publishers, 1997.

117. Rabinowitz HM. *Race Relations in the Urban South, 1865–1890*, p. 129.

118. Rabinowitz HN. *Race Relations in the Urban South, 1865–1890*, p. 129.

119. Rabinowitz HN. *Race Relations in the Urban South, 1865–1890*, p. 133.

120. Rabinowitz HN. *Race Relations in the Urban South, 1865–1890*, p. 138.

121. Rabinowitz HN. *Race Relations in the Urban South, 1865–1890*, p. 151.

122. Rabinowitz HN. *Race Relations in the Urban South, 1865–1890*; Starr P. *The Social Transformation of American Medicine*; Mohr CL. *On the Threshold of Freedom*; Bremner RH. *The Public Good*; White HA. *The Freedmen's Bureau in Louisiana*; Summerville J. *Educating Black Doctors.*

123. Sardell A. *The U.S. Experiment in Social Medicine: The Community Health Center Program, 1956–1986.* Pittsburgh, PA: The University of Pittsburgh Press, 1988, p. 23.

124. Sardell A. *The U.S. Experiment in Social Medicine*, pp. 23–49; Rosenberg CE. *The Care of Strangers*; Katz MB. *In the Shadow of the Poorhouse: A Social History of Welfare in America.* New York: Basic Books, 1986, rev. and updated ed., 1996; Novotny A, Smith C, eds. *Images of Healing.*

125. Sardell A. *The U.S. Experiment in Social Medicine*, p. 23.

126. Sardell A. *The U.S. Experiment in Social Medicine*, p. 238; Rabinowitz HN. *Race Relations in the Urban South, 1865–1890*; Bullough B, Bullough VL. *Poverty, Ethnic Identity, and Health Care*; Rosenberg CE. *The Care of Strangers*; Roberts MJ, Clyde AT. *Your Money or Your Life*; Starr P. *The Social Transformation of American Medicine*; Wisner E. *Social Welfare in the South: From Colonial Times to World War I.* Baton Rouge: Louisiana State University Press, 1970.

127. Wilson FA, Neuhauser D. *Health Services in the United States.* 2nd Ed. Cambridge, MA: Ballinger Publishing Company, 1982, p. 239.

128. Rosen G. The idea of social medicine in America. *Canadian Medical Association Journal* 1949; 61:316–323.

129. Rosen G. The idea of social medicine in America.

130. Sardell A. *The U.S. Experiment in Social Medicine*; Morais HM. *The History of the Negro in Medicine*; Hine DC. *Black Women in White*; *The New Grolier Multimedia Encyclopedia*, MPC Version, Release 6, s.v. United States history.

131. Starr P. *The Social Transformation of American Medicine*, pp. 343–347; Bennett JT, DiLorenzo TJ. *Unhealthy Charities: Hazardous to Your Health and Wealth.* New York: Basic Books, 1994; Wilson FA, Neuhauser D. *Health Services in the United States*; Patterson JT. *The Dread Disease: Cancer and Modern American Culture.* Cambridge, MA: Harvard University Press, 1987; Neverdon-Morton C. *Afro-American Women of the South and the Advancement of the Race, 1895–1925.* Knoxville: The University of Tennessee Press, 1989, pp. 109, 110, 181; Hine DC. *Black Women in White*, pp. 19, 20.

132. Lee PR, Benjamin AE. Governmental and legislative control and direction of health services in the United States. In: Holland WW, Detels R, Knox G. *Oxford Textbook of Public Health.* 2nd ed. (Vol. 1). Oxford: Oxford University Press, 1991, pp. 217–230.

133. Bremner RH. *The Public Good*, pp. 142–143.

134. White HA. *The Freedmen's Bureau in Louisiana*, p. 100.

135. Lee PR, Benjamin AE. Governmental and legislative control and direction of health services in the United States; White HA. *The Freedmen's Bureau in Louisiana*; Bremner RH. *The Public Good.*

136. Starr P. *The Social Transformation of American Medicine*; Lyons AS, Petrucelli RJ. *Medicine: An Illustrated History.* New York: Harry N. Abrams, 1978; Novotny A, Smith C, eds. *Images of Healing*; Ludmerer KM. *Learning to Heal*, p. 11.

137. Stevens RA. *American Medicine and the Public Interest*, p. 31.

138. Stevens R. *American Medicine and the Public Interest*, pp. 30–33; Ginzberg E. *The Medical Triangle*; Starr P. *The Social Transformation of American Medicine*, pp. 127–134; Sonnedecker G. *Kremers and Undang's History of Pharmacy.* Rev. 4th ed. Philadelphia: J.B. Lippincott Company, 1976; Lyons AS, Petrucelli RJ. *Medicine: An Illustrated History*; Jordan WC. Voodoo Medicine. In: RA Williams, ed. *Textbook of Black-Related Diseases.* New York: McGraw-Hill, 1975, pp. 715–738; Armstrong D, Armstrong EM. *The Great American Medicine Show: Being an Illustrated History of Hucksters, Healers, Health Evangelists and Heroes from Plymouth Rock to the Present.* New York: Prentice Hall, 1991.

139. Starr P. *The Social Transformation of American Medicine*; Lyons AS, Petrucelli RJ. *Medicine: An Illustrated History*; Novotny A, Smith C, eds. *Images of Healing*; Armstrong D, Armstrong EM. *The Great American Medicine Show.*

140. Starr P. *The Social Transformation of American Medicine*, pp. 127–134; Armstrong D, Armstrong EM. *The Great American Medicine Show*; Lyons AS, Petrucelli RJ. *Medicine: An Illustrated History*; Novotny A, Smith C, eds. *Images of Healing*; Curtis JL. *Blacks, Medical Schools, and Society.* Ann Arbor: The University of Michigan Press, 1971; Morais HM. *The History of the Negro in Medicine.*

141. Starr P. *The Social Transformation of American Medicine*, p. 129.

142. Haller JS Jr. *American Medicine in Transition 1840–1910.* Urbana: University of Illinois Press, 1981, pp. 267–276; Starr P. *The Social Transformation of American Medicine*, pp. 127–134; Lyons AS, Petrucelli RJ. *Medicine: An Illustrated History*; Novotny A, Smith C, eds. *Images of Healing*; Armstrong D, Armstrong EM. *The Great American Medicine Show.*

143. Haller JS Jr. *American Medicine in Transition 1840–1910*, p. 245.

144. Haller JS Jr. *American Medicine in Transition 1840–1910*, pp. 245–246.

145. Wilson FA, Neuhauser D. *Health Services in the United States.* 2nd ed., pp. 99–136; Starr P. *The Social Transformation of American Medicine*; Haller JS Jr. *American Medicine in Transition 1840–1910*, pp. 245–247; Morais HM. *The History of the Negro in Medicine*; Rosen G. *The Structure of American Medical Practice 1875–1941.* Philadelphia: University of Pennsylvania Press, 1983.

146. Wilson FA, Neuhauser D. *Health Services in the United States.* 2nd ed., pp. 257–272. Breeden, JD. Science and medicine, pp. 1337–1343. In: Wilson CR, Ferris W, eds. *Encyclopedia of Southern Culture.* Chapel Hill: The University of North Carolina Press, 1989; Fee E. History and development of public health, pp. 10–30. In: Sutchfield FD, Keck CW. *Principles of Public Health Practice.* Albany, NY: Delmar Publishers, 1997.

147. Starr P. *The Social Transformation of American Medicine*; Morais HM. *The History of the Negro in Medicine*; Byrd WM, Clayton LA. An American health dilemma.

148. Shryock RH. *The Development of Modern Medicine*; Starr P. *The Social Transformation of American Medicine*; Ackerknecht EH. *A Short History of Medicine.* rev. ed. Baltimore: The Johns Hopkins University Press, 1982.

149. Starr P. *The Social Transformation of American Medicine*; Stevens R. *American Medicine and the Public Interest*; Rosen G. *The Structure of American Medical Practice 1875–1941*; Cobb WM. *The First Negro Medical Society*; Woodson CG. *The Negro Professional Man and the Community*. Washington, DC: The Association for the Study of Negro Life and History, 1934.

150. Starr P. *The Social Transformation of American Medicine*, p. 69.

151. Starr P. *The Social Transformation of American Medicine*; Stevens R. *American Medicine and the Public Interest*; Rosen G. *The Structure of American Medical Practice 1875–1941*.

152. Stevens R. *American Medicine and the Public Interest*, p. 24.

153. Rosen G. *The Structure of American Medical Practice 1875–1941*, p. 20.

154. Stevens R. *American Medicine and the Public Interest*; Rosen G. *The Structure of American Medical Practice 1875–1941*; Ludmerer KM. *Learning to Heal: The Development of American Medical Education*. New York: Basic Books, 1985; Starr P. *The Social Transformation of American Medicine*.

155. Ludmerer KM. *Learning to Heal*, p. 11.

156. Ludmerer KM. *Learning to Heal*, p. 14.

157. Stevens R. *American Medicine and the Public Interest*; Rosen G. *The Structure of American Medical Practice 1875–1941*; Ludmerer KM. *Learning to Heal*; Starr P. *The Social Transformation of American Medicine*; Morais HM. *The History of the Negro in Medicine*; Curtis JL. *Blacks, Medical Schools, and Society*; Walsh MR. *"Doctors Wanted: No Women Need Apply": Sexual Barriers in the Medical Profession, 1835–1975*. New Haven, CT: Yale University Press, 1977.

158. Ludmerer KM. *Learning to Heal*; Starr P. *The Social Transformation of American Medicine*.

159. Ludmerer KM. *Learning to Heal*, p. 47.

160. Rothstein WG. *American Medical Schools and the Practice of Medicine*. New York: Oxford University Press, 1987, p. 104.

161. Ludmerer KM. *Learning to Heal*; Epps CH Jr., Johnson DG, Vaughan AL. Black medical pioneers: African-American "firsts" in academic and organized medicine: Part one. *Journal of the National Medical Association* 1993; 85:629–644; Rothstein WG. *American Medical Schools and the Practice of Medicine*; Stevens R. *American Medicine and the Public Interest*; Starr P. *The Social Transformation of American Medicine*.

162. Starr P. *The Social Transformation of American Medicine*, p. 81.

163. Burrow JG. *The American Medical Association: Voice of American Medicine*. Baltimore: N.P., 1963, p. 12.

164. Starr P. *The Social Transformation of American Medicine*, p. 102.

165. Ludmerer KM. *Learning to Heal*; Rothstein WG. *American Medical Schools and the Practice of Medicine*; Stevens R. *American Medicine and the Public Interest*, pp. 35, 58–59; Starr P. *The Social Transformation of American Medicine*; Dowling HF. *City Hospitals: The Undercare of the Underprivileged*; Morais HM. *The History of the Negro in Medicine*; Cobb WM. *The First Negro Medical Society*, pp. 6, 21; Tocqueville A de. *Democracy in America*. New York: Harper Perennial, 1988, pp. 667–668; Wolinsky H. Healing wounds: Lonnie R. Bristow steps up to head the American Medical Association, one of the nation's premier—and most rigidly segregated—professional groups. *Emerge* July/August 1994; 10(5):42.

166. Starr P. *The Social Transformation of American Medicine*, p. 81.

167. Ludmerer KM. *Learning to Heal*, p. 44.

168. Ludmerer KM. *Learning to Heal*; Rothstein WG. *American Medical Schools and the Practice of Medicine*; Stevens R. *American Medicine and the Public Interest*; Starr P. *The Social Transformation of American Medicine*; Walsh MR. "*Doctors Wanted: No Women Need Apply*"; Rosenberg CE. *The Care of Strangers*; Savitt TL. *Medicine and Slavery*; Bullough B, Bullough VL. *Poverty, Ethnic Identity, and Health Care*; Jones JH. *Bad Blood: The Tuskegee Syphilis Experiment.* New York: The Free Press, 1981.

169. Vogel MJ. *The Invention of the Modern Hospital*, p. 110.

170. Vogel MJ. *The Invention of the Modern Hospital*; Starr P. *The Social Transformation of American Medicine*; Rosenberg CE. *The Care of Strangers.*

171. Du Bois WEB. *The Philadelphia Negro: A Social Study.* New York: Schocken Books, 1967; Brawley B. *A Social History of the American Negro*; Frazier EF. *The Negro in the United States*; Logan RW. *The Negro in American Life and Thought*; Logan RW. *The Betrayal of the Negro*; Higginbotham AL, Jr. *Shades of Freedom*; Morais HM. *The History of the Negro in Medicine*; Vogel MJ. *The Invention of the Modern Hospital*; Starr P. *The Social Transformation of American Medicine.*

172. Buckler H. *Daniel Hale Williams: Negro Surgeon.* New York: Pitman Publishing, 1954; Perry JE. *Forty Cords of Wood: Memoirs of a Medical Doctor.* Jefferson City, MO: Lincoln University Press, 1947; Morais HM. *The History of the Negro in Medicine*; Woodson CG. *The Negro Professional Man and the Community.*

173. Morais HM. *The History of the Negro in Medicine*; Cobb WM. The Black American in medicine; Byrd WM. Medical associations. In: Salzman J, Smith DL, West C, eds. *Encyclopedia of African-American Culture and History* (5 vols.). New York: Macmillan Library Reference USA, 1996, pp. 1747–1749; Byrd WM, Clayton LA. An American health dilemma; Du Bois WEB. *The Souls of Black Folk: Essays and Sketches.* Chicago: A. C. McClurg, 1903, unabridged rep. ed., New York: Dodd, Mead, and Company, 1979.

174. Cobb WM. Alexander Thomas Augusta, quote p. 328.

175. Cobb WM. Alexander Thomas Augusta; Robinson HS. Anderson Ruffin Abbot, M.D., 1837–1913. *Journal of the National Medical Association* 1980; 72:713–716; Morais HM. *The History of the Negro in Medicine*; Cornish DT. *The Sable Arm.*

176. White HA. *The Freedmen's Bureau in Louisiana*, p. 100.

177. White HA. *The Freedmen's Bureau in Louisiana*; Ward GC, Burns R, Burns K. *The Civil War*; Morais HM. *The History of the Negro in Medicine*; Bremner RH. *The Public Good.*

178. White HA. *The Freedmen's Bureau in Louisiana*; Morais HM. *The History of the Negro in Medicine*; Bremner RH. *The Public Good*; Numbers RL. *Almost Persuaded: American Physicians and Compulsory Health Insurance, 1912–1920.* Baltimore: The Johns Hopkins University Press, 1978, pp. 10–13.

179. Low WA, Clift VA, eds. *Encyclopedia of Black America*, p. 834; Shryock RH. A medical perspective on the Civil War; Cobb WM. Alexander Thomas Augusta; Haller JS Jr. *Outcasts from Evolution*, pp. 29–30; Baxter JH. *Statistics, Medical and Anthropological, of the Provost Marshal-General's Bureau.*

180. White HA. *The Freedmen's Bureau in Louisiana*, p. 100.

181. White HA. *The Freedmen's Bureau in Louisiana*, p. 100.

182. White HA. *The Freedmen's Bureau in Louisiana*; Morais HM. *The History of the Negro in Medicine*; Bremner RH. *The Public Good.*

183. Jones JH. *Bad Blood.* p. 19.

184. Morais HM. *The History of the Negro in Medicine*; Summerville J. *Educating Black Doctors*; Bremner RH. *The Public Good*; White HA. *The Freedmen's Bureau in Louisiana*.

185. Morais HM. *The History of the Negro in Medicine*, p. 31.

186. Cobb WM. *Medical Care and the Plight of the Negro*, p. 7.

187. Morais HM. *The History of the Negro in Medicine*; Epps CH Jr., Johnson DG, Vaughan AL. Black medical pioneers; Cobb WM. *Progress and Portents for the Negro in Medicine*.

188. Morais HM. *The History of the Negro in Medicine*, p. 43.

189. Cobb WM. The Black American in medicine; Morais HM. *The History of the Negro in Medicine*, pp. 40–43; Epps HR. The Howard University medical department in the Flexner era: 1910–1929. *Journal of the National Medical Association* 1989; 81:885.

190. Cobb WM. *The First Negro Medical Society*, p. 9.

191. Morais HM. *The History of the Negro in Medicine*; Flexner A. *Medical Education in the United States and Canada: A Report to the Carnegie Foundation for the Advancement of Teaching*. New York: Carnegie Foundation for the Advancement of Teaching, 1910; Travella S. Black hospitals struggling to survive: Of more than 200 medical centers, only 8 are left, p. 12. *Health: A Weekly Journal of Medicine, Science and Society, The Washington Post*, September 11, 1990; Kaufman M, Galishoff S, Savitt TL, eds. *Dictionary of American Medical Biography*; Organ CH, Kosiba MM. eds. *A Century of Black Surgeons: The U.S.A. Experience* (2 Vols.). Norman, OK: Transcript Press; Buckler H. *Daniel Hale Williams: Negro Surgeon*.

192. Reitzes DC. *Negroes and Medicine*. Cambridge, MA: Harvard University Press, 1958, p. 197.

193. Reitzes DC. *Negroes and Medicine*, pp. 196, 197–200; Cobb WM. Charles Burleigh Purvis (1842–1929); Morais HM. *The History of the Negro in Medicine*; Cobb WM. *The First Negro Medical Society*, pp. 7, 10–12; Brawley B. *A Social History of the American Negro*; Logan RW. *The Negro in American Life and Thought*; Logan RW. *The Betrayal of the Negro*.

194. Cobb WM. *The First Negro Medical Society*, p. 10.

195. Cobb WM. *The First Negro Medical Society*, p. 11.

196. Cobb WM. *The First Negro Medical Society*, pp. 10–12; Cobb WM. *Progress and Portents for the Negro in Medicine*; Cobb WM. Alexander Thomas Augusta; Cobb WM. Charles Burleigh Purvis (1842–1929); Ullman V. *Martin R. Delany: The Beginnings of Black Nationalism*. Boston: Beacon Press, 1971; Morais HM. *The History of the Negro in Medicine*; Savitt TL. The education of Black physicians at Shaw University, 1882–1918. In Crow J, Hatley FJ, eds. *Black Americans in North Carolina and the South*. Chapel Hill: University of North Carolina Press, 1984, pp. 160–188; Savitt TL. Entering a white profession: Black physicians in the new south, 1880–1920. *Bulletin of the History of Medicine* 1987; 61:507–540.

197. Cobb WM. Alexander Thomas Augusta, p. 328.

198. Cobb WM. Alexander Thomas Augusta, p. 328.

199. Cobb WM. Alexander Thomas Augusta, p. 328.

200. Cobb WM. Alexander Thomas Augusta, p. 327.

201. Cobb WM. *The First Negro Medical Society*, pp. 10–12; Cobb WM. *Progress and Portents for the Negro in Medicine*; Cobb WM. Alexander Thomas Augusta; Cobb WM. Charles Burleigh Purvis (1842–1929); Ullman V. *Martin R. Delany: The Beginnings of Black Nationalism*; Morais HM. *The History of the Negro in Medicine*; Wolinsky H.

Healing wounds; Brawley B. A *Social History of the American Negro*; Logan RW. *The Negro in American Life and Thought*; Logan RW. *The Betrayal of the Negro*.

202. Cobb WM. *The First Negro Medical Society*, pp. 14–15.

203. Cobb WM. *The First Negro Medical Society*, pp. 10–12; Cobb WM. *Progress and Portents for the Negro in Medicine*; Cobb WM. Alexander Thomas Augusta; Cobb WM. Charles Burleigh Purvis (1842–1929); Ullman V. *Martin R. Delany: The Beginnings of Black Nationalism*; Morais HM. *The History of the Negro in Medicine*.

204. Cobb WM. *The First Negro Medical Society*, pp. 10–12; Cobb WM. *Progress and Portents for the Negro in Medicine*; Cobb WM. Alexander Thomas Augusta; Cobb WM. Charles Burleigh Purvis (1842–1929); Morais HM. *The History of the Negro in Medicine*; Epps HR. The Howard University medical department in the Flexner era; Savitt TL. Abraham Flexner and the black medical schools. In: Barzansky EM, Gevitz N, eds. *Flexner and the 1990s; Medical Education in the 20th Century*. N.P., 1989, p. 23; Manning KR. *Black Apollo of Science*; Byrd WM, Clayton LA. A *Black Health Trilogy*.

205. Morais HM. *The History of the Negro in Medicine*, pp. 40–48; Meharry Medical College. Hubbard and Sneed. *Bulletin of Meharry Medical College: 80th Anniversary Issue*: 11; Summerville J. *Educating Black Doctors*, pp. 12–20; Braden ME. *John Braden: A Pioneer in Negro Education*; Roman CV. *Meharry Medical College: A History*; Meharry F. *History of the Meharry Family in America*. Lafayette, IN: Lafayette Printing, 1925.

206. Morais HM. *The History of the Negro in Medicine*, p. 48.

207. Morais HM. *The History of the Negro in Medicine*, p. 48.

208. Morais HM. *The History of the Negro in Medicine*; Cobb WM. Henry Fitzbutler, 1842–1901. *Journal of the National Medical Association* 1952; 44:403–407; Savitt TL. Lincoln University medical department—a forgotten 19th century Black medical school. *Journal of the History of Medicine and Allied Sciences* 1985; 40:42–65; Summerville J. *Educating Black Doctors*; Roman CV. *Meharry Medical College: A History*.

209. Morais HM. *The History of the Negro in Medicine*, p. 42.

210. Roman CV. *Meharry Medical College: A History*; Summerville J. *Educating Black Doctors*; Meharry Medical College. *Bulletin of Meharry Medical College: 80th Anniversary Issue*. Savitt TL. Entering a white profession: Black physicians in the new south, 1880–1920. *Bulletin of the History of Medicine* 1987; 61:507–540; Savitt TL. Lincoln University medical department—a forgotten 19th century Black medical school; Cobb WM. Henry Fitzbutler, 1842–1901; Morais HM. *The History of the Negro in Medicine*, p. 42; Roman CV. *Meharry Medical College: A History*; Meharry F. *History of the Meharry Family in America*; Braden ME. *John Braden: A Pioneer in Negro Education*.

211. Savitt TL. The education of Black physicians at Shaw University, 1882–1918; McBride E. Inequality in the availability of Black physicians. *New York State Journal of Medicine* 1985; 85:139–142; Morais HM. *The History of the Negro in Medicine*; Cobb WM. John Andrew Kenney, M.D., 1874–1950. *Journal of the National Medical Association* 1956; 48:75.

212. Starr P. *The Social Transformation of American Medicine*, p. 112.

213. Starr P. *The Social Transformation of American Medicine*; Rothstein WG. *American Physicians in the 19th Century: From Sects to Science*. Baltimore, MD: The Johns Hopkins University Press, 1972; Brawley B. A *Social History of the American Negro*; Morais HM. *The History of the Negro in Medicine*; Cobb WM. Henry Fitzbutler, 1842–1901; Savitt TL. The education of Black physicians at Shaw University, 1882–1918; Savitt TL. Lincoln University medical department—a forgotten 19th century Black medical school.

214. Morais HM. *The History of the Negro in Medicine*; Bousfield MO. An account of physicians of color in the United States; Cobb WM. Nathan Francis Mossell, M.D., 1856–1946. *Journal of the National Medical Association* 1954; 46:118–130; Lynk MV. *Sixty Years of Medicine, or The Life and Times of Dr. Miles V. Lynk: An Autobiography*. Memphis: Twentieth Century Press, 1951; Cobb WM. Henry Fitzbutler, 1842–1901.

215. Byrd WM, Clayton LA. An American health dilemma; Byrd WM, Clayton LA. *A Black Health Trilogy*; Morais HM. *The History of the Negro in Medicine*; Cobb WM. The Black American in medicine.

216. Morais HM. *The History of the Negro in Medicine*, p. 80.

217. Cobb WM. Nathan Frances Mossell, M.D., 1856–1946.

218. Starr P. *The Social Transformation of American Medicine*, p. 11.

219. Morais HM. *The History of the Negro in Medicine*; Cobb WM. *The First Negro Medical Society*; Cobb WM. Nathan Francis Mossell, M.D., 1856–1946; Perry JE. *Forty Cords of Wood*; Summerville J. *Educating Black Doctors*; Savitt TL. Entering a white profession.

220. Chatman JA. *The Lone Star State Medical, Dental, and Pharmaceutical History*. N.P.: Lone Star State Medical, Dental, and Pharmaceutical Association, 1956; Cobb WM. Monroe Alpheus Majors, 1864–. *Journal of the National Medical Association* 1955; 47:139–141; Cobb WM. *The First Negro Medical Society*; Morais HM. *The History of the Negro in Medicine*; Byrd WM. The NMA founding date laid to rest [Letter to the Editor]. *Journal of the National Medical Association* 1993; 85:99; Cobb WM. Miles Vandahrust Lynk. *Journal of the National Medical Association* 1952; 44:475–476; Lynk MV. *Sixty Years of Medicine, or The Life and Times of Dr. Miles V. Lynk: An Autobiography*. Memphis: Twentieth Century Press, 1951; Boyd RF. Dr. R.F. Boyd of Nashville, Tenn., President of the American Association of Colored Physicians and Surgeons. *The Washington Bee* October 3, 1896; National Medical Association. Dr. I. Garland Penn. *Journal of the National Medical Association* 1930; 22:171–172; Chase HS. "Shelling the citadel of race prejudice": William Calvin Chase and the Washington "Bee", 1882–1921. In Rosenberg FC, ed. *Records of the Columbia Historical Society of Washington, D.C. 1973–1974*. Washington, DC: Columbia Historical Society of Washington, DC, 1976, pp. 371–391.

221. Konold DE. *A History of American Medical Ethics: 1847–1912*. Madison: University of Wisconsin Press, 1962, p. 52.

222. Konold DE. *A History of American Medical Ethics: 1847–1912*, p. 56.

223. Konold DE. *A History of American Medical Ethics: 1847–1912*, p. 52; Morais HM. *The History of the Negro in Medicine*; Perry JE. *Forty Cords of Wood*; Summerville J. *Educating Black Doctors*; Savitt TL. Entering a white profession; Lynk MV. *Sixty Years of Medicine, or The Life and Times of Dr. Miles V. Lynk*.

224. Savitt TL. Entering a white profession, quote p. 517.

225. Perry JE. *Forty Cords of Wood*, pp. 159–160.

226. Bullough B, Bullough VL. *Poverty, Ethnic Identity, and Health Care*; Cameron S, Wisdom EJ. Iron in his blood. *AIM for Racial Harmony and Peace* 1988; 15:10–11; Cobb WM. John Edward Perry, M.D., 1870–; Cobb WM. Miles Vandahrust Lynk; Lynk MV. *Sixty Years of Medicine, or The Life and Times of Dr. Miles V. Lynk*; Perry JE. *Forty Cords of Wood*; Manning KR. *Black Apollo of Science*; Byrd WM. R. F. Boyd: To serve this present age; Townsend AM. The medical profession of greater Nashville. *Nashville Globe* September 4, 1908.

227. Cobb WM. Robert Fulton Boyd. *Journal of the National Medical Association* 1953; 45:233–234, 233.

228. Cobb WM. Robert Fulton Boyd; Haley JT. Dr. Robert Fulton Boyd. In *The Afro-American Encyclopedia.* Nashville, TN: Haley and Florida, 1896, pp. 59–62; Cameron S, Wisdom EJ. Iron in his blood; Summerville J. *Educating Black Doctors;* Roman CV. *Meharry Medical College: A History;* Death of Robert Fulton Boyd. *The Meharry News* 1913; 11:9–10; Rabinowitz HN. *Race Relations in the Urban South, 1865–1890;* Perry JE. *Forty Cords of Wood;* Manning KR. *Black Apollo of Science;* Byrd WM. R. F. Boyd: To serve this present age; Roman CV. *Meharry Medical College: A History;* Morais HM. *The History of the Negro in Medicine;* Boyd RF. What are the causes of the great mortality among the Negroes in the cities of the south, and how is that mortality to be lessened? In: Culp DW, ed. *Twentieth Century Negro Literature.* Naperville, IL: J. L. Nichols, 1902, pp. 215–220; Boyd RF. Mercy Hospital. *Journal of the National Medical Association* 1909; 1:43; Jones JH. *Bad Blood;* Organ CH, Kosiba MM. eds. *A Century of Black Surgeons;* Starr P. *The Social Transformation of American Medicine;* Byrd WM. The NMA founding date laid to rest; Kaufman M, Galishoff S, Savitt TL, eds. *Dictionary of American Medical Biography* (Vol. 1), pp. 86–87; Wilson OH, Christie A. Early history of medical education in Nashville. *Journal of the Tennessee Medical Association* 1969; 62:819–829; Hunt S. The Flexner report and Black academic medicine; Summerville J. Formation of a black medical profession in Tennessee, 1880–1920; Jacobson TC. *Making Medical Doctors: Science and Medicine at Vanderbilt Since Flexner.* Tuscaloosa: The University of Alabama Press, 1987.

229. Bousfield MO. An account of physicians of color in the United States, pp. 61–84, 74–75.

230. Savitt TL. Entering a white profession.

231. Savitt TL. Entering a white profession; Perry JE. *Forty Cords of Wood;* Lynk MV. *Sixty Years of Medicine, or The Life and Times of Dr. Miles V. Lynk;* Haley JT. Dr. Robert Fulton Boyd; Byrd WM. R. F. Boyd: To serve this present age; Bousfield MO. An account of physicians of color in the United States; Buckler H. *Daniel Hale Williams: Negro Surgeon.*

232. Ackerknecht EH. *A Short History of Medicine;* Lyons AS, Petrucelli RJ. *Medicine: An Illustrated History;* Shryock RH. *The Development of Modern Medicine;* Morais HM. *The History of the Negro in Medicine.*

233. Jones JH. *Bad Blood,* pp. 20–21.

234. Jones JH. *Bad Blood,* pp. 21–22.

235. Jones JH. *Bad Blood,* p. 24.

236. Dowling HF. *City Hospitals: The Undercare of the Underprivileged;* Jones JH. *Bad Blood,* p. 24; Rosenberg CE. *The Care of Strangers;* Morais HM. *The History of the Negro in Medicine;* Ryan W. *Blaming the Victim.*

237. Brandt AM. Racism and research: The case of the Tuskegee syphilis study. *Hastings Center Report* 1978; 8:21–29.

238. Jones JH. *Bad Blood,* p. 23.

239. Jones JH. *Bad Blood,* p. 23.

240. Brandt AM. Racism and research: The case of the Tuskegee syphilis study. In: Leavitt JW, Numbers RL, eds. *Sickness and Health in America: Readings in the History of Medicine and Public Health.* Madison: The University of Wisconsin Press, 1985, pp. 331–343; quote p. 332.

241. Brandt AM. Racism and research: The case of the Tuskegee syphilis study; Haller JS Jr. *Outcasts from Evolution;* Jones JH. *Bad Blood;* Morais HM. *The History of the Negro in Medicine;* Rydell RW. *All the World's a Fair: Visions of Empire at American International Expositions, 1876–1916.* Chicago: The University of Chicago Press, 1984.

242. Haller JS Jr. *Outcasts from Evolution*, p. 40.

243. Brandt AM. Racism and Research: The Case of the Tuskegee Syphilis Study; Fredrickson GM. *The Black Image in the White Mind*, pp. 228–282; Reed J. Scientific racism. In Wilson CR, Ferris W, eds. *Encyclopedia of Southern Culture*, pp. 1358–1360; Jones JH. *Bad Blood*; Haller JS Jr. *Outcasts from Evolution*; Chase A. *The Legacy of Malthus: The Social Costs of the New Scientific Racism*. New York: Knopf, 1980.

244. Haller JS Jr. *Outcasts from Evolution*, p. 41.

245. Jones JH. *Bad Blood*, p. 16.

246. Jones JH. *Bad Blood*, p. 17.

247. Greenberg DS. Black health: Grim statistics. *Lancet* 1990; 355:780–781; Dula A. Toward an African-American perspective on bioethics. *Journal of Health Care for the Poor and Underserved* 1991; 2:259–269; Washington HA. Of men and mice: Human guinea pigs: Unethical testing targets Blacks and the poor. *Emerge* October 1994; 1(6):24; Robinson LS. Dialogue: Curbing a sick practice: Energy Secretary Hazel O'Leary focuses on government accountability in testing. *Emerge* October 1994; 1(6):20; Duster R. *Backdoor to Eugenics*. New York: Routledge, 1990; Chase A. *The Legacy of Malthus*; Shea S, Fullilove MT. Entry of black and other minority students in US medical schools: Historical perspectives and recent trends. *New England Journal of Medicine* 1985; 313:933–940; Byrd WM, Clayton LA. An American health dilemma; Charatz-Litt C. A chronicle of racism.

248. Cobb WM. *The First Negro Medical Society*; Cobb WM. *Medical Care and the Plight of the Negro*; Cobb WM. *Progress and Portents for the Negro in Medicine*; Curtis JL. *Blacks, Medical Schools, and Society*; Morais HM. *The History of the Negro in Medicine*.

249. Dickerson DC. "The Black Physician." Paper presented at the Black Health: Historical Perspectives and Current Issues Conference. Department of the History of Medicine, University of Wisconsin-Madison, April 6, 1990; Ullman V. *Martin R. Delany: The Beginnings of Black Nationalism*; Morais HM. *The History of the Negro in Medicine*; Woodson CG. *The Negro Professional Man and the Community*; Summerville J. Formation of a black medical profession in Tennessee, 1880–1920. *Journal of the Tennessee Medical Association* October 1983: 644–646; Cobb WM. *The First Negro Medical Society*; Cobb WM. *Medical Care and the Plight of the Negro*; Cobb WM. *Progress and Portents for the Negro in Medicine*; Curtis JL. *Blacks, Medical Schools, and Society*.

250. Greenberg DS. Black health: Grim statistics; National Center for Health Statistics. *Health Status of the Disadvantaged Chartbook/1990*. Hyattsville, MD: Public Health Service, 1991; Clayton LA, Byrd WM. The African American cancer crisis, part I: The problem. *Journal of Health Care for the Poor and Underserved* 1993; 4:83–101; Byrd WM, Clayton LA. The African-American cancer crisis, part II: A prescription. *Journal of Health Care for the Poor and Underserved* 1993; 4:102–116; Morais HM. *The History of the Negro in Medicine*; Bullough B, Bullough VL. *Poverty, Ethnic Identity, and Health Care*; Washington HA. Of men and mice; Robinson LS. Dialogue: Curbing a sick practice.

⋊ Select Bibliography

Abercrombie TJ, Barbey B. When the Moors ruled Spain. *National Geographic,* July 1988, 86–119. Photographs (in color) by Bruno Barbey. Map; Calendar of Events.

Ackerknecht EH. *A Short History of Medicine.* Revised Edition. Baltimore, Maryland: The Johns Hopkins University Press, 1982.

Adorno TW, Else F, Levinson DJ, Sanford RN. *The Authoritarian Personality.* Abbreviated Edition. New York: W.W. Norton and Company, 1982.

Allen GE. Eugenics comes to America. 441–475. In: Jacoby R, Glauberman N, eds. *The Bell Curve Debate: History, Documents, Opinions.* New York: Times Books Division of Random House, 1995.

Allport GW. *The Nature of Prejudice.* Reading, Massachusetts: Addison-Wesley Publishing Company, 1979.

Aly G, Chroust P, Pross C. *Cleansing the Fatherland: Nazi Medicine and Racial Hygiene.* Baltimore, Maryland: The Johns Hopkins University Press, 1994.

The American Anti-Slavery Society. *American Slavery As It Is: Testimony of a Thousand Witnesses. The Anti-Slavery Examiner,* 1839 (No. 6), New York: The American Anti-Slavery Society, 1839.

American Cancer Society. *Cancer and the Socioeconomically Disadvantaged.* Atlanta, Georgia: American Cancer Society, 1990.

Annas GJ, Grodin MA, eds. *The Nazi Doctors and the Nuremberg Code: Human Rights in Human Experimentation.* New York: Oxford University Press, 1992.

Arad Y, ed. *The Pictorial History of the Holocaust.* New York: Macmillan Publishing Company, 1990.

Arato A, Gebhardt E, eds. *The Essential Frankfurt School Reader*. New York: Continuum, 1982.

Armstrong D, Armstrong EM. *The Great American Medicine Show: Being an Illustrated History of Hucksters, Healers, Health Evangelists, and Heroes from Plymouth Rock to the Present*. New York: Prentice Hall, 1991.

Armstrong, M. *Fanny Kemble: A Passionate Victorian*. New York: The Macmillan Company, 1938.

Asante MK. *The Afrocentric Idea*. Philadelphia: Temple University Press, 1987.

Asante MK. *Afrocentricity*. Trenton, New Jersey: Africa World Press, 1988.

Asante MK. Kemet, *Afrocentricity and Knowledge*. Trenton, New Jersey: Africa World Press, 1990.

Asante MK. Putting Africa at the center. *Newsweek* 1991 (September 23); 118:46.

Asante MK. Roots of the truth: Repelling attacks on Afrocentrism. *Emerge* (July–August, No. 9) 1996; 7:66.

Auletta K. *The Underclass*. New York: Random House, 1982. Paperback Edition. New York: Vintage Books, 1983.

Bagdikian BH. *The Media Monopoly*. Boston: Beacon Press, 1983.

Bancroft F. *Slave Trading in the Old South*. New York: Frederick Ungar Publishing Company, 1959.

Banton M, Harwood J. *The Race Concept*. New York: Praeger Publishers, 1975.

Banton M. *Racial Theories*. Cambridge: Cambridge University Press, 1987.

Barbeau AE, Henri F. *The Unknown Soldiers: Black American Troops in World War I*. Philadelphia: Temple University Press, 1974.

Barzun J. Race: *A Study in Modern Superstition*. N.P., 1937. *Race: A Study in Superstition*. Revised Edition. New York: Harper and Row Publishers, 1965.

Baxter JH. *Statistics, Medical and Anthropological, of the Provost Marshal-General's Bureau, Derived from Records of the Examination for Military Service in the Armies of the United States during the Late War of the Rebellion, of Over a Million Recruits, Drafted Men, Substitutes, and Enrolled Men*. Two volumes. Washington, D.C.: N.P., 1875.

Beardsley EH. A *History of Neglect: Health Care for Blacks and Mill Workers in the Twentieth-Century South*. Knoxville: The University of Tennessee Press, 1987.

Beecher HK. Ethics and clinical research. *New England Journal of Medicine* 1966; 274:1354–1360.

Begley S, Chideya F, Wilson L. Out of Egypt, Greece: Seeking the roots of Western civilization on the banks of the Nile. *Newsweek* 1991 (September 23); 118:49–50.

Beider RE. Science Encounters the Indian, 1820–1880: The Early Years of American Ethnology. Norman: University of Oklahoma Press, 1986.

Bender GA. *Great Moments in Medicine*. Detroit: Northwood Institute Press, 1966.

Bennett JT, DiLorenzo TJ. *Unhealthy Charities: Hazardous to Your Health and Wealth*. New York: Basic Books, 1994.

Bennett L. *Before the Mayflower: A History of the Negro in America, 1619–1964*. Revised Edition. Chicago: Johnson Publishing Company, 1961. Paperback Edition. Baltimore, Maryland: Penguin Books, 1966.

Bernal M. *Black Athena: The Afroasiatic Roots of Classical Civilization*. Volume 1. The Fabrication of Ancient Greece 1785–1985. New Brunswick, New Jersey: Rutgers University Press, 1987.

Bernal M. Black Athena: *The Afroasiatic Roots of Classical Civilization.* Volume 2. *The Archaeological and Documentary Evidence.* New Brunswick, New Jersey: Rutgers University Press, 1991.

Bernstein RB, Rice KS. *Are We to Be a Nation? The Making of the Constitution.* Cambridge, Massachusetts: Harvard University Press, 1987.

Berry LH. *I Wouldn't Take Nothin' for My Journey: Two Centuries of an Afro-American Minister's Family.* Chicago: Johnson Publishing Company, 1981.

Blanton WB. *Medicine in Virginia in the Seventeenth Century.* Richmond, Virginia: The William Byrd Press, 1930.

Blanton WB. *Medicine in Virginia in the Eighteenth Century.* Richmond, Virginia: Garrett and Massie, 1931.

Blassingame JW. *The Slave Community: Plantation Life in the Antebellum South.* New York: Oxford University Press, 1972.

Blassingame JW. *Black New Orleans, 1860–1880.* Chicago: The University of Chicago Press, 1973.

Blendon RJ, Aiken LH, Freeman HE, Corey CR. Access to medical care for Black and White Americans: A matter of continuing concern. *Journal of the American Medical Association* 1989; 262:278–281.

Blendon RJ, Edwards JN, eds. *System in Crisis: The Case for Health Care Reform.* Volume 1. *The Future of American Health Care.* New York: Faulkner and Gray, 1991.

Blendon RJ, Hyams TS, eds. *Reforming the System: Containing Health Care Costs in an Era of Universal Coverage.* Volume 2. *The Future of American Health Care.* New York: Faulkner and Gray, 1991.

Bogdanich W. *The Great White Lie: Dishonesty, Waste, and Incompetence in the Medical Community.* New York: Simon and Schuster, 1991.

Boles JB. *Black Southerners 1619–1869.* Lexington: The University of Kentucky Press, 1984.

Boorstin DJ. *The Discoverers.* Volume 1. *Time.* New York: Random House, Inc., 1983. Two-Volume Illustrated Deluxe Edition. New York: Harry N. Abrams, 1991.

Boorstin DJ. *The Discoverers.* Volume 2. *The Earth and the Seas.* New York: Random House, Inc., 1983. Two-Volume Illustrated Deluxe Edition. New York: Harry N. Abrams, 1991.

Boorstin DJ. The equality of the human species. 111–123. In: Boorstin DJ. *Hidden History: Exploring our Secret Past.* New York: Harper and Row Publishers, 1987. Paperback Edition. New York: Vintage Books, 1989.

Bousfield MO. An account of physicians of color in the United States. *Bulletin of the History of Medicine* 1945; 17:61–84.

Boyd RF. Dr. RF. Boyd of Nashville, Tenn., President of the American Association of Colored Physicians and Surgeons. *The Washington Bee,* October 3, 1896.

Boyd RF. What are the causes of the great mortality among the Negroes in the cities of the South, and how is that mortality to be lessened? 215–220. In: Culp DW, ed. *Twentieth Century Negro Literature.* Naperville, Illinois: JL. Nichols, 1902.

Boyd RF. Mercy Hospital. *Journal of the National Medical Association* 1909; 1:43.

Braden ME. *John Braden: A Pioneer in Negro Education.* Morristown, Tennessee: Triangle Press, 1935.

Bradsher K. As 1 million leave ranks of insured, debate heats up. *The New York Times,* August 27, 1995, 1.

Brandt AM. Racism and research: The case of the Tuskegee Syphilis Study. 331–343. In: Leavitt JW, Numbers RL, eds. *Sickness and Health in America: Readings in the History of Medicine and Public Health.* Madison: The University of Wisconsin Press, 1985.

Brawley B. *A Social History of the American Negro: Being a History of the Negro Problem in the United States Including a History and Study of the Republic of Liberia.* New York: Macmillan Company, 1921. Paperback Edition. London: Collier-Macmillan Ltd., 1970.

Breeden JO. Science and medicine. 1337–1343. In: Wilson CR, Ferris W. eds. *Encyclopedia of Southern Culture.* Chapel Hill: The University of North Carolina Press, 1989.

Breitman R. *The Architect of Genocide: Himmler and the Final Solution.* New York: Alfred A. Knopf, 1991.

Bremner RH. *The Public Good: Philanthropy and Welfare in the Civil War Era.* New York: Alfred A. Knopf, 1980.

Brinkley A. *The Unfinished Nation: A Concise History of the American People.* New York: Alfred A. Knopf, 1993.

Brown ER. *Rockefeller Medicine Men: Medicine and Capitalism in America.* Berkeley: University of California Press, 1979.

Buckler H. Daniel Hale Williams: *Negro Surgeon.* New York: Pitman Publishing Corporation, 1954.

Bullough B, Bullough VL. *Poverty, Ethnic Identity, and Health Care.* New York: Appleton-Century-Crofts, 1972.

Bullough VL. *The Development of Medicine As a Profession: The Contribution of the Medieval University to Modern Medicine.* New York: Hafner Publishing Company, 1966.

Burke J. Fit to rule. 239–273. In: Burke J. *The Day the Universe Changed.* Boston: Little, Brown, and Company, 1985.

Burns R, Ades L. *The Way West: The Way the West Was Lost and Won, 1845–1893.* A six-hour documentary series [videotape] for *The American Experience,* Boston: WGBH Educational Foundation, 1995.

Byne W. Debate: Is homosexuality biologically influenced? The biological evidence challenged. *Scientific American* 1994 (May, No. 5); 270:43, 50.

Byrd WM. Peer Review: *The Perversion of a Process.* Report prepared for the Subcommittee on Civil Rights of the House Committee on the Judiciary. 99th Congress, 2nd Session, 1986.

Byrd WM. Inquisition, peer review, and black physician survival. *Journal of the National Medical Association* 1987; 79:1027–1029.

Byrd WM. Robert F. Boyd: A life of triumph. *Meharry Alumni Magazine* 1988; 9:17.

Byrd WM. Race, biology, and health care: Reassessing a relationship. *Journal of Health Care for the Poor and Underserved* 1990; 1:278–292.

Byrd WM. *Documentary Report: Negro Diseases and Physiological Peculiarities.* Nashville, Tennessee: Cancer Control Research Unit, Meharry Medical College, July 12, 1990. In: Byrd WM, Clayton LA. A *Black Health Trilogy* [videotape and 188-page documentary report]. Washington, D.C.: The National Medical Association and the African American Heritage and Education Foundation; 1991. Revised Edition. Washington, D.C.: The National Medical Association, 1994.

Byrd WM. The Letter to the Editor: The NMA Founding Date Laid to Rest. *Journal of the National Medical Association* 1993; 85:99.

Byrd WM, Clayton LA. The "slave health deficit": Racism and health outcomes. *Health/PAC Bulletin* 1991; 21:25–28.

Byrd WM, Clayton LA. A *Black Health Trilogy* [videotape and 188-page documentary report]. Washington, D.C.: The National Medical Association and the African American Heritage and Education Foundation; 1991.

Byrd WM, Clayton LA. An American health dilemma: A history of blacks in the health system. *Journal of the National Medical Association* 1992; 84:189–200.

Byrd WM, Clayton LA. Designing a New Health Care System for the United States. Unpublished Document. Boston: Harvard School of Public Health, 1992.

Byrd WM, Clayton LA. The African-American cancer crisis, part 2: A prescription. *Journal of Health Care for the Poor and Underserved* 1993; 4:102–116.

Byrd WM. Medical associations. 1747–1749. In: Salzman J, Smith DL, West C. eds. *Encyclopedia of African-American Culture and History*. 5 Volumes. New York: Macmillan Library Reference USA, Simon and Schuster Macmillan, 1996.

Byrd WM, Clayton LA. Health System Component Analysis: A Health Policy Analytic Tool. A documentary report prepared for Summit '93: Regional Summits on Health Care Reform, Department HPM, Harvard School of Public Health, November 1993.

Cameron S, Wisdom EJ. Iron in his blood. *AIM for Racial Harmony and Peace* 1988; 15:10–11.

Campbell RB. *An Empire for Slavery: The Peculiar Institution in Texas, 1821–1865*. Baton Rouge: Louisiana State University Press, 1989.

Caplan AL, ed. *When Medicine Went Mad: Bioethics and the Holocaust*. Totowa, New Jersey: Humana Press, 1992.

Chandler DL. In shift, many anthropologists see race as social construct. *The Boston Sunday Globe*, May 11, 1997, p. A30.

Chandler WB. Of gods and men: Egypt's old kingdom. 117–182. In: Van Sertima I. *Egypt Revisited: Journal of African Civilizations*. New Brunswick, New Jersey: Transaction Publishers, 1989.

Chandler WB. The Moor: Light of Europe's Dark Age. 144–175. In: Van Sertima I, ed. *African Presence in Early Europe*. New Brunswick: Transaction Publishers, 1990.

Chang K. UM professor questions lack of diversity in genome project. *The Baltimore Sun*, February 22, 1997, Maryland Section.

Charatz-Litt C. A chronicle of racism: The effects of the White medical community on Black health. *Journal of the National Medical Association* 1992; 84:717–725.

Chase A. *The Legacy of Malthus: The Social Costs of the New Scientific Racism*. New York: Alfred A. Knopf, 1980.

Chase HS. "Shelling the citadel of race prejudice": William Calvin Chase and the Washington "Bee", 1882–1921. 371–391. In Rosenberger, FC, ed. *Records of the Columbia Historical Society of Washington, D.C. 1973–1974*. Washington, D.C.: Columbia Historical Society of Washington, D.C., 1976.

Chatman JA. *The Lone Star State Medical, Dental, and Pharmaceutical History*. N.P.: Lone Star State Medical, Dental, and Pharmaceutical Association, 1956.

Chicago Tribune. *The American Millstone: An Examination of the Nation's Permanent Underclass*. Chicago: Contemporary Books, 1986.

Chomsky N. *Deterring Democracy*. New York: Hill and Wang, 1991. Paperback Edition, 1992.

Chomsky N. *Profit over People: Neoliberalism and Global Order*. New York: Seven Stories Press, 1999.

Christianson EH. Medicine in New England. 101–153. In: Numbers RL, ed. *Medicine in the New World: New Spain, New France, and New England*. Knoxville: The University of Tennessee Press, 1987.

Churchill LR. Rationing *Health Care in America: Perceptions and Principles of Justice*. Notre Dame, Indiana: University of Notre Dame Press, 1987.

Clayton LA, Byrd WM. The African American cancer crisis, Part 1: The Problem. *Journal of Health Care for the Poor and Underserved* 1993; 4: 83–101.

Clayton LA, Byrd WM. Race, a major health status and outcome variable, 1980–1999: With some historical perspectives. *Journal of the National Medical Association*. In press 2000.

Cobb WM. *The First Negro Medical Society: A History of the Medico-Chirurgical Society of the District of Columbia*. Washington, D.C.: The Associated Publishers, 1939.

Cobb WM. *Medical Care and the Plight of the Negro*. New York: The National Association for the Advancement of Colored People, 1947.

Cobb WM. *Progress and Portents for the Negro In Medicine*. New York: The National Association for the Advancement of Colored People, 1948.

Cobb WM. Dr. David J. Peck: First Negro to graduate from an American medical school. *Bulletin of the Medico-Chirurgical Society of the District of Columbia* 1949; 6(2):3.

Cobb WM. Alexander Thomas Augusta. *Journal of the National Medical Association* 1952; 44:327–329.

Cobb WM. Henry Fitzbutler, 1842–1901. *Journal of the National Medical Association* 1952; 44:403–407.

Cobb WM. James McCune Smith. *Journal of the National Medical Association* 1952; 44:160–162.

Cobb WM. Martin Robison Delany. *Journal of the National Medical Association* 1952; 44:232–238.

Cobb WM. Miles Vandahrust Lynk. *Journal of the National Medical Association* 1952; 44:475–476.

Cobb WM. Charles Burleigh Purvis (1842–1929). *Journal of the National Medical Association* 1953; 45:79–82.

Cobb WM. Robert Fulton Boyd. *Journal of the National Medical Association* 1953; 45: 233–234.

Cobb WM. Nathan Francis Mossell, M.D., 1856–1946. *Journal of the National Medical Association* 1954; 46:118–130.

Cobb WM. Monroe Alpheus Majors, 1864–. *Journal of the National Medical Association* 1955; 47:139–141.

Cobb WM. William Wells Brown, M.D., (1816–1884). *Journal of the National Medical Association* 1955; 47:207–211.

Cobb WM. John Andrew Kenney, M.D., 1874–1950. *Journal of the National Medical Association* 1956; 48:75.

Cobb WM. John Edward Perry, M.D., 1870–. *Journal of the National Medical Association* 1956; 48:292–296.

Cobb WM. "Dr." James Still—New Jersey pioneer. *Journal of the National Medical Association* 1963; 55:196–199.

Cobb WM. 1981. The Black American in Medicine. *Journal of the National Medical Association* 73 (Suppl. 1):1183–1244.

Cogan T. *The Works of the Late Professor Camper on the Connexion between the Science of Anatomy and the Arts of Drawing, Painting, Statuary: Containing a Treatise on the Natural Difference of Features in Persons of Different Countries and Periods of Life; And on Beauty, With a New Method of Sketching Heads, National Features, and Portraits of Individuals, with Accuracy, Illustrated with Seventeen Plates, Explanatory of the Professor's Leading Principles.* Two Books. A New Edition. London: J. Hearne, 1821.

Cohen IB. *Album of Science: From Leonardo to Lavoisier, 1450–1800.* New York: Charles Scribner's Sons, 1980.

Coon CS. *The Origin of Races.* New York: Alfred A. Knopf, 1962.

Coon CS. *The Living Races of Man.* New York: Alfred A. Knopf, 1965.

Cooper-Patrick L, Gallo JJ, Gonzales JJ, Vu HT, Powe NR, Nelson C, et al. Race, gender, and partnership in the patient–physician relationship. *Journal of the American Medical Association* 1999; 282:583–589.

Cornelius LJ. Limited access to health care continues in minority groups. *National Medical Association News,* March–April 1993, 1.

Cornish DT. *The Sable Arm: Negro Troops in the Union Army, 1861–1865.* New York: W. W. Norton and Company, 1966.

Cose E. *The Rage of a Privileged Class.* New York: HarperCollins Publishers, 1993.

Cose E. *Color-Blind: Seeing Beyond Race in a Race-Obsessed World.* New York: Harper-Collins Publishers, 1997.

Count EW. The biological basis of human sociality. *American Anthropologist* 1958; 60:1049–1085.

Cray E. *In Failing Health: The Medical Crisis and the A.M.A.* Indianapolis, Indiana: The Bobbs-Merrill Company, 1970.

Curry LP. *The Free Black in Urban America, 1800–1850: The Shadow of the Dream.* Chicago: The University of Chicago Press, 1981.

Curtin PD. *The Atlantic Slave Trade: A Census.* Madison: The University of Wisconsin Press, 1969.

Curtis JL. *Blacks, Medical Schools, and Society.* Ann Arbor: The University of Michigan Press, 1971.

David PA, Gutman HG, Sutch R, Temin P, Wright G. *Reckoning with Slavery: A Critical Study in the Quantitative History of American Negro Slavery.* New York: Oxford University Press, 1976.

Davidson B. *The African Slave Trade.* Revised and Expanded Edition. Boston: Atlantic Monthly Press Book, Little, Brown, and Company, 1961.

Davidson B. Africa. An Eight-Part Series [videotapes]. Produced by Mitchell Beazley Television, RM Arts/Channel Four co-production in association with the Nigerian Television Authority, 1984.

Davidson B. The ancient world and Africa: Whose roots? *Race and Class* 1987; Volume 29, No.2.

Davis DB. *The Problem of Slavery in Western Culture.* Ithaca, New York: Cornell University Press, 1966.

Davis DB. *The Problem of Slavery in the Age of Revolution, 1770–1823.* Ithaca: Cornell University Press, 1975.

Davis DB. *Slavery and Human Progress.* New York: Oxford University Press, 1984.

Davis K, Lillie-Blanton M, Lyons B, Mullan F, Powe N, Rowland D. Health care for black Americans: The public sector role. 213–247. In: Willis DP, ed. *Health Policies and Black Americans.* New Brunswick, New Jersey: Transaction Publishers, 1989.

Death of Robert Fulton Boyd. *The Meharry News* 1913; 11:9–10.

Degler CN. *In Search of Human Nature: The Decline and Revival of Darwinism in American Social Thought.* New York: Oxford University Press, 1991.

De Tocqueville A. *Democracy in America.* 2 Volumes. Ed. JP Mayer. Trans. G Lawrence. New York: Harper and Row Publishers, 1966. Paperback Edition. New York: Harper Perennial, 1988.

Devisse J. *The Image of the Black in Western Art.* Part 2. *From the Early Christian Era to the Age of Discovery. 1. From the Demonic Threat to the Incarnation of Sainthood.* Cambridge, Massachusetts: The Menil Foundation, distributed by the Harvard University Press, 1979.

Devisse J, Mollat M. *The Image of the Black in Western Art.* Part 2. *From the Early Christian Era to the Age of Discovery. 2. Africans in the Christian Ordinance of the World (Fourteenth to the Sixteenth Century.* Cambridge, Massachusetts: The Menil Foundation, distributed by the Harvard University Press, 1979.

Dickerson DC. The black physician. Paper presented at the Black Health: Historical Perspectives and Current Issues Conference. Department of the History of Medicine, University of Wisconsin–Madison, April 6, 1990.

Diop CA. *The African Origin of Civilization: Myth or Reality,* ed. and trans. M Cook. Westport, Connecticut: Lawrence Hill and Company, 1974.

Diop CA. Origin of the ancient Egyptians. 27–57. In: Mokhtar G, ed. *General History of Africa. II: Ancient Civilizations of Africa.* Published under the auspices of the UNESCO International Scientific Committee for the Drafting of a General History of Africa, Berkeley: University of California Press, 1981.

Diop CA. *Civilization or Barbarism: An Authentic Anthropology,* trans. Ngemi YM, ed. Salemson HJ and de Jager M. Westport, Connecticut: Lawrence Hill Books, 1991.

Dor-Ner Z, Sheller WG. *Columbus and the Age of Discovery.* New York: William Morrow and Company, 1991.

Dow GF. Slave *Ships and Slaving.* Salem, Massachusetts: Marine Research Society, 1927. Reprint Edition. Toronto: Coles Publishing Company Limited, 1980.

Dowling HF. City Hospitals: *The Undercare of the Underprivileged.* Cambridge, Massachusetts: Harvard University Press, 1982.

Doyle DH. *Nashville in the New South, 1880–1930.* Knoxville: The University of Tennessee Press, 1985.

Drake SC. *Black Folk Here and There: An Essay in History and Anthropology.* Volume 1. Los Angeles: Center for Afro-American Studies, University of California, 1987.

Drake SC. *Black Folk Here and There: An Essay in History and Anthropology.* Volume 2. Los Angeles: Center for Afro-American Studies, University of California, 1990.

Dreyfuss J, Lawrence C. *The Bakke Case: The Politics of Inequality.* New York: Harcourt Brace Jovanovich, 1979.

Du Bois WEB. *The Suppression of the African Slave Trade to the United States of America, 1638–1870.* N.P., 1896. Reprint. Baton Rouge: Louisiana State University Press, 1969.

Du Bois WEB. *Mortality among Negroes in Cities.* Proceedings of the Conference for Investigation of City Problems. Atlanta, Georgia: Atlanta University Publications, 1896.

Du Bois WEB. *Social and Physical Conditions of Negroes in Cities*. Proceedings of the Second Conference for the Negro City Life. Atlanta, Georgia: Atlanta University Publications, 1897.

Du Bois WEB. *The Philadelphia Negro: A Social Study*. N.P. 1899. Reprint. New York: Schocken Books, 1967.

Du Bois WEB. *The Souls of Black Folk: Essays and Sketches*. Chicago: AC. McClurg, 1903. Unabridged Reprint Edition. New York: Dodd, Mead, and Company, 1979.

Du Bois WEB. *The Health and Physique of the Negro American*. A Social Study Made under the Direction of the Eleventh Atlanta Conference. Atlanta, Georgia: Atlanta University Publications, 1906.

Du Bois WEB. *The Negro*. New York: Henry Holt and Company, 1915. Reprint Edition. London: Oxford University Press, 1970.

Du Bois WEB. *Black Reconstruction in America: An Essay Toward a History of the Part Which Black Folk Played in the Attempt to Reconstruct Democracy in America, 1860–1880*. N.P.: Harcourt, Brace and Company, 1935. Reprint Edition. Cleveland, Ohio: Meridian Books, The World Publishing Company, 1964.

Duffy J. State's Rights Medicine. 1355–1356. In: Wilson CR, Ferris W, eds. *The Encyclopedia of Southern Culture*. Chapel Hill: The University of North Carolina Press, 1989.

Dula A. Toward an African-American perspective on bioethics. *Journal of Health Care for the Poor and Underserved* 1991; 2:259–269.

Dunglison R. *Human Physiology with Three Hundred and Sixty-Eight Illustrations*. Two Volumes, Sixth Edition. Philadelphia: Lea and Blanchard, 1846.

Duster T. *Backdoor to Eugenics*. New York: Routledge, 1990.

Edelman MW. *Families in Peril: An Agenda for Social Change*. Cambridge, Massachusetts: Harvard University Press, 1987.

Edelman MW. *The State of America's Children Yearbook 1995*. Washington, D.C.: Children's Defense Fund, 1995.

Elkins SM. *Slavery: A Problem in American Institutional and Intellectual Life*. 3rd ed. Chicago: The University of Chicago Press, 1976.

Enthoven AC. The history and principles of managed competition. *Health Affairs* (Suppl. 1993): 24–48.

Epps HR. The Howard University Medical Department in the Flexner era: 1910–1929. *Journal of the National Medical Association* 1989; 81:885.

Epps CH Jr., Johnson DG, Vaughan AL. Black medical pioneers: African-American "firsts" in academic and organized medicine: Part I. *Journal of the National Medical Association* 1993; 85:629–644.

Epps CH Jr., Johnson DG, Vaughan AL. Black medical pioneers: African-American "firsts" in academic and organized medicine: Part II. *Journal of the National Medical Association* 1993; 85:703–720.

Escarce JJ, Epstein KR, Colby DC, Schwartz JS. Racial differences in the elderly's use of medical procedures and diagnostic tests. *American Journal of Public Health* 1993; 83:948–954.

Estes JW. *The Medical Skills of Ancient Egypt*. Canton, Massachusetts: Science History Publications/USA, a Division of Watson Publishing International, 1989.

Everett S. *The Slaves: An Illustrated History of the Monstrous Evil*. New York: G.P. Putnam's Sons, 1978.

Ewbank DC. History of Black mortality and health before 1940. 100–128. In: Willis DP, ed. *Health Policies and Black Americans*. New Brunswick, New Jersey: Transaction Publishers, 1989.

Falk LA. Black abolitionist doctors and healers, 1810–1885. *Bulletin of the History of Medicine* 1980; 54:253–272.

Farley R. *Growth of the Black Population: A Study of Demographic Trends*. Chicago: Markham Publishing Company, 1970.

Farley R, Allen WR. *The Color Line and the Quality of Life in America*. New York: Oxford University Press, 1989.

Faust DG. Slavery in the American experience. 1–19 [11]. In: Campbell EDC Jr., Rice K., eds. *Before Freedom Came: African-American Life in the Antebellum South*. Charlottesville, Virginia: The Museum of the Confederacy, Richmond, and the University Press of Virginia, 1991.

Fausto-Sterling A. Anatomy. *Encyclopedia of African American Culture and History*. Eds. Salzman J, Smith DL, West C. 5 Volumes. New York: Macmillan Library Reference USA, 1996.

Feagin JR, Feagin CB. *Racial and Ethnic Relations*. Sixth Edition. Upper Saddle River, New Jersey: Prentice Hall, 1999.

Feagin JR, Spikes MP. *Living with Racism: The Black Middle-Class Experience*. Boston: Beacon Press, 1994.

Feagin JR, Vera H. *White Racism: The Basics*. New York: Routledge, 1995.

Fee E. History and development of public health. 10–30. In: Sutchfield FD, Keck CW. *Principles of Public Health Practice*. Albany, New York: Delmar Publishers, 1997.

Fee E. The origins and development of public health in the United States. 35–72. In: Detels R, Holland WW, McEwen J, Omenn GS, eds. *Oxford Textbook of Public Health*. Volume 1. *The Scope of Public Health*. Third Edition. New York: Oxford University Press, 1997.

Finch CS. The Black roots of Egypt's glory. 138–143. In: Van Sertima I, ed. *Great Black Leaders: Ancient and Modern*. New Brunswick, New Jersey: Transaction Publishers, 1988.

Finch CS. Imhotep the physician: Archetype of the great man. 213–231. In: Van Sertima I, ed. *Great Black Leaders: Ancient and Modern*. New Brunswick, New Jersey: Transaction Publishers, 1988.

Finch CS. Science and symbol in Egyptian medicine: Commentaries on the Edwin Smith papyrus. 325–351. In: Van Sertima I, ed. *Egypt Revisited: Journal of African Civilizations*. New Brunswick, New Jersey: Transaction Publishers, 1989.

Finch CS. Science and symbol in Egyptian medicine: Commentaries on the Edwin Smith papyrus. 325–351. In: Van Sertima I, ed. *Egypt Revisited: Journal of African Civilizations*. New Brunswick, New Jersey: Transaction Publishers, 1989.

Finch CS. *The African Background to Medical Science: Essays in African History, Science and Civilizations*. London: Karnak House, 1990.

Finch CS. *Africa and the Birth of Science and Technology: A Brief Overview*. Decatur, Georgia: Khenti Publications, 1992.

Finch CS. *Echoes of the Old Darkland: Themes from the African Eden*. Decatur, Georgia: Khenti Publications, 1994.

Fineberg KS, Peters JD, Willson JR, Kroll DA. *Obstetrics/Gynecology and the Law*. Ann Arbor, Michigan: Health Administration Press, 1984.

Finley M. *Ancient Slavery and Modern Ideology*. Great Britain: Chatto and Windus Ltd., 1980. Paperback Edition. New York: Pelican Books of the Penguin Group, 1983.

Fish JM. Mixed blood. *Psychology Today* 1995 (November–December, No. 6); 28:55.

Fitzhugh G. *Cannibals All! or, Slaves without Masters*. Richmond, Virginia: A. Morris, 1854. Reprint Edition. Cambridge, Massachusetts: The Belknap Press of Harvard University Press, 1960.

Fitzhugh G. *A Sociology for the South; or, The Failure of Free Society*. Richmond, Virginia: A. Morris, 1854.

Flexner A. *Medical Education in the United States and Canada: A Report to the Carnegie Foundation for the Advancement of Teaching*. New York: Carnegie Foundation for the Advancement of Teaching, Bulletin No. 4, 1910.

Fogel RW. *Without Consent or Contract: The Rise and Fall of American Slavery*. New York: W.W. Norton and Company, 1989.

Franklin JH. *From Slavery to Freedom: A History of Negro Americans*. Third Edition. New York: Alfred A. Knopf, 1967. Reprint Edition. New York: Vintage Books, 1969.

Franklin JH. *A Southern Odyssey: Travelers in the Antebellum North*. Baton Rouge: Louisiana State University Press, 1976.

Frazier EF. *The Negro in the United States*. Revised Edition. New York: The Macmillan Company, 1957.

Fredrickson GM. *The Inner Civil War: Northern Intellectuals and the Crisis of the Union*. New York: N.P., 1965.

Fredrickson GM, Knobel DT. History of Prejudice and Discrimination. 829–847. In: Thernstrom S, Orlov A, Handlin O, eds. *Harvard Encyclopedia of American Ethnic Groups*. Cambridge, Massachusetts: The Belknap Press of Harvard University Press, 1980.

Fredrickson GM. *The Black Image in the White Mind: The Debate on Afro-American Character and Destiny, 1871–1914*. New York: Harper and Row Publishers, 1971. Reprint Edition. Middletown, Connecticut: Wesleyan University Press, 1987.

Fuchs VR. *The Health Economy*. Cambridge, Massachusetts: Harvard University Press, 1986.

Gans HJ. *The War against the Poor: The Underclass and Antipoverty Policy*. New York: Basic Books, 1995.

Gates HL. Beware of the new pharaohs. *Newsweek*, September 23, 1991; 118:47.

Gay P. *Age of Enlightenment. Great Ages of Man: A History of the World's Cultures*. New York: Time Incorporated, 1965.

Genovese ED. *The Political Economy of Slavery: Studies in the Economy and Society of the Slave South*. New York: Vintage Books, 1965.

Genovese ED. *From Rebellion to Revolution: Afro-American Slave Revolts in the Making of The New World*. Baton Rouge, Louisiana: Louisiana State University Press, 1979. Paperback Edition. New York: Vintage Books, 1981.

Genovese ED. *The World the Slaveholders Made: Two Essays in Interpretation*. New York: Pantheon Books, 1969. Paperback Edition. Middletown, Connecticut: Wesleyan University Press, 1988.

Gilman SL. *Freud, Race, and Gender*. Princeton, New Jersey: Princeton University Press, 1993.

Ginzberg E. The monetarization of medical care. *New England Journal of Medicine* 1984; 310:1162–1165.

Ginzberg E. The destabilization of health care. *New England Journal of Medicine* 1986; 315:757–767.

Ginzberg E. *The Medical Triangle: Physicians, Politicians, and the Public*. Cambridge, Massachusetts: Harvard University Press, 1990.

Ginzberg E. Improving health care for the poor: Lessons from the 1980s. *Journal of the American Medical Association* 1994; 271:464–467.

Ginzberg E, personal interview, July 8, 1995.

Ginzberg E, Dutka AB. *The Financing of Biomedical Research*. Baltimore, Maryland: The Johns Hopkins University Press, 1989.

Glasgow DG. *The Black Underclass: Poverty, Unemployment, and Entrapment of Ghetto Youth*. London: Jossey-Bass Limited, 1980. Paperback Edition. New York: Vintage Books, 1981.

Glazer N, Ueda R. Policy against prejudice and discrimination. 847–858. In: Thernstrom S, Orlov A, Handlin O, eds. *Harvard Encyclopedia of American Ethnic Groups*. Cambridge, Massachusetts: The Belknap Press of Harvard University Press, 1980.

Goldberg DT. The social formation of racist discourse. 295–318. In: Goldberg DT, ed. *Anatomy of Racism*. Minneapolis: University of Minnesota Press, 1990.

Gordon M. *Slavery in the Arab World*. New York: New Amsterdam Books, 1989.

Gossett TF. *Race: The History of an Idea in America*. Dallas, Texas: Southern Methodist University Press, 1963. Reprint Edition. New York: Schocken Books, 1965.

Gould SJ. *Ever since Darwin: Reflections in Natural History*. New York: W.W. Norton and Company, 1977.

Gould SJ. *The Panda's Thumb: More Reflections in Natural History*. New York: W.W. Norton and Company, 1980.

Gould SJ. Wide hats and narrow minds. 145–151. In: Gould SJ. *The Panda's Thumb: More Reflections in Natural History*. New York: W.W. Norton and Company, 1980.

Gould SJ. *The Mismeasure of Man*. New York: W.W. Norton and Company, 1981.

Gould SJ. Bound by the great chain. 281–291. In: Gould SJ. *The Flamingo's Smile: Reflections in Natural History*. New York: W.W. Norton and Company, 1985.

Gould SJ. *The Flamingo's Smile: Reflections in Natural History*. New York: W.W. Norton and Company, 1985.

Gould SJ. The Hottentot Venus. 291–305. In: *The Flamingo's Smile: Reflections in Natural History*. New York: W.W. Norton and Company, 1985.

Gould SJ. To show an ape. 263–280. In: Gould SJ. *The Flamingo's Smile: Reflections in Natural History*. New York: W.W. Norton and Company, 1985.

Gratus J. *The Great White Lie: Slavery, Emancipation, and Changing Racial Attitudes*. New York: Monthly Review Press, 1973.

Greenberg DS. Black health: Grim statistics. *The Lancet* 1990; 355:780–781.

Grolier Electronic Publishing, Inc. United States history. In: *The New Grolier Multimedia Encyclopedia*. Release 6, MPC Version. Novato, California: The Software Toolworks, Inc., 1993.

Guthrie D. *A History of Medicine*. Philadelphia: J.B. Lippincott Company, 1946.

Gutman H, Sutch R. Victorians All? The Sexual Mores and Conduct of Slaves and Their Masters. 134–162. In: David PA, Gutman HG, Sutch R, Temin P, Wright G. *Reckoning with Slavery*. New York: Oxford University Press, 1976.

Hacker A. *Two Nations: Black and White, Separate, Hostile, Unequal*. New York: Ballantine Books, 1992. Expanded and Updated Edition. 1995.

Haeger K. *The Illustrated History of Surgery*. New York: Bell Publishing Company, 1988.

Haley JT. Dr. Robert Fulton Boyd. 59–62. In *The Afro-American Encyclopedia*. Nashville, Tennessee: Haley and Florida, 1896.

Haller JS Jr. *Outcasts from Evolution: Scientific Attitudes of Racial Inferiority, 1859–1900*. New York: McGraw-Hill Book Company, 1971.

Haller JS Jr. *American Medicine in Transition 1840–1910*. Urbana: University of Illinois Press, 1981.

Haller JS Jr., Haller RM. *The Physician and Sexuality in Victorian America*. University of Illinois Press, 1974. Reprint Edition. New York: W.W. Norton and Company, 1977.

Haller MH. *Eugenics: Hereditarian Attitudes in American Thought*. New Brunswick, New Jersey: Rutgers University Press, 1963.

Hanft RS, Fishman LE, Evans W. *Blacks and the Health Professions in the 80s: A National Crisis and a Time for Action*. Prepared for the Association of Minority Health Professions Schools, N.P., 1983.

Harding S, ed. *The "Racial Economy" of Science: Toward a Democratic Future*. Bloomington: Indiana University Press, 1993.

Harding V. *There Is a River: The Black Struggle for Freedom in America*. New York: Harcourt Brace Jovanovich, 1981. Reprint Edition. New York: Vintage Books, 1983.

Harmer RM. *American Medical Avarice*. New York: Abelard-Schuman, 1975.

Harris JE. *Africans and Their History*. Revised and Updated Edition. New York: New American Library, 1972.

Harris JE, ed. *Global Dimension of the African Diaspora*. Second Edition. Washington, D.C.: Howard University Press, 1993.

Harrison DD, Cooke CW. An elucidation of factors influencing physicians' willingness to perform elective female sterilization. *Obstetrics and Gynecology* 1988; 72:565–569.

Haynes MA. The gap in health status between Black and White Americans. In the *Textbook of Black-Related Diseases*. Edited by Williams RA, 1–30. New York: McGraw-Hill Book Company, 1975.

Health Policy Advisory Center. The emerging health apartheid in the United States. *Health/PAC Bulletin* 1991; 21:3–4.

Hearnshaw LS. *Cyril Burt Psychologist*. Ithaca, New York: Cornell University Press, 1979.

Herman ES, Chomsky N. *Manufacturing Consent: The Political Economy of the Mass Media*. New York: Pantheon Books, 1988.

Herrnstein RJ, Murray C. *The Bell Curve: Intelligence and Class Structure in American Life*. New York: The Free Press, 1994.

Herskovits MJ. *Franz Boas: The Science of Men in the Making*. New York: Charles Scribner's Sons, 1953.

Higginbotham AL, Jr. *In the Matter of Color: Race and the American Legal Process, The Colonial Period*. New York: Oxford University Press, 1978.

Higginbotham AL, Jr. *Shades of Freedom: Racial Politics and Presumptions of the American Legal Process*. New York: Oxford University Press, 1996.

Hine DC. *Black Women in White: Racial Conflict and Cooperation in the Nursing Profession, 1890–1950*. Bloomington: Indiana University Press, 1989.

Hine DC. Tubman, Harriet Ross (c. 1821–1913). 1176–1180. In: Hine DC, ed. *Black Women in America: An Historical Encyclopedia*. 2 Volumes. Brooklyn, New York: Carlson Publishing, 1993.

Honour H. *The Image of the Black in Western Art. Part IV. From the American Revolution to World War I. 1. Slaves and Liberators.* Cambridge, Massachusetts: The Menil Foundation, distributed by Harvard University Press, 1989.

Honour H. *The Image of the Black in Western Art. Part IV. From the American Revolution to World War I. 2. Black Models and White Myths.* Cambridge, Massachusetts: The Menil Foundation, distributed by Harvard University Press, 1989.

Horkheimer M. Traditional and critical theory. 188–243. In: Horkheimer M. *Critical Theory.* New York: Herder and Herder, 1972.

Horsman R. *Race and Manifest Destiny: The Origins of American Racial Anglo-Saxonism.* Cambridge, Massachusetts: Harvard University Press, 1981.

Horsman R. *Josiah Nott of Mobile: Southerner, Physician, and Racial Theorist.* Baton Rouge: Louisiana State University Press, 1987.

Hubbard GW. Yesterday, today and tomorrow. *Journal of the National Medical Association* 1909; 1:133–135.

Hubbard GW. Meharry Medical College—Dean Hubbard. *Journal of the National Medical Association* 1915; 7:324–325.

Hubbard R, Wald E. *Exploding the Gene Myth: How Genetic Information Is Produced and Manipulated by Scientists, Physicians, Employers, Insurance Companies, Educators, and Law Enforcers.* Boston: Beacon Press, 1993.

Huggins NI. *Black Odyssey: The Afro-American Ordeal in Slavery.* New York: Pantheon Books, Inc., 1977. Reprint Edition. New York: Random House, Vintage Books Division, 1979.

Hughes L, Meltzer M, Lincoln CE. Revised Fifth Edition. *A Pictorial History of Blackamericans.* New York: Crown Publishers, 1983.

Hughes L, Meltzer M, Lincoln CE, Spencer JM. Revised Sixth Edition. *A Pictorial History of Blackamericans.* New York: Crown Publishers, 1995.

Hunt S. The Flexner report and Black academic medicine: An assignment of place. *Journal of the National Medical Association* 1993; 85:151–155.

Hunt SB. The Negro as a soldier. *Quarterly Journal of Psychological Medicine* 1867 (October); 1:175.

Hunt SB. The Negro as a soldier. *London Anthropological Review* 1869, 42–43.

Hutchins RM, ed. *Great Books of the Western World.* Vol. 49. *Darwin. The Descent of Man and Selection in Relation to Sex.* by Charles Darwin. Chicago: University of Chicago Press, 1952.

Illich I. *Medical Nemesis: The Expropriation of Health.* New York: Pantheon Books, Inc., 1976. Paperback Edition. Toronto: Bantam Books, 1977.

Jaco EG. *Patients, Physicians, and Illness: A Sourcebook in Behavioral Science and Health.* Third Edition. New York: The Free Press, 1979.

Jacobson TC. *Making Medical Doctors: Science and Medicine at Vanderbilt Since Flexner.* Tuscaloosa: The University of Alabama Press, 1987.

James CLR. *The Black Jacobins: Toussaint L'Ouverture and the San Domingo Revolution.* Second Revised Edition. New York: Vintage Books, 1963.

James GGM. *Stolen Legacy: Greek Philosophy Is Stolen Egyptian Philosophy.* New York: Philosophical Library, 1954. Reprint Edition. Newport News, Virginia: United Brothers Communication Systems, 1989.

Jaynes GD, Williams RM. eds. *A Common Destiny: Blacks and American Society.* Washington, D.C.: National Academy Press, 1989.

Jencks C. *Rethinking Social Policy: Race, Poverty, and the Underclass*. Cambridge, Massachusetts: Harvard University Press, 1992.

Jhally S, Lewis J. *Enlightened Racism: The Cosby Show, Audiences, and the Myth of the American Dream*. Boulder, Colorado: Westview Press, 1992.

Johnson C, Smith P. *Africans in America: America's Journey through Slavery*. New York: Harcourt Brace and Company, 1998.

Johnson H, Broder DS. *The System: The American Way of Politics at the Breaking Point*. Boston: Little, Brown, and Company, 1996.

Jones JH. *Bad Blood: The Tuskegee Syphilis Experiment*. New York: The Free Press, 1981. New and Expanded Edition, 1993.

Jones MJ, Whitney DC, eds. *The World Book Encyclopedia*. Chicago: Field Enterprises, Inc., 1957. S.v. History of the United States, by Mowry GE, 8329.

Jones MJ, Whitney DC, eds. *The World Book Encyclopedia*. Chicago: Field Enterprises, Inc., 1957. S.v. Reconstruction, by Hicks JD, 6830.

Jordan WC. Voodoo Medicine. 715–738. In: Williams RA, ed. *Textbook of Black-Related Diseases*. New York: McGraw-Hill, 1975.

Jordan WD. *White over Black: American Attitudes toward the Negro, 1550–1812*. New York: W.W. Norton and Company, 1968.

Joyner C. The World of the Plantation Slaves. 50–99. In: Campbell EDC Jr, Rice K., eds. *Before Freedom Came: African-American Life in the Antebellum South*. Charlottesville, Virginia: The Museum of the Confederacy, Richmond, and the University Press of Virginia, 1991.

Katz J. *Experimentation with Human Beings: The Authority of the Investigator, Subject, Professions, and State in the Human Experimentation Process*. New York: Russell Sage Foundation, 1972.

Katz MB. *In the Shadow of the Poorhouse: A Social History of Welfare in America*. New York: Basic Books, 1986. Revised and Updated Edition, 1996.

Katz WL. *Breaking the Chains: African-American Slave Resistance*. New York: Atheneum, 1990.

Kaufman M, Galishoff S, Savitt TL, eds. *Dictionary of American Medical Biography*. Two Volumes. Westport, Connecticut: Greenwood Press, 1984.

Kaus M. *The End of Equality*. New York: Basic Books, 1992.

Kenney JA. *The Negro in Medicine*. Tuskegee, Alabama: Tuskegee Institute Press, 1912.

Kenney JA. Second annual oration on surgery. *Journal of the National Medical Association*, 1941; 33:203–214.

Kerner O. *Report of the National Advisory Commission on Civil Disorders*. New York: E.P. Dutton and Company, 1968. Paperback Edition. New York: Bantam Books, 1968.

Kevles DJ. *In the Name of Eugenics: Genetics and the Uses of Human Heredity*. Berkeley: University of California Press, 1985.

Kinder DR, Sanders LM. *Divided by Color: Racial Politics and Democratic Ideals*. Chicago: The University of Chicago Press, 1996.

King G, Bendel R. A statistical model estimating the number of African American physicians in the United States. *Journal of the National Medical Association* 1995; 84:264–272.

King JC. *The Biology of Race*. Revised Edition. Berkeley: University of California Press, 1981.

King M, Wilson AC. Evolution at two levels in humans and chimpanzees. *Science* April 11, 1975; 188(4184);107–116.

Kiple KF, King VH. *Another Dimension to the Black Diaspora: Diet, Disease, and Racism.* Cambridge: Cambridge University Press, 1981.

Klein HS. *The Middle Passage: Comparative Studies in the Atlantic Slave Trade.* Princeton, New Jersey: Princeton University Press, 1978.

Kluger R. *Simple Justice: The History of* Brown v. Board of Education *and Black America's Struggle for Equality.* New York: Alfred A. Knopf, 1976. Paperback Edition. New York: Vintage Books, 1977.

Knowles LL, Prewitt K. *Institutional Racism in America.* Englewood Cliffs, New Jersey: Prentice-Hall, 1969.

Kochanek KD, Jeffrey DM, Rosenberg HM. Why did Black life expectancy decline from 1984 through 1989 in the United States? *American Journal of Public Health* 1994; 84:938–944.

Komaromy M, Grumbach K, Drake M. The role of Black and Hispanic physicians in providing health care for underserved populations. *New England Journal of Medicine* 1996; 334:1305–1314.

Konner M. *Medicine at the Crossroads: The Crisis in Health Care.* New York: Pantheon Books, 1993.

Konold DE. *A History of American Medical Ethics: 1847–1912.* Madison: The University of Wisconsin Press, 1962.

Kosa J, Zola IK, eds. *Poverty and Health: A Sociological Analysis.* Revised Edition. Cambridge, Massachusetts: Harvard University Press, 1975.

Kovel J. *White Racism: A Psychohistory.* New York: Random House, 1970. Reprint Edition. New York: Columbia University Press, 1984.

Kozol J. *Savage Inequalities: Children in America's Schools.* New York: Crown Publishers, 1991.

Kragh H. *An Introduction to the Historiography of Science.* Cambridge: Cambridge University Press, 1987, Paperback Edition, 1989, 1–40.

Kurtis B. *Slavery's Buried Past,* A documentary video segment for *The New Explorers,* Boston, WGBH, December 18, 1996.

Lane-Poole S. *The Story of the Moors in Spain.* N.P. 1886. Reprint Edition. Baltimore, Maryland: Black Classic Press, 1990.

Lee PR, Benjamin AE. Governmental and legislative control and direction of health services in the United States. 217–230. In: Holland WW, Detels R, Knox G, eds. *Oxford Textbook of Public Health.* Volume 1. *Influences of Public Health.* Second Edition. Oxford: Oxford University Press, 1991.

Lefkowitz M. *Not Out of Africa: How Afrocentrism Became an Excuse to Teach Myth As History.* New York: Basic Books, 1996.

Leiris M. Race and culture. In: *Race and History.* Paris: United Nations Educational, Scientific and Cultural Organization, 1951.

Lemann N. *The Promised Land: The Great Black Migration and How It Changed America.* New York: Alfred A. Knopf, 1991.

Lemann N. Taking affirmative action apart. *The New York Times Magazine,* June 11, 1995; Section 6, 36.

Lemann N. The structure of success in America. *The Atlantic Monthly* 1995 (August, No. 2); 276:41.

Lemann N. The great sorting. *The Atlantic Monthly* 1995 (September, No. 3); 276:84.

LeVay S, Hamer DH. Debate: Is homosexuality biologically influenced? Evidence for a biological influence in male homosexuality. *Scientific American* 1994 (May, No. 5); 270:43.

Levin J, Levin W. *The Functions of Discrimination and Prejudice*. Second Edition. New York: Harper and Row Publishers, 1982.

Lévi-Strauss C. Race and history. In: *Race and History*. Paris: United Nations Educational, Scientific and Cultural Organization, 1951.

Lewin R. *In the Age of Mankind*. Washington, D.C.: Smithsonian Books, 1988.

Lewis B. The African diaspora and the civilization of Islam. 37–56. In: Kilson ML, Rothberg RI, eds. *The African Diaspora: Interpretive Essays*. Cambridge, Massachusetts: Harvard University Press, 1976.

Lewis B. *Race and Slavery in the Middle East: An Historical Enquiry*. New York: Oxford University Press, 1990.

Lewis JH. Contribution of an unknown Negro to anesthesia. *Journal of the National Medical Association* 1931; 23:23–24.

Lewis JH. *The Biology of the Negro*. Chicago: The University of Chicago Press, 1942.

Lewontin RC, Rose S, Kamin LJ. *Not in Our Genes: Biology, Ideology, and Human Nature*. New York: Pantheon Books, 1984.

Lifton RJ. *The Nazi Doctors: Medical Killing and the Psychology of Genocide*. New York: Basic Books, 1986.

Lifton RJ, Eric Markusen. *The Genocidal Mentality: Nazi Holocaust and Nuclear Threat*. New York: Basic Books, 1990.

Logan RW. *The Negro in American Life and Thought: The Nadir, 1877–1901*. New York: Macmillan Publishing Company, 1954. *The Betrayal of the Negro: From Rutherford B. Hayes to Woodrow Wilson*. Enlarged, Revised, Paperback Edition. London: Collier Macmillan Ltd., 1965.

Lorenz K. *Evolution and Modification of Behavior*. Chicago: The University of Chicago Press, 1965.

Lovejoy AO. *The Great Chain of Being: A Study of the History of an Idea*. Cambridge, Massachusetts: Harvard University Press, 1936. Reprint Paperback Edition. 1964.

Low WA, Clift VA. eds. *Encyclopedia of Black America*. New York: McGraw-Hill. Reprint Edition. New York: Da Capo Press, 1981.

Luce HR. *Life's Picture History of Western Man*. New York: Time Incorporated, 1951.

Ludmerer KM. *Learning to Heal: The Development of American Medical Education*. New York: Basic Books, 1985.

Lundberg GD. National health care reform: An aura of inevitability is upon us. *Journal of the American Medical Association* 1991; 265:2566–2567.

Lurie E. *Louis Agassiz: A Life in Science*. Chicago: The University of Chicago Press, 1960.

Lynk MV. *Sixty Years of Medicine, or The Life and Times of Dr. Miles V. Lynk: An Autobiography*. Memphis, Tennessee: Twentieth Century Press, 1951.

Lyons AS, Petrucelli RJ. *Medicine: An Illustrated History*. New York: Harry N. Abrams, 1978.

Magee MJ. The old slave house. 49–54. In: Magee MJ. *Cavern of Crime*. Smithland, Kentucky: The Livingston Ledger, 1973.

Magnusson M, ed. *Cambridge Biographical Dictionary*. Cambridge: Cambridge University Press, 1990.

Majno G. *The Healing Hand: Man and Wound in the Ancient World*. Cambridge, Massachusetts: Harvard University Press, 1975.

Malone TE, Johnson KW. *Report of the Secretary's Task Force on Black and Minority Health*. Washington, D.C.: U.S. Department of Health and Human Services, 1986.

Mangano JJ. Young adults in the 1980s: Why mortality rates are rising. *Health PAC/Bulletin* 1991; 21:19–24.

Manning KR. *Black Apollo of Science: The Life of Ernest Everett Just*. New York: Oxford University Press, 1983.

Manning KR. Folk medicine. 1002–1003. In: Salzman J, Smith DL, West C. eds. *Encyclopedia of African-American Culture and History*. 5 Volumes. New York: Macmillan Library Reference USA, Simon and Schuster Macmillan, 1996.

Mannix DP, Cowley M. *Cargoes: The Atlantic Slave Trade, 1518–1865*. New York: Viking Press, 1962.

Manson-Bahr PEC, Bell DR. *Manson's Tropical Diseases*. Nineteenth Edition. London: Baillière Tindall, 1987.

Manton KG, Patrick CH, Johnson KW. Health differentials between blacks and whites: Recent trends in mortality and morbidity. 129–199. In: Willis DP, ed. *Health Policies and Black Americans*. New Brunswick, New Jersey: Transaction Publishers, 1989.

Marable M. *Race, Reform. and Rebellion: The Second Reconstruction in Black America, 1945–1990*. Revised Second Edition. Jackson: University Press of Mississippi, 1991.

Marshall PJ, Williams G. *The Great Map of Mankind: Perceptions of New Worlds in the Age of Enlightenment*. Cambridge, Massachusetts: Harvard University Press, 1982.

Marshall TH. *Citizenship, Social Class, and Other Essays*. Cambridge: Cambridge University Press, 1950.

Massey DS, Denton NA. *American Apartheid: Segregation and the Making of the Underclass*. Cambridge, Massachusetts: Harvard University Press, 1993.

Mayr E. *The Growth of Biological Thought: Diversity, Evolution, and Inheritance*. Cambridge, Massachusetts: The Belknap Press of Harvard University Press, 1982.

Mazrui AA. *The Africans*. A Nine-Part Series [videotapes]. Sponsored by the Annenberg/CPB Project, Washington, D.C.: WETA and the BBC, 1986.

Mazrui AA. *The Africans: A Triple Heritage*. Boston: Little, Brown, and Company, 1986.

McBride D. Inequality in the availability of Black physicians. *New York State Journal of Medicine* 1985; 85:139–142.

McCord C, Freeman HP. Excess mortality in Harlem. *New England Journal of Medicine* 1990; 322:173–177.

McGregor DK. *Sexual Surgery and the Origins of Gynecology: J. Marion Sims, His Hospital, and His Patients*. New York: Garland Publishing, 1989.

McManus EJ. *A History of Negro Slavery in New York*. Syracuse, New York: Syracuse University Press, 1966.

McNeill WH. *Plagues and Peoples*. New York: Doubleday, 1976. Paperback Edition. New York: Anchor Books, 1989.

MD Magazine. Afro-American Asclepius. *MD Magazine* 1963 (April), 202–205.

Meadows J. *The Great Scientists*. New York: Oxford University Press, 1987.

Meharry F. *History of the Meharry Family in America*. Lafayette, Indiana: Lafayette Printing Company, 1925.

Meharry Medical College. Black Medical History Archive Collection. Meharry Medical College Library, Kresge Learning Resources Center, Meharry Medical College, Nashville, Tennessee.

Meharry Medical College. Hubbard and Sneed. 11. In the *Bulletin of Meharry Medical College: 80th Anniversary Issue*. Nashville, Tennessee: Meharry Medical College, 1956.

Mellon J, ed. *Bullwhip Days: The Slaves Remember*. New York: Weidenfeld and Nicolson, 1988.

Milner R. *The Encyclopedia of Evolution: Humanity's Search for its Origins*. New York: Facts on File, 1990.

Moeller DW. *Environmental Health*. Cambridge, Massachusetts: Harvard University Press, 1992.

Mohr CL. *On the Threshold of Freedom: Masters and Slaves in Civil War Georgia*. Athens: The University of Georgia Press, 1986.

Montagu A. *Race, Science and Humanity*. New York: Van Nostrand Reinhold, 1963.

Morais HM. *The History of the Negro in Medicine*. Under auspices of The Association for the Study of Negro Life and History. New York: Publishers Company, 1967.

Morton SG. *Crania Americana or, A Comparative View of the Skulls of Various Aboriginal Nations of North and South America to which is prefixed An Essay on the Varieties of the Human Species*. Philadelphia: J. Dobson, Chestnut Street, 1839.

Moynihan DP. *The Negro Family: The Case for National Action*. Washington, D.C.: U.S. Department of Labor, 1965.

Muir H, ed. *Larousse Dictionary of Scientists*. New York: Larousse, 1994.

Myrdal G. *An American Dilemma: The Negro Problem and Modern Democracy*. New York: Harper and Row Publishers, 1944.

National Center for Health Statistics. *Health Status of the Disadvantaged Chartbook/1990*. Hyattsville, Maryland: U.S. Public Health Service, 1991.

National Center for Health Statistics. Advance report of final mortality statistics, 1989. Monthly vital statistics report; Volume 40 No. 8 suppl. 2. Hyattsville, Maryland: U.S. Public Health Service, 1992.

National Center for Health Statistics. *Prevention profile. Health United States, 1991*. Hyattsville, Maryland: U.S. Public Health Service, 1992.

National Center for Health Statistics. *Health United States, 1994*. Hyattsville, Maryland: U.S. Public Health Service, 1995.

National Center for Health Statistics. *Health United States, 1995*. Hyattsville, Maryland: U.S. Public Health Service, May 1996.

National Medical Association. Dr. I. Garland Penn. *Journal of the National Medical Association* 1930; 22:171–172.

Nelkin D, Tancredi L. *Dangerous Diagnostics: The Social Power of Biological Information*. New York: Basic Books, 1989.

Neverdon-Morton C. *Afro-American Women of the South and the Advancement of the Race, 1895–1925*. Knoxville: The University of Tennessee Press, 1989.

Newman DK, Amidei NJ, Carter BL, Day D, Kruvant WJ, Russell JS. Second-Class Medicine. 187–235. In: *Protest, Politics, and Prosperity: Black Americans and White Institutions, 1940–75*. New York: Pantheon Books, 1978.

Newsome F. Black contributions to the early history of Western medicine. *Journal of the National Medical Association* 1979; 71:189–193.

Nichols CH. *Many Thousands Gone: The Ex-Slaves' Account of their Bondage and Freedom*. Leiden, Netherlands: E.J. Brill, 1963. Paperback Edition. Bloomington: Indiana University Press.

Nisbet R. *Prejudices: A Philosophical Dictionary*. Cambridge, Massachusetts: Harvard University Press, 1982.

Nott JC, Gliddon GR. *Types of Mankind or, Ethnological Researches*. Philadelphia: Lippincott, Grambo and Company, 1854.

Novotny A, Smith C. eds. *Images of Healing: A Portfolio of American Medical and Pharmaceutical Practice in the 18th, 19th, and Early 20th Centuries*. New York: Macmillan Publishing Company, 1980.

Nuland SB. *Doctors: The Biography of Medicine*. New York: Alfred A. Knopf, 1988.

Numbers RL. *Almost Persuaded: American Physicians and Compulsory Health Insurance, 1912–1920*. Baltimore: The Johns Hopkins University Press, 1978.

Numbers RL, ed. *Medicine in the New World: New Spain, New France, and New England*. Knoxville: The University of Tennessee Press, 1987.

Oakes J. *The Ruling Race: A History of American Slaveholders*. New York: Alfred A. Knopf, 1982. Reprint Edition. New York: Vintage Books, 1983.

Oates SB. Children of darkness. *American Heritage* 1973 (October, No. 6); 24:42.

O'Bannion LC. Are African-American doctors being locked out? The down side of managed care. *National Medical Association News* 1995 (Winter), 1.

Omi M, Winant H. *Racial Formation in the United States: From the 1960s to the 1980s*. London: Routledge and Kegan Paul, 1986.

Omi M, Winant H. *Racial Formation in the United States: From the 1960s to the 1990s*. Second Edition. New York: Routledge, 1994.

O'Reilly K. *Nixon's Piano: Presidents and Racial Politics from Washington to Clinton*. New York: The Free Press, 1995.

Orfield G, Eaton SE. *Dismantling Desegregation: The Quiet Reversal of* Brown v. Board of Education. The Harvard Project on School Desegregation. New York: The New Press, 1996.

Organ CH, Kosiba MM, eds. *A Century of Black Surgeons: The U.S.A. Experience*. 2 Volumes. Norman, Oklahoma: Transcript Press.

Outlaw L. Toward a critical theory of race. 58–82. In: Goldberg DT, ed. *Anatomy of Racism*. Minneapolis: University of Minnesota Press, 1990.

Owens LH. *This Species of Property: Slave Life and Culture in the Old South*. Oxford: Oxford University Press, 1976.

Painter NI. Truth, Sojourner (c. 1799–1883). 1172–1180. In: Hine DC, ed. *Black Women in America: An Historical Encyclopedia*. 2 Volumes. Brooklyn, New York: Carlson Publishing, 1993.

Parkinson W. *This Gilded African: Toussaint L'Overture*. London: Quartet Books, 1980.

Parsons T. *The Social System*. Glencoe, Illinois: The Free Press, 1951.

Patterson JT. *The Dread Disease: Cancer and Modern American Culture*. Cambridge, Massachusetts: Harvard University Press, 1987.

Patterson O. *Slavery and Social Death: A Comparative Study*. Cambridge, Massachusetts: Harvard University Press, 1982.

Patterson O. *Rituals of Blood: Consequences of Slavery in Two American Centuries*. Washington, D.C.: Civitas/Counterpoint, 1999.

Perry JE. *Forty Cords of Wood: Memoirs of a Medical Doctor*. Jefferson City, Missouri: Lincoln University Press, 1947.

Pettigrew TF. Prejudice. 820–829. In: Thernstrom S, Orlov A, Handlin O, eds. *Harvard Encyclopedia of American Ethnic Groups*. Cambridge, Massachusetts: The Belknap Press of Harvard University Press, 1980.

Phillips UB. *American Negro Slavery: A Survey of the Supply, Employment and Control of Negro Labor As Determined by the Plantation Regime*. N.P.: D. Appleton and Company, 1918. Paperback Edition. Baton Rouge: Louisiana State University Press, 1966.

Pieterse JN. *White on Black: Images of Africa and Blacks in Western Popular Culture*. New Haven, Connecticut: Yale University Press, 1992.

Pimienta-Bey JV. Moorish Spain: Academic source and foundation for the rise and success of western European universities in the middle ages. 182– 247. In: Van Sertima I, ed. *Golden Age of the Moor*. New Brunswick, New Jersey: Transaction Publishers, 1992.

Pinkney A. *The Myth of Black Progress*. Cambridge, England: Cambridge University Press, 1984.

Polednak AP. Poverty, residential segregation, and Black/White mortality ratios in urban areas. *Journal of Health Care for the Poor and Underserved* 1993; 4:363–373.

Pope-Hennessy J. *Sins of the Fathers: A Study of the Atlantic Slave Traders, 1441–1807*. New York: Alfred A Knopf, Inc., 1967. Reprint Edition. New York: Capricorn Books, 1969.

Porter DB. David Ruggles, 1810–1849; Hydropathic practitioner. Parts 1, 2. *Journal of the National Medical Association* 1957; 49:67–72; 49:130–134.

Porter DB. Ruggles, David. 536–538. In Logan RW, Winston MR, eds. *Dictionary of American Negro Biography*. New York: W.W. Norton and Company, 1982.

Proctor RN. *Racial Hygiene: Medicine under the Nazis*. Cambridge, Massachusetts: Harvard University Press, 1988.

Prothrow-Stith D. Division of Public Health Practice: Strategic Planning Document. Harvard School of Public Health, Boston, Massachusetts, 1997.

Rabinowitz HN. *Race Relations in the Urban South, 1865–1890*. New York: Oxford University Press, 1978.

Randall VR. Racist health care: Reforming an unjust health care system to meet the needs of African-Americans. *Health Matrix: Journal of Law–Medicine* 1993 (Spring, No. 1); 3:127–194.

Randall VR. Does Clinton's health care reform proposal ensure (e)qual(ity) of health care for ethnic Americans and the poor? *Brooklyn Law Review* 1994 (Spring, No. 1); 60:167–237.

Randall VR. Slavery, segregation and racism: Trusting the health care system ain't always easy! An African American perspective on bioethics. *Saint Louis University Public Law Review* 1996 (No. 2); 15:191–235.

Ransford O. *Bid the Sickness Cease: Disease in the History of Black Africa*. London: John Murray (Publishers) Ltd., 1983.

Reed J. Scientific racism. 1358–1360. In Wilson CR, Ferris W, eds. *Encyclopedia of Southern Culture*. Chapel Hill: The University of North Carolina Press, 1989.

Reilly K. *The West and the World: A Topical History of Civilization*. New York: Harper and Row Publishers, 1980.

Reiser RJ, Dyck AJ, Curran WJ, eds. Final report of the Tuskegee Syphilis Study Ad Hoc Advisory Panel. 316–321. In: *Ethics in Medicine: Historical Perspectives and Contemporary Concerns*. Cambridge, Massachusetts: MIT Press, 1977.

Reitzes DC. *Negroes and Medicine*. Cambridge, Massachusetts: Harvard University Press, published for the Commonwealth Fund, 1958.

Researchers say race isn't base for scientific study. *Fort Worth Star-Telegram*, February 20, 1995, Section A-7.

Reuter EB. *The American Race Problem*. Revised Third Edition. Revision and Preface by Masuoka J. New York: Thomas Y. Crowell Company, 1970.

Reynolds V, Falger V, Vine I, eds. *The Sociobiology of Ethnocentrism: Evolutionary Dimensions of Xenophobia, Discrimination, Racism and Nationalism*. London: Croom Helm Ltd., 1987.

Rice MF, Jones W. Public policy compliance/enforcement and black American health: Title VI of the civil rights act of 1964. 98–115. In: Jones W Jr., Rice MF, eds. *Health Care Issues in Black America: Policies, Problems, and Prospects*. New York: Greenwood Press, 1987.

Riggs MT. *Ethnic Notions*. Berkeley, California: Berkeley Art Center, produced in cooperation with KQED, San Francisco, 1987. Filmstrip.

Riggs MT. *Color Adjustment*. San Francisco: The American Film Institute and the California Council for the Humanities, produced in cooperation with KQED, San Francisco, 1991. Filmstrip.

Riley HD. Moore, Samuel P. (1813–1889) Confederate surgeon. 1374–1375. In: Wilson CR, Ferris W. eds. *Encyclopedia of Southern Culture*. Chapel Hill: The University of North Carolina Press, 1989.

Risse GB. Medicine in New Spain. 12–63. In: Numbers RL, ed. *Medicine in the New World: New Spain, New France, and New England*. Knoxville: The University of Tennessee Press, 1987.

Roberts J. *The Triumph of the West*. Boston: Little, Brown, and Company, 1985.

Roberts J. *The Triumph of the West* (videotape). A multipart documentary produced by the BBC, 1985.

Roberts JM. *History of the World*. New York: Alfred A. Knopf, 1976. Revised, Reprint, Edition. *The Penguin History of the World*. London: Penguin Books, Ltd., 1990.

Roberts MJ, Clyde AT. *Your Money or Your Life: The Health Care Crisis Explained*. New York: Main Street Books published by Doubleday, 1993.

Robert Wood Johnson Foundation. Special Report Number One, The Foundation's Minority Medical Training Programs: Minority Applicants to Medical School Are Better Qualified Today than in Mid-'70s, Yet Less Likely to Be Accepted. Princeton, New Jersey: Robert Wood Johnson Foundation, 1987.

Robinson HS. Anderson Ruffin Abbott, MD. 1837–1913. *Journal of the National Medical Association* 1980; 72:713–716.

Robinson LS. Dialogue: Curbing a sick practice: Energy Secretary Hazel O'Leary focuses on government accountability in testing. *Emerge* 1994 (October, No. 1); 6:20.

Rogers JA. *World's Great Men of Color*. Vol. 1. New York: Collier Macmillan Publishers, 1972.

Rogers JA. *Nature Knows No Color Line: Research into the Negro Ancestry in the White Race*. St. Petersburg, Florida: Helga M. Rogers, 1952. Third Edition. St. Petersburg, Florida: Helga M. Rogers, 1980.

Roman CV. *Meharry Medical College: A History*. Nashville, Tennessee: Sunday School Publishing Board of the National Baptist Convention, 1934.

Rosen G. The idea of social medicine in America. *Canadian Medical Association Journal* 1949; 61:316–323.

Rosen G. *The Structure of American Medical Practice 1875–1941*. Philadelphia: University of Pennsylvania Press, 1983.

Rosenbaum S, Layton C, Liu J. *The Health of America's Children*. Washington, D.C.: Children's Defense Fund, 1991.

Rosenberg CE. *The Care of Strangers: The Rise of America's Hospital System*. New York: Basic Books, 1987.

Rossetti L. *The University of Padua: An Outline of Its History*. Trieste, Italy: Edizioni LINT Trieste, 1983.

Rothman DJ. Our brother's keepers. *American Heritage* 1972 (December, No. 1); 24:38.

Rothstein WG. *American Physicians in the 19th Century: From Sects to Science*. Baltimore, Maryland: The Johns Hopkins University Press, 1972.

Rothstein WG. *American Medical Schools and the Practice of Medicine*. New York: Oxford University Press, 1987.

Rowland Hogue CJ, Hargraves MA. Class, race, and infant mortality in the United States. *American Journal of Public Health* 1993; 83:9–12.

Rush B. Observations intended to favour a supposition that the Black color (as it is called) of the Negroes is derived from the leprosy. American Philosophical Society, *Transactions* (1799); 4:289–297.

Russell JH. *The Free Negro in Virginia, 1619–1865*. Baltimore: Johns Hopkins Press, 1913. Reprint Paperback Edition. New York: Dover Publications, Inc., 1969.

Russett CE. *Sexual Science: The Victorian Construction of Womanhood*. Cambridge, Massachusetts: Harvard University Press, 1989.

Ryan W. *Blaming the Victim*. New York: Vintage Books, 1971. Revised, Updated Edition. New York: Vintage Books, 1976.

Ryan W. *Equality*. New York: Pantheon Books, 1981.

Rydell RW. *All the World's a Fair: Visions of Empire at American International Expositions, 1876–1916*. Chicago: The University of Chicago Press, 1984.

Sack K. Public hospitals around the country cut basic service. *The New York Times*, August 20, 1995, 1.

Sanders R. *Lost Tribes and Promised Lands: The Origins of American Racism*. Boston: Little, Brown, and Company, 1978.

Sardell A. *The U.S. Experiment in Social Medicine: The Community Health Center Program, 1956–1986*. Pittsburgh: The University of Pittsburgh Press, 1988.

Savitt TL. The use of Blacks for medical experimentation and demonstration in the old south. *Journal of Southern History* 1982; 48:331–348.

Savitt TL. The education of Black physicians at Shaw University, 1882–1918. 160–188. In Crow J, Hatley FJ, eds. *Black Americans in North Carolina and the South*. Chapel Hill: University of North Carolina Press, 1984.

Savitt TL. Black health on the plantation: Masters, slaves, and physicians. 313–330. In: Leavitt JW, Numbers RL, eds. *Sickness and Health in America: Readings in the History of Medicine and Public Health*. Madison: The University of Wisconsin Press, 1985.

Savitt TL. Lincoln University medical department—a forgotten 19th century Black medical school. *Journal of the History of Medicine and Allied Sciences* 1985; 40:42–65.

Savitt TL. Entering a white profession: Black physicians in the new South, 1880–1920. *Bulletin of the History of Medicine* 1987; 61:507–540.

Savitt TL. *Medicine and Slavery: The Diseases and Health Care of Blacks in Antebellum Virginia.* Urbana: University of Illinois Press, 1987.

Savitt TL. Abraham Flexner and the Black medical schools. 65–81. In: Barzansky EM, Gevitz N, eds. *Beyond Flexner: Medical Education in the 20th Century.* New York: Greenwood Press, 1992.

Sawyer D. The Tuskegee Study. [videotape segment], *Prime Time*, ABC television network, February 6, 1992.

Schiebinger L. *The Mind Has No Sex? Women in the Origins of Modern Science.* Cambridge, Massachusetts: Harvard University Press, 1989.

Schlosser E. The prison-industrial complex. *The Atlantic Monthly*, December 1998, 51.

Schulman KA, Berlin JA, Harless W, Kerner JF, Sistrunk SS, Gersh BJ, et al. The effect of race and sex on physician recommendations for cardiac catheterization. *New England Journal of Medicine* 1999; 340:618–626.

Schuman H, Steeh C, Bobo L, Krysan M. *Racial Attitudes in America: Trends and Interpretations.* Revised Edition. Cambridge, Massachusetts: Harvard University Press, 1997.

Shea S, Fullilove MT. Entry of black and other minority students in US medical schools: Historical perspectives and recent trends. *New England Journal of Medicine* 1985; 313:933–940;

Sheridan RB. *Doctors and Slaves: A Medical and Demographic History of Slavery in the British West Indies, 1680–1834.* Cambridge: Cambridge University Press, 1985.

Shipman P. *The Evolution of Racism: Human Differences and the Use and Abuse of Science.* New York: Simon and Schuster, 1994.

Shryock RH. A medical perspective on the civil war. 90–108. In: Shryock RH. *Medicine in America: Historical Essays.* Baltimore, Maryland: The Johns Hopkins Press, 1966.

Shryock RH. Medical sources and the social historian. 275–297. In: Shryock RH. *Medicine in America: Historical Essays.* Baltimore, Maryland: The Johns Hopkins Press, 1966.

Shryock RH. *The Development of Modern Medicine: An Interpretation of the Social and Scientific Factors Involved.* Madison: The University of Wisconsin Press, 1974.

Sidel VW, Sidel R, eds. *Reforming Medicine: Lessons of the Last Quarter Century.* New York: Pantheon Books, 1984.

Sigerist HE. *The Great Doctors: A Biographical History of Medicine.* New York: W.W. Norton and Company, 1933. Reprint Edition. New York: Dover Publications, 1971.

Sigerist HE. An outline of the development of the hospital. *Bulletin of the Institute of the History of Medicine* 1936; 4:573–581.

Simone TM. *About Face: Race in Postmodern America.* Brooklyn, New York: Autonomedia, 1989.

Sindler AP. *Bakke, DeFunis, and Minority Admissions: The Quest for Equal Opportunity.* New York: Longman, 1978.

Sirasi NG. *Medieval and Early Renaissance Medicine: An Introduction to Knowledge and Practice.* Chicago: The University of Chicago Press, 1990.

Skocpol T. *Boomerang: Health Care Reform and the Turn against Government.* New York: W.W. Norton and Company, 1997.

Smedley A. *Race in North America: Origin and Evolution of a Worldview.* Second Edition. Boulder, Colorado: Westview Press, 1999.

Smith DB. *Health Care Divided: Race and Healing a Nation*. Ann Arbor: The University of Michigan Press, 1999.

Smith JA. A lecture introductory to the Second Course of Anatomical Instruction in the College of Physicians and Surgeons for the State of New York . . . *New-York Medical and Philosophical Journal and Review* (1809); 1:32–48.

Smith SS; Jordan WD, ed. *An Essay on the Causes of the Variety of Complexion and Figure in the Human Species*. 1810. Reprint, Cambridge, Massachusetts: The Belknap Press of Harvard University Press, 1965.

Sniderman PM, Piazza T. *The Scar of Race*. Cambridge, Massachusetts: The Belknap Press of Harvard University Press, 1993.

Sniderman PM, Carmines EG. *Reaching Beyond Race*. Cambridge, Massachusetts: Harvard University Press, 1997.

Snowden FM Jr. *Blacks in Antiquity: Ethiopians in the Greco-Roman Experience*. Cambridge, Massachusetts: The Belknap Press of Harvard University Press, 1970.

Sonnedecker G. *Kremers and Undang's History of Pharmacy*. Revised Fourth Edition. Philadelphia: J.B. Lippincott Company, 1976.

Stafford BM. *Body Criticism: Imaging the Unseen in Enlightenment Art and Medicine*. Cambridge, Massachusetts: The MIT Press, 1991.

Stampp KM. *The Peculiar Institution: Slavery in the Ante-Bellum South*. New York: Alfred A. Knopf, 1956. Reprint Edition. New York: Vintage Books, 1956.

Stanford University. Health care in America: Armageddon on the horizon? *Stanford Law and Policy Review* 1991 (Fall); 3:1–260.

Stannard DE. *American Holocaust: Columbus and the Conquest of the New World*. New York: Oxford University Press, 1992.

Stanton W. *The Leopard's Spots: Scientific Attitudes toward Race in America, 1815–1859*. Chicago: The University of Chicago Press, 1960.

Starr P. *The Social Transformation of American Medicine*. New York: Basic Books, 1982.

Starr P, Zelman WA. Bridge to compromise: Competition under a budget. *Health Affairs* (Supplement 1993): 7–23.

Steckel RH. Slave mortality: analysis of evidence from plantation records. *Social Science History* 1979; 3:86–114.

Steinberg S. *The Ethnic Myth: Race, Ethnicity, and Class in America*. N.P.: Atheneum Publishers, 1981. Updated and Expanded Edition. Boston: Beacon Press, 1989.

Steinberg S. *Turning Back: The Retreat from Racial Justice in American Thought and Policy*. Boston: Beacon Press, 1995.

Sterling D. *The Making of an Afro-American: Martin Robison Delany, 1812–1885*. Garden City, New York: Doubleday and Company, 1971.

Stevens RA. *American Medicine and the Public Interest*. New Haven, Connecticut: Yale University Press, 1971.

Stigler SM. *The History of Statistics: The Measurement of Uncertainty before 1900*. Cambridge, Massachusetts: The Belknap Press of Harvard University Press, 1986.

Still J. *Early Recollections and Life of Dr. James Still, 1812–1885*. Facsimile Edition. Medford, New Jersey: Medford Historical Society, 1971.

Stocking GW. *Race, Culture, and Evolution: Essays in the History of Anthropology*. Chicago: The University of Chicago Press, 1982.

Stone N, ed. *The Times Atlas of World History*. Third Edition. Maplewood, New Jersey: Hammond Incorporated, 1989.

Strait G, DiIanni D. *The Deadly Deception*, A documentary video segment for *Nova*, Boston, WGBH, 1993.

Stringer C, McKie R. *African Exodus: The Origins of Modern Humanity*. London: Jonathan Cape Ltd., 1996. First American Edition. New York: A John Macrae Book, Henry Holt and Company, 1997.

Sullivan LW. The status of blacks in medicine. *New England Journal of Medicine* 1983; 309:807–809.

Summerville J. *Educating Black Doctors: A History of Meharry Medical College*. University: The University of Alabama Press, 1983.

Summerville J. Formation of a black medical profession in Tennessee, 1880–1920. *Journal of the Tennessee Medical Association* 1983 (October); 644–646.

Survey: 60 million experience lapses in health coverage. *Physician's Financial News*, January 15, 1995, 2.

Sutch R. The care and feeding of slaves. 231–301. In: David PA, Gutman HG, Sutch R, Temin P, Wright G. *Reckoning with Slavery: A Critical Study in the Quantitative History of American Negro Slavery*. New York: Oxford University Press, 1976.

Swinton DH. The economic status of African Americans: "Permanent" poverty and inequality. In: Dewart J, ed. *The State of Black America 1991*. New York: National Urban League, 1991.

Swinton DH. The economic status of African Americans: Limited ownership and persistent inequality. In: Tidwell BJ, ed. *The State of Black America 1992*. New York: National Urban League, 1992.

Swinton DH. The economic status of African Americans during the Reagan-Bush era: Withered opportunities, limited outcomes, and uncertain outlook. 135–200. In: Tidwell BJ, ed. *The State of Black America 1993*. New York: National Urban League, 1993.

Takaki RY. *Iron Cages: Race and Culture in Nineteenth-Century America*. New York: Alfred A. Knopf, 1979.

Tannenbaum F. *Slave and Citizen: The Negro in the Americas*. New York: Alfred A. Knopf, 1946. Paperback Edition. New York: Vintage Books, N.D.

Taylor MW. *Harriet Tubman: Antislavery Activist*. New York: Chelsea House Publishers, 1991, 10, 84–86.

Terkel S. *Race: How Blacks and Whites Think and Feel about the American Obsession*. New York: The New Press, 1992.

Terry RW. *For Whites Only*. Grand Rapids, Michigan: William B. Eerdmans, 1970. Paperback, Revised, Reprint Edition. Grand Rapids, Michigan: William B. Eerdmans, 1992.

Thomas H. *The Slave Trade: The Story of the Atlantic Slave Trade: 1440–1870*. New York: Simon and Schuster, 1997.

Thomas SB, Quinn SC. Public health then and now: The Tuskegee syphilis study, 1932 to 1972: Implications for HIV education and AIDS risk education programs in the Black community. *American Journal of Public Health* 1991; 81:1498–1504.

Thomas VG. Explaining health disparities between African-American and white populations: Where do we go from here? *Journal of the National Medical Association* 1992; 84:837–840.

Thorwald J. *Science and Secrets of Early Medicine: Egypt, Babylonia, India, China, Mexico, Peru*. New York: Harcourt, Brace and World, 1962.

Tierney J, Wright L, Springen K. The search for Adam and Eve: Scientists claim to have found our common ancestor—a woman who lived 200,000 years ago and left resilient genes that are carried by all of mankind. *Newsweek,* January 11, 1988; 61:46.

Tosteson DC. An open letter from the Dean to the Harvard community: Letter from second-year students: Letter from HMS Third World Caucus. *Harvard Medical Area Focus,* January 9, 1992, 8–13.

Townsend AM. The medical profession of greater Nashville. *Nashville Globe,* September 4, 1908.

Travella S. Black hospitals struggling to survive: Of more than 200 medical centers, only 8 are left. 12. In: *Health: A Weekly Journal of Medicine, Science and Society, The Washington Post,* September 11, 1990, p. 1.

Tucker WH. *The Science and Politics of Racial Research.* Urbana: University of Illinois Press, 1994.

Tunley R. *The American Health Scandal.* New York: Harper and Row Publishers, 1966.

Turner PA. *Ceramic Uncles and Celluloid Mammies: Black Images and Their Influence on Culture.* New York: Anchor Books, 1994.

Tyler RC, Murphy LR, eds. *The Slave Narratives of Texas.* Austin, Texas: The Encino Press, 1974.

Ullman V. *Martin R. Delany: The Beginnings of Black Nationalism.* Boston: Beacon Press, 1971.

UNESCO. *The Race Question in Modern Science.* New York: Whiteside, Inc., and William Morrow and Company, 1956.

U.S. Bureau of the Census. *Negro Population of the United States: 1790–1915* (1918).

U.S. Bureau of the Census. *Negroes in the United States 1920–32* (1935).

U.S. Bureau of the Census. *Statistical Abstract of the United States, 1993.* U.S. Department of Commerce. Washington, D.C.: U.S. Government Printing Office, 1992.

U.S. Congress, House/Senate. *Health Security Act.* 103rd Congress, 1st session, H.R.3600/S.1757. *Congressional Record.* November 1993.

U.S. Department of Health and Human Services. *Health in America: 1776–1976.* Washington, D.C.: U.S. Health Resources Administration, DHEW Pub. No. (HRA) 76–616, 1976.

U.S. Department of Health and Human Services. *Report of the Secretary's Task Force on Black and Minority Health.* Volume 1. *Executive Summary.* Washington, D.C.: U.S. Government Printing Office, August 1985.

U.S. Department of Health and Human Services. *Report of the Secretary's Task Force on Black and Minority Health.* Volume 2. *Crosscutting Issues in Minority Health.* Washington, D.C.: U.S. Government Printing Office, August 1985.

U.S. Department of Health and Human Services. *Report of the Secretary's Task Force on Black and Minority Health.* Volume 3. *Cancer.* Washington, D.C.: U.S. Government Printing Office, January 1986.

U.S. Department of Health and Human Services. *Report of the Secretary's Task Force on Black and Minority Health.* Volume 4. *Cardiovascular and Cerebrovascular Diseases. Part 1.* Washington, D.C.: U.S. Government Printing Office, January 1986.

U.S. Department of Health and Human Services. *Report of the Secretary's Task Force on Black and Minority Health.* Volume 4. *Cardiovascular and Cerebrovascular Diseases. Part 2.* Washington, D.C.: U.S. Government Printing Office, January 1986.

U.S. Department of Health and Human Services. *Report of the Secretary's Task Force on Black and Minority Health.* Volume 5. *Homicide, Suicide, and Unintentional Injuries.* Washington, D.C.: U.S. Government Printing Office, January 1986.

U.S. Department of Health and Human Services. *Report of the Secretary's Task Force on Black and Minority Health.* Volume 6. *Infant Mortality and Low Birth Weight.* Washington, D.C.: U.S. Government Printing Office, January 1986.

U.S. Department of Health and Human Services. *Report of the Secretary's Task Force on Black and Minority Health.* Volume 7. *Chemical Dependency Diabetes.* Washington, D.C.: U.S. Government Printing Office, January 1986.

U.S. Department of Health and Human Services. *Report of the Secretary's Task Force on Black and Minority Health.* Volume 8. Hispanic Health Issues: Inventory of DHHS Programs: Survey of Non-Federal Community. Washington, D.C.: U.S. Government Printing Office, January 1986.

U.S. Department of Health and Human Services. *Health Status of the Disadvantaged Chartbook/1990.* Washington, D.C.: U.S. Department of Health and Human Services, Public Health Service, Publication No. (HRSA) HRS-P-DV 90–1.

U.S. Department of Health and Human Services. *Cultural Competence for Evaluators: A Guide for Alcohol and Other Drug Abuse Prevention Practitioners Working with Ethnic/Racial Communities.* Rockville, Maryland: Office for Substance Abuse Prevention, Alcohol, Drug Abuse, and Mental Health Administration, DHHS Publication No. (ADM)92–1884, 1992.

Van den Berghe PL. *Race and Racism: A Comparative Perspective.* New York: Wiley, 1967.

Van Sertima I. *They Came before Columbus.* New York: Random House, 1976.

Van Sertima I. Race and origin of the Egyptians. 2–8. In: Van Sertima I, ed. *Egypt Revisited: Journal of African Civilizations.* New Brunswick, New Jersey: Transaction Publishers, 1989.

Veatch RM. Benefitting mentally retarded children by giving them hepatitis. 274–277. In: Veatch RM. *Case Studies in Medical Ethics.* Cambridge, Massachusetts: Harvard University Press, 1977.

Veatch RM. *A Theory of Medical Ethics.* New York: Basic Books, 1981.

Vercoutter J, Leclant J, Snowden FM Jr., Desanges J. *The Image of the Black in Western Art.* Part 1. *From the Pharaohs to the Fall of the Roman Empire.* Cambridge, Massachusetts: The Menil Foundation, distributed by the Harvard University Press, 1976.

Viola HJ, Margolis C. *Seeds of Change: A Quincentennial Commemoration.* Washington, D.C.: Smithsonian Institution Press, 1991.

Vlach JM. Plantation landscapes of the antebellum South. 21–49. In: Campbell EDC Jr., Rice K., eds. *Before Freedom Came: African-American Life in the Antebellum South.* Charlottesville, Virginia: The Museum of the Confederacy, Richmond, and the University Press of Virginia, 1991.

Vogel MJ. *The Invention of the Modern Hospital: Boston 1870–1930.* Chicago: The University of Chicago Press, 1980.

Wade RC. *Slavery in the Cities: The South 1820–1860.* London: Oxford University Press, 1964.

Wade WC. *The Fiery Cross: The Ku Klux Klan in America.* New York: Simon and Schuster, 1987.

Walinsky A. The crisis of public order. *The Atlantic Monthly* 1995 (July, No. 1); 276:39.

Walker HE. *The Negro in the Medical Profession.* Publications of the University of Virginia Phelps-Stokes Fellowship Papers. N.P. University of Virginia, 1949.

Walsh MR. *Doctors Wanted No Women Need Apply: Sexual Barriers in the Medical Profession, 1835–1975.* New Haven, Connecticut: Yale University Press, 1977.

Wanniski J. Behind the curve: Journalists who accept the findings of *The Bell Curve* are "benevolent racists." *Forbes MediaCritic* 1995 (Spring, No. 3); 2:86.

Ward GC, Burns R, Burns K. *The Civil War.* New York: Alfred A. Knopf, 1990.

Warner JH. The idea of southern medical distinctiveness: Medical knowledge and practices in the Old South. 179–205. In: Numbers RL, Savitt TL, eds. *Science and Medicine in the Old South.* Baton Rouge: Louisiana State University Press, 1989.

Warner JH. A southern medical reform: The meaning of the antebellum argument for southern medical education. 206–225. In: Numbers RL, Savitt TL, eds. *Science and Medicine in the Old South.* Baton Rouge: Louisiana State University Press, 1989.

Washington H. The widening gap in race-based pollution. *Emerge*, July–August 1995, 19.

Washington HA. Of men and mice: Human guinea pigs: Unethical testing targets Blacks and the poor. *Emerge* 1994 (October, No. 1): 6:24.

Wassermann HP. *Ethnic Pigmentation: Historical, Psychological, and Clinical Aspects.* New York: American Elsevier Publishing Company, 1974.

Watkins TH, A low comedy for high stakes: The taking of California. *American Heritage* 1973 (February, No. 2); 24:4.

Weisbord RG. *Genocide? Birth Control and the Black American.* Westport, Connecticut: Greenwood Press, 1975.

Wendt H. *From Ape to Adam: The Search for the Ancestry of Man.* Indianapolis, Indiana: The Bobbs-Merrill Company, 1972.

West C. *Race Matters.* Boston: Beacon Press, 1993. Paperback Reprint Edition. New York: Vintage Books, 1994.

White DG. Female slaves in the plantation South. 101–121. In: Campbell EDC Jr., Rice K., eds. *Before Freedom Came: African-American Life in the Antebellum South.* Charlottesville, Virginia: The Museum of the Confederacy, Richmond, and the University Press of Virginia, 1991.

White HA. *The Freedmen's Bureau in Louisiana.* Baton Rouge: Louisiana State University Press, 1970.

Whol S. *The Medical Industrial Complex.* New York: Harmony Books, 1984.

Williams E. *Capitalism and Slavery.* Chapel Hill: The University of North Carolina Press, 1944. Paperback Edition. Chapel Hill: University of North Carolina Press, 1994.

Williams E. *From Columbus to Castro: The History of the Caribbean.* New York: Vintage Books, 1970.

Wilson EO. *Sociobiology: The New Synthesis.* Cambridge, Massachusetts: Harvard University Press, 1975.

Wilson FA, Neuhauser D. *Health Services in the United States.* Second Edition. Cambridge, Massachusetts: Ballinger Publishing Company, 1982.

Wilson OH, Christie A. Early history of medical education in Nashville. *Journal of the Tennessee Medical Association* 1969; 62:819–829.

Wilson V. *The Book of the Presidents.* Brookeville, Maryland: American History Research Associates, 1962.

Wilson WJ. *The Declining Significance of Race: Blacks and Changing American Institutions.* Chicago: The University of Chicago Press, 1978. Second Edition. Chicago: The University of Chicago Press, 1980.

Wilson WJ. *The Truly Disadvantaged: The Inner City, the Underclass, and Public Policy.* Chicago: The University of Chicago Press, 1987.

Wilson WJ. *When Work Disappears: The World of the New Urban Poor.* New York: Alfred A. Knopf, 1996.

Winchell A. *Preadamites; or A Demonstration of the Existence of Men before Adam; together with a Study of their Condition, Antiquity, Racial Affinities, and Progressive Dispersion over the Earth.* Chicago: S.C. Griggs and Company, 1880.

Wing KR, Rose MG. Health facilities and the enforcement of civil rights. 243–267. In: Roemer R, McKray G, eds. *Legal Aspects of Health Policy: Issues and Trends.* Westport, Connecticut: Greenwood Press, 1980.

Wisner E. *Social Welfare in the South: From Colonial Times to World War I.* Baton Rouge: Louisiana State University Press, 1970.

Wolff EN. *Top Heavy: A Study of the Increasing Inequality of Wealth in America.* New York: The Twentieth Century Fund Press, 1995.

Wolinsky H. Healing wounds: Lonnie R. Bristow steps up to head the American Medical Association, one of the nation's premier—and most rigidly segregated—professional groups. *Emerge* 1994 (July–August, No. 10); 5:42.

Wood PH. *Black Majority: Negroes in Colonial South Carolina from 1670 through the Stono Rebellion.* New York: Alfred A. Knopf, 1974. Paperback Edition. New York: W.W. Norton and Company, 1975.

Woodson, CG. *The Negro Professional Man and the Community.* Washington, D.C.: The Association for the Study of Negro Life and History, 1934.

Young RJC. *Colonial Desire: Hybridity in Theory, Culture and Race.* London: Routledge, 1995.

Ziegler P. *The Black Death.* N.P.: John Day Company, Inc., 1969. Paperback Edition. New York: Harper and Row Publishers, 1971.

Zinn H. *A People's History of the United States.* New York: Harper and Row Publishers, 1980. Paperback Edition. New York: Harper Perennial, 1990.

)(A Note on Sources

One of the major limiting factors in modern scholarship has been overspecialization. This fragmentation prevents planners from coming to grips with large issues and may be partially responsible for recent U.S. failures in domestic planning, economic planning, and government. It certainly bedevils the current attempts at health policy planning. In response to this challenge, this study has been built upon an eclectic data base. Good sources translate into good results and sound conclusions. Therefore, models, hypotheses, and quantitative pronouncements in this study meet the criteria of being logically consistent and thoroughly grounded in facts. Based on these principles, it is not likely that one will go too far afield. With this in mind, a short overview on sources utilized—including a brief sampling—will reveal the "bloodlines" of this book.

By the utilization of first-rate documentation, this study does not intend to be handicapped by requiring specialty-level expertise in order to express itself, have an opinion, or form conclusions in a particular discipline. Therefore, one of the strengths of this study is the use of information from many fields. A brief survey of the academic terrain we traveled, with some of the books that served as our signposts, follows.

The medical literature was a major source of information for this study. Medical journals such as the *New England Journal of Medicine*, the *Journal of Health Care for the Poor and Underserved*, the *Lancet*, the *Journal of the American Medical Association*, the *Journal of the National Medical Association*, and many others were freely utilized. Medical textbooks such as *William's Obstetrics, The Textbook of Black-Related Diseases, Manson's Tropical Diseases,* and *Cancer: Principles and Practice of Oncology* were also sources.

Works from the realm of public health were another resource we tapped. Examples of a few noted references used include the *American Journal of Public Health* and the *Oxford Textbook of Public Health.* Harvard School of Public Health professor Deborah Prothrow-Stith's important public health study on violence, *Deadly Consequences,* and Dade Moeller's contemporary work based on his broad experiences at Harvard, *Environmental Health,* were also utilized.

The sociological literature was a consistent source of useful material. Some of the classical literature in this field we utilized were W. E. B. Du Bois's *The Atlanta University Studies,* Benjamin Brawley's *A Social History of the American Negro,* Gunnar Myrdal's epochal *An American Dilemma,* E. Franklin Frazier's *The Negro Family in the United States,* and Amidei Newman and colleagues' *Protest, Politics, and Prosperity: Black Americans and White Institutions, 1940–75.* Some of the modern period works dealing with late-twentieth-century problems are Michael Harrington's classic *The Other America,* Frances Fox Piven and Richard A. Cloward's *Regulating the Poor,* Stephen Steinberg's *The Ethnic Myth,* William Julius Wilson's *The Truly Disadvantaged* and *When Work Disappears,* Reynolds Farley and Walter R. Allen's *The Color Line and the Quality of Life in America,* Alphonse Pinkney's *The Myth of Black Progress,* and Douglas Glasgow's *The Black Underclass.* Recent cutting-edge works in the field include Andrew Hacker's *Two Nations: Black and White, Separate, Hostile, Unequal;* Ellis Cose's *The Rage of a Privileged Class* and *Color Blind;* Joe R. Feagin and Melvin Spikes's *Living with Racism: The Black Middle-Class Experience;* Sniderman and Piazza's *The Scar of Race;* Christopher Jencks's *Rethinking Social Policy: Race, Poverty, and the Underclass;* and Douglas A. Massey and Nancy A. Denton's *American Apartheid: Segregation and the Making of the Underclass.* From the young field of medical sociology we utilized Paul Starr's Pulitzer prize–winning *The Social Transformation of American Medicine,* Stanley Whol's *The Medical Industrial Complex,* Edward Beardsley's *A History of Neglect: Health Care for Blacks and Mill Workers in the Twentieth-Century South,* Rosemary Stevens's *American Medicine and the Public Interest,* Charles Rosenberg's *The Care of Strangers: The Rise of America's Hospital System,* and James H. Jones's riveting examination of the Tuskegee study, *Bad Blood.*

Studies from the fields of philosophy and ethics as related to "racial thought" include Michael Banton's *Racial Theories;* Lucius Outlaw's landmark article "Toward a Critical Theory of Race," included in David Theo Goldberg's *Anatomy of Racism;* Cornel West's *Race Matters;* and Timothy Simone's *About Face: Race in Postmodern America.* Reference works in the field such as *The Oxford Companion to Philosophy* and *The Cambridge Dictionary of Philosophy* were freely utilized.

Studies focused on "racial thought" in general and scientific racism in particular were invaluable. Classic works in the field such as Michael Banton and

J. Harwood's *The Race Concept*; William Stanton's *The Leopard's Spots: Scientific Attitudes toward Race in America, 1815–1859*; Winthrop Jordan's *White over Black: American Attitudes toward the Negro, 1550–1812*; Thomas F. Gossett's *Race: The History of an Idea in America*; Ronald Sanders's *Lost Tribes and Promised Lands: The Origins of American Racism*; George M. Fredrickson's *The Black Image in the White Mind: The Debate on Afro-American Character and Destiny, 1871–1914*; and John S. Haller Jr.'s *Outcasts from Evolution: Scientific Attitudes of Racial Inferiority, 1859–1900* were the foundation of much of the inquiry. Related works dealing specifically with race and class issues and eugenics such as Demel J. Kevles's *In the Name of Eugenics*, Mark H. Haller's *Eugenics: Hereditarian Attitudes in American Thought*, and Weisbord's *Genocide? Birth Control and the Black American* were especially valuable. Only a few examples of the more recent outpourings of scholarly literature on scientific racism and "racial thought" can be mentioned. A few are Stephen J. Gould's *The Mismeasure of Man*; Allan Chase's *The Legacy of Malthus: The Social Costs of the New Scientific Racism*; R. C. Lewontin, Steven Rose, and Leon Kamin's *Not in Our Genes: Biology, Ideology, and Human Nature*; Pat Shipman's *The Evolution of Racism: Human Differences and the Use and Abuse of Science*; and Reginald Horsman's *Race and Manifest Destiny: The Origins of American Racial Anglo-Saxonism*.

From the health policy and management literature we utilized journals such as *Health Affairs*, the *Stanford Law and Policy Review*, and the *International Journal of Health Services*. Recently books in the field like Eli Ginzberg's *The Medical Triangle* and *The Road to Reform: The Future of Health Care in America*, and Robert Blendon's *System in Crisis: The Case for Health Care Reform* and *Reforming the System: Containing Health Care Costs in an Era of Universal Coverage* served as resources. Landmark references dealing with the recent failed health reform were Haynes Johnson and David Broder's *The System: The American Way of Politics at the Breaking Point* and Theda Skocpol's *Boomerang: Health Care Reform and the Turn against Government*.

Political science research, especially that focusing on the Black and African American experience, provided sociocultural insights, understanding, and depth to the work. These include Frantz Fanon's *The Wretched of the Earth*, Harold Cruse's *Plural but Equal*, and Haynes Walton's *The Political Philosophy of Martin Luther King, Jr.*

Historical works served as the bedrock upon which much of the study was conducted. This too was consistent with the basic premises and goals and objectives laid out for this work, which strives to perform a history-based descriptive and structural analysis of the U.S. health system from an African American perspective. Works were culled from the areas of general history, medical history, and the history of science. Some rare primary references utilized were C. V. Roman's classic *Meharry Medical College: A History*, John A. Kenney's rare and significant *The Negro in Medicine*, Samuel George Morton's *Crania Americana*:

A Comparative View of the Skulls of Various Aboriginal Nations of North and South America to which is prefixed an Essay on the Varieties of the Human Species, W. Montague Cobb's The First Negro Medical Society: A History of the Medico-Chirurgical Society of the District of Columbia, Robley Dunglison's Human Physiology with Three Hundred and Sixty-Eight Illustrations, and Josiah Clark Nott and George Gliddon's Types of Mankind or, Ethnological Researches. Some eclectic historical references focusing on Blacks and antiquity included the Menil Foundation and Harvard's multivolume The Image of the Black in Western Art, St. Clair Drake's Black Folk Here and There, and Martin Bernal's Black Athena. Ancient historical foundations were provided by Sir Moses Finley's Ancient Slavery and Modern Ideology, and Joseph E. Harris's Africans and Their History. General historical works that are more readily available are J. Mark Roberts's The Triumph of the West and the History of the World, Lerone Bennett's Before the Mayflower, Ronald Takaki's Iron Cages, W. E. B. Du Bois's The Suppression of the African Slave Trade, and John Hope Franklin's From Slavery to Freedom. They were extremely useful. Works focusing specifically on American history such as Alan Brinkley's The Unfinished Nation: A Concise History of the American People, and Howard Zinn's A People's History of the United States were also necessary to complete the undertaking. Specialized works focusing on African Americans such as Manning Marable's Race, Reform, and Rebellion: The Second Reconstruction in Black America, 1945–1990 and Nicholas Leamann's The Promised Land: The Great Black Migration and How It Changed America were extremely useful.

General medical historical works that proved useful were Albert S. Lyons and R. Joseph Petrucelli's epochal Medicine: An Illustrated History; Douglas Guthrie's A History of Medicine; Castiglioni's A History of Medicine; Jurgen Thorwald's Science and Secrets of Early Medicine: Egypt, Babylonia, India, China, Mexico, Peru; W. B. Blanton's Medicine in Virginia in the Seventeenth Century and Medicine in Virginia in the Eighteenth Century; George A. Bender's Great Moments in Medicine; and Guido Majno's The Healing Hand. There were a few medical history works that included significant information about the African American experience in the health system. Some of these include Herbert Morais's The History of the Negro in Medicine, Harry F. Dowling's City Hospitals, and James Summerville's Educating Black Doctors. Other medical history works such as Todd Savitt's classic Medicine and Slavery: The Diseases and Health Care of Blacks in Antebellum Virginia, Richard Sheridan's Doctors and Slaves: A Medical and Demographic History of Slavery in the British West Indies, 1680–1834, and William Postell's The Health of Slaves on Southern Plantations contained huge amounts of information on Blacks in the health system and proved to be immensely valuable.

Though epidemiologic information about African Americans was culled from works as disparate as Leslie Howard Owen's This Species of Property: Slave Life and Culture in the Old South, and Edward Byron Reuter's The American

Race Problem, much was gained from the formal literature. Epidemiologically oriented works like Oliver Ransford's *Bid the Sickness Cease: Disease in the History of Black Africa*, Reynolds Farley's *Growth of the Black Population*, Abraham and David Lilienfeld's *Foundations of Epidemiology*, and Charles H. Hennekens's *Epidemiology in Medicine* were all useful in different ways. Douglas Ewbank's landmark article, "History of Black Mortality and Health Before 1940," in *Health Policies and Black Americans*, edited by D. P. Willis, proved especially valuable as a rare source quantitatively evaluating the African American health experience over time. Ewbanks also applied the latest statistical methodology to old data and resurrected some unutilized data bases on the subject.

Health policy monographs provided historical and contemporary perspective regarding the U.S. health system. Works covering earlier periods included Ronald Numbers's *Almost Persuaded: American Physicians and Compulsory Health Insurance, 1912–1920*; E. Richard Brown's *Rockefeller Medicine Men: Medicine and Capitalism in America*; Daniel S. Hirshfield's *The Lost Reform: The Campaign for Compulsory Health Insurance in the United States 1932 to 1943*; Ed Cray's *In Failing Health: The Medical Crisis and the A.M.A.*; B. Bullough and Vern L. Bullough's *Poverty, Ethnic Identity, and Health Care*; and Barbara Ehrenreich and John Ehrenreich's *The American Health Empire: Power, Profits, and Politics*. Contemporary perspectives were gained by researching Victor Sidel and Ruth Sidel's *Reforming Medicine: Lessons of the Last Quarter Century*; Eli Ginzberg's *The Medical Triangle: Physicians, Politicians, and the Public*; and Walt Bogdanich's *The Great White Lie: Dishonesty, Waste, and Incompetence in the Medical Community*.

Periodicals proved to be particularly useful. Some of the most important newspapers include the *New York Times*, the *Boston Globe*, the *Dallas Morning News*, the *Washington Post*, and the *Detroit News*. Relevant information from magazines such as *The New Republic*, *Emerge*, *The Atlantic Monthly*, *The Crisis*, *Ebony*, *Time*, and *Newsweek* was also used.

Public documents were invaluable. Some of the more prominent ones include *The Report of the Secretary's Task Force on Black and Minority Health*; *Health United States, 1991–1996*; and *The Health Status of Minorities and Low Income Groups*.

Research foundation, community organization, and voluntary health organization documents and reports were useful. Some of the important ones utilized include the American Cancer Society's *Cancer Facts and Figures*, the Children's Defense Fund's *America's Children in Poverty*, the Twentieth Century Fund report *Top Heavy: A Study of Increasing Inequality of Wealth in America*, and the National Urban League's *The State of Black America*.

Psychiatric and behavioral science references proved to be a mother lode of information, especially about the dynamics of prejudice in Western society in general, in U.S. society in particular, and in the learned professions. Classic works such as T. W. Adorno, Else Frankel-Brunswik, Daniel J. Levinson, and R

Nevitt Sanford's *The Authoritarian Personality*, and Gordon Allport's *The Nature of Prejudice*, lived up to their reputations. Some particularly valuable modern works were Joel Kovel's *White Racism: A Psychohistory*; Robert Jay Lifton's *The Nazi Doctors*; Robert Jay Lifton and Eric Markusen's *The Genocidal Mentality*; Frances Cress Welsing's *The Isis Papers*; Patricia Turner's *Ceramic Uncles and Celluloid Mammies: Black Images and Their Influence on Culture*; Robert Terry's revised edition of *For Whites Only*; and Robert Guthrie's *Only the Rat was White*.

Medical ethics works proved to be extremely valuable in lending perspective, condemning past blunders, and proposing health system solutions grounded in medical ethical principles. Some especially useful ones include *A Theory of Medical Ethics*, by Robert M. Veatch, Joel Reiser's *Ethics in Medicine*, and Larry Churchill's *Rationing Health Care in America*.

An unexpected gold mine of information on African American health proved to be biographical literature. Some of the outstanding sources were J. Edward Perry's *Forty Cords of Wood: Memoirs of a Medical Doctor*; Fawn Brody's *Thomas Jefferson*; Helen Buckler's *Daniel Hale Williams: Negro Surgeon*; and Kenneth Manning's epochal *Ernest Everett Just: Black Apollo of Science*. Deeper insights into the growth of scientific racism and Black patient abuse were also obtained from biographical works such as Reginald Horsman's *Josiah Nott of Mobile: Southerner, Physician, and Racial Theorist*, and Deborah Kuhn McGregor's *Sexual Surgery and the Origins of Gynecology: J. Marion Sims, His Hospital, and His Patients*.

Determining the legal status of African Americans throughout their sojourn in North America was critical. Sound legal scholarship with some relevant health care ramifications was available in A. Leon Higginbotham Jr.'s classics *In the Matter of Color: Race and the American Legal Process, The Colonial Period*, and *Shades of Freedom: Racial Politics and Presumptions of the American Legal Process*. Richard Kluger's magisterial *Simple Justice: The History of* Brown v. Board of Education *and Black America's Struggle for Equality* also proved invaluable in adding legal context to the African American experience.

✗ *Index*

⟩⟨ Credits

---

p. 38, Figure 1.1 From *The Nature of Prejudice* by Gordon Allport. Copyright © 1979, 1958, 1954. Reprinted by permission of Perseus Books Publishers, a member of Perseus Books, L.L.C.

p. 39, Figure 1.2 From *The Nature of Prejudice* by Gordon Allport. Copyright © 1979, 1958, 1954. Reprinted by permission of Perseus Books Publishers, a member of Perseus Books, L.L.C.

p. 55, Figure 1.3 From Henry Fairfield Osborn, produced for the American Museum, 1923, and William King Gregory, *Our Face from Fish to Man*, 1929.

p. 57, Figure 1.4 From Julien Joseph Virey, *The Natural History of the Negro*, 1837.

p. 59, Figure 1.5 From Alexander Winchell, *Preadamites: or, A Demonstration of the Existence of Men Before Adam; together with a Study of Their Condition, Antiquities, and Progressive Dispersion over the Earth*, 1880.

p. 76, Figure 1.6 From Guido Majno, *The Healing Hand: Man and Wound in the Ancient World*, 1975.

p. 107, Table 1.2 From Sanford B. Hunt, "The Negro As a Soldier," *The Anthropological Review*, 1869. Courtesy of National Library of Medicine.

p. 182, Figure 2.1 Reprinted with permission of the Mansell Collection/Time Inc.

p. 183, Figure 2.2 Courtesy of the Library of Congress.

p. 197, Table 3.1 Curtin, Philip D. *The Atlantic Slave Trade* © 1969. Reprinted by permission of the University of Wisconsin Press.

p. 197, Table 3.2 Curtin, Philip D. *The Atlantic Slave Trade* © 1969. Reprinted by permission of the University of Wisconsin Press.

p. 203, Figure 3.1 Reproduced by kind permission of the President and Council of the Royal College of Surgeons of England.

p. 210, Figure 4.1 Reprinted with permission from the Library Company of Philadelphia.

p. 235, Figure 4.2   Reprinted by permission of Louisiana State University Press from *The Health of Slaves on Southern Plantations*, by William D. Postell. Copyright © 1951 by Louisiana State University Press.

p. 263, Figure 5.1   Reprinted with permission from the Chicago Historical Society.

p. 267, Figure 5.2   From *An Account of the New York Hospital*. New York: Mahlon Day, 1820. Courtesy of Charles Rosenberg.

p. 268, Figure 5.3   Courtesy of the Library of Congress.

p. 273, Figure 5.4   Reprinted by permission of Parke Davis & Company.

p. 282, Figure 5.5   John Goldblatt.

p. 285, Table 5.1   Reprinted with kind permission of Todd L. Savitt.

p. 286, Table 5.2   Reprinted by permission of Transaction Publishers.

p. 293, Figure 5.6   Courtesy of the Boston Medical Library in the Francis A. Countway Library of Medicine, Rare Book Room, Boston, Massachusetts.

p. 301, Table 5.5   From Robley Dunglison, *Human Physiology*, 1841.

p. 306, Figure 5.7   From *A Pictorial History of the Negro in America* by Langston Hughes and Milton Meltzer. Copyright © 1968 by Milton Meltzer and The Estate of Langston Hughes. Used by permission of Crown Publishers, a division of Random House, Inc.

p. 309, Figure 5.8   From *Harper's Weekly*.

p. 313, Figure 5.9   From *Blacks at Harvard: A Documentary History of African-American Experience at Harvard and Radcliffe*. New York: New York University Press, 1993, by permission of the editor.

p. 331, Figure 6.1   Ernest Haeckel, *Anthropologie*, 1874. Courtesy of The American Museum of Natural History.

p. 332, Figure 6.2   Adolf von Menzel. Hamburg, Hamburg Kunsthalle.

p. 333, Figure 6.3   Courtesy of the National Archives.

p. 343, Figure 6.5   From F. T. Miller, *The Photographic History of the Civil War*. New York: Review of Reviews Co., 1911.

p. 372, Figure 6.6   From W. N. Hartshorn, *An Era of Progress and Promise 1863–1910: The Religion, Moral, and Educational Development of the American Negro Since His Emancipation*, 1910.

p. 373, Figure 6.7   Courtesy of the Prints and Photographs Division, Library of Congress.

p. 390, Figure 6.8   Reprinted by permission of the Morland-Springarn Research Center, Howard University.

p. 393, Figure 6.9   From F. T. Miller, *The Photographic History of the Civil War*. New York: Review of Reviews Co., 1911.